Management of Open Globe Injuries

Seanna Grob · Carolyn Kloek
Editors

Management of Open Globe Injuries

Springer

Editors
Seanna Grob
Department of Ophthalmology
Harvard Medical School
Massachusetts Eye and Ear
Boston, MA
USA

Carolyn Kloek
Department of Ophthalmology
Harvard Medical School
Massachusetts Eye and Ear
Boston, MA
USA

ISBN 978-3-030-10196-1 ISBN 978-3-319-72410-2 (eBook)
https://doi.org/10.1007/978-3-319-72410-2

This Springer imprint is published by Springer Nature, under the registered company Springer International Publishing AG
The registered company address is: Gewerbestrasse 11, 6330 Cham, Switzerland

Contents

Editors, Associate Editors, and Contributors

Editors

Seanna Grob, M.D., M.A.S. Department of Ophthalmology, Harvard Medical School, Massachusetts Eye and Ear, Boston, MA, USA

Carolyn Kloek, M.D. Department of Ophthalmology, Harvard Medical School, Massachusetts Eye and Ear, Boston, MA, USA

Associate Editors

Christopher M. Andreoli, M.D. Vitreoretinal Surgery, Atrius Health and Department of Ophthalmology, Harvard Medical School, Massachusetts Eye and Ear, Boston, MA, USA

Yewlin E. Chee, M.D. Vitreoretinal Surgery, Department of Ophthalmology, University of Washington, Seattle, WA, USA

Dean Eliott, M.D. Vitreoretinal Surgery, Department of Ophthalmology, Harvard Medical School, Massachusetts Eye and Ear, Boston, MA, USA

Matthew F. Gardiner, M.D. Emergency Ophthalmology Services, Department of Ophthalmology, Harvard Medical School, Massachusetts Eye and Ear, Boston, MA, USA

Alice C. Lorch, M.D., M.P.H. Department of Ophthalmology, Harvard Medical School, Massachusetts Eye and Ear, Boston, MA, USA

Joan W. Miller, M.D. Department of Ophthalmology, Harvard Medical School, Massachusetts Eye and Ear and Massachusetts General Hospital, Boston, MA, USA

John B. Miller, M.D. Vitreoretinal Surgery, Department of Ophthalmology, Harvard Medical School, Massachusetts Eye and Ear, Boston, MA, USA

Roberto Pineda, M.D. Cornea and Refractive Surgery, Department of Ophthalmology, Harvard Medical School, Massachusetts Eye and Ear, Boston, MA, USA

Ankoor S. Shah, M.D., Ph.D. Department of Ophthalmology, Harvard Medical School, Boston Children's Hospital and Massachusetts Eye and Ear, Boston, MA, USA

Tomasz P. Stryjewski, M.D. Department of Ophthalmology, Harvard Medical School, Massachusetts Eye and Ear and Massachusetts General Hospital, Boston, MA, USA

Katherine E. Talcott, M.D. Vitreoretinal Surgery, Wills Eye Hospital, Philadelphia, PA, USA

Angela Turalba, M.D. Glaucoma Service, Department of Ophthalmology, Harvard Medical School, Massachusetts Eye and Ear, Boston, MA, USA

Peter B. Veldman, M.D. Cornea and Refractive Surgery, Department of Ophthalmology and Visual Science, University of Chicago, Chicago, IL, USA

Yoshihiro Yonekawa, M.D. Vitreoretinal Surgery, Harvard Medical School, Massachusetts Eye and Ear and Boston Children's Hospital, Boston, MA, USA

Contributors

Grayson W. Armstrong, M.D., M.P.H. Department of Ophthalmology, Harvard Medical School, Massachusetts Eye and Ear, Boston, MA, USA

Durga S. Borkar, M.D. Department of Ophthalmology, Harvard Medical School, Massachusetts Eye and Ear, Boston, MA, USA

Alison Callahan, M.D. Oculoplastic Surgery, Department of Ophthalmology, Tufts Medical Center, Boston, MA, USA

Ashley A. Campbell, M.D. Oculoplastic Surgery, Department of Ophthalmology, Johns Hopkins University School of Medicine, Baltimore, MD, USA

Catherine J. Choi, M.D. Bascom Palmer Eye Institute, University of Miami, Miami, FL, USA

Jonathan C. Chou, M.D. Department of Ophthalmology, Harvard Medical School, Massachusetts Eye and Ear, Boston, MA, USA

Liza M. Cohen, M.D. Department of Ophthalmology, Harvard Medical School, Massachusetts Eye and Ear, Boston, MA, USA

Lisa A. Cowan, M.D., Ph.D. Southern California Permanente Medical Group, Bakersfield, CA, USA

Mohammad Dahrouj, M.D., Ph.D. Department of Ophthalmology, Harvard Medical School, Massachusetts Eye and Ear, Boston, MA, USA

J. Daniel Diaz, M.D. Department of Ophthalmology, Harvard Medical School, Massachusetts Eye and Ear, Boston, MA, USA

Emma Davies, M.D. Cornea and Refractive Surgery, Department of Ophthalmology, Harvard Medical School, Massachusetts Eye and Ear, Boston, MA, USA

Avni P. Finn, M.D., M.B.A. Department of Ophthalmology, Duke Eye Center, Duke Medical School, Durham, NC, USA

Eric D. Gaier, M.D., Ph.D. Department of Ophthalmology, Harvard Medical School, Massachusetts Eye and Ear, Boston, MA, USA

Isaiah Giese, M.D. Department of Ophthalmology, Harvard Medical School, Massachusetts Eye and Ear, Boston, MA, USA

Natalie Homer, M.D. Department of Ophthalmology, Harvard Medical School, Massachusetts Eye and Ear, Boston, MA, USA

Benjamin Jastrzembski, M.D. Department of Ophthalmology, Harvard Medical School, Massachusetts Eye and Ear, Boston, MA, USA

Karen W. Jeng-Miller, M.D., M.P.H. Department of Ophthalmology, Harvard Medical School, Massachusetts Eye and Ear, Boston, MA, USA

Daniel Learned, M.D. Department of Ophthalmology, Harvard Medical School, Massachusetts Eye and Ear, Boston, MA, USA

Daniel R. Lefebvre, M.D., F.A.C.S. Oculoplastic Surgery, Department of Ophthalmology, Harvard Medical School, Massachusetts Eye and Ear, Boston, MA, USA

Michael Lin, M.D. Department of Ophthalmology, Harvard Medical School, Massachusetts Eye and Ear, Boston, MA, USA

Kristine Lo, M.D. Department of Ophthalmology, Harvard Medical School, Massachusetts Eye and Ear, Boston, MA, USA

K. Matthew McKay, M.D. Department of Ophthalmology, Harvard Medical School, Massachusetts Eye and Ear, Boston, MA, USA

Shizuo Mukai, M.D. Vitreoretinal Surgery, Department of Ophthalmology, Harvard Medical School, Massachusetts Eye and Ear, Boston, MA, USA

Huy V. Nguyen, M.D. Department of Ophthalmology, Harvard Medical School, Massachusetts Eye and Ear, Boston, MA, USA

Victoria S. North, M.D. Department of Ophthalmology, Harvard Medical School, Massachusetts Eye and Ear, Boston, MA, USA

Thanos D. Papakostas, M.D. Department of Ophthalmology, Harvard Medical School, Massachusetts Eye and Ear, Boston, MA, USA

Safa Rahmani, M.D., M.S. Department of Ophthalmology, Harvard Medical School, Massachusetts Eye and Ear, Boston, MA, USA

Rohini Rao, M.D. Department of Ophthalmology, Harvard Medical School, Massachusetts Eye and Ear, Boston, MA, USA

Veena Rao, M.D. Glaucoma Service, Department of Ophthalmology, Harvard Medical School, Massachusetts Eye and Ear, Boston, MA, USA

Edith R. Reshef, M.D. Department of Ophthalmology, Harvard Medical School, Massachusetts Eye and Ear, Boston, MA, USA

Miin Roh, M.D., Ph.D. Department of Ophthalmology, Harvard Medical School, Massachusetts Eye and Ear, Boston, MA, USA

Elizabeth J. Rossin, M.D., Ph.D. Department of Ophthalmology, Harvard Medical School, Boston, MA, USA

Lucia Sobrin, M.D., M.P.H. Uveitis Service, Department of Ophthalmology, Harvard Medical School, Massachusetts Eye and Ear, Boston, MA, USA

James A. Stefater, M.D., Ph.D. Department of Ophthalmology, Harvard Medical School, Massachusetts Eye and Ear, Boston, MA, USA

Zeba A. Syed, M.D. Department of Ophthalmology, Harvard Medical School, Massachusetts Eye and Ear, Boston, MA, USA

Marisa Gobuty Tieger, M.D. Department of Ophthalmology, Harvard Medical School, Massachusetts Eye and Ear, Boston, MA, USA

Danielle Trief, M.D., M.Sc. Cornea and Refractive Surgery, Columbia University Medical Center, New York City, NY, USA

Cindy Ung, M.D. Department of Ophthalmology, Harvard Medical School, Massachusetts Eye and Ear, Boston, MA, USA

Demetrios Vavvas, M.D., Ph.D. Vitreoretinal Surgery, Department of Ophthalmology, Harvard Medical School, Massachusetts Eye and Ear, Boston, MA, USA

Jay Wang, M.D. Department of Ophthalmology, Harvard Medical School, Massachusetts Eye and Ear, Boston, MA, USA

Yvonne Wang, M.D. Department of Ophthalmology, Harvard Medical School, Massachusetts Eye and Ear, Boston, MA, USA

Natalie Wolkow, M.D., Ph.D. Department of Ophthalmology, Harvard Medical School, Massachusetts Eye and Ear, Boston, MA, USA

David Wu, M.D., Ph.D. Vitreoretinal Surgery, Harvard Medical School, Massachusetts Eye and Ear, Boston, MA, USA

Michael K. Yoon, M.D. Oculoplastic Surgery, Department of Ophthalmology, Harvard Medical School, Massachusetts Eye and Ear, Boston, MA, USA

Lucy H. Young, M.D., Ph.D. Vitreoretinal Surgery, Department of Ophthalmology, Harvard Medical School, Massachusetts Eye and Ear, Boston, MA, USA

Tavé van Zyl, M.D. Department of Ophthalmology, Harvard Medical School, Massachusetts Eye and Ear, Boston, MA, USA

Introduction

According to the American Academy of Ophthalmology, an estimated 2.4 million eye injuries occur in the United States annually. An open globe injury is a severe form of ocular trauma in which a full-thickness defect develops in the wall of the eye, threatening not only the vision but also the quality of life of those affected. Our understanding of how to best address eye trauma has progressed substantially over time, and we now have significantly improved visual outcomes for patients in many cases when evidence-based treatment protocols are utilized.

Our experience in treating open globe injuries is based on our work at Massachusetts Eye and Ear, which serves as a major referral center for eye trauma and ophthalmic emergencies throughout New England. It is one of only a few hospitals in the United States that has a dedicated ophthalmology Emergency Department open around the clock; we are the initial point of evaluation for many patients with severe eye trauma.

Each year, Mass. Eye and Ear ophthalmologists surgically repair over a hundred open globe injuries and care for countless patients with nonsurgical eye trauma. Our trauma and emergency care teams also partner with clinicians at other Boston hospitals in the care of emergent and inpatient multisystem trauma, furthering their understanding of eye trauma principles. While each open globe injury is unique, we have developed frameworks and principles based on the vast experience and research of Mass. Eye and Ear's Ophthalmology team, which we use to guide management of patients with these injuries.

We are proud to have published, since 2010, an annual report on our medical and surgical quality and outcomes across our subspecialty areas, including open globe repair. Dedicated to our mission of eradicating blinding diseases and disorders, we hope to advance the standards for transparency and benchmarks in our discipline by spearheading the discussion and working toward ever better outcomes. Our ophthalmologists have spoken nationally and internationally on these topics and have published numerous articles describing our excellent outcomes and experience in eye trauma. We welcome the opportunity to educate and be educated in efforts to protect, preserve, and restore vision.

We are thrilled to present to you *Management of Open Globe Injuries*, in which we draw on the extensive experience of the Mass. Eye and Ear Eye Trauma Service and Emergency Department to present cases that highlight key principles in the management of open globe injuries.

We hope this text serves as a valuable resource for those who are called upon to care for patients with open globe injuries.

Boston, MA, USA — Joan W. Miller, M.D.
Boston, MA, USA — Carolyn Kloek, M.D.
Boston, MA, USA — Seanna Grob, M.D., M.A.S.

Part I
Management of Open Globe Injuries

Chapter 1
Classification of Open Globe Injuries

Edith R. Reshef and Matthew F. Gardiner

1.1 Introduction

As in any field of medicine, it is important to have a consistent, systematic approach to the evaluation of ocular trauma in order to provide the best possible care and ensure optimal clinical outcomes. When evaluating such injuries, utilization of a common language amongst providers, which includes a standardized terminology and classification system, is crucial to avoid ambiguity and confusion. In the mid-1990s, a concerted effort was made to classify eye injuries which has led to improved communication between practitioners, as well as the creation of more consistent, unambiguous clinical research in the field. Here, we provide a brief summary of these definitions, classification schemes, and prognostic predictors of ocular trauma.

1.2 Definitions: The Birmingham Eye Trauma Terminology

Ocular trauma can result in a wide variety of injuries affecting all parts of the globe. Some injuries which look deceptively benign may have devastating implications, while others which appear ominous initially may have a good prognosis. When trying to objectively describe eye injuries, the different presentations, mechanisms of injury, and affected ocular tissues make for potentially inaccurate communication between providers. In the past when there was no common syntax to describe ocular trauma, different terms were used to describe the same injury, or any one term could mean different things to different people.

E. R. Reshef, M.D. (✉) • M. F. Gardiner, M.D.
Department of Ophthalmology, Harvard Medical School, Massachusetts Eye and Ear, Boston, MA, USA

S. Grob, C. Kloek (eds.), *Management of Open Globe Injuries*,
https://doi.org/10.1007/978-3-319-72410-2_1

Table 1.1 Terms and definitions in BETT

Term	Definition	Explanation
Eye wall	Sclera and cornea	Though the eye wall has three layers posterior to the limbus, clinical and practical purposes dictate that violation of only the most external tissue is to be considered
Closed globe injury	No full-thickness wound of eye wall	The cornea and the sclera are not breached through and through
Open globe injury	Full-thickness wound of the eye wall	The cornea and/or sclera is breached through and through
Contusion	No wound of the eye wall	The damage may be due to direct energy delivery/shock wave by the object (e.g., choroidal rupture), or to changes in the shape of the globe (e.g., angle recession)
Lamellar laceration	Partial-thickness wound of the eye wall	Partial-thickness wound of the eye wall
Rupture	Full-thickness wound of the eye wall, caused by a large blunt object	Since the eye is filled with incompressible liquid, the impact results in instant intraocular pressure (IOP) elevation. The eye wall yields at its weakest point (rarely at the impact site, rather, for instance, along an old cataract wound); the actual wound is produced by an inside-out mechanism, and tissue prolapse is almost unavoidable
Laceration	Full-thickness wound of the eye wall, caused by a sharp object	The wound is at the impact site and is created by an outside-in mechanism; since IOP elevation is unavoidable, tissue prolapse is common
Penetrating injury	An entrance wound is present	If more than one wound is present, each must have been caused by a different object
Intraocular foreign body	One or more foreign objects are present	Technically a penetrating injury, but grouped separately because of different clinical implications (management, prognosis)
Perforating Injury	Both an entrance and an exit wound are present	The two wounds are caused by the same agent

After Kuhn, F. Ocular Traumatology, 2008. Terminology of Mechanical Injuries: the Birmingham Eye Trauma Terminology, page 7. Copyright ©, reproduced with permission from Springer Nature

The need for consistent language led to the development of the Birmingham Eye Trauma Terminology (BETT), a standardized language that is widely used today to describe ocular trauma (Table 1.1) [1–3]. This system enables more coherent communication between clinicians and unambiguous transmission of clinical data which allows us to better analyze outcomes and more accurately predict visual prognosis.

1.2.1 Open vs. Closed Globe Injury

The first step in classifying ocular trauma is to differentiate between an open and a closed globe. As BETT uses the wall of the eye as the frame of reference, the integrity of the sclera and cornea differentiates between open and closed globe injuries. An open globe injury is classified as any full-thickness wound whereas a partial-thickness injury to the eye, regardless of the extent of the trauma, is classified as closed globe injury.

1.2.2 Mechanism of Injury (Type)

The next step in evaluating globe injury (open or closed) is to determine whether the force was delivered via a blunt or sharp object. In open globe trauma, injuries due to blunt objects are called ruptures, whereas injuries from sharp objects are called lacerations. Lacerations are further classified based on the entry and exit wounds in the following way:

1. Penetrating injury: If the entry wound and exit wound are the same
2. Perforating injury: If the entry wound and exit wound are different and caused by the same object
3. Intraocular foreign body (IOFB): If the entry wound is present but the object (or part of it) remains in the eye (Fig. 1.1)

In closed globe injury, damage from a blunt object is called a contusion, whereas trauma from a sharp object causing a partial thickness wound is called a lamellar laceration (Fig. 1.2).

Inevitably, some injuries remain difficult to classify. For example, a bullet that is retained in the vitreous will technically be defined as an IOFB because there is an entry wound. However, because a bullet may confer blunt injury as well it may create features consistent with rupture elsewhere in the eye. In these situations, the ophthalmologist can either describe the injury as "mixed" (in this case, IOFB with rupture), or can refer to the most severe element of the injury.

1.3 Anatomical Location of Injury (Zone)

Once the nature (open vs. closed globe) and mechanism of injury have been defined, the anatomical location (or zone) of the injury should be determined, as this will help to complete the classification of the injury. The anatomic region of an ocular injury is a critical part of the initial ophthalmic exam, because it provides prognostic information. There are two different classification systems depending on whether the injury is an open or closed globe injury—both classifications include three "zones".

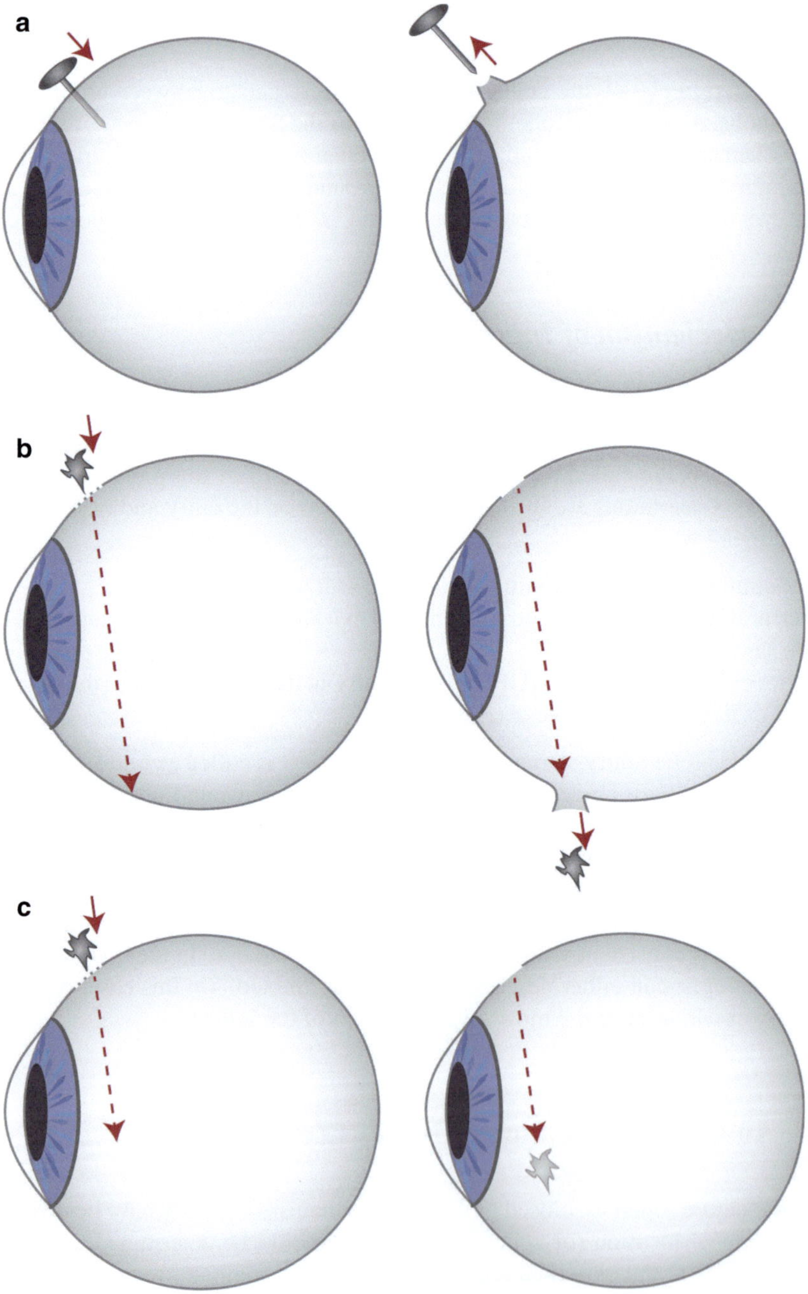

Fig. 1.1 Classification of lacerations. Penetrating injuries (**a**) have the same entry and exit wound, perforating injuries (**b**) have different entry and exit wounds which are caused by the same object, and intraocular foreign bodies (**c**) have an entry wound with the object remaining in the eye (This figure was published in Ocular Trauma, Banta, J. Page 43, Copyright © Elsevier 2007, reproduced with permission from Elsevier Saunders.)

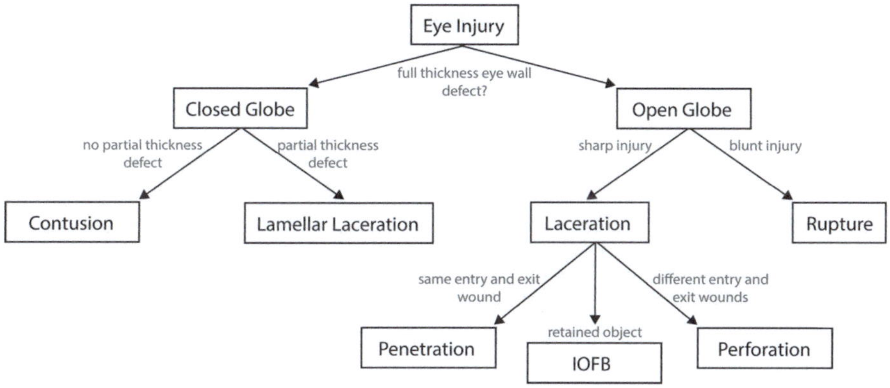

Fig. 1.2 Guideline to classifying ocular trauma in BETT. Flow diagram of injury types/guide to classifying injuries (After Kuhn, F. Ocular Traumatology, 2008. Classification of Mechanical Eye Injuries, page 8. Copyright ©, reproduced with permission from Springer Nature.)

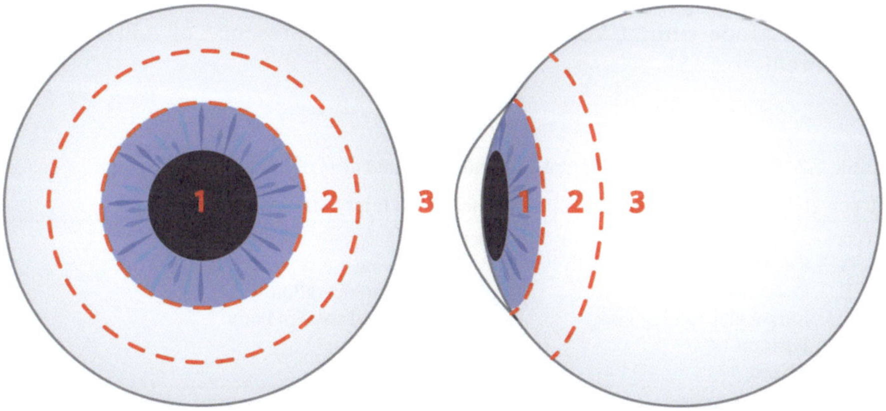

Fig. 1.3 Zones of injury for open globe. Zone I includes the cornea and limbus, Zone II spans from the limbus to 5 mm posterior into the sclera, and Zone III includes the area more than 5 mm posterior to the limbus. (Reproduced with permission from: Andreoli CM, Gardiner MF. Open globe injuries: Emergent evaluation and initial management. In: UpToDate, Post TW (Ed), UpToDate, Waltham, MA. (Accessed on 5/30/2017.) Copyright © 2017 UpToDate, Inc. For more information visit www.uptodate.com.)

For open globe injuries, Zone I injuries involve the cornea and limbus. Zone II injuries involve the anterior 5 mm of the sclera. Zone III injuries include full-thickness lacerations or ruptures that extend more than 5 mm posterior to the limbus (Fig. 1.3).

For closed globe injuries, Zone I includes the most external structures of the bulbar conjunctiva, sclera, and cornea. Zone II involves deeper blunt injuries of the anterior segment, including the lens and zonules. Zone III refers to the posterior segment including the vitreous, retina, optic nerve, choroid, and ciliary body).

1.4 Putting it All Together: Classification System

A clinical classification system was developed in 1997 based on four factors which help to determine prognosis and the likely final visual outcome (Table 1.2) [4, 5]. Two different classification systems exist—one for open globe injuries and one for closed globe injuries, however, both classifications are based on the same following four factors:

1. Type: the mechanism of injury
2. Grade: the initial visual acuity
3. Pupil: presence or absence of afferent pupillary defect
4. Zone: the anatomic location of the injury

Therefore, once the nature (open vs. closed globe) and mechanism (type) of injury have been defined, the initial ophthalmologic exam should include visual acuity (grade), evaluation for afferent pupillary defect (pupil), and the anatomic location of the injury (zone). All four of these factors have been shown to have prognostic value in estimating the final visual outcome, however, grade (initial visual acuity) and pupil (presence of APD) are the most predictive [5].

Table 1.2 Classification of open globe injuries (left) and closed globe injuries (right)

Open globe injury classification	Closed globe injury classification
Type: A. Rupture B. Penetrating C. Intraocular foreign body D. Perforating E. Mixed	Type: A. Contusion B. Lamellar laceration C. Superficial foreign body D. Mixed
Grade (Visual Acuity): A. ≥20/40 B. 20/50 to 20/100 C. 19/100 to 5/200 D. 4/200 to light perception E. No light perception	Grade (Visual Acuity): A. ≥20/40 B. 20/50 to 20/100 C. 19/100 to 5/200 D. 4/200 to light perception E. No light perception
Pupil: Positive: relative afferent pupillary defect present in affected eye Negative: relative afferent pupillary defect absent in affected eye	Pupil: Positive: relative afferent pupillary defect present in affected eye Negative: relative afferent pupillary defect absent in affected eye
Zone (See Fig. 1.2) I. Isolated to cornea and limbus II. Limbus to 5 mm posterior into the sclera III. Posterior to 5 mm from the limbus	Zone (See Fig. 1.2) I. External (limited to bulbar conjunctiva, sclera, cornea) II. Anterior segment (includes anterior chamber, iris, angle, lens, and pars plicata) III. Posterior segment (all internal structures posterior to lens capsule, including ciliary body, choroid, vitreous, retina, optic nerve)

After Kuhn, F. Ocular Traumatology, Classification of Mechanical Eye Injuries, 2008. Page 14,

1.5 Prognosis: The Ocular Trauma Score

After a serious eye injury, patients and family are most concerned about the eye's future potential. Patients will often ask 'Will I go blind?' or 'Will my vision recover?' Though it may be difficult to know the final visual acuity after all healing and surgical rehabilitation is complete, it is important for the clinician to have basic prognostic information at the initial evaluation. Though primary enucleation is generally discouraged except in cases where the eye cannot be closed, the clinician should convey realistic expectations for recovery.

Over the years, studies have examined which factors have the biggest influence on final visual acuity following ocular trauma [5–13]. The largest study to date, done in 2002 by Kuhn et al., identified six factors that have the highest prognostic significance: initial visual acuity, as well as five anatomical factors (rupture, endophthalmitis, perforating injury, retinal detachment, and APD). A scoring system has been developed whereby each of these six factors is assigned a point value whose sum helps predict the patient's visual acuity after recovery. This system, called the Ocular Trauma Score (OTS), provides a simple, easy-to-calculate quantitative prognostic score based on a limited number of variables all of which are determined during the initial evaluation of the injury. It can be easily referenced, and can provide reliable prognostic information—one study quoting a 77% likelihood of predicting the patient's final visual outcome within +/− one visual category [14, 15] (Table 1.3).

Table 1.3 Calculating the Ocular Trauma Score

Step 1: Determining the raw points

Variable	Raw points
Initial vision:	
NLP	60
LP/HM	70
1/200–19/200	80
20/200–20/50	90
≥20/40	100
Rupture	−23
Endophthalmitis	−17
Perforating injury	−14
Retinal detachment	−11
Afferent pupillary defect	−10

Step 2: Conversion of raw points into the OTS, and identification of the likely visual outcome (%)

Sum of raw points	OTS	NLP (%)	LP/HM (%)	1/200–19/200 (%)	20/200–20/50 (%)	≥20/40 (%)
0–44	1	74	15	7	3	1
45–65	2	27	26	18	15	15
66–80	3	2	11	15	31	41
81–91	4	1	2	3	22	73
92–100	5	0	1	1	5	94

After Kuhn, F. Ocular Traumatology, 2008. Predicting the Severity of an injury: The Ocular Trauma Score, page 20. Copyright ©, reproduced with permission from Springer Nature
NLP: no light perception, LP: light perception, HM: hand motion, OTS: ocular trauma score

1.6 Summary

1. It is important to have a systematic approach, consistent terminology, and uniform classification system when evaluating ocular trauma.
2. The Birmingham Eye Trauma Terminology (BETT) provides the accepted ocular traumatology definitions, and should always be used amongst providers to avoid confusion.
3. The classification system that includes type, grade, pupil, and zone provides a straightforward method of evaluating eye injuries and carries important prognostic information.
4. The Ocular Trauma Score (OTS) can be calculated immediately following the initial eye exam/surgery. It is a reliable prognostic tool, and should be used during decision-making and patient counseling.

References

1. Kuhn F, Pieramici DJ. Ocular trauma: principles and practice. New York: Thieme; 2002.
2. Kuhn F. Ocular traumatology. Berlin: Springer; 2008.
3. Banta JT. Ocular trauma. Philadelphia: Elsevier Saunders; 2007.
4. Pieramici DJ, Sternberg P, Aaberg TM, et al. A system for classifying mechanical injuries of the eye (Globe). Am J Ophthalmol. 1997;123:820–31.
5. Pieramici DJ, Au Eong K-G, Sternberg P, Marsh MJ. The prognostic significance of a system for classifying mechanical injuries of the eye (globe) in open-globe injuries. J Trauma. 2003;54:750–4.
6. Williams DF, Mieler WF, Abrams GW, Lewis H. Results and prognostic factors in penetrating ocular injuries with retained intraocular foreign bodies. Ophthalmology. 1988;95:911–6.
7. Joseph E, Zak R, Smith S, Best WR, Gamelli RL, Dries DJ. Predictors of blinding or serious eye injury in blunt trauma. J Trauma. 1992;33:19–24.
8. Bastiaensen LA. The visual prognosis of a perforation of the eyeball: a retrospective study. Doc Ophthalmol Adv Ophthalmol. 1981;50:213–31.
9. Sternberg P, de Juan E, Michels RG, Auer C. Multivariate analysis of prognostic factors in penetrating ocular injuries. Am J Ophthalmol. 1984;98:467–72.
10. Abu El-Asrar AM, Al-Amro SA, Khan NM, Kangave D. Visual outcome and prognostic factors after vitrectomy for posterior segment foreign bodies. Eur J Ophthalmol. 2000;10:304–11.
11. De Souza S, Howcroft MJ. Management of posterior segment intraocular foreign bodies: 14 years' experience. Can J Ophthalmol. 1999;34:23–9.
12. Esmaeli B, Elner SG, Schork MA, Elner VM. Visual outcome and ocular survival after penetrating trauma. A clinicopathologic study. Ophthalmology. 1995;102:393–400.
13. Hutton WL, Fuller DG. Factors influencing final visual results in severely injured eyes. Am J Ophthalmol. 1984;97:715–22.
14. Kuhn F, Maisiak R, Mann L, Morris R, Witherspoon CD. The OTS: predicting the final vision in the injured eye. In: Kuhn F, Piermici DJ, editors. Ocular trauma: principles and practice. New York: Thieme; 2002. p. 9–13.
15. Kuhn F, Morris R, Mester V, Witherspoon CD, Mann L. Predicting the severity of an eye injury: the ocular trauma score (OTS). In: Ocular traumatology. Berlin: Springer; 2008. p. 17–22.

Chapter 2
Pre-Operative Management of Open Globe Injury

Victoria S. North and Matthew F. Gardiner

2.1 Evaluation of the Ocular Trauma Patient

2.1.1 General Evaluation

In approaching a patient with suspected ocular trauma, it is essential to assess for life-threatening injuries first. Vitals signs should be checked, mental status assessed, and a brief physical exam performed. If there are any concerning signs or symptoms such as hemodynamic instability, neurologic deficits, or respiratory distress, the patient should be triaged to the appropriate emergency department or trauma center. After life-threatening conditions are assessed and treated, the clinician can then proceed with a detailed ophthalmologic history and physical exam. If an open globe is suspected, an ophthalmologist should be contacted immediately for emergent evaluation.

2.1.2 History [1–3]

The clinician should obtain a detailed history of present illness (HPI). It is important to determine the exact timing of the eye injury, as surgical repair should be planned within 24 hours. The time the patient last ate should also be noted for surgical planning, and the patient should be instructed not to eat until an open globe has been ruled out or until after surgical repair. The patient should be asked about the presence of any symptoms such as pain, changes in vision, diplopia or photophobia. Details regarding the mechanism of injury are especially important, as certain

V. S. North, M.D. (✉) • M. F. Gardiner, M.D.
Department of Ophthalmology, Harvard Medical School, Massachusetts Eye and Ear, Boston, MA, USA

S. Grob, C. Kloek (eds.), *Management of Open Globe Injuries*,
https://doi.org/10.1007/978-3-319-72410-2_2

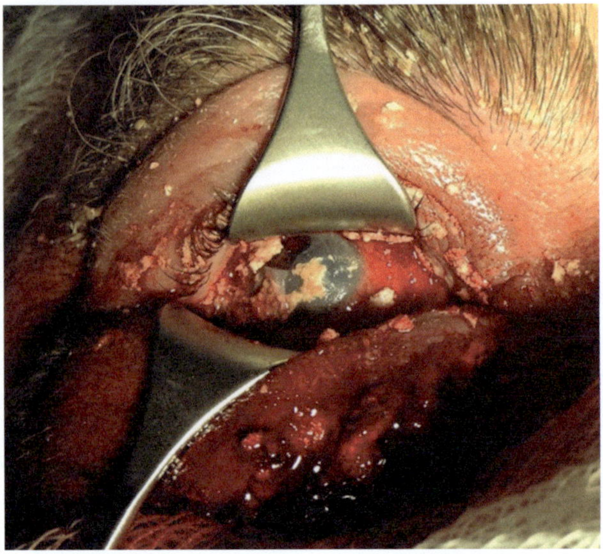

Fig. 2.1 Open globe injury after a blast injury with plaster material covering the ocular surface, requiring careful and expeditious removal of all material (as shown here), copious irrigation, and urgent surgical exploration and repair of the ruptured globe

features such as a high velocity projectile, injury with a sharp object, or high impact blunt trauma are suggestive of high-risk trauma. If a retained foreign body is suspected, details about the material composition, size, and shape of the object are useful. If chemical injury is suspected, immediate irrigation is essential and should precede a more detailed history and physical exam (Fig. 2.1). Irrigation in the setting of an open globe injury should be done only with sterile liquids and with extreme care to prevent extrusion of intraocular contents. Whenever possible, collateral information from witnesses should be obtained. An ocular history should be taken, including prior functional status and visual acuity (VA), eye conditions, medications, prior surgeries, and whether contact lenses or glasses were worn at the time of injury. Finally, it is important to obtain a basic medical history including medication allergies, tetanus immunization status, prior surgeries, active medications, and timing of last meal.

2.1.3 Physical Examination [1–3]

The ophthalmologic exam in trauma patients is often challenging due to the subject's significant pain and anxiety. General principles for examining such patients include minimizing manipulation of the eye (e.g. by deferring formal extraocular muscle testing) and avoiding any application of pressure to the globe or measurement of intraocular pressure whenever open globe injury is suspected. Topical medications such as tetracaine and fluorescein should also be avoided until open globe injury can be ruled out. If medicines must be applied, they should be from new, unopened bottles. In addition, all foreign bodies should be left in place until the comprehensive work-up is complete and definitive management is planned, as it might be best to

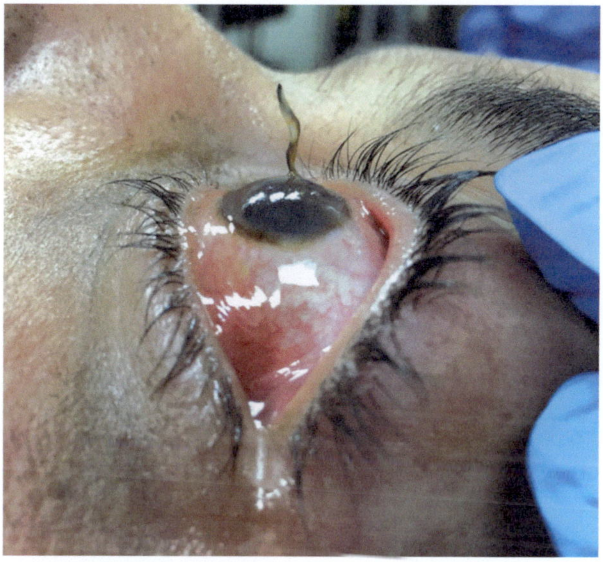

Fig. 2.2 Pre-operative photograph showing a metal wire protruding from the cornea that was removed intraoperatively in a controlled setting. The patient underwent removal of the foreign body and corneal repair as well as lensectomy and vitrectomy

remove the foreign bodies in the operating room under controlled conditions. (Fig. 2.2).

The first step of the physical exam is a general inspection of the head, face, eyes and eyelids, noting any ecchymoses, edema, or lacerations. Inspection should begin externally and progress internally. Ptosis and exophthalmos or enophthalmos should be measured and recorded. Periorbital soft-tissue and bony deformities such as crepitus or a "step-off" should also be noted, as these may be suggestive of an orbital or other facial fractures. Once attention is directed to the eye itself, first note any gross deformity with significant volume loss, large corneal lacerations, or prolapsed uvea. Sometimes, the full extent of injury can be masked and may require a more thorough examination. Subconjunctival hemorrhage can hide scleral lacerations, and intraocular hemorrhages can limit complete dilated fundus examination.

Visual acuity (VA) is a key component of the exam and is especially important in determining a baseline against which future exams can be compared. Testing each eye separately, VA can be assessed with a Snellen chart or near vision card, and refractive error should be accounted for either with glasses or by using a pinhole. If the patient's vision is too poor for the Snellen method, VA should be assessed via counting fingers, hand motion, or light perception as able. If vision is noted to be no light perception, this should be checked repeatedly, often by more than one physician, to confirm the finding pre-operatively. Visual fields can be tested to confrontation.

Pupils should be examined for direct and consensual responses to light, and a swinging flashlight test used to assess for a relative afferent pupillary defect (rAPD). This defect is present upon paradoxical dilation when light is shone into the eye. In general, a dilated pupil can indicate traumatic mydriasis, iris sphincter damage, direct damage to the third nerve, or secondary third nerve compression from

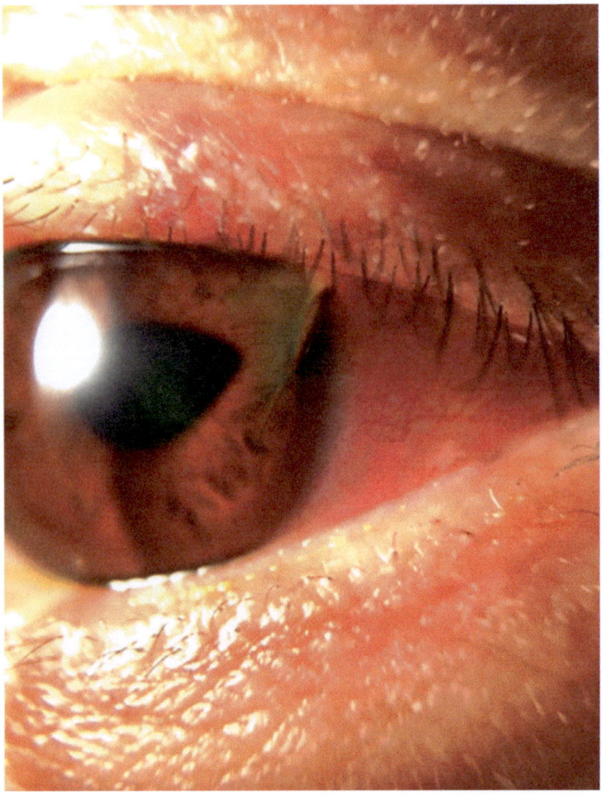

Fig. 2.3 Pre-operative photograph showing a peaked pupil towards the area of the corneal laceration laterally

increased intracranial pressure. A peaked pupil is a classic clinical finding seen in many open globe injuries and may be the first abnormality noted in children who cannot cooperate with a slit lamp examination (Fig. 2.3). Assessing color vision and red saturation can be useful adjunctive tools when time permits.

Intraocular pressure (IOP) should be checked following ocular trauma, but testing should be deferred until an open globe injury is ruled out. Importantly, a normal IOP does not exclude the possibility of an open globe injury, and IOP can be either high or low in the setting of trauma. High IOP can result from aqueous humor outflow obstruction either from anterior chamber inflammation, hyphema, angle closure, or an anteriorly dislocated lens. Low IOP can occur with open globe injury, ciliary body injury, cyclodialysis, or retinal detachment.

The conjunctiva, cornea, and anterior segment are best examined with a slit-lamp. The conjunctiva should be inspected for the presence of chemosis, subconjunctival hemorrhage, emphysema, foreign bodies, lacerations, or abrasions. Three hundred and sixty degree bullous subconjunctival hemorrhage is concerning for a posterior rupture in the setting of associated vitreous hemorrhage (Fig. 2.4). Eyelid eversion for complete inspection should only be performed once open globe injury has been excluded. All layers of the cornea should be examined closely, with special attention given to the presence of abrasions, edema, or lacerations. A Seidel test is useful for

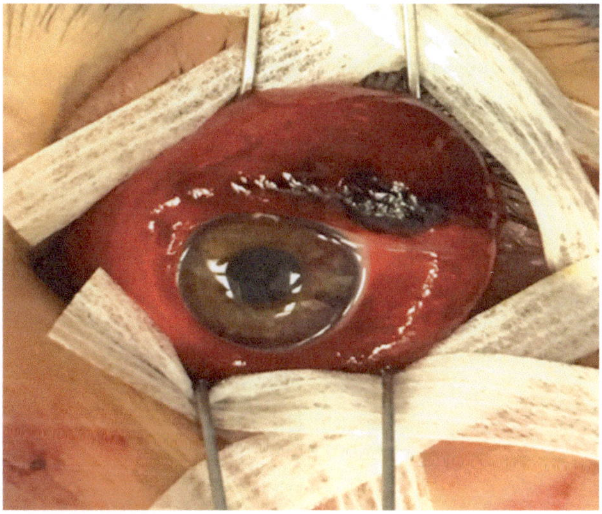

Fig. 2.4 Pre-operative external photograph of a soft globe with bullous 360° subconjunctival hemorrhage found to have a large Zone III rupture globe

evaluating for full-thickness corneal lacerations: fluorescein is carefully applied and the eye is examined under blue light—in cases of a full-thickness laceration, aqueous flowing from the anterior chamber will appear as a clear stream of fluid parting the yellow dye, indicating a positive Seidel test. It is important to assess the depth of the anterior chamber as well as the presence of cell, flare, hyphema, hypopyon, vitreous or foreign bodies. In the absence of an open globe injury, gonioscopy is a useful tool for close examination of the anterior chamber angle. However, in the setting of an open globe, gonioscopy may place too much pressure on a vulnerable globe and should be performed post-operatively to assess trauma to the angle structures. The iris should be inspected for breaks and pupil irregularities—here direct illumination or retroillumination can be helpful. Iris defects may be a key finding in cases of intraocular foreign bodies and should increase the examiner's suspicion for a posterior foreign body. Finally, the lens should be inspected for position, clarity, intralenticular foreign bodies, and integrity of the lens capsule, as post-traumatic changes such as subcapsular opacities and pigmentary alterations can occur (e.g. a Vossius ring of brown pigment on anterior lens capsule).

Complete ophthalmologic exam includes evaluation of the posterior segment, thus nearly all open globe patients should undergo a careful dilated examination pre-operatively. Exceptions to dilation include: cases of intracranial injury or hemorrhage that require close pupillary examination to monitor neurological status, a free-floating anterior chamber foreign body that may fall posteriorly if the pupil is dilated, or a foreign body through and through the iris where dilation risks moving the foreign body and causing further damage. In these cases, the pupils should be dilated as soon as possible, such as after the foreign body is removed in the operating room. The posterior segment should be evaluated for the presence of intraocular foreign bodies, hemorrhage, retinal trauma, or other issues prior to surgery as certain findings may change the initial operative plan or pre-operative discussion with the

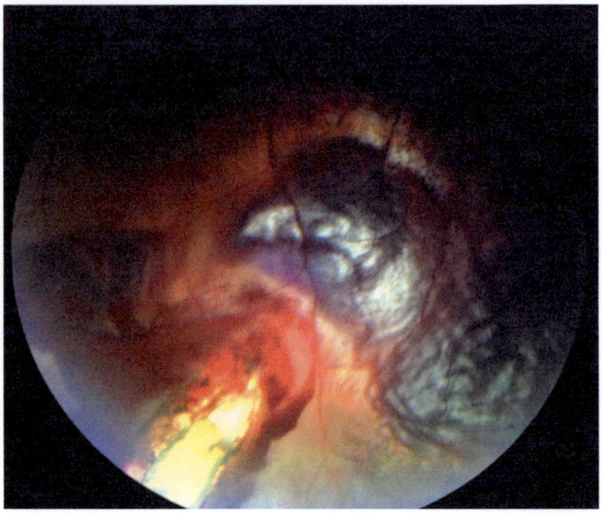

Fig. 2.5 Fundus photograph showing an inferior scleral laceration from a perforating injury with surrounding preretinal and subretinal hemorrhage. Note the foreign body within the scleral laceration

patient (Fig. 2.5). Scleral depression is not recommended as it can risk causing further damage and extrusion of intraocular contents. In many cases of ocular trauma, funduscopic exam may be limited by significant intraocular hemorrhage, an edematous, hazy cornea, or a traumatic cataract. Therefore, we often rely on adjunctive studies such as computed tomography (CT) scans to assist with the evaluation of open globe injuries and to rule out intraocular metallic foreign bodies or other associated facial or head trauma.

2.1.4 Clinical Features of Open Globe Injuries [1–3]

Though an open globe injury can present with a myriad of clinical features, certain findings are strongly associated and should prompt the clinician to pursue additional work-up. These are summarized in Table 2.1. They include markedly decreased visual acuity and pupil irregularities such as a peaked or eccentric pupil and a rAPD (Fig. 2.3). Low IOP is classic, though normal or even high IOP does not exclude the possibility of an open globe injury. However, IOP generally should be deferred if open globe is suspected prior to surgical repair. Similarly, discrepancy in anterior chamber depths is characteristic of open globes, but the defect may be either an abnormally deep (posterior laceration or rupture) or abnormally shallow chamber (anterior laceration or rupture) (Fig. 2.6). Extrusion of intraocular structures such as vitreous and uvea is highly specific for an open globe. Hemorrhagic chemosis, especially if present for 360°, may be suggestive as well (Fig. 2.4). Finally, irregularities such as corneal or scleral tenting and a positive Seidel test are clinical features that may indicate an open globe injury has occurred.

Table 2.1 Common physical findings in open globe injuries

Open globe injury: common physical findings
• Markedly decreased visual acuity
• Eccentric or peaked pupil
• Relative afferent pupillary defect
• Low intraocular pressure
• Shallow or abnormally deep anterior chamber
• Extrusion of vitreous
• External prolapse of uvea or other intraocular structures
• Hemorrhagic chemosis or subconjunctival pigment, especially in 360° pattern
• Tenting of cornea or sclera at puncture site
• Positive Seidel test

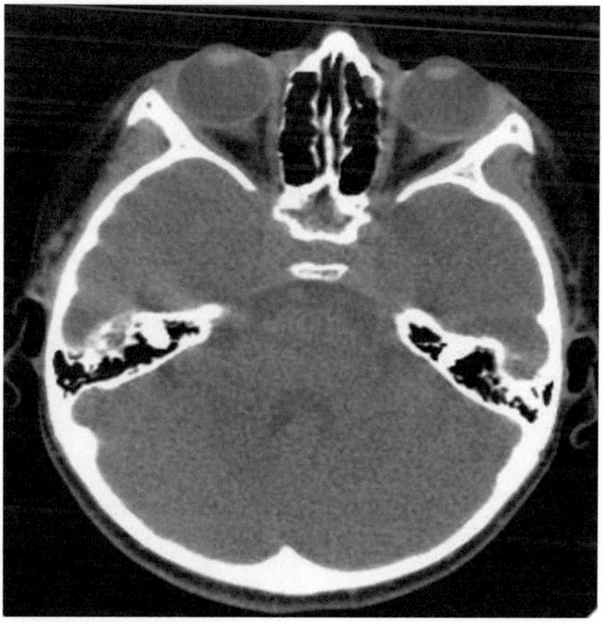

Fig. 2.6 Axial CT image showing a shallow anterior chamber on the right compared to the left in the setting of a Zone I open globe injury of the right eye

2.2 Imaging of Open Globe Injuries

2.2.1 Orbital CT

Computed tomography (CT) is the preferred imaging modality for trauma patients and should be ordered on almost all patients with suspected open globe injury. In cases of suspected open globe injury, non-contrast CT scan of the orbits with thin (i.e. 1–2 mm) axial and coronal cuts should be obtained [3]. If head trauma is suspected, orbital CT can be extended to evaluate the brain as well. CT findings suggestive of open globe injury include change in globe contour or scleral irregularity (Fig. 2.7), obvious volume loss, an absent or dislocated lens (Fig. 2.8), vitreous hemorrhage (Fig. 2.7), retinal detachment, large discrepancy in the depth of the anterior chambers (Fig. 2.6), and the presence of an intraocular foreign body (Figs. 2.9 and 2.10) or intraocular gas (Fig. 2.11) [4, 5]. Several studies evaluating the sensitivity and specificity of CT findings in diagnosing patients with open globe injury have demonstrated sensitivity between 56 and 76% and specificity ranging

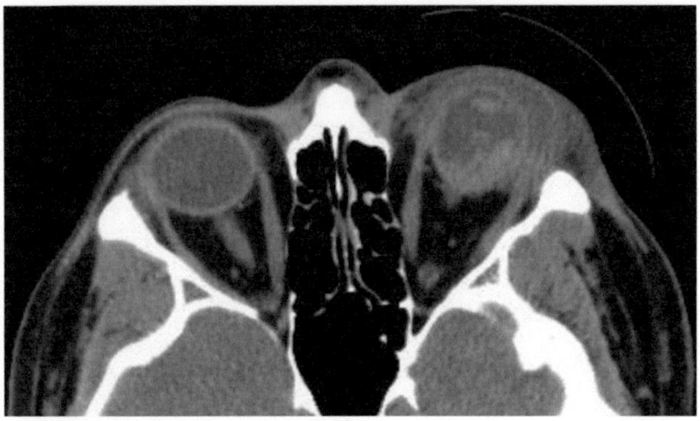

Fig. 2.7 Axial CT image of a severe Zone III injury demonstrating irregularity of the globe contour of the left eye with intraocular hemorrhage

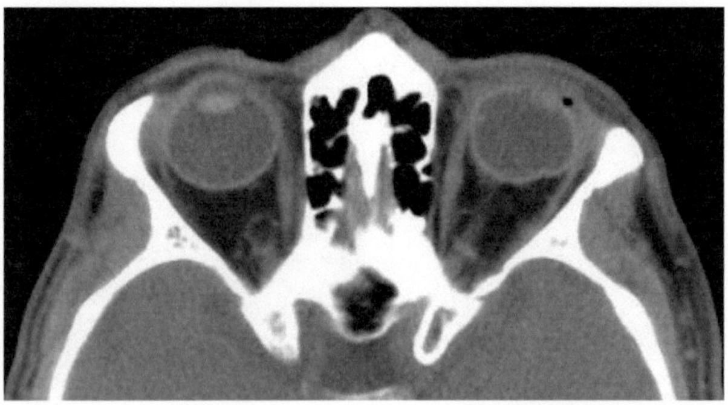

Fig. 2.8 Axial CT image showing a normal appearing globe and lens of the right eye and a left globe with irregular scleral contour and an absent lens

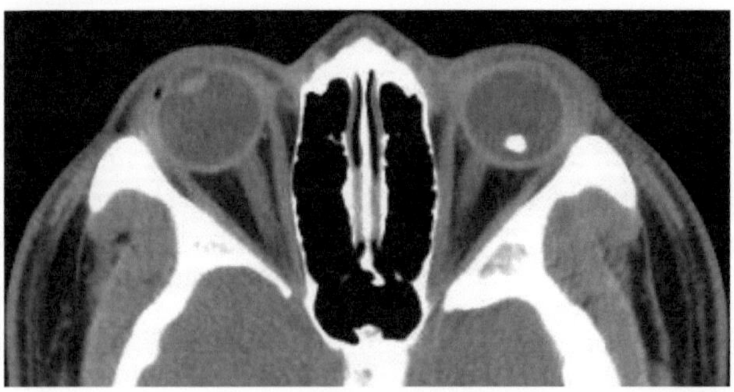

Fig. 2.9 Axial CT image showing an intraocular foreign body in the left eye located in the vitreous

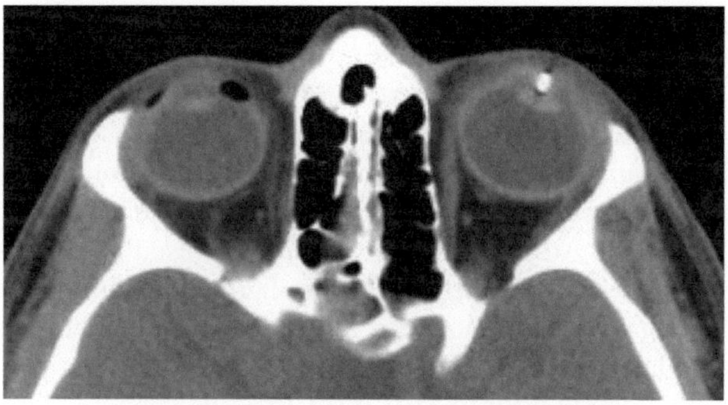

Fig. 2.10 Axial CT image showing an intraocular foreign body in the left eye penetrating the cornea into the anterior chamber

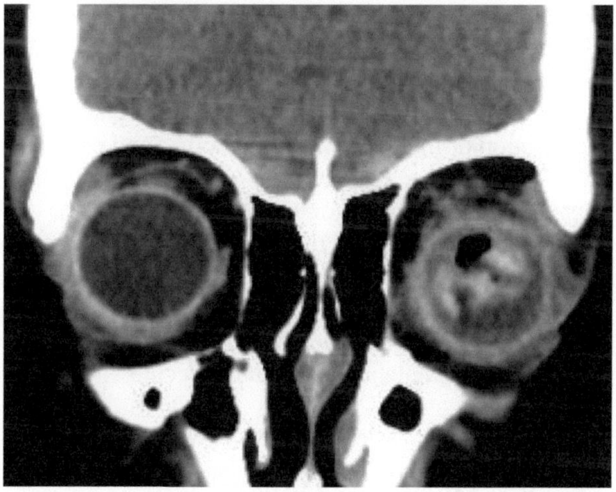

Fig. 2.11 Coronal CT image showing intraocular gas and hemorrhage in the left eye in the setting of a perforating open globe injury

from 79 to 100% [4–6]. These studies conclude that CT is not sensitive enough to be solely relied upon for diagnosis of all open globe injuries, but that it is a useful diagnostic tool when combined with history and physical exam. In addition, CT is relatively inexpensive, quick, can be used when a metallic foreign body is suspected, and produces less motion artifact than other imaging modalities.

2.2.2 *Other Imaging Modalities [1–3]*

Orbital CT imaging is the gold-standard imaging study for evaluating open globe injuries. We recommend ordering this on almost all patients with suspected open globe injury to rule out intraocular foreign body, evaluate for location of posterior rupture, and exclude other periocular trauma such as orbital fractures. However, in rare circumstances it may not be ideal. In particular, its use is contraindicated in pregnant women. Additionally, CT may not provide sufficient information about organic or non-metallic intraocular foreign bodies.

Magnetic resonance imaging (MRI) has an overall higher resolution of soft tissues in the orbit and brain. It can be helpful in diagnosing vascular lesions and other intracranial processes and can be used in pregnant women. However, MRI done initially in open globe injuries before CT or X-ray to rule out a metallic intraocular foreign body can be risky and is not recommended. MRI is also much more expensive and slower to obtain than CT, limiting its use in emergency situations. Additionally, MRI cannot be used in patients with pacemakers or other devices. It is suboptimal for visualizing bony structures, such as associated orbital or facial fractures, and may not be available at all medical centers.

Plain film (i.e. X-ray) can be useful to screen for the presence of a metallic foreign body prior to MRI if CT imaging cannot be done. In centers where CT and MRI are unavailable, plain film can help determine the presence and the general location of intraocular or intraorbital foreign bodies and orbital fractures. However, it is not as detailed as CT imaging, is not useful in identifying radiolucent material, and cannot visualize soft tissues well.

Finally, ultrasonography such as a B-scan can be useful to determine the presence and location of intraocular foreign bodies and can also provide general information about the posterior segment when funduscopic exam is limited. However, B-scan imaging requires direct contact with the eyelids or eye and places pressure on the globe. Therefore, it is not recommended in the setting of open globe injury prior to open globe exploration and repair. It is especially helpful after globe repair in determining the presence of retinal detachments, posterior capsule violation, lens dislocation, etc. B-scan imaging also requires experienced personnel and may not be practical or available at all medical centers.

2.3 Pre-Operative Management

2.3.1 General Management [1–3]

After life-threatening injuries have been assessed and treated, management of a suspected open globe injury should focus on preventing further damage, controlling symptoms, and providing infection prophylaxis (Table 2.2). Immediate ophthalmology consultation is indicated for any case of suspected open globe injury, and in preparation for possible surgical intervention these patients should take nothing by mouth (NPO status). Further injury to the eye should be prevented with strict bed rest with the head of the bed at 30° and no heavy lifting or strenuous activity. All services should avoid any unnecessary manipulation of the eye, and the ophthalmologist should make sure to inform other services of the status of the eye and the importance of not manipulating it or the periocular area in general. The open globe should be kept covered with a protective shield (e.g. a Fox shield) at all times to ensure that neither the patient nor other providers inadvertently put pressure on the eye, as this could cause extrusion of intraocular contents. Additionally, eye drops should be avoided unless an ophthalmologist deems them safe, and foreign bodies should not be removed until additional work-up or consultation is obtained.

Table 2.2 Key steps in the pre-operative management of open globe injuries

Open globe injury: pre-operative management
• Assess and treat life-threatening injuries first
• Immediate ophthalmology consultation if open globe suspected
• Obtain imaging (non-contrast CT of orbits with thin axial and coronal cuts)
• Ensure nothing by mouth (NPO)
• Avoid manipulating eye or applying pressure to globe
• Only use a new bottle for any necessary eye drops for an ophthalmic exam
• Determine time of injury to help plan for open globe repair within 24 hour of injury
• Do not attempt to remove foreign object
• Cover affected eye with a shield
• Strict bed rest with head of bed elevated 30°
• Aggressive treatment of nausea to avoid vomiting (e.g. IV ondansetron or metoclopramide)
• Treat anxiety (e.g. IV lorazepam) and pain (e.g. IV morphine) as needed
• Begin IV antibiotics
– Vancomycin (15 mg/kg, or approximately 1 g q12 hour × 4 doses)
– Ceftazidime (1 g q8 hour × 6 doses)
• Administer tetanus prophylaxis depending on immunization status and nature of wound
• Ensure definitive management by ophthalmologist

Symptom control should be achieved with intravenous (IV) medications whenever possible. Aggressive treatment of nausea is especially important in order to prevent vomiting and the associated increase in IOP, as this can lead to extrusion of ocular contents. Severe pain is typically managed with IV morphine or similar medications. It is also helpful to treat anxiety, both for the patient's comfort and for ease of examination. With children and intoxicated or otherwise uncooperative adults, it may be necessary to perform an exam under anesthesia to ensure a safe and thorough inspection. If intubation is required, it is typically recommended that the anesthesiologist avoid agents that have the potential to increase IOP, including high dose ketamine (e.g. 6 milligrams per kilogram or mg/kg) and succinylcholine. Lower doses of ketamine (e.g. 3 mg/kg) have not been shown to increase IOP, and premedication with dexmedetomidine when succinylcholine is used may lessen the rise in IOP [7, 8]. However, given these limitations, other agents such as midazolam for sedation and rocuronium for paralysis are preferred whenever possible. In addition, the type of laryngoscope used may also influence IOP, and the anesthesiologist should be aware of potential differences [9].

Life-threatening surgeries will take precedence over open globe injury repair, such as intracrainial hemorrhage requiring craniotomy and decompression. However, other non-emergent surgeries, especially those that may place pressure on the globe (such as facial or orbital fracture repair) should be postponed until after globe repair and preferably until the globe has had time to heal. It is important this information is relayed to other consulting services and a detailed plan for patient care is determined based on the severity and urgency of the patient's other injuries. In severe traumas, a multi-specialty surgery may occur to address all of the emergent/urgent surgical issues.

2.3.2 Antibiotics

Antibiotics are routinely used in the setting of open globe injury to prevent the development of post-traumatic endophthalmitis. The incidence of endophthalmitis in the absence of prophylactic antibiotic use is estimated at 10–11% [10]. Lacerations, delay from time of injury to presentation, the presence of an intraocular foreign body, and primary intraocular lens placement are all associated with a higher risk of developing post-traumatic endophthalmitis, whereas early primary repair, intraocular tissue prolapse and self-sealing of wounds are associated with lower risk [10–12].

The most common organisms isolated in culture-positive cases of endophthalmitis after trauma are gram-positive cocci (including Enterococcus, coagulase-negative staphylococci and *Staphylococcus aureus*), followed by Bacillus species and fungi [13, 14]. As cultures are not routinely obtained for open globe patients, the antibiotic regimen of choice should be broad with especially strong gram-positive coverage. Typically, IV vancomycin (15 mg/kg or approximately 1 gram (g) every 12 hours for 4 doses) and a third-generation cephalosporin such as ceftazidime (50 mg/kg or 1 g every 8 hours for 6 doses) are used for a minimum of 48 hours. Given that trauma patients may move between multiple areas of the emergency department and hospital, we find it useful to place a checklist in the patient's chart to ensure all doses are given. In patients with a penicillin or beta-lactam allergy, a fluoroquinolone such as ciprofloxacin can be used instead of ceftazidime. Prophylactic fungal coverage is not routinely used unless there are high-risk features such as intraocular organic foreign material.

The rate of endophthalmitis with IV antibiotic prophylaxis is very low—one study looking at patients treated with IV vancomycin and cefepime reported an incidence of 0.9% [11]. Similarly, another large case series in which patients were treated with 48 hours of IV vancomycin and ceftazidime saw an incidence of 0.9% [12]. Some recent studies have suggested oral regimens alone may be non-inferior to IV regimens [15, 16]. For instance, one study saw the development of endophthalmitis in 2–3% of patients treated with prophylactic antibiotics, and this did not differ significantly between those treated with a primarily IV regimen (IV cefazolin with oral ciprofloxacin) and those treated with oral antibiotics alone (oral cefuroxime and oral ciprofloxacin) [15]. However, our practice is to use IV vancomycin and a third-generation cephalosporin given the patients' NPO status, a desire to prevent nausea and vomiting, and the fact that most patients will be hospitalized for the 48 hour period.

2.3.3 Tetanus Prophylaxis

Though uncommon, there are case reports of post-traumatic endophthalmitis caused by *Clostridium tetani* [17]. In addition, animal models have shown clinical tetanus can develop in unimmunized mice when *Clostridium tetani* or its toxin is introduced into the anterior chamber, but not in immunized mice or in experiments involving non-perforating injury models [18]. These studies support the administration of prophylaxis against tetanus following perforating ocular injuries, especially when immunization status is unknown or not up to date, but not in cases of uncomplicated corneal abrasions or other types of non-perforating ocular injuries [18]. In our practice, patients with penetrating eye injury are assessed for tetanus immunization status, and tetanus booster and/or tetanus immune globulin are administered on a case-by-case basis [17].

2.4 Conclusion

- A detailed yet expedited history and ophthalmologic exam should be obtained after assessing and treating life-threatening injuries. The HPI should include mechanism of injury and details of any suspected foreign bodies.
- Clinical features of open globe injuries include markedly decreased visual acuity, peaked or eccentric pupil, relative afferent pupillary defect, low intraocular pressure, extrusion of intraocular structures, hemorrhagic chemosis, and corneal or scleral irregularities.
- Pre-operative assessment should include thorough external inspection, slit lamp exam, and CT scan of the orbits with thin cuts.
- Pre-operative management should center on minimizing further damage (strict bed rest, avoiding unnecessary manipulation of the eye, covering with a protective shield), aggressive symptom control, and infection prophylaxis with intravenous (IV) antibiotics and tetanus immunization when indicated.

References

1. Moraczewski AL. History and examination of the injured eye. In: Banta JT, editor. Ocular trauma. Philadelphia: W B Saunders; 2007. p. 19–38.
2. Harlan JB Jr, Ng EWM, PIeramici DJ. Evaluation. In: Kuhn F, Pieramici DJ, editors. Ocular trauma: principles and practice. New York: Thieme; 2002. p. 52–69.
3. Harlan JB, Pieramici DJ. Evaluation of patients with ocular trauma. Ophthalmol Clin North Am. 2002;15(2):153–61.
4. Arey ML, Mootha VV, Whittemore AR, Chason DP, Blomquist PH. Computed tomography in the diagnosis of occult open-globe injuries. Ophthalmology. 2007;114(8):1448–52.
5. Yuan WH, Hsu HC, Cheng HC, et al. CT of globe rupture: analysis and frequency of findings. AJR Am J Roentgenol. 2014;202(5):1100–7.
6. Joseph DP, Pieramici DJ, Beauchamp NJ. Computed tomography in the diagnosis and prognosis of open-globe injuries. Ophthalmology. 2000;107(10):1899–906.
7. Nagdeve NG, Yaddanapudi S, Pandav SS. The effect of different doses of ketamine on intraocular pressure in anesthetized children. J Pediatr Ophthalmol Strabismus. 2006;43(4):219–23.
8. Mowafi HA, Aldossary N, Ismail SA, Alqahtani J. Effect of dexmedetomidine premedication on the intraocular pressure changes after succinylcholine and intubation. Br J Anaesth. 2008;100(4):485–9.

9. Karaman T, Dogru S, Karaman S, et al. Intraocular pressure changes: the McGrath video laryngoscope vs the Macintosh laryngoscope; a randomized trial. J Clin Anesth. 2016;34:358–64.
10. Zhang Y, Zhang MN, Jiang CH, Yao Y, Zhang K. Endophthalmitis following open globe injury. Br J Ophthalmol. 2010;94(1):111–4.
11. Huang JM, Pansick AD, Blomquist PH. Use of intravenous vancomycin and cefepime in preventing endophthalmitis after open globe injury. J Ocul Pharmacol Ther. 2016;32(7):437–41.
12. Andreoli CM, Andreoli MT, Kloek CE, Ahuero AE, Vavvas D, Durand ML. Low rate of endophthalmitis in a large series of open globe injuries. Am J Ophthalmol. 2009;147(4):601–8.
13. Long C, Liu B, Xu C, Jing Y, Yuan Z, Lin X. Causative organisms of post-traumatic endophthalmitis: a 20-year retrospective study. BMC Ophthalmol. 2014;14:34.
14. Relhan N, Albini TA, Pathengay A, Kuriyan AE, Miller D, Flynn HW. Endophthalmitis caused by Gram-positive organisms with reduced vancomycin susceptibility: literature review and options for treatment. Br J Ophthalmol. 2016;100(4):446–52.
15. Du Toit N, Mustak S, Cook C. Randomised controlled trial of prophylactic antibiotic treatment for the prevention of endophthalmitis after open globe injury at Groote Schuur Hospital. Br J Ophthalmol. 2017;101(7):862–7. https://doi.org/10.1136/bjophthalmol-2016-309736. Epub 2016 Oct 28.
16. Tabatabaei SA, Soleimani M, Behrooz MJ, Sheibani K. Systemic oral antibiotics as a prophylactic measure to prevent endophthalmitis in patients with open globe injuries in comparison with intravenous antibiotics. Retina. 2016;36(2):360–5.
17. Iyer MN, Kranias G, Daun ME. Post-traumatic endophthalmitis involving Clostridium tetani and Bacillus spp. Am J Ophthalmol. 2001;132(1):116–7.
18. Benson WH, Snyder IS, Granus V, Odom JV, Macsai MS. Tetanus prophylaxis following ocular injuries. J Emerg Med. 1993;11(6):677–83.

Chapter 3
Pre-Operative Counseling and Intraoperative Considerations and Instruments

Seanna Grob, Angela Turalba, and Alice C. Lorch

3.1 Introduction

There are a number of steps that are important prior to taking the patient to the operating room for open globe repair. The prior chapter discusses the details of the patient exam, imaging, and medical management of the patient pre-operatively. However, there are additional steps that can foster a good doctor-patient relationship and lead to a successful open globe repair. These include pre-operative patient counseling and detailed discussion, pre-operative surgical planning, and instrument set-up in the operating room.

3.2 Pre-Operative Counseling

Once an open globe is confirmed, then a detailed discussion with the patient is crucial. Prior to starting the discussion, patients should be asked if they would like to include any other family members or friends in the conversation. Each surgeon will develop his or her own style in discussing these injuries with patients and families. In this chapter we outline some tips and guidelines based on our experience.

The main goal pre-operatively is to educate the patient and set expectations. If the extent of their injury, the course of care, and all of the possibilities are discussed with the patient in detail prior to globe repair, then the patient will never be too surprised with each step of treatment or any turn of events in the post-operative course.

S. Grob, M.D., M.A.S. (✉) • A. Turalba, M.D. • A. C. Lorch, M.D., M.P.H.
Department of Ophthalmology, Harvard Medical School, Massachusetts Eye and Ear, Boston, MA, USA

S. Grob, C. Kloek (eds.), *Management of Open Globe Injuries*,
https://doi.org/10.1007/978-3-319-72410-2_3

Start by telling the patient that they have an open globe injury, which refers to an injury that has a full-thickness cut or opening in the eye. It is helpful to describe the exam findings to the patient. Make sure to try and use basic terminology as much as possible. A typical explanation might include "there is a full-thickness cut in the cornea or the clear front part of the eye" or, "there are some contents from the inside of the eye that are on the outside of the eye". If there is a concern for posterior rupture, then it is important to tell the patient that the exam and imaging is consistent with an open globe injury and the recommendation is to explore the globe and "find the cut to sew it shut."

It is important to emphasize that the primary goal of the first surgery is to close the eye. Depending on the clinical exam on presentation, we also often emphasize that this will be just the first surgery and likely the patient will require other surgeries to save the eye or achieve the best possible visual and/or aesthetic outcome. Future surgeries could include, but are not limited to, repair of retinal detachment, vitrectomy for vitreous hemorrhage, traumatic cataract removal, repair of pupillary defects, placement of intraocular lens, penetrating keratoplasty, or other refractive surgeries to improve corneal astigmatism. Especially if there is a significant posterior rupture, then the patient will likely require at least one retinal surgery. There may be circumstances where other steps can be addressed in the primary surgery, such as foreign body removal, lensectomy, or vitrectomy, but often, the main goal of the first surgery is just to repair the globe and follow up surgeries are discussed after globe repair when the eye has had a chance to heal.

Do not understate the severity of the injury. If the patient presents with low vision and an afferent pupillary defect, make sure the patient and family understand the poor prognosis prior to open globe repair, including the possibility of losing all vision. Patients presenting with no light perception vision rarely recover any vision [1, 2]. When a patient presents with no light perception vision, it is recommended that this is checked and rechecked by the ophthalmologist. It may also be helpful for more than one person to document that this was the patient's vision in the patient's medical record. This finding should be discussed in detail with the patient. For patients with severe open globes, but light perception on presentation, discussing with the patient that their ability to see light might go away over the subsequent days due to the severity of the trauma to the eye and/or retina even with a successful open globe repair surgery can help set expectations. Often, patients are very stressed and anxious about the injury and as such are uncertain about whether they see light on presentation. It is worth taking time to confirm visual acuity.

Even for patients who come in with good vision and a Zone I open globe, it is important to tell the patient that their vision could worsen after repair of the globe and scarring or healing of the cornea. Additionally, immediately after the repair, a patient's vision can significantly decline from corneal edema and astigmatism from the newly placed sutures, so it is important to warn the patient of this change. Open globe patients are also at risk for infection and other potential issues like retinal detachments or glaucoma down the line. Thus, it is important to not understate the severity of the injury during the initial discussion and emphasize the likelihood of long term follow up after this injury.

For corneal wounds, it can also be helpful to prepare the patient for the potential complications that are associated with corneal wounds, such as wound leaks.

Complex stellate wounds or corneal wounds with retained foreign bodies may be more challenging to close and more prone to leaking. Discussing the process of checking for leaks and the steps for dealing with leaks pre-operatively can also help prepare the patient for post-operative issues.

If a traumatic cataract is seen or there is possible concern for one, it is important to review the plan for management of traumatic cataract with the patient. For cataracts without lens capsule violation, it is important to tell the patient that their vision may not improve after the repair, since the cataract will still be affecting their vision (unless it can be safely removed primarily). For patients with lens capsule involvement, it is important to review the different potential options and treatment courses. Sometimes, if the view is clear and it is safe to remove the cataract during the primary globe repair, then this will be the plan. However, commonly the view to the lens is obstructed after repair of a large corneal laceration and it's safer to remove the lens at a later date. This later date could be a few days to a week depending on if there is significant prolapse of lens material, inflammation, and/or an elevated intraocular pressure. This could also be weeks to even months later if there is minimal prolapse of lens material and controlled intraocular pressure and inflammation. This discussion could prepare the patient for the number of different possibilities and make the discussion later, much easier.

If there is concern for an open globe, but it cannot be confirmed due to patient cooperation (e.g. child or anxious adult), then it is important to discuss with the patient and/or family the importance of going to the operating room for an examination under anesthesia. In these cases, it is important to have patient consent for a number of different possibilities that could arise in the operating room. Consent for examination under anesthesia with possible exploration and repair of ruptured globe and all associated procedures. This could include repair of facial lacerations, canalicular laceration, lensectomy, removal of foreign body, or vitrectomy. If there are injuries that you are more concerned about, make sure to take more time to discuss these possibilities. Alternatively, especially in the setting of children, it can be helpful to make sure the family stays around the hospital and can be easily contacted from the operating room after the examination under anesthesia is complete. Then the exam findings and the surgical plan can be discussed with the family at that time prior to proceeding.

If the vision is no light perception and has been confirmed more than once, then it is reasonable to discuss the options of globe repair versus enucleation or evisceration with the patient. We have found that most patients want to try and save their eye even if it means they might never see out of it again. Some patients at least would like to give the eye a chance with the globe repair and find out the visual result on follow up exam. Some patients chose to proceed with enucleation shortly after globe repair due to a blind and painful eye, but other patients prefer to keep their eye even without light perception and the known risk of sympathetic ophthalmia. This is a patient's choice and if they would like to save the globe, this should at least be attempted. There is a huge psychological component to losing an eye after enucleation that needs to be considered [3]. Many patients are happy to have "saved" their eye even if it is no light perception.

The patient should also be informed about the potential complications related to open globe injuries. As mentioned above, risks discussed should include infection or endophthalmitis, bleeding, retinal detachment, corneal scarring, cataract, vision loss, loss of the eye, and of need for more surgery. Additionally, the risk of sympathetic ophthalmia should be discussed with the patient. Studies show the incidence of sympathetic ophthalmia being less than 1% and ranging from 0 to 0.37% [4–10]. Often even when patients hear about this condition, they still are interested in saving their eye.

After you feel the patient has been adequately informed about the surgical procedure and plan and the potential future issues, then you can proceed with having the patient sign the surgical consent for open globe exploration and repair.

3.3 Pre-Operative Planning

Writing out the steps of your planned open globe repair prior to going to the operating room can be helpful. This can really organize your surgical plan and also help determine what sutures and surgical instruments are needed.

For corneal wounds, it is useful to draw out the corneal wound as soon as you examine the patient. Corneal edema will worsen overtime and if you are not proceeding to the operating room immediately and the surgery is going the following morning or there are no immediate openings in the operating room, the appearance of the corneal wound will change with time. Additionally, it can be helpful to think through suture placement in a complex corneal wound paying attention to aligning the limbus and the apices of a stellate corneal laceration first.

Example plan for Zone I Corneal Laceration

1. Paracentesis directed towards the corneal laceration
2. Inject filtered air +/− balanced salt solution to fill the anterior chamber
3. Place 10-0 nylon sutures to align the limbus or apices first
4. Place 10-0 nylon sutures to align the remainder of the corneal wound
5. Use an iris spatula to ensure no iris in the corneal wound while placing sutures
6. Inject filtered air as needed through the paracentesis to maintain anterior chamber depth
7. Consider using a cyclodialysis spatula to gently sweep iris out of the wound if necessary
8. After corneal wound repaired, replace filtered air with balanced salt solution in the anterior chamber
9. Rotate suture knots and replace loose or tight sutures as needed
10. Check corneal wound for leaks with fluorescein strip
11. If does not leak, then suture the paracentesis and bring the eye to normal pressure and check paracentesis for leak
12. If leaks, then replace/change sutures where leak located and recheck with fluorescein strip
13. If continues to leak after placing and replacing sutures, then consider corneal glue (make sure to have necessary supplies) or if slow leak, then consider a bandage contact lens

Writing out the steps for posterior ruptures is also helpful. Reminding yourself about how to hook and isolate muscles in case you need to do this to expose the rupture site is also important, particularly if not part of usual practice.

Pre-operative planning is also helpful in order to know which instruments and equipment you will need for globe repair. This allows the operating room staff to have everything you need readily available. Then, they will not need to be running around looking for things intraoperatively. Below you will see the common instruments we use for our globe repairs.

3.4 Intraoperative Considerations and Instruments

3.4.1 Surgical Instruments

Pre-operative preparation is especially important for a successful open globe repair. Our operating room staff is very familiar with open globe repairs, surgical preferences, and eye surgery in general. However, when operating at a main operating room or a place less familiar with eye surgery cases, it is essential to know your own equipment and the instruments you will need and communicate this effectively to the staff.

Below is an example of our common operating room table set up for open globe repairs (Fig. 3.1).

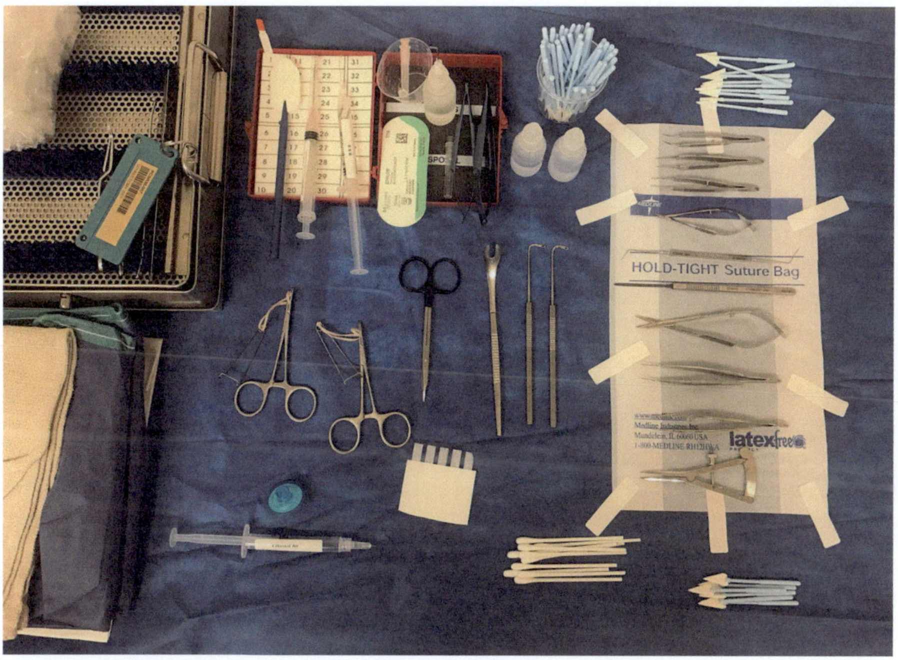

Fig. 3.1 Common instrument set up for open globe repair

List of commonly used instruments includes:

Eye drape
Thin Steri strips
Jaffe eyelid speculums with rubber bands and hemostats x 2
Paracentesis blade
Castroviejo 0.12 forceps × 2
Colibri forceps
Blunt Wescott scissors
Curved Stevens scissors
Iris spatula
Cyclodialysis spatula
Fine needle holders
Tying forceps: one bent and one straight
Vannas scissors
Caliper
Gass muscle hooks
Schepens retractor
Filtered air
Weck-Cels and Q-tips
Sterile irrigating balanced salt solution ×2–3 bottles and irrigating cannula
Balanced salt solution in a syringe with a 30-gauge cannula
Sutures

Jaffe eyelid speculums or similar are especially important for retracting the eyelids, while keeping pressure off of the globe. The commonly used eyelid speculums may place unwanted pressure on the globe causing extrusion of intraocular contents. Jaffe speculums lift the eyelids up and off of the globe. The ones we use are below (Fig. 3.2) and a rubber band is attached to the end and then secured in place with a hemostat attached to the surgical drape. Thin Steri strips™ can be placed over the eyelashes and eyelid margin on the upper and lower eyelid after the eye drape is placed to retract the eyelashes out of the field. Then the Jaffe eyelid speculums can be placed.

An iris spatula is an especially useful tool in open globe repair. It can be used by the assistant to hold iris or other uveal tissue out of the wound and the suture pass while the surgeon continues to suture.

Filtered air is also a key component of corneal laceration repair (Fig. 3.3). It keeps the anterior chamber formed and the wound dry while suturing the cornea. It has to be injected intermittently during repair as the air will continue to leak through the corneal wound until it is completely closed. Viscoelastic or sodium hyaluronate may also be helpful to keep the iris back from the cornea or when doing a traumatic cataract extraction.

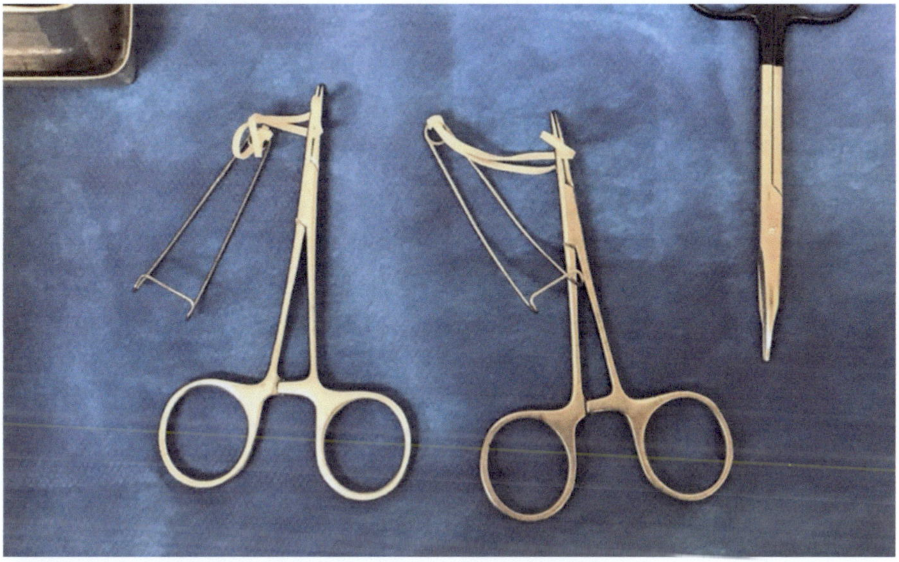

Fig. 3.2 Jaffe eyelid speculums for the upper and lower eyelid with attached rubber bands and hemostats

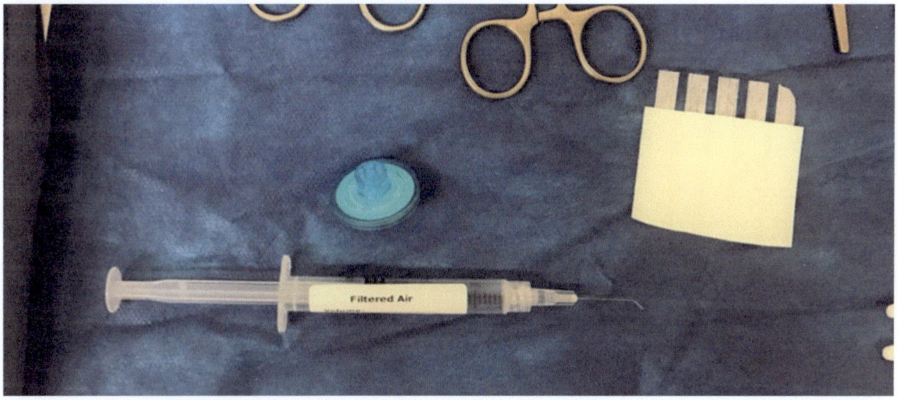

Fig. 3.3 Filtered air on a 30-gauge cannula

The Schepens orbital retractor (Fig. 3.4) is a useful instrument for retracting for posterior rupture repairs. Thin malleable retractors that often come in a separate malleable set are also helpful for posterior rupture exposure.

Gass muscle hooks with an oval hole (often used for retinal detachment/scleral buckle surgery) are used for isolating muscles (Fig. 3.4). A 2-0 silk suture is passed

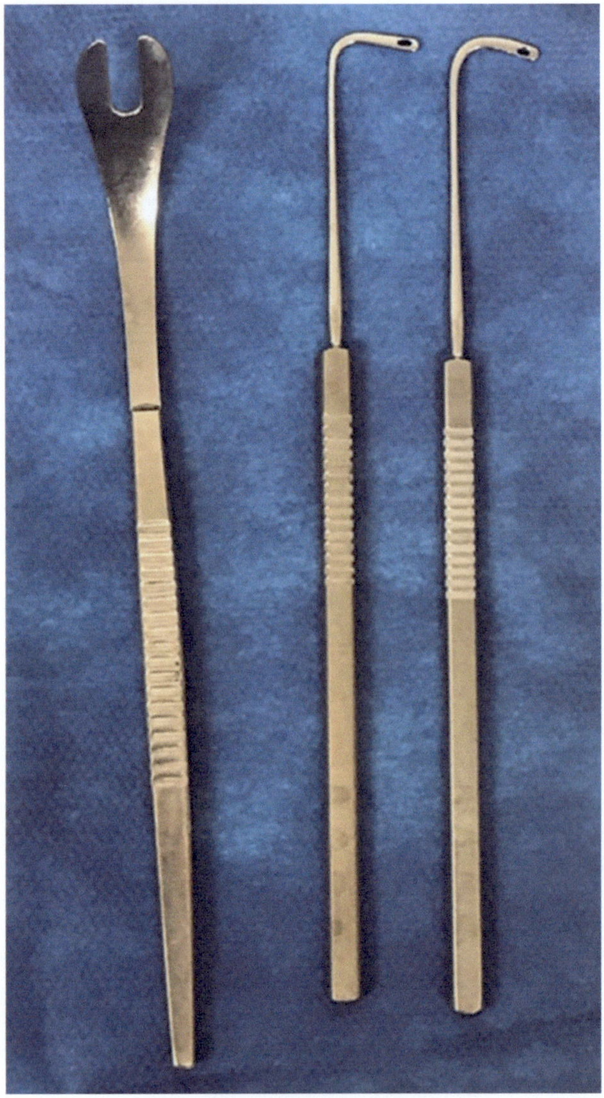

Fig. 3.4 Gass muscle hooks (right) are helpful for hooking and isolating the extraocular muscles and a Schepens retractor which can be helpful for exposing posterior ruptures

through the hole and the muscle is hooked and then the 2-0 silk suture is pulled through to wrap around the muscle insertion site. The suture can then be used to move and retract the globe and can also be used to explore posterior to the muscle insertion to look for posterior ruptures or extension of wounds.

Weck-cels® (Beaver-Visitec International, Inc., Waltham, MA) and balanced salt solution are often used generously. An assistant can use these regularly to clear heme off of the eye to help visualize the wound and to keep the cornea from drying out.

Depending on the open globe rupture, additional instruments may be necessary. Microsurgical technology set (MST set) may be needed to secure an anterior chamber foreign body or fashion a capsulorrhexis from a violated anterior capsule. The retina intraocular foreign body forceps may be helpful as well and are larger than the ones in the MST set. The phacoemulsification machine would need to be set up for a traumatic cataract, and cataract surgery instruments available as well as a vitrector if doing a primary vitrectomy and/or lensectomy. Remember to check the microscope prior to starting the case to make sure it is set up how you like and working appropriately. Also ask the scrub tech whether the correct sterile microscope handles are available and are sterile as well.

Finally, a subconjunctival injection of cefzolin and dexamethasone at the conclusion of the repair is given. This is done away from the location of the laceration or rupture. The concentration we use for subconjunctival injections is Cefazolin 100 mg/0.5 ml and Dexamethasone 400 mcg/0.1 ml. This might not be available at all hospitals.

If you work at an eye hospital, often a cataract surgery set and a vitrectomy set include the necessary surgical instruments. An eyelid or oculoplastics set can be added if there are eyelid or facial lacerations that need to be addressed. If you are covering a hospital on call, you may need to figure out what sets they have and what is available in them. Some hospitals have specific eye trauma sets available.

3.4.2 Sutures

The most commonly used sutures in open globe repair include a 10-0 nylon for corneal wound repair, 9-0 nylon for limbus realignment, and an 8-0 nylon for scleral wound repair (Fig. 3.5). We prefer these sutures on a spatulated needle. An 8-0 Vicryl suture is used to close the conjunctiva after a peritomy or to repair conjunctival lacerations.

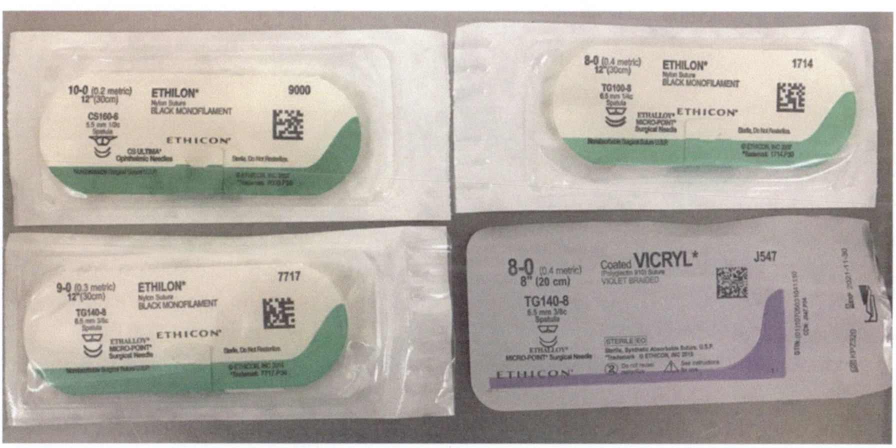

Fig. 3.5 Common sutures for open globe repair 10-0, 9-0, and 8-0 nylon sutures and an 8-0 Vicryl suture

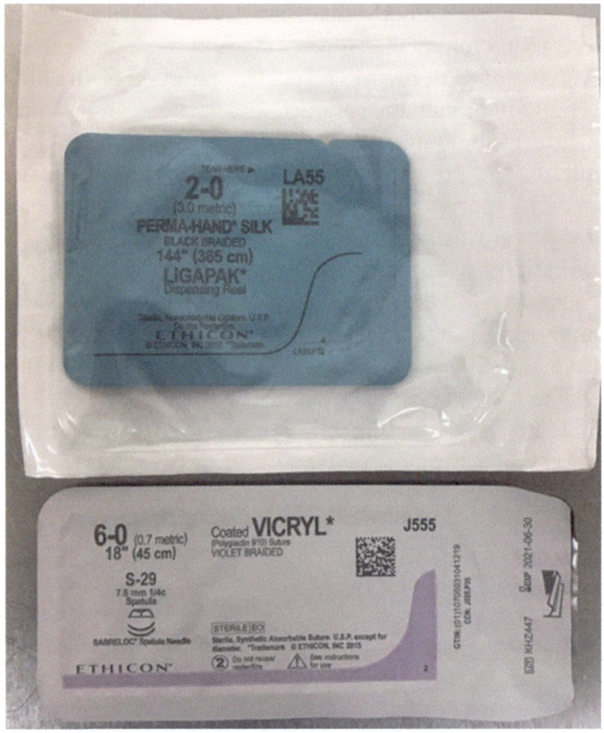

Fig. 3.6 Sutures for muscle isolation including a 2-0 silk suture on a reel and a 6-0 Vicryl double-armed suture on a spatulated needle

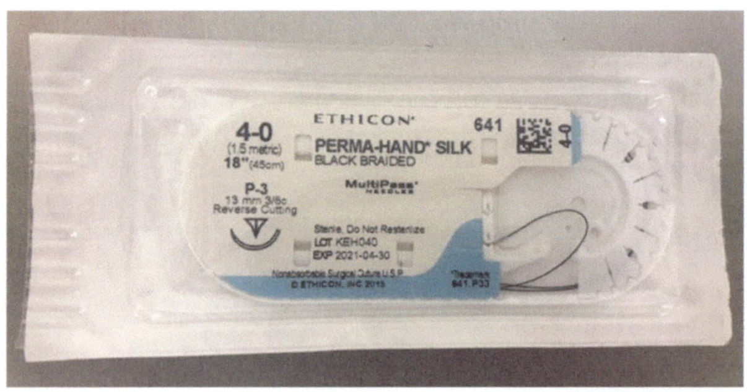

Fig. 3.7 4-0 silk suture for eyelid retraction

A 2-0 silk suture on a reel (or without a needle) are used for passing through a Gass muscle hook and hooking and securing the extraocular muscles during open globe exploration and repair (Fig. 3.6). A 6-0 Vicyl double-armed suture on a spatulated needle is used for imbricating the edge of the muscle near the muscle insertion if it needs to be disinserted for exposure of the rupture site for repair (Fig. 3.6).

A 4-0 silk suture can be helpful in cases where there are significant eyelid lacerations and marginal eyelid lacerations that do not allow a Jaffe lid speculum to stay in place. The suture can be passed through the eyelid margin and retracted with a hemostat or other (Fig. 3.7).

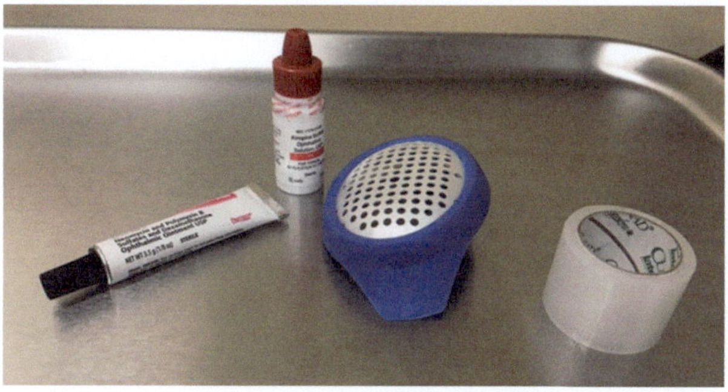

Fig. 3.8 Post-operatively place a drop of atropine and antibiotic ointment (dexamethasone, neomycin, and polymixin B ophthalmic ointment shown here) in the surgical eye. Then gently tape the eyelids closed with a thin Steri-strip, tape a sterile eye pad over the eyelids, and then tape a fox shield (shown here) over the eye pad. The eye pad is removed the following day, but the fox shield should be covering and protecting the eye at all times

3.4.3 Post-Operative Supplies

After globe repair, a drop of atropine and also some antibiotic ophthalmic ointment can be placed in the surgical eye. Then gently tape the eyelids shut with a thin Steri-strip and then tape a sterile eye pad over the closed eyelids followed by a protective fox shield (Fig. 3.8).

References

1. Han YS, Kavoussi SC, Adelman RA. Visual recovery following open globe injury with initial no light perception. Clin Ophthalmol. 2015;9:1443–8.
2. Salehi-Had H, et al. Visual outcomes of vitreoretinal surgery in eyes with severe open-globe injury presenting with no-light-perception vision. Graefes Arch Clin Exp Ophthalmol. 2009;247(4):477–83.
3. Ye J, et al. Vision-related quality of life and appearance concerns are associated with anxiety and depression after eye enucleation: a cross-sectional study. Plos One. 2015;10(8):e0136460.
4. Andreoli CM, et al. Low rate of endophthalmitis in a large series of open globe injuries. Am J Ophthalmol. 2009;147(4):601–8. e2.
5. Zhang Y, et al. Development of sympathetic ophthalmia following globe injury. Chin Med J. 2009;122(24):2961–6.
6. Chang GC, Young LH. Sympathetic ophthalmia. Semin Ophthalmol. 2011;26(4-5):316–20.
7. Savar A, et al. Enucleation for open globe injury. Am J Ophthalmol. 2009;147(4):595–600.e1.
8. Rofail M, Lee GA, O'Rourke P. Prognostic indicators for open globe injury. Clin Exp Ophthalmol. 2006;34(8):783–6.
9. Rahman I, et al. Open globe injuries: factors predictive of poor outcome. Eye (Lond). 2006;20(12):1336–41.
10. Casson RJ, Walker JC, Newland HS. Four-year review of open eye injuries at the Royal Adelaide Hospital. Clin Exp Ophthalmol. 2002;30(1):15–8.

Chapter 4
Post-Operative Management

Seanna Grob, Angela Turalba, and Alice C. Lorch

4.1 Introduction

Post-operative care is just as important as a good open globe repair for the best visual acuity and aesthetic outcome. It is crucial that the patients are followed closely and referred promptly to subspecialty services when necessary. Patients may need coaching and special attention to help them through the post-operative clinical course, whether excellent or poor outcomes are expected.

4.2 Follow Up Schedule

In our protocol, the patient is admitted after open globe repair to complete the 48 hours of intravenous (IV) antibiotics (see Chap. 2 for antibiotic schedule) [1]. Depending on how many doses of antibiotics they received prior to the repair, the patient may stay inpatient for approximately 24–48 hours. Outside hospitals are instructed to start IV antibiotics as soon as an open globe is suspected, and as such the length of stay can be minimized.

At the end of surgical repair, a subconjunctival injection of cefazolin and dexamethasone is administered away from the area of injury and atropine and antibiotic ointment are placed on the eye. An eye patch with fox shield is placed over the surgical eye and is left in place until the following day. No drops are put in the eye overnight and the patient is told to rest.

The patient is seen daily while they are an inpatient. In multi-trauma cases where the patient has to remain inpatient for longer due to recovery or surgical intervention

S. Grob, M.D., M.A.S. (✉) • A. Turalba, M.D. • A. C. Lorch, M.D., M.P.H.
Department of Ophthalmology, Harvard Medical School, Massachusetts Eye and Ear, Boston, MA, USA

S. Grob, C. Kloek (eds.), *Management of Open Globe Injuries*,
https://doi.org/10.1007/978-3-319-72410-2_4

from other traumas, the examinations can be spread out after the patient is seen on post-operative day 1, but the patient is monitored regularly.

A simplified schedule for follow up is:

1. *Post-operative Day 1 Visit*
2. *Post-operative Week 1 Visit*
3. *Post-operative Week 3–4 Visit*
4. *Post-operative Week 5–6 Visit (consider starting corneal suture removal)*
5. *Post-operative Week 12 (contact lens evaluation and trauma follow up)*

The above schedule is obviously modified for more or less frequent visits, including subspecialty visits, depending on the nature of the injury and surgery. (Example: Figs. 4.1a, b and 4.2—See later chapter for full discussion of this case).

This schedule changes for pediatric patients; corneal sutures are removed in this patient population earlier, often in the operating room.

Our simplified schedule for pediatric follow up is:

1. *Post-operative Day 1 Visit*
2. *Post-operative Week 1 Visit (often co-evaluation with a pediatric ophthalmologist)*
3. *Post-operative Week 3–4 Visit (often co-evaluation with a pediatric ophthalmologist)*
4. *Post-operative Week 4–5 Removal of corneal sutures in the operating room*
5. *Post-operative Week 5–6 Follow up with pediatric ophthalmologist and close follow up after this for glasses, contacts, amblyopia prevention or management, et cetera.*

We will review a more detailed summary of our plan of the follow up visits below.

4.3 Post-Operative Day 1

On the post-operative day 1 visit, the eye patch is removed and the eye is examined thoroughly. This includes a complete ophthalmic examination. Care should be taken to evaluate:

1. *Eyelids and periorbital area if any lacerations repaired or any changes overnight.*
2. *The conjunctiva for good closure and scleral coverage after surgical repair for any scleral lacerations or ruptures.*
3. *The sclera for good contour and closure after repair.*
4. *The cornea for good closure if a corneal laceration was repaired, that the sutures are intact, and there are no leaks (Seidel test).*
5. *Anterior chamber for depth, as a shallow or flat chamber might suggest a wound leak, as well as for inflammation, fibrin, hyphema, or hypopyon, etc.*

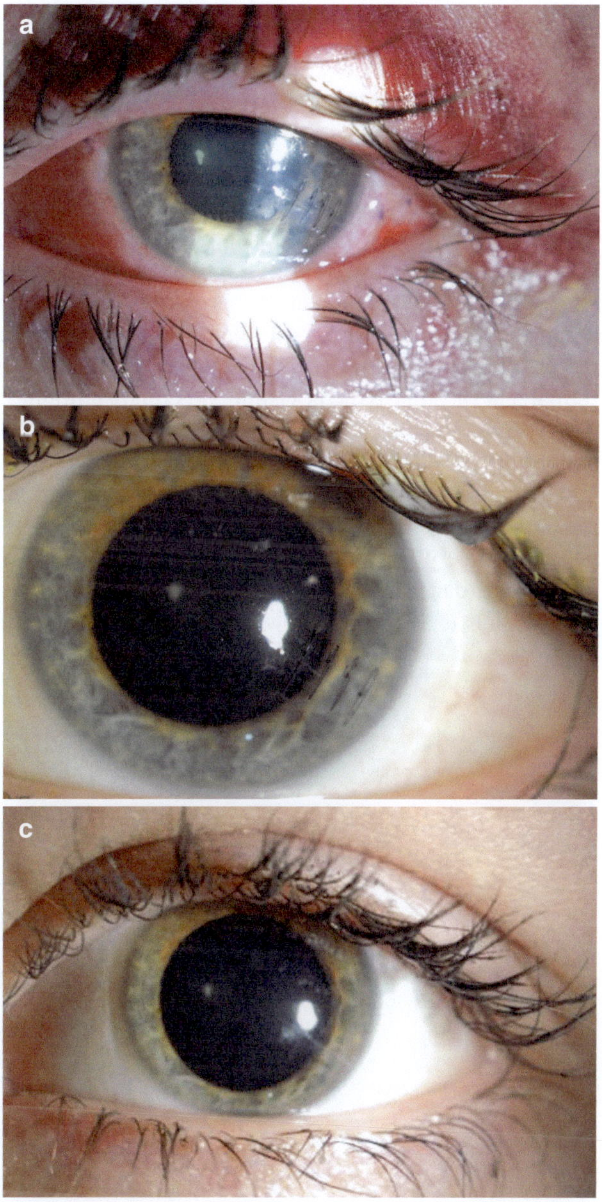

Fig. 4.1 (**a**) Post-operative day one after corneal laceration repair of the left eye. (**b**) Post-operative month 1 after open globe repair with all corneal sutures in place. Sutures were subsequently removed around 6 weeks post-operatively. (**c**) Slit lamp photograph approximately 6 weeks after suture removal

6. *Iris for any trauma or hemorrhage.*
7. *Lens for cataract, lens capsule damage, lens material in the anterior chamber, etc.*
8. *Vitreous for hemorrhage, vitreous debris, endophthalmitis, etc.*
9. *Posterior exam for hemorrhages, edema, retinal tears, retinal detachments, etc.*

On post-operative day 1, per our protocol, eye drops are started. The patient is initially started on prednisolone acetate 1% one drop 6 times daily, gatifloxicin one drop 4 times daily, and atropine 1% one drop daily. This is adjusted if the patient has allergies to any of these medications or if there is concern for infection or other issue.

If there is no view posteriorly due to a dense traumatic cataract, significant corneal edema, or vitreous hemorrhage, or there is concern for a retinal issue, the patient will get a detailed B-scan ultrasound to evaluate the retina and posterior segment usually before discharge (Fig. 4.2). This is done in the imaging department by a skilled ultrasound technician. If there is any concern for retinal trauma or posterior hemorrhage, the patient should then be scheduled to see a retina specialist around the post-operative week 1 time. However, if there is a clear view posteriorly and a retinal tear or other issue is visible, this referral might be arranged more quickly.

Additionally, we have a thorough discussion with the patient about the surgery and the intraoperative findings. After surgical exploration and repair, there is a better understanding of the severity of the injury and this can then be conveyed to the patient. There might also be more clarity about what the treatment course will be post-operatively and this can also be discussed with the patient. Patients also are often very distraught on initial presentation to the hospital and repetition of expectations is helpful to allow processing of relevant information.

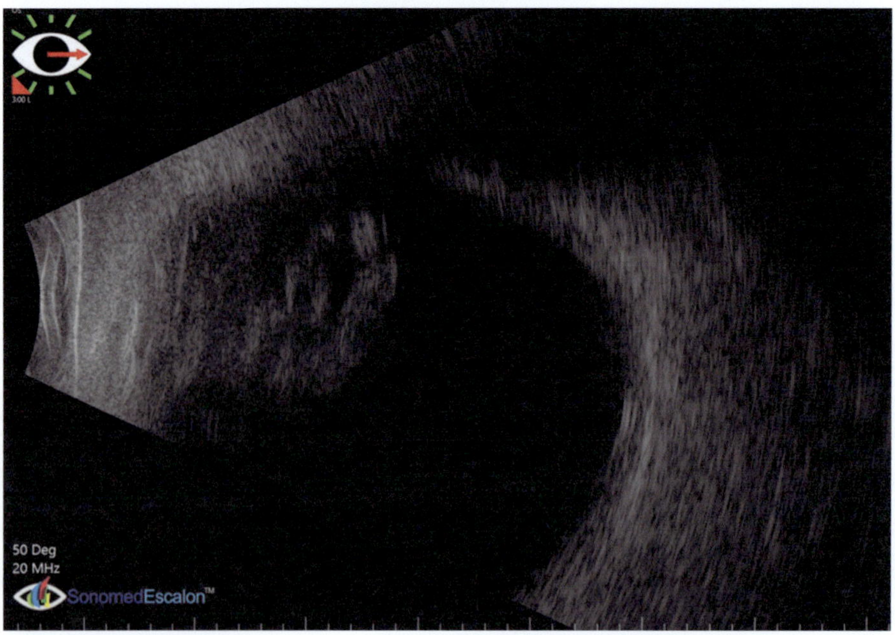

Fig. 4.2 B-scan ultrasound after open globe repair showing the lens tilting posteriorly into the vitreous without evidence of retinal detachment

Patients are also instructed to wear a fox shield at all times including while sleeping. This is intended to prevent any further trauma to the eye and also as a reminder to the patient to not rub or touch the eye. Specifically discuss the importance of not rubbing the eye as this can delay healing and eye rubbing should also be something to ask the patient about if the healing process is not proceeding as would be expected.

Patients are also instructed not to do any heavy lifting, strenuous exercise, or swimming over the following 6 weeks or while the corneal sutures are in place. This can be very challenging for some patients, for example those working in construction. We often recommend the patient stay out of work while the eye is healing, unless they are involved in a desk job and there is no strenuous activity involved. There are several cases in which patients did not follow these recommendations and experienced delayed wound healing or wound dehiscence.

Return precautions are reviewed carefully with the patient. Patients are told to return immediately for evaluation if worsening pain, changes in vision, flashes, floaters, or any other concerning changes.

Patients may need psychological support during the period immediately after their injury. This should be addressed both by asking the patients about their emotional reaction, but also offering referral to a psychologist or psychiatrist. In our hospital, we have developed a multi-disciplinary eye trauma team that includes social work and a psychologist for management of the emotional component of healing from these injuries.

All of our patients are initially seen by a social worker who sees the patient while they are an inpatient receiving IV antibiotics. The social worker will help discuss financial support, insurance coverage for those without insurance, psychological support, screen for domestic violence and assist with finding a safe place to stay, and also will find shelter for those that are homeless. The social workers can also help get the patient connected to the Commission for the Blind and Visually Impaired and other helpful programs for the patient. If the patient is from out of state, the social worker can also help coordinate care at another facility. They also are very helpful with coordinating follow up visits for those that have difficulty traveling (patients that don't drive and don't have family members that can help, etc.) or for finding nursing facilities where patients can stay to ensure they get the necessary eye drops and eye care.

Many open globe injuries are work-related injuries. These patients may require special assistance with worker's compensation paperwork after their surgery and over subsequent visits. Some require submission of each follow up visit note to document progress of the patient. Usually worker's compensation sends specific paperwork with the patient or sends it directly to the physician's office. Additionally, open globe injuries from motor vehicle accidents or assaults may result in litigation and lawyers may contact the surgeon requesting details about the severity of the injuries, level of vision loss, and permanent affects from the trauma. Often notes and medical documents are all processed through the medical records department, however, if the patient needs specific paperwork filled out, it is important to help whenever possible.

4.4 Post-Operative Drops

The patient is initially started on prednisolone acetate 1% one drop 6 times daily, gatifloxicin one drop 4 times daily, and atropine 1% one drop daily on post-operative day 1. This regimen is continued for 1 week. At the post-operative week one appointment the gatifloxicin is stopped and the prednisolone is decreased to one drop 4 times daily and the atropine is usually continued. The patient then follows up in 2–3 weeks and at that time a taper for the prednisolone is initiated. This could include a weekly taper (one drop 4 times a day for one week, then one drop 3 times a day for 1 week, then one drop 2 times a day for 1 week, then one drop once a day for 1 week, then stop) or a more rapid taper depending on the clinical examination. The continuation of atropine should depend on whether any residual intraocular hemorrhage or inflammation exists.

The above regimen is used for typical cases, but should be adjusted based on the patient and clinical exam. If there is concern for a corneal infection or ulcer then antibiotic drops may need to be given every hour and fortified topical antibiotics may need to be started. Occasionally in this context, prednisolone should be stopped.

4.5 Follow Up Visits

The post-operative visit schedule is usually followed closely to the summary above. Patients should have a complete ophthalmic examination at each of the follow up visits. Corneal wounds should be monitored closely to ensure they are healing appropriately and a Seidel test should be checked at each follow up visit. Patients with new flashes and floaters should be carefully examined for new retinal issues. The eye should be monitored for signs of infection, including a corneal suture abscess or ulcer or endophthalmitis (Fig. 4.3). Coordinated care with other specialties should be monitored to confirm the patient is getting the appropriate follow up – examples may include care for facial fractures with oculoplastics or facial plastics or head and neck surgery, care for retinal detachments or other retinal pathology by a retina specialist, etc.

Patients will be seen more frequently if there is concern for endophthalmitis, uncontrolled intraocular pressure, lens capsule violation, corneal ulcer, or infection. Frequent follow up can sometimes be a challenge for patients, as some patients are traveling long distances to get specialty eye care, and some patients do not have an easy means of transportation, or rely on family or friends for a ride. It is important to discuss this issue with the patient to help figure out the best possible plan for follow up to ensure the patient gets the appropriate care. Coordinating visits with subspecialty services to minimize the number of trips the patient has to make can also be helpful. Appointments can also be coordinated with a local ophthalmologist closer to the patient.

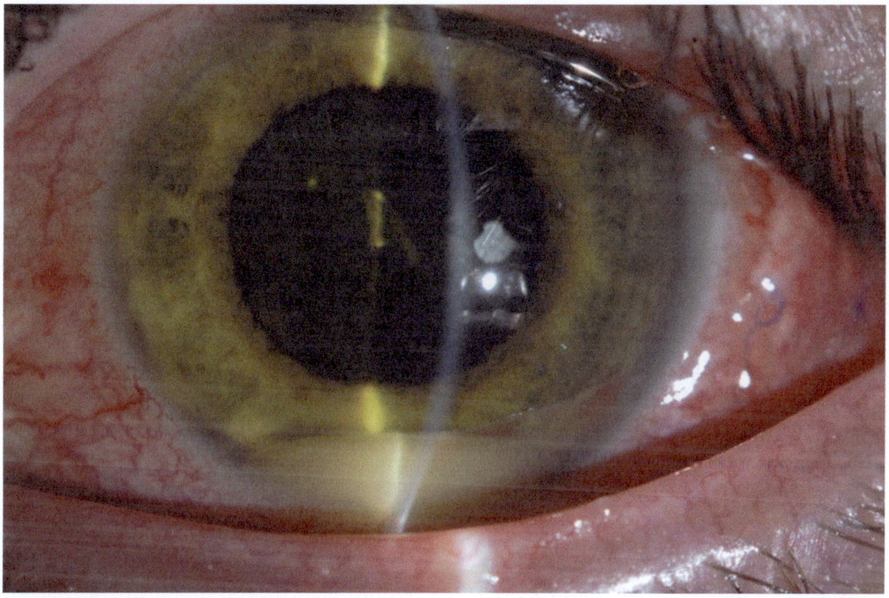

Fig. 4.3 Slit lamp photography after open globe repair showing a hypopyon concerning for endophthalmitis

If a patient is no light perception after surgical repair, the patient is given the option of referral to oculoplastics for enucleation versus close monitoring. The controversy around urgent enucleation is discussed in another chapter. Patients with an eye that is no light perception and significantly painful will often consider enucleation and patients are referred to oculoplastics. Patients who have a relatively comfortable eye often want to save their eye even with the discussion of the risk of sympathetic ophthalmia. Fortunately, we have treatments for this condition now and it is rare, so patients are given the option.

All patients should get a refraction either while inpatient or at the one week post-operative visit and a prescription for polycarbonate protective glasses. These are important to protect the injured eye in the post-operative period, but also now the non-injured, "good" eye. All patients should be encouraged to get these glasses and to wear them at all times during the day and then to wear the fox shield at night. Patients without a need for corrective glasses are given a prescription for plano polycarbonate glasses to wear. These can often be purchased online as well for a cheaper price. Patients may need a specific note from an ophthalmologist saying that the plano polycarbonate glasses are medically necessary in order to get them covered by insurance. Patients are also counseled to use protective goggles with any work that could injure the eye at all times in the future. For pediatric patients, it is important to spend time counseling the parent(s) about the importance of protective eyewear and the use of polycarbonates and safety glasses. Some parents will ensure their child is wearing the glasses at all times and others will need encouragement and education.

Suture removal often is initiated around 6 weeks. A more detailed discussion about suture removal occurs in the chapters with corneal injuries. With complex corneal wounds, the initiation of suture removal may occur after 6 weeks and suture removal may take place over several visits with 2–3 weeks in between each visit. All corneal sutures should be removed at some point to prevent corneal neovascularization and scarring. However, if these findings are not seen, then the sutures can be watched carefully and taken out slowly.

After all corneal sutures are removed, the patient can follow up with a contact lens specialist within 4–6 weeks. Our contact lens service recommends 6 weeks to ensure any epithelial defects from suture removal have healed and that the cornea has relaxed to its resting position after suture removal (so ideally once the contact lens is prescribed, the prescription will not change). The trauma service usually sees the patient the same day as this initial contact lens evaluation to see how the patient tolerates the lens and the best-corrected visual acuity at that time.

After the eye has stabilized, the post-operative follow up visits can be spread out to every few months and then yearly. At one of the follow up visits, a gonioscopy examination should be completed to evaluate for angle recession or synechiae that could increase the risk of glaucoma in the future. Patients who had uveal tissue exposure as part of their injury or surgery should also be reminded of the risk of sympathetic ophthalmia on follow up visits and told to return immediately if they experience any vision changes in the non-traumatized eye.

Imaging can be helpful throughout the course of open globe repair and recovery. We often get an intraoperative photo and follow up slit lamp photos on subsequent visits. These can be a great education tool for the patient, showing them the progress from their initial presentation. They can be helpful for subspecialty services following the patient as well so they also can follow the progress of the patient.

4.6 Subspecialty Care

Patients are often following with another subspecialty service. Patients are either being seen by a retina specialist for treatment of retinal issues, oculoplastics specialist for management of fractures or evaluation for enucleation, a glaucoma specialist for management of intraocular pressure, a corneal specialist for pupilloplasty or iris- sutured intraocular lens, or an optometrist for contact lens evaluation.

Patients with concern for retinal trauma are referred to a retina specialist within the first 1–2 weeks. If surgery is necessary for repair of a retinal detachment, drainage of choroidals, or removal of vitreous hemorrhage and membranes, it is often done within the first 1–3 weeks after the initial open globe repair. This gives the eye a chance to recover from the initial repair such that the eye will remain formed during the retinal surgery. If there is an intraocular foreign body, this is immediately referred to retina on initial presentation for open globe repair and removal of the intraocular foreign body.

It can be helpful to the patient to keep track of their subspecialty doctors and confirm that the patient has seen the necessary specialists, as patients may be confused by the schedule or misunderstand the importance of each follow up.

Reference

1. Andreoli CM, et al. Low rate of endophthalmitis in a large series of open globe injuries. Am J Ophthalmol. 2009;147(4):601–608.e2.

Chapter 5
Controversies in Open Globe Injury Management

Marisa Gobuty Tieger, Carolyn Kloek, and Alice C. Lorch

5.1 Antibiotic Prophlaxis for Open Globe Injury (OGI)

An OGI exposes intraocular contents to pathogens and increases susceptibility for infection [2]. Endophthalmitis is a feared complication of OGI which typically results in a devastating impact on vision. The rate of endophthalmitis following OGI has been reported between 0.9–7.2% [3] and has been found to be higher within a subgroup of patients with intraocular foreign bodies (IOFB,) ranging from 8.1–28% [4, 5]. As a result, antibiotic prophylaxis has become common practice. However, there are no standard guidelines for antibiotic selection. The leading causative bacteria in posttraumatic endophthalmitis is streptococcus, followed by coagulase negative staphylococcus, and bacillus [6]. Gram positive organisms have been reported to cause 61–75% of post-operative endophthalmitis, gram negative organisms 7.7–10% [7], and 5.5–8.3% attributed to fungal infections [6, 7]. Accordingly, an antibiotic should be selected to provide broad bacterial coverage for both gram positive and negative organisms. Ideally, an antibiotic with maximal vitreous penetrance should be selected, but there is limited research available on vitreous penetration for most systemically administered antibiotics [3].

Multiple antibiotic regimens have been proposed. Available mechanisms of delivery include IV, oral, and intraocular (intravitreal or intracameral) antibiotics. The intravenous (IV) antibiotics with adequate vitreous penetration include fluoroquinolones, ceftazidime, and vancomycin [3]. Combinations including

Expert Opinions by: Christopher Andreoli, M.D., Michael Yoon, M.D., Lucia Sobrin, M.D., M.P.H., Alice Lorch M.D., Peter Veldman, M.D., Dean Eliott M.D.

M. G. Tieger, M.D. (✉) • A. C. Lorch, M.D., M.P.H.
Department of Ophthalmology, Harvard Medical School, Massachusetts Eye and Ear, Boston, MA, USA

C. Kloek, M.D.
Department of Ophthalmology, Harvard Medical School, Massachusetts Eye and Ear, Boston, MA, USA

S. Grob, C. Kloek (eds.), *Management of Open Globe Injuries*,
https://doi.org/10.1007/978-3-319-72410-2_5

gentamicin with cefazolin [8], vancomycin with ceftazidime have been used in clinical trials [9, 10]. Oral fluoroquinolones are also thought to provide adequate vitreous penetration although studies suggest that ciprofloxacin is the only one to achieve the MIC90 for pseudomonas coverage [3]. Oral antibiotic regimens that have been used in clinical trials include ciprofloxacin (750 mg every 12 hours) and oral cefuroxime (250 mg every 12 hours) [11]. Intravitreal agents have also been used in various clinical trials; these combinations have included vancomycin with ceftazidime [2] and clindamycin with gentamicin [8].

MEE follows a standardized protocol for patients with open globe injuries which includes 48 hours of IV vancomycin (1 g every 12 hours for 4 total doses) and ceftazidime (1 g every 8 hours for 6 total doses) along with intraoperative subconjunctival cefazolin and post-operative topical gatifloxacin eye drops. Over a 7-year period the rate of endophthalmitis was found to be 0.9% [9]. This is one of the lowest reported rates of post-traumatic endophthalmitis in the non-military community and likely reflects the value of a standardized and broad spectrum protocol for the management of OGI. Recently, two randomized control trials evaluated oral versus IV antibiotics as well as oral and IV versus oral alone. Tabatabaei et al. performed a prospective study comparing prophylactic IV ceftazidime (1 g every 8 hours) and vancomycin (1 g every 12 hours) to oral ciprofloxacin (750 mg every 12 hours) for 3 days duration. There was no statistically significant difference in the rate of endophthalmitis between the two groups (2.1% in the IV group and 2.2% in the oral group) [10]. A second study by du Toit et al. compared prophylactic IV cefazolin (1 g every 8 hours) with oral ciprofloxacin (750 mg every 12 hours) to oral ciprofloxacin (750 mg every 12 hours) and oral cefuroxime (250 mg every 12 hours) for 3 days. This study also found no statistically significant difference in the rate of endophthalmitis between the two groups (2.0% in the IV and oral group and 2.7% in the oral only group) [11]. The benefits of eliminating the need for intravenous therapy include the reduced cost of treatment and a reduction in the complications associated with IV access [10, 11]. However, it is difficult to adopt the findings of these studies, as the reported endophthalmitis rates are higher than those we have found with a standard IV regimen [9].

An additional, more direct mode of antibiotic delivery is intravitreal antibiotic injection. Intravitreal antibiotic injection is limited in practice due to possible complications including vitreous hemorrhage, retinal breaks, and detachment [2]. There is also a risk of drug toxicity, particularly with gentamicin and now vancomycin with recent description of hemorrhagic occlusive retinal vasculitis (HORV). The efficacy in endophthalmitis prophylaxis was evaluated in a study of 70 eyes comparing intravitreal and systemic IV antibiotics to IV antibiotics alone. The antibiotics administered included intravitreal ceftazidime and vancomycin with IV ciprofloxacin compared to IV ciprofloxacin. The rate of endophthalmitis was 6.25% in the intravitreal group compared to 18.42% in the IV therapy group [2]. An additional study by Soheilian et al. evaluated the use of prophylactic intravitreal or intracameral gentamicin and clindamycin compared to placebo injection in 346 eyes. All patients received intravenous gentamicin sulfate (3–5 mg/kg) every 8 hours and cefazolin (50 mg/kg) every 6 hours for 5 days. The rate of endophthalmitis was 2.3% in the control group and 0.3% in the intravitreal/intracameral group ($p = 0.04$). The benefit was only seen in those with an intraocular foreign body (IOFB) and intravitreal injection was found to be superior to intracameral injection [8]. Given the risks of intravitreally injected medications in the context of limited proven benefit, our team rarely gives intravitreal injections unless there is an IOFB or suspicion for endophthalmititis.

5.1.1 *Expert Opinion Written by Christopher Andreoli M.D.*

Antibiotic prophylaxis for prevention of endophthalmitis remains standard of care for this type of injury, however the details of the prophylaxis are varied and somewhat controversial. Most advocate for systemic therapy, however agent and route (intravenous vs. oral) varies. Some groups advocate for intraocular antibiotics in all cases, some in cases with intraocular foreign bodies only, and others not at all. Most recommendations include post-operative topical antibiotics.

We advocate for repair of these injuries following a standardize protocol within 24 hours of injury including systemic antibiotic prophylaxis. Our standard protocol includes 48 hours of intravenous therapy (usually ceftazidime and vancomycin) with consideration of intravitreal antiobiotics in cases with IOFB [9] or frank signs of intraocular infection on presentation. Patient are discharged on topical antibiotic therapy for 1 week.

5.2 Primary Enucleation, Evisceration, and Repair in No Light Perception Eyes

The evolution of surgical management of OGIs and the development of new techniques over the years has vastly altered the appropriate standard of care. Today, primary closure is almost always attempted for OGIs, often combined with subsequent surgeries, such as vitrectomy, to achieve the best possible visual potential. Primary enucleation or evisceration is reserved for cases in which recovery of function is thought to be impossible and there is a patient-oriented motivation for removal.

Currently, the majority of enucleations in the United States are performed for eye trauma (41%) followed by tumors [12, 13]. The benefits of primary enucleation include minimizing the need for future anesthesia and prevention of sympathetic ophthalmia. Indications for primary enucleation after an OGI include the inability to repair due to unrecognizable ocular contents, avulsion or transection of the optic nerve, and inability of the patient to undergo multiple surgeries [1, 14–17]. Ruptured eyes are more likely to undergo enucleation compared to those with lacerations [17]. When it is determined that an eye merits primary enucleation due the extent of its injury, other patient-oriented factors must be considered. Ideally, the fellow eye should be normal, and the patient alert and cooperative for consent [13] with full understanding that removal of the traumatized eye precludes return of any level of vision [13].

An alternative to enucleation, evisceration, includes removal of intraocular contents while sparing the scleral shell [18]. The benefits of evisceration include improved cosmetic outcomes, ease of operation, improved mobility post-operatively, faster recovery, definitive placement of the implant with respect to extraocular muscles, and minimization of psychological complications post-operatively [13, 18–24]. Unlike enucleation, evisceration does not reduce the theoretic risk of sympathetic ophthalmia [25–28]. Of note, du Toit et al. reported 491 primary eviscerations in the setting of penetrating trauma with no reports of sympathetic ophthalmia. However, given that the incidence of sympathetic ophthalmia is low (0.3%) [17], this study is not conclusive [20].

The rates of primary enucleation have steadily decreased since the mid-twentieth century. Pieramici et al. reported a primary enucleation rate of 30% of OGIs between 1970–1981 which decreased to 24% between 1985 and 1993 [29]. In OGIs occurring after 2006, Soni et al. reported a rate of primary enucleation of 7% [30]. The decreasing frequency of enucleations is likely due to improved surgical techniques as well as available management options for sympathetic ophthalmia.

Recent studies have shown visual improvement post-operatively in patients presenting with NLP after OGI, making the decision for enucleation or evisceration even more controversial. In 2008, Schmidt et al. reported 6/33 (18%) eyes presenting with NLP that had visual recovery [31]. In 2009, Salehi-Had et al. reported 12 of 57 (21%) NLP eyes with visual recovery after primary repair with an average of 3.75 days for vision recovery [14]. In 2011, Feng et al. reported that 18 of 33 NLP eyes (55%) after OGI recovered light perception or better, with five eyes having better than 20/200 vision [32]. In 2012, Agrawal et al. reported visual improvement in NLP eyes after OGI in 9/27 (33%) [33]. In 2013, an additional report found that 17 of 73 (23%) NLP eyes had improvement to light perception or better after primary repair [30]. In a 2015 report by Han et al., 4/25 (16%) patients with OGI that were NLP regained vision after primary repair and vitreoretinal surgery [15]. In 2016, Chee et al. reported a case of an OGI with NLP vision prior to primary repair as well on POD1 and POD10, but improvement in vision to 20/50 after external drainage of choroidals and repair of a total funnel retinal detachment [34] .

Based on the observed improvement in visual acuity after primary repair and often subsequent surgeries, it is useful to assess which factors are prognostic indicators of visual improvement in NLP eyes after OGI. The ocular trauma score (OTS), published in 2002, is a set of criteria that aid in determining the likelihood of visual recovery in eye injuries [35]. The factors included in the calculation include pre-operative visual acuity, presence of rupture, endophthalmitis, perforating injury, retinal detachment, and relative afferent pupillary defect. A separate prognostic model (open globe outcome classification tree) was developed to help predict vision survival after OGI in 2007 and found that the absence of a relative afferent pupillary defect (RAPD) served as the best predictor of vision preservation.

Patients with open globe injuries are often in significant distress or in other ways incapacitated and as such visual acuity testing pre-operatively can be inaccurate. Therefore, although expected improvement in patients with NLP vision is often minimal, it is important to consider the possibility before proceeding to primary removal of the eye.

5.2.1 *Expert Opinion Written by Michael K. Yoon M.D.*

The management of open globe injuries with no light perception vision remains a challenge. In cases where there is no identifiable globe, or if the ocular fragments that remain are insufficient for open globe closure, then primary removal of the eye or ocular remnants is quite clear. However, in cases with no light perception and sufficient tissue for closure and repair, opinions vary. I recommend primary globe repair in these cases with appropriate antibiotic treatment. From a psychosocial point of view, this allows patients who have suffered a severe trauma an opportunity to understand their injury and feel that reasonable efforts were made to allow for possible recovery. Eye removal is associated with higher levels of anxiety and depression [36] and a majority may develop phantom eye syndrome [37]. Medically, the primary fear of ophthalmologists is developing sympathetic ophthalmia. While this rare inflammatory condition is always considered, enucleation or evisceration as a preventative measure is unproven [38, 39] (and has never been demonstrated to be protective). Finally, enucleation surgery carries long-term risk of anophthalmic socket syndrome, implant migration, and implant extrusion all requiring additional surgery for repair. While the loss of vision is a devastating event for any patient as well as a professional disappointment for ophthalmologists, maintaining a non-functioning organ can offer benefit to the patient's physical and psychosocial wellbeing.

5.3 Enucleation for Prevention of Sympathetic Ophthalmia

Sympathetic ophthalmia (SO) is a bilateral granulomatous panuveitis that occurs in the non-injured eye as a consequence of the exposure of ocular antigens due to injury of the other eye. These injuries occur most often in the setting of trauma or surgery and result in an autoimmune T cell mediated response in the non-injured eye [18, 19]. The presentation ranges from 2 weeks to 10 years but data suggests that 83% present within 1 year from the time of injury [40]. Symptoms include decreased vision, redness, and photophobia. Common exam findings included anterior chamber cells and flare, as well as vitritis, keratic precipitates and Dalen-Fuchs nodules [40].

Given the pathophysiology of this disease, it is thought that enucleation of an injured eye with exposed uvea could decrease future risk of sympathetic ophthalmia. As a result, it traditionally has been common practice for eyes with open globe injuries that had no light perception vision to be enucleated within two weeks of the injury to prevent development of SO [17]. The current practice has shifted as a result of improved surgical techniques allowing for visual improvement in low vision or NLP eyes post-operatively, and improved treatment options for SO. There are multiple studies that have evaluated NLP eyes following OGI after primary repair in which no cases of SO were observed [15, 30, 32, 33]. The rate of SO following OGI was most recently reported as

0.3% (2 of 660 open globe injuries). In this study, the 2 patients reported to have SO were adequately treated with systemic immunosuppression with corticosteroids and retained vision [17].

The treatment for SO has improved dramatically with the utilization of steroids and other immunosuppressants. Within the 89 cases identified in the medline search, the most common treatment reported was systemic steroids, which were used in 95% of cases described. Other treatments used included topical steroids and intraocular steroid injections. In addition, immunomodulators were used in 76% of cases and of these the most commonly used medications included methotrexate followed by cyclosporine and azathioprine. With the utilization of available treatments, 70% of these patients experienced improved visual acuity from their initial encounter [40]. In a separate report with 11 eyes diagnosed with sympathetic ophthalmia secondary to trauma, 64% obtained vision equal to or better than 20/25 [41].

5.3.1 Expert Opinion: Lucia Sobrin, M.D., M.P.H.

There is a long-standing teaching in ophthalmology that enucleation within two weeks of an open globe injury can prevent sympathetic ophthalmia (SO). This approach was first advocated based on a small case series in the 1930s [42–44]. In particular, Dr. Joy reported on six eyes removed before any signs of SO in fellow eye: one eye was enucleated within 2 weeks and the patient had a benign course with preservation of 20/15 vision while the other 5 eyes were enucleated 26 or more days after injury and all of them developed SO with hands motion vision or worse in the sympathizing eye [44]. A review of 63 cases from MEE found that the shortest interval to development of SO was 17 days from day of inciting event [45]. Based on this observation, the study concluded: "*... enucleation must be done within two weeks of the injury if sympathetic ophthalmia is to be prevented.*" However, this series also includes a patient who developed SO despite having enucleation within the first two weeks of injury [45]. This suggests the immune response may already be triggered but the disease subclinical at the time of enucleation, even when done within two weeks of the injury. There are also reports, albeit rare, of the onset of SO within two weeks of the injury and as early as nine days after injury [44, 46, 47].

Given this information, our current approach is to only consider enucleation for eyes that have been confirmed to have no light perception vision as there are instances, when SO does develop, where the inciting eye ends with better vision than the sympathizing eye. For patients with no light perception after trauma and surgical repair, we inform them of the very small risk of SO and that there is some data to suggest early removal of the eye may diminish, but not eliminate, the risk of SO. Several days are often required for the patient to come to terms with the injury and decide to proceed with enucleation. If he or she does choose enucleation, we expedite scheduling of the surgery so it occurs in the shortest interval possible. After enucleation, we still review symptoms of SO closely with the patient, emphasizing that there is still a small chance it could occur despite early enucleation.

5.4 Primary Lensectomy and Intraocular Lens Implantation

Lens damage has been reported to occur in 30% of OGIs [48]. This can lead to complications including phacoanaphylaxis, phacomorphic glaucoma, and intumescent cataract [48, 49]. Surgical options in the setting of lens violation include removal during primary repair or removal during a second operation after the corneal edema resolves (see later cases for a more detailed discussion on management of open globes with lens violation).

Leaving a patient aphakic rather than implanting an intraocular lens (IOL) at the time of primary repair remains controversial, mostly due to the risk of infection with implanting a foreign body and the difficulty in determining the IOL power [50]. Andreoli et al. found that primary intraocular lens placement was a risk factor for endophthalmitis in a study of 675 OGIs. In these cases, only those with definite lens capsule disruption underwent lensectomy (111 cases) and only cases with adequate visualization for measurements had an IOL placed (6 of 111 cases) [9]. In addition, many patients may still require contact lenses for correction of corneal astigmatism after insertion of an IOL due to the significant corneal surface irregularity [50]. Therefore, it may not be beneficial in patients with large corneal lacerations to implant an IOL, as the corneal contour can change significantly throughout the healing process.

The benefits to implanting an IOL at the time of primary repair include reducing the number of operations involved in visual rehabilitation and anesthesia required for these surgeries as well as faster rehabilitation and improvement in the binocular function [49]. Rabsamen et al. published a report in 1995 describing the outcomes of 14 patients that underwent primary repair of corneal laceration, lens extraction and primary insertion of an IOL within 12 hours of presentation and 48 hours of injury. Patients with an IOFB were included in addition to those requiring PPV. Posterior IOL was placed in all patients (6 in in the capsular bag). The IOL measurements were obtained from the non-injured eye. The final refraction was +/−1.5D in 11/14 patients [50]. A more recent study in 2008 evaluated 9 patients with open globe injuries and 4 of the 9 underwent primary closure, lensectomy, placement of an intraocular lens, and vitrectomy within 48 hours from the time of injury. These patients all received a sulcus PCIOL using measurements obtained from the fellow eye. The final refraction was +/−1D in 4/9 patients with one patients final refraction −4.00 and attributed to the scleral buckle [49].

5.4.1 Expert Opinion Written by Alice Lorch M.D.

Although the majority of our open globe patients develop a traumatic cataract, regardless of the zone of injury, we only consider primary lens removal in the setting of frank lens capsular violation with extrusion of lenticular contents. This is most commonly seen in the setting of a corneal laceration. This is performed not for visual recuperation, but instead because lenticular contents inside the anterior chamber must be removed to prevent significant post-operative inflammation and associated elevation of intraocular pressure. Primary lensectomy should be performed after closure of the corneal wound and generally is performed with a vitrector, given unknown status of the zonules or posterior capsule in these cases. This is easier with younger patients as their lens is softer; with older patients and denser lenses, phacoemulsification is sometimes necessary and can be performed with caution after initial anterior vitrectomy. We leave patients aphakic after primary lensectomy; this is out of concern for infection, but also because we have had great success by our optometrists with prescribing aphakic contact lenses. Leaving a patient aphakic allows them the option of secondary lens implantation in a controlled setting at a later date and allows for more accurate lens measurements after the corneal sutures have been removed and the corneal curvature stabilized. Many patients opt to remain aphakic with a contact lens.

Of note, in eyes with a traumatic cataract with lens violation but also concern for posterior rupture, a primary closure is initially performed, closely followed by pars plana vitrectomy and lensectomy by a retina specialist.

We generally wait to remove traumatic cataracts without capsular violation until full recovery of the corneal laceration. This is usually about 2 months after initial injury at which time all sutures have been removed and biometry can be performed. Of note, we caution patients who undergo cataract surgery for a traumatic cataract that many will still need a contact lens after the surgery for maximum refractive improvement due to corneal irregularity. We work closely with our contact lens optometry service with this aim.

5.5 Full vs. Partial Thickness Corneal Sutures

The closure of corneal lacerations in the setting of open globe injuries is performed with either full-thickness or partial thickness sutures. Many surgeons have preference for one of the two closure options, but there are no clinical trials that have been performed to show a clear benefit of either option. Considerations include the risk of infection with full-thickness sutures as well as the risk of uneven depth of partial thickness sutures leading to poor corneal wound closure. More research is needed in this area to further determine the best surgical approach.

5.5.1 Expert Opinion Written by Peter Veldman M.D.

Traditionally, corneal lacerations (as well as penetrating keratoplasties) have been closed utilizing either full-thickness or partial thickness suturing (attempting to approximate 90% stromal depth), with preference for either being largely passed from surgical mentor to mentee. While each approach has a long track record of successful corneal wound closure, the potential relative advantages of full-thickness suturing include a more anatomically correct tissue alignment (both anteriorly and posteriorly), faster corneal deturgesence, as well as faster visual rehabilitation. I believe that these advantages are particularly relevant in the management of traumatic corneal lacerations, in which there may be irregular and asymmetrical wounds, including asymmetry in stromal hydration/thickness on opposing sides of the same wound. It is not hard to imagine that a surgeon under the challenging circumstances of a trauma closure might place partial thickness suture passes at varying depths. Unfortunately, even a 20% mismatch in suture depth (70% vs. 90% depth) can lead to profound corneal edema and delayed stromal clearance due to the resultant exposed corneal stroma (~100–150 μm in this case) as a result of a mismatch of the internal aspect of the cornea. This mismatch not only delays and limits visual rehabilitation, but may compromise the ability to safely perform necessary procedures such as vitrectomy or secondary lens extraction due to the resultant edema and poor surgical visibility. Skeptics of full-thickness corneal suturing have suggested an increased risk of infection due to the presence of a full-thickness tract into the eye, however through a combination of re-epithelialization, healing at the level of the Descemet membrane and relatively short intervals to suture removal in trauma, this has not proven to be an issue in my experience. Additionally, surgeons should take reassurance based upon the experience of senior colleagues who have spent distinguished careers utilizing full-thickness suturing techniques in penetrating keratoplasty without a notable rise in post-operative infection rates. Of course these questions and concerns would be best answered by a randomized controlled trial comparing partial and full-thickness suturing. Unfortunately, that study has not been done.

My current practice involves the utilization of either technique, as dictated by the clinical scenario. When I encounter a relatively symmetrical wound without significant edema or asymmetry, typically a sharp injury, I will close using attempted 90% depth suturing. On the other hand, if the wound involves notable stromal edema, particularly if that edema is asymmetrical on either side of the wound, I will utilize full-thickness sutures, placing them as vertically as possible on either side of the wound (box suture technique). I believe that in my hands, doing so facilitates better anterior and posterior stromal alignment and earlier corneal deturgescence than would be possible were I to utilize partial thickness suturing. Finally, a hybrid of the two techniques involving initial placement of full-thickness sutures in order to achieve anatomically correct re-approximation followed by partial thickness suturing (with or without the eventual removal of the full-thickness passes) may also prove useful in certain scenarios.

5.6 Repair of Posterior Ruptures

The repair of posterior lacerations and ruptures is complicated by the lack of research to support primary closure versus closure by secondary intention. Some of the controversies surrounding this repair include the risk of endophthalmitis, sympathetic ophthalmia, extrusion of retinal contents, and posterior leaks during vitrectomy.

5.6.1 Expert Opinion Written by Dean Eliott M.D.

There are varying opinions regarding closure of posterior lacerations and ruptures among different specialties in ophthalmology. Some ophthalmologists advocate for complete closure to lower the risk of endophthalmitis. This should not be a primary consideration given the posterior location and the barrier of the conjunctiva and the rapid closure of the wound by scar tissue. Studies have shown that in full-thickness scleral wounds, connective tissue extends through the full-thickness of the wound by day 3 and the wound is undetectable by ultrasound on day 7 [51]. An additional consideration is the prevention of a posterior leak while performing a vitrectomy following the open globe repair. I have encountered a leak as a result of incomplete closure twice throughout my career but in my opinion this is preferential to the risk of incarcerated retina and vitreous. A theoretical consideration is the risk of sympathetic ophthalmia with leaving open globes unrepaired but this risk is minimal and treatments are available.

The risk with repairing posterior ruptures and lacerations is the pressure exerted on the globe while attempting to gain access to the posterior structures. The increased pressure can lead to the extrusion of vitreous and retina and ultimately incarceration. Incarcerated retina will then need to be resected which limits visual potential. In my practice, I would suture and repair any laceration/rupture that does not require aggressive manipulation of the globe or removal of the extraocular muscles. Ruptures or lacerations with an exit site that extend into posterior Zone III would preferentially close by secondary intention. Ultimately the surgical technique used to repair posterior ruptures and lacerations should depend on the surgeon's comfort and preference, as complete wound closure and incomplete closure are both acceptable techniques.

References

1. Negrel AD, Thylefors B. The global impact of eye injuries. Ophthalmic Epidemiol. 1998;5:143–69.
2. Narang S, Gupta V, Gupta A, et al. Role of prophylactic intravitreal antibiotics in open globe injuries. Indian J Ophthalmol. 2003;51:39–44.
3. Lorch A, Sobrin L. Prophylactic antibiotics in posttraumatic infectious endophthalmitis. Int Ophthalmol Clin. 2013;53:167–76.
4. Mieler WF, Ellis MK, Williams DF, et al. Retained intraocular foreign bodies and endophthalmitis. Ophthalmology. 1990;97:1532.
5. Banker TP, McClellan AJ, Wilson BD, et al. Culture-positive endophthalmitis after open globe injuries with and without retained intraocular foreign bodies. Ophthalmic Surg Lasers Imaging Retina. 2016;48(8):632–7.
6. Chhabra S, Kunimoto DY, Kazi L, et al. Endophthalmitis after open globe injury: microbiologic spectrum and susceptibilities of isolates. Am J Ophthalmol. 2006;142:852–4.
7. Bhagat N, Nagori S, Zarbin M. Post-traumatic Infectious Endophthalmitis. Surv Ophthalmol. 2001;56:214–51.
8. Soheilian M, Rafati N, Mohebbi MR, et al. Prophylaxis of acute posttraumatic bacterial endophthalmitis: a multicenter, randomized clinical trial of intraocular antibiotic injection, report 2. Arch Ophthalmol. 2007;125(4):460–5.

9. Andreoli CM, Andreoli MT, Kloek CE, et al. Low rate of endophthalmitis in a large series of open globe injuries. Am J Ophthalmol. 2009;147(4):601–8.
10. Tabatabaei SA, Soleimani M, Behrooz MJ, et al. Systemic oral antibiotics as a prophylactic measure to prevent endopthalmitis in patients with open globe injuries in comparison with intravenous antibiotics. Retina. 2016;36:360–5.
11. Du toit N, Mustak S, Cook C. Randomized controlled trial of prophylactic antibiotic treatment for the prevention of endophthalmitis after open globe injury at Groote Schuur Hospital. Br J Ophthalmol. 2017;101:862–7.
12. Saeed MU, Chang BY, Khandwala M, et al. Twenty year review of histopathological findings in enucleated/eviscerated eyes. J Clin Pathol. 2006;59(2):153–5.
13. Moshfeghi DM, Moshfeghi AA, Finger PT. Enucleation. Surv Ophthalmol. 2000;44:277–301.
14. Salehi-Had H, Andreoli CM, Andreoli MT, et al. Visual outcomes of vitreoretinal surgery in eyes with severe open-globe injury presenting with no-light-perception vision. Graefes Arch Clin Exp Ophthalmol. 2009;247:477–83.
15. Han YS, Kavoussi SC, Adelman RA. Visual recovery following open globe injury with initial no light perception. Clin Ophthalmol. 2015;9:1443–8.
16. Bhagat N, Turbin R, Langer P, et al. Approach to management of eyes with no light perception after open globe injury. J Ophthalmic Vis Res. 2016;11(3):313–8.
17. Savar A, Andreoli MT, Kloek CE, et al. Enucleation for open globe injury. Am J Ophthalmol. 2009;147:595–600.
18. McAlinden C, Saldanha M, Laws D. Evisceration for the management of ocular trauma. BMJ Case Rep. https://doi.org/10.1136/bcr-2013-201235.
19. Zheng C, Wu AY. Enucleation versus evisceration in ocular trauma: a retrospective review and study of current literature. Orbit. 2013;32(6):356–61.
20. du Toit N, Motala MI, Richards J, et al. The risk of sympathetic ophthalmia following evisceration for penetrating eye injuries at Groote Schuur Hospital. Br J Ophthalmol. 2008;92: 61–3.
21. O'Donnell BA, Kersten R, McNab A, et al. Enucleation versus evisceration. Clin Experiment Ophthalmol. 2005;33(1):5–9.
22. Nakra T, Simon GJ, Douglas RS, et al. Comparing outcomes of enucleation and evisceration. Ophthalmology. 2006;113(12):2270–5.
23. Tari AS, Malihi M, Kasaee A, et al. Enucleation with hydroxyapatite implantation versus evisceration plus scleral quadrisection and alloplastic implantation. Ophthal Plast Reconstr Surg. 2009;25(2):130–3.
24. Ababneh OH, AboTaleb EA, Abu Ameerh MA, et al. Enucleation and evisceration at a tertiary care hospital in a developing country. BMC Ophthalmol. 2015;15:120.
25. Frost WA. What is the best method of dealing with a lost eye? Br Med J. 1887;1(1378):1153–4.
26. Ruedemann AD Jr. Sympathetic ophthalmia after evisceration. Am J Ophthalmol. 1964;57:770–90.
27. Green WR, Maumenee AE, Sanders TE, et al. Sympathetic uveitis following evisceration. Trans Am Acad Ophthalmol Otolaryngol. 1972;76(3):625–44.
28. Friedlin J, Pak J, Tessler HH, et al. Sympathetic ophthalmia after injury in the Iraq War. Ophthal Plast Reconstr Surg. 2006;22(2):133–4.
29. Pieramici DJ, MacCumber MW, Humayun MU, et al. Open-globe injury. Update on types of injuries and visual results. Ophthalmology. 1996;103(11):1798–803.
30. Soni NG, Bauza AM, Son JH, et al. Open globe ocular trauma: functional outcome of eyes with no light perception at initial presentation. Retina. 2013;33(2):380–6.
31. Schmidt GW, Broman AT, Hindman HB. Vision survival after open globe injury predicted by classification and regression tree analysis. Ophthalmology. 2008;115(1):202–9.
32. Feng K, Hu YT, Ma Z. Prognostic indicators for no light perception after open-globe injury: eye injury vitrectomy study. Am J Ophthalmol. 2011;152(4):654–662.e2.
33. Agrawal R, Wei HS, Teoh S. Predictive factors for final outcome of severely traumatized eyes with no light perception. BMC Ophthalmol. 2012;12:16.
34. Chee YE, Kanoff JM, Eliott D. Remarkable visual recovery after severe open globe injury. Am J Ophthalmol Case Rep. 2016;3:34–5.

35. Kuhn F, Maisiak R, Mann L, et al. The Ocular Trauma Score (OTS). Ophthalmol Clin North Am. 2002;15(2):163–5.
36. Ye J, Lou L, Jin K, et al. Vision-related quality of life and appearance concerns are associated with anxiety and depression after eye enucleation: a cross-sectional study. PLoS One. 2015;10(8):e0136460.
37. Hope-Stone L, Brown SL, Heimann H, et al. Phantom eye syndrome: patient experiences after enucleation for uveal melanoma. Ophthalmology. 2015;122(8):1585–90.
38. Lubin JR, Albert DM, Weinstein M. Sixty-five years of sympathetic ophthalmia: a clinicopathologic review of 105 cases. Ophthalmology. 1980;87(2):109–21.
39. Cunningham ET, Kilmartin D, Agarwal M, Zierhut M. Sympathetic ophthalmia. Ocular Immun Inflamm. 2017;25(2):149–51.
40. Castiblanco CP, Adelman RA. Sympathetic ophthalmia. Graefes Arch Clin Exp Ophthalmol. 2009;247:289–302.
41. Aziz HA, Flynn HW, Young RC. Sympathetic ophthalmia: clinicopathologic correlation in a consecutive case series. Retina. 2015;35(8):1696–703.
42. Dor L. La guérison des deux yeux dans l'ophtalmie sympathique. Arch d'Opht. 1931;48:811.
43. Fuchs A. Arch Oftal B. Aires. 1932;7:67.
44. Joy HH. A survey of cases of sympathetic ophthalmia occurring in New York State. Arch Ophthalmol. 1935;14(5):733–41.
45. Irvine R. Sympathetic ophthalmia: a clinical review of 63 cases. Arch Ophthalmol. 1940;24:149–67.
46. Stafford WR. Sympathetic ophthalmia. Report of a case occurring ten and one-half days after injury. Arch Ophthamol. 1965;74:521–4.
47. Nettleship E. Trans Ophthal Soc UK. 1886;170.
48. Muga R, Maul E. The management of lens damage in perforating corneal lacerations. Br J Ophthalmol. 1978;62(11):784–7.
49. Assi A, Chacra CB, Cherfan G. Combined lensectomy, vitrectomy, and primary intraocular lens implantation in patients with traumatic eye injury. Int Ophthalmol. 2008;28(6):387–94.
50. Rubsamen PE, Irvin WD, McCuen BW, et al. Primary intraocular lens implantation in the setting of penetrating ocular trauma. Ophthalmology. 1995;102(1):101–7.
51. Hikichi T, Yoshida A, Hasegawa T, Ohnishi M, Sato T, Muraoka S. Wound healing of scleral self-sealing incision: a comparison of ultrasound biomicroscopy and histology findings. Graefes Arch Clin Exp Ophthalmol. 1998;236(10):775–8.

Part II
Case-Based Approach to Open Globe Injuries

Chapter 6
Case 1: Linear Corneal Laceration from Scissors

Natalie Wolkow, Ankoor S. Shah, and Seanna Grob

6.1 History of Present Illness

A 6-year-old, healthy girl presented with concern for an open globe injury of the right eye.

- The patient was at home cutting out paper shapes for a card for her mother and father, when she poked her eye with the pair of scissors that she was using.
- Initial evaluation at another hospital revealed normal visual acuity and a grossly normal-appearing eye except for an irregularly-shaped right pupil. Given this finding, she was transferred to Massachusetts Eye and Ear (MEE) for an urgent ophthalmologic examination.
- She had minimal pain and denied blurry vision.

Electronic Supplementary Material The online version of this chapter (https://doi.org/10.1007/978-3-319-72410-2_6) contains supplementary material, which is available to authorized users.

N. Wolkow, M.D., Ph.D. (✉) • S. Grob, M.D., M.A.S.
Department of Ophthalmology, Harvard Medical School, Massachusetts Eye and Ear, Boston, MA, USA
e-mail: natalie_wolkow@meei.harvard.edu

A. S. Shah, M.D., Ph.D.
Department of Ophthalmology, Harvard Medical School, Boston Children's Hospital and Massachusetts Eye and Ear, Boston, MA, USA

S. Grob, C. Kloek (eds.), *Management of Open Globe Injuries*,
https://doi.org/10.1007/978-3-319-72410-2_6

6.2 Initial Trauma Evaluation

6.2.1 Visual Acuity (Without Correction)

OD: 20/20 – 3
OS: 20/25 + 1

6.2.2 Pupils

OD: Tear-drop shaped, no afferent pupillary defect by reverse
OS: Round, no afferent pupillary defect

6.2.3 External Examination

Normal

6.2.4 Slit Lamp Examination

	OD	OS
Lids and lashes	Normal	Normal
Sclera and conjunctiva	Trace injection	Normal
Cornea	4-mm, inferior, horizontal laceration, with iris plugging the wound, Seidel positive	Normal
Anterior chamber	Shallow inferiorly	Normal
Iris	Vertically oblong pupil, with iris plugging corneal wound	Normal
Lens	Normal	Normal
Vitreous	Normal	Normal

6.2.5 Dilated Examination

Macula/Nerve OD: Normal
Periphery OD: Normal
Macula/Nerve: OS: Normal
Periphery OS: Normal

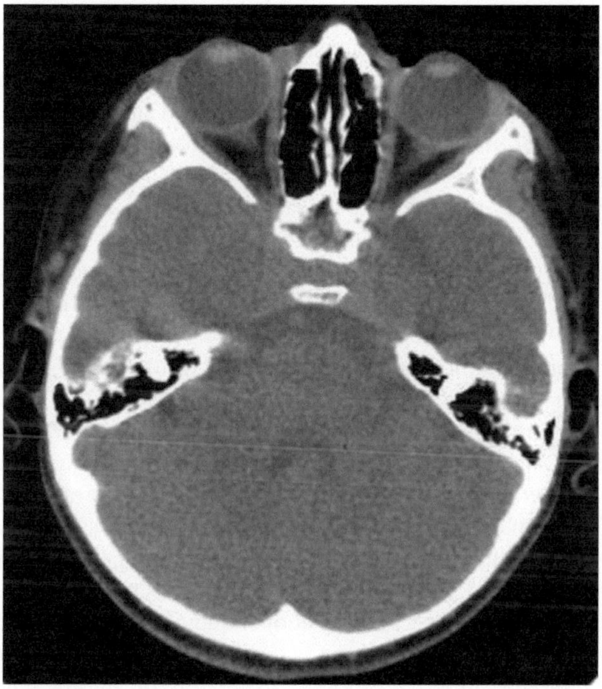

Fig. 6.1 Axial, non-contrast computed tomography (CT) scan of the orbits demonstrating no intraocular foreign body and a slightly shallow anterior chamber in the right eye compared to the left eye

6.2.6 Radiographic Imaging

Computed tomography (CT) of the orbits was remarkable for a shallower anterior chamber on the right than the left. There was no evidence of an intraocular foreign body (Fig. 6.1).

6.3 Surgeon's Initial Assessment and Pre-operative Plan

This patient had a Zone I open globe injury of the right eye with iris incarceration in the wound, requiring surgical repair.

This case raises five important areas of discussion, including (1) evaluation and management of children presenting with potential open globe injuries, (2) setting appropriate post-operative expectations in patients who present with excellent pre-operative visual acuity, (3) repair of simple Zone I lacerations, (4) management of corneal wounds with iris incarceration, and (5) post-operative care of children with open globe injuries.

Open globe injuries are common in children. At MEE, the eye trauma service sees 10-20 children each year who present with open globe injuries from pencils, scissors, toys and other common household objects. Children may sustain injuries from almost any type of situation, from being poked in the eye by a stick when stooping down to look at a turtle by the side of the road, to poking oneself in the eye at night with a pocket knife that was stealthily stashed away under a pillow, to a rock thrown at a friend while playing [like in Case 4 (Chap. 9)], to a pen thrown across a classroom.

Some children may present with white and quiet appearing eyes, with excellent visual acuity and few signs of ocular injury, requiring careful examination and attention to detail to find evidence of globe injury. As in this case, one of the first signs of an open globe injury may be an abnormal, peaked or displaced pupil. This finding should raise suspicion for occult injury requiring further investigation of a possible open globe injury.

Some children, such as the patient in the current case, are quite mature for their age and very cooperative, allowing for an excellent pre-operative evaluation and assessment. Oftentimes, however, it may be almost impossible to determine the extent of the ocular injury, or even if there is indeed an open globe injury present. The child might be scared, anxious, or in pain from the injury, which may make an examination difficult. Forcing a child to cooperate with an examination by restraint may only make matters worse if there is an open globe injury, as straining may place pressure on the globe promoting expulsion of intraocular contents. In situations of suspected ocular trauma or open globe injury in an uncooperative child, we recommend proceeding to an examination under anesthesia (EUA), where the extent of ocular injury can be assessed thoroughly in a controlled and calm environment. Unfortunately, if an examination cannot be completed prior to an EUA, one may encounter injuries intraoperatively that were not expected, so one should be prepared to discuss the varied possibilities and scenarios with the parents or care-givers. Consent should be obtained from the parents, and should include examination of both eyes under anesthesia, as well as globe exploration and repair of open globe injury if one is found. If other injuries are suspected, consent may need to include possible repair of eyelid lacerations or possible need for lensectomy or other procedures. Discussing the possibility of various injuries and obtaining consent for repair of the different possible injuries avoids having to obtain additional consent intraoperatively from the parents if an open globe injury is confirmed. It is helpful to ensure that one has the correct cellular telephone number(s) of the parents or caregivers, so that if anything needs to be discussed intraoperatively after the EUA, they may be easily contacted.

Anesthesia in children can be concerning and worrisome to parents, as there have been reports of neuro-developmental changes in young animals exposed to anesthesia, as well as some studies reporting long-term neuro-developmental and behavioral effects in children undergoing repeated general anesthesia [1, 2]. Other large retrospective studies, however, have not found substantial neuro-developmental changes in children undergoing general anesthesia [2, 3]. As pain can also have detrimental effects on neuro-development, the risks and benefits of anesthesia must be weighed. We are of the opinion that in situations of a possible open globe injury, the benefits of an EUA usually outweigh the potential risks of missing an open globe injury and risking vision loss. Moreover, most parents are relieved to have a thorough examination performed under sedation, as an examination with an uncooperative child can also be very traumatic for the parents or caregivers as well.

The risks of radiation from CT scans of the head in children also are of concern to some parents. Meta-analyses and reviews have found that a CT scan of the head in childhood is associated with a slight increase in the incidence of brain malignancy [4]. Because of these studies, use of weaker, pediatric doses of radiation are recommended if a child is to have a CT scan [5]. Our standard approach in all cases of eye trauma is to obtain a CT scan of the orbits to rule-out fractures and intraocular and intraorbital foreign bodies as this could completely change the surgical management of the ocular trauma. Also, a retained intraocular foreign body can be detrimental to vision in the long term.

Clues that may alert one to a possible open globe injury in a child include a history of injury with a sharp object, including pencils, sticks, scissors, knives, or glass, or a history of being hit with a projectile object at high speed, including a toy thrown across a room, a BB from a BB gun, or a dart. Open globe injuries should also be suspected in children who have significant discomfort and are reluctant to open their eyes. Conjunctival lacerations or subconjunctival foreign bodies should alert one to a possible deeper injury. In children with white and quiet eyes and good visual acuity, other clues may include an irregularly-shaped pupil or an iris transillumination defect. If there is an iris transillumination defect, traumatic cataract and lens capsule involvement should be suspected.

In some situations, an injury may be suspicious for possible child abuse. A strange or inconsistent history pertaining to the mechanism of injury that is inappropriate to the child's age can be suggestive of abuse. Marks or injuries on other parts of the body may also be suggestive. The ophthalmologist should consciously be aware of the possibility of child abuse, make sure to note and document any other visible injuries, and ask for appropriate consultation as needed. At MEE, all patients with open globe injuries are seen by a social worker to help assess for these types of situations.

Our current case is notable for a presenting visual acuity of 20/20 and minimal eye pain. In situations of excellent pre-operative visual acuity, the patient must be strongly counseled that the purpose of surgery for an open globe injury is to close the eye in order to prevent infection and to preserve the eye. Patients should be warned that sutures induce astigmatism, that their vision will be blurrier post-operatively, and that this may be the case until sutures are removed or indefinitely if corneal scarring affects their vision. They should be given some hope, however, by reminding them that good pre-operative visual acuity is a strong predictor of good post-operative visual acuity in open globe injuries [6], and often if the laceration is not in the central pupillary axis, the final visual result can be excellent.

Like adults, children with open globe injuries should receive 48 hours of intravenous antibiotics. Children's antibiotic doses are based on weight, so it is important that a child be weighed upon presentation. Our institution typically doses vancomycin at 10–15 mg/kg/dose every 6 hours and ceftazidime at 30–50 mg/kg/

dose every 8 hours. We recommend checking vancomycin dosing after the fourth dose of the drug to ensure therapeutic levels, and we adjust subsequent levels as needed. It is prudent to check pediatric dosing with the hospital pharmacy and/or an infectious disease specialist. Additionally, in all trauma cases, a tetanus immunization is updated. Most children will be up-to-date based on their pediatric immunization regimen; however, there is a substantial population of children who have not received immunizations, so an immunization history should be obtained and verified.

When repairing an open globe injury in the operating room, an initial assessment to determine the extent of injury is the first step. Then it is helpful to create a paracentesis with a 15° or a microvitreoretinal blade as an entry port to introduce balanced saline solution or filtered air to maintain the anterior chamber during surgical repair. For cataract surgery, surgeons often use 0.12 forceps on the opposite side of the globe for stability as the paracentesis is being created, or a Fine-Thorton fixation ring. These fixation approaches, however, should typically not be used for open globe injuries because too much pressure is placed on the soft globe. Instead, 0.12 forceps should be used to grasp the sclera at the limbus just posterior to the location of placement of the paracentesis, and a very gentle and controlled push-pull movement is performed to complete a paracentesis on a soft globe. If the chamber is flat, often the paracentesis blade needs to be directed down towards the iris to prevent a very long paracentesis track through the corneal stroma. In these cases, the blade cannot be fully inserted into the anterior chamber otherwise it might puncture the lens, and one may need to adjust and increase the size of the paracentesis by cutting sideways while coming out of the wound. It is also important to direct the paracentesis towards the laceration (instead of towards the center of the eye), to make it easier to perform manipulations near the wound, such as removing incarcerated iris.

If the injury is confirmed to be a simple linear Zone I corneal laceration, 10–0 nylon sutures are used to close the wound with the sutures aligned perpendicular to the wound. They should be evenly spaced and sufficiently long to appropriately align the wound edges. Short sutures may be difficult to rotate, but the surgeon may elect to place them if he or she is trying to avoid a suture pass through the pupillary axis or the central cornea.

When there is suspicion of iris incarceration in the corneal wound, filling the anterior chamber with filtered air may help confirm if this is indeed the case (please see Video 6.1 of this case). When there is no iris incarceration, the anterior chamber will fill with a uniform air bubble under the laceration. If incarceration is present, a portion of the anterior chamber may not fill completely and will remain shallow (see Video 6.1 of this case). In such cases, an iris spatula or cyclodialysis spatula should be used to sweep the trapped iris from the wound to reposition it into the eye, and then the anterior chamber should be re-inflated with filtered air. Sometimes it may be difficult to place initial sutures as the anterior chamber will not maintain form. Once initial sutures are placed, however, and the anterior chamber is more stable, one can sweep under the wound with a cyclodialysis spatula to ensure that iris is not caught in the wound. A small amount of cohesive viscoelastic may be used to keep the iris away from the cornea as well, but we recommend using sparingly because it can prolapse through the corneal wound and coat the sutures, making suturing and wound closure more difficult.

6.4 Surgical Exploration and Repair: Operative Note

Risks, benefits, and alternatives were discussed and informed consent was obtained from the parents. In the pre-operative area, the patient was identified, and the right eye was marked. The patient was brought into the operating room where a time out was performed and general anesthesia was induced. The patient was prepared and draped in the usual sterile ophthalmic fashion. Jaffe lid speculae were used to retract the eyelids to minimize pressure on the globe. The right eye was inspected under the microscope. There was a 4-mm, shelved-appearing, horizontal, full-thickness corneal laceration at 6 o'clock, approximately 2 mm from the limbus. The wound appeared full-thickness centrally with possible pigment and iris in the wound and partial thickness nasally and temporally. The iris was dilated and overall round, other than the extension of iris to the wound. The anterior chamber was formed, without hyphema, and the lens appeared intact.

The surgical approach was superior. A paracentesis was made at 9 o'clock with a 15° super-sharp blade. Filtered air was injected through the paracentesis. It was noted to fill incompletely at 6 o'clock, suggesting iris entrapment. A cyclodialysis spatula was used to sweep the iris at the 6 o'clock position under the wound. After this maneuver, the wound appeared to have less pigment and additional injected filtered air filled the anterior chamber completely and evenly. Next, three 10–0 nylon sutures were placed vertically, perpendicular to the wound to close the laceration. The filtered air was replaced with balanced saline solution. The wound was tested with a fluorescein strip and found to be Seidel negative. The paracentesis was hydrated with balanced saline solution. Subconjunctival cefazolin-dexamethasone was injected. The drapes and speculae were removed. Both eyes were then examined with a 20D lens, and the optic nerves and retinas were found to be normal. Atropine drops and neomycin sulfate-polymixin b sulfate and dexamethasone ophthalmic ointment were then instilled in the right eye and the right eye was patched. The patient tolerated the procedure well, without complications.

6.4.1 Surgical Exploration and Repair: Pearls

- It is useful to make a paracentesis at the start of the case when repairing an open globe injury involving the cornea. This allows the surgeon to have control of the anterior chamber and inject filtered air or balanced saline solution as needed throughout the repair.

- Iris incarceration in a corneal wound should be released by deepening the anterior chamber with filtered air, by sweeping gently under the wound with a cyclodialysis spatula, or by repositioning it into the anterior chamber with an iris spatula.
- For simple linear Zone I corneal lacerations, 10–0 nylon sutures should be used and placed perpendicular to the wound at approximately 80–95% depth in the corneal stroma. This topic of depth of suturing in corneal lacerations is discussed more in Chap. 5 - Controversies.

6.4.2 Surgical Video

Please see Video 6.1

6.5 Post-Operative Course

The patient was admitted to MEE for 48 hours of intravenous antibiotics. On post-operative day 1, her visual acuity was 20/200 pinhole improvement to 20/70 in the operative eye, intraocular pressure was 11 mmHg, and the anterior chamber was formed. She was started on the usual post-operative drops of prednisolone acetate 1% six times daily, atropine ophthalmic 1% once daily, and gatifloxacin 0.5% four times daily.

On post-operative week 1, her visual acuity was 20/50 with pinhole testing. Gatifloxacin and atropine were stopped, and a weekly prednisolone taper was initiated, 4× per day for 1 week, 3× per day for 1 week, 2× per day for 1 week, 1× per day for 1 week and then stop. Additionally, the patient and her family received strict instructions to start patching the left eye for at least 1 hour per day while reading or watching television for amblyopia therapy. Sample patches were provided (Fig. 6.2).

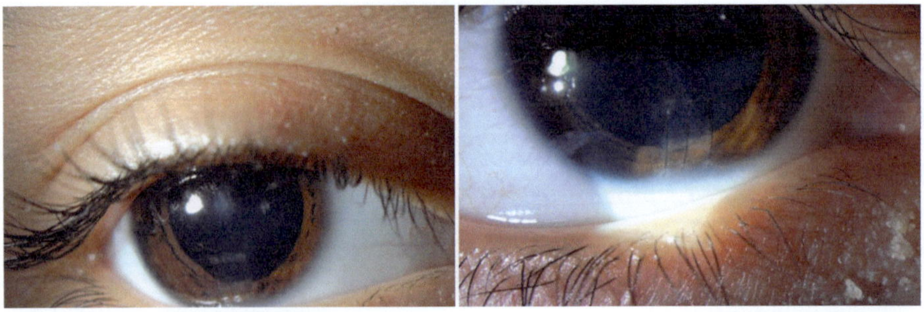

Fig. 6.2 Anterior segment photographs at post-operative week 1, demonstrating the inferior horizontal corneal laceration with three vertical evenly-spaced corneal sutures

At the post-operative month 1 visit, she was doing well, with visual acuity 20/25 with pinhole. Suture removal was scheduled for the following week in the operating room.

6.6 Suture Removal: Operative Note

The risks, benefits, and alternatives were discussed with the patient and her father pre-operatively, and the father consented to proceed with removal of the corneal sutures of the right eye. The patient was brought to the operating room where the anesthesia team proceeded with mask anesthesia. A careful time-out procedure was observed, and the correct patient and the eye were identified. A drop of 5% povidone and gatifloxacin were placed in the right eye. A 15° blade was used to remove the three corneal sutures. The wound was checked with fluorescein after the sutures were removed. There was a small leak from the last suture track that did not completely resolve after waiting. There was no leak from the main wound even with provocation. A bandage contact lens was placed due to the slow leak along with gatifloxacin four times daily in the right eye.

6.7 Post-suture Removal Course

Post-suture removal, she continued on gatifloxacin 4× per day until the post-operative week 6 visit. At that visit, the bandage contact lens was removed, and the corneal wounds were Seidel negative. Visual acuity was 20/15–1 without correction in the right eye. The patient was instructed to follow-up in 2 weeks with Pediatric ophthalmology for further care, where visual acuity remained similar. A slight irregularity to the retinoscopic reflex was noted from the corneal wound inducing irregular astigmatism. Since irregular astigmatism can be amblyogenic, close follow-up care was advised, but the patient did not return. We generally recommend that children in the amblyopic age range follow-up every 3–4 months initially and then gradually be spaced to every 6 months until the age of 8 to ensure there is no induced amblyopia with time.

6.8 Final Trauma Evaluation

6.8.1 Final Visual Acuity

OD: 20/15
OS: 20/15
Cycloplegic Refraction

OD: +0.75 +0.25 x55 (irregular retinoscopic reflex)
OS: +1.00 diopters sphere

6.8.2 Pupils

OD: Round, no afferent pupillary defect
OS: Round, no afferent pupillary defect

6.8.3 Slit Lamp Examination

	OD	OS
Lids and Lashes	Normal	Normal
Sclera and Conjunctiva	Normal	Normal
Cornea	4-mm, inferior, horizontal corneal scar	Normal
Anterior Chamber	Normal	Normal
Iris	Normal	Normal
Lens	Normal	Normal
Vitreous	Normal	Normal

6.8.4 Dilated Examination

Macula/Nerve OD: Normal
Periphery OD: Normal
Macula/Nerve: OS: Normal
Periphery OS: Normal (Fig. 6.3)

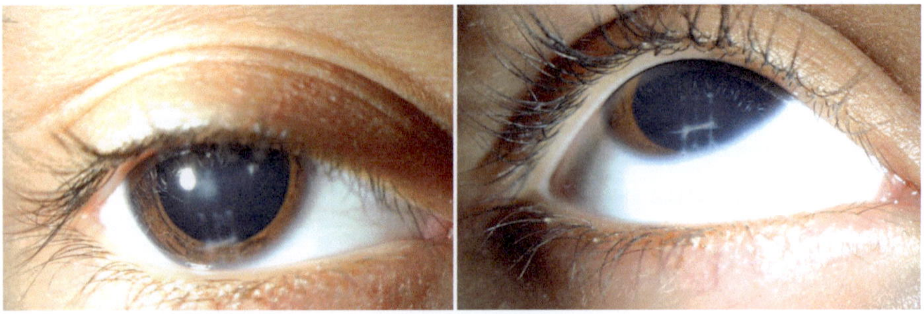

Fig. 6.3 Anterior segment photographs at post-operative week 6, which is 1 week post suture removal, demonstrating the scarring from the corneal laceration and the corneal sutures. Her visual acuity at this visit was 20/15 in the surgical eye

6.9 Review and Lessons Learned

Children with potential open globe injuries need a thorough examination. Open globe injuries may be present even in situations where the visual acuity is 20/20 and there is no pain. If an adequate examination is not possible in the clinic setting, an EUA is warranted. Open globe injuries should be suspected in children when there is a history of injury with a sharp object, or when a peaked pupil, iris transillumination defect or conjunctival laceration is seen on examination.

Patients with good pre-operative visual acuity should be warned that their immediate post-operative vision will be much worse due to astigmatism induced by sutures or corneal edema that develops due to suture placement. The clinician should stress that the goal of surgery is closure of the eye to prevent infection and to preserve the globe. However, we often discuss with patients that one predictor of a good final visual acuity is the pre-operative visual acuity [6], so the fact that this patient presented with 20/20 vision was an indication that she would do well post-operatively. The 10–0 nylon sutures should be used and placed perpendicular to the wound at approximately 85–90% depth in the corneal stroma. A paracentesis should be made directed towards the wound to assist with release of iris from the wound and anterior chamber depth maintenance.

Post-operative amblyopia therapy is essential in children with open globe injuries to maintain their best visual potential [please see Case 4 (Chap. 9) for a more complete discussion of amblyopia therapy in children with open globe injuries].

Post-operatively, most children with open globe injuries do not complain of significant discomfort, and acetaminophen (Tylenol) is typically sufficient for pain relief, with an occasional narcotic dose needed in the first post-operative day. Children are usually started on similar post-operative eye drops as adults, prednisolone six times daily, gatifloxacin four times daily, and atropine once daily.

Since children heal more rapidly than adults, and also begin to develop corneal scarring early on, suture removal is typically performed earlier than in adults. In adults, sutures are typically removed starting at 6 weeks post repair. In children, one may consider suture removal starting from four weeks post injury. In our patient, sutures were removed 5 weeks after open globe repair. Then, we typically see the patient on post-operative day 1, week 1, and once again the week before suture removal to assess for proper wound healing before taking the patient to the operating room.

Suture removal in children, and also in uncooperative adults, typically requires anesthesia in the operating room setting. Anesthesia is only needed for a few minutes in these cases, and can often be provided with mask anesthesia. However, some anesthesiologists prefer a laryngeal mask airway (LMA). After sedation, antibiotic drops and 5% povidone iodine are instilled, sutures are quickly removed, and the wound is tested to ensure that it is Seidel negative. Antibiotic drops are instilled after all sutures are removed. In most cases, we try to remove all of the sutures while in the operating room to prevent any additional trips to the operating room and additional anesthesia. This means that for longer wounds, one may elect to wait an extra week or two prior to suture removal to ensure that the wound has healed and all sutures can be removed at once. If, however, the wound does not seem stable while removing sutures, it is wise to stop any further removal, and instead schedule for additional time in the operating room in a few weeks after the wound has had more time to heal.

6.10 Key Learning Points

- If there is any suspicion for an open globe injury or other ocular trauma in a child, and the child is not cooperative for an adequate examination in the clinic or emergency department, there should be low threshold for performing an examination under anesthesia.
- Open globe injuries may present without pain and with excellent visual acuity.
- Antibiotic dosing in a child is different than in adults, and it is helpful to communicate with the hospital pharmacist or infectious disease specialist to determine appropriate dosing.
- CT imaging is necessary even in pediatric patients to rule out an intraocular foreign body or other facial trauma.
- In linear corneal lacerations, it is important to place the sutures perpendicular to the wound.
- Sutures should be removed more quickly in children than in adults to minimize scarring and neovascularization. Sutures in children are removed under anesthesia in the operating room often approximately 4–5 weeks after repair.
- Patching therapy is an essential part of post-operative management of children, who are still at risk for amblyopia.

References

1. Mann GE, Kahana M. The uncomfortable reality … We simply do not know if general anesthesia negatively impacts the neurocognitive development of our small children. Int J Pediatr Otorhinolaryngol. 2015;79(9):1379–81.
2. Jevtovic-Todorovic V. General anesthetics and neurotoxicity. How much do we know? Anesthesiol Clin. 2016;34:439–51.
3. Graham MR, Brownell M, Chateau DG, Dragan RD, Burchill C, Fransoo RR. Neurodevelopmental assessment in kindergarten in children exposed to general anesthesia before the age of 4 years: a retrospective matched cohort study. Anesthesiology. 2016;125(4):667–77.
4. Chen JX, Kachniarz B, Gilani S, Shin JJ. Risk of malignancy associated with head and neck CT in children. Otolaryngol Head Neck Surg. 2014;151(4):554–66.
5. Hartin CW Jr, Jordan JM, Gemme S, Glick PL, Caty MG, Ozgediz DE, Bass KD. Computed tomography scanning in pediatric trauma: opportunities for performance improvement and radiation safety. J Surg Res. 2013;180(2):226–31.
6. Kuhn F, Maisiak R, Mann L, Mester V, Morris R, Witherspoon CD. The Ocular Trauma Score (OTS). Ophthalmol Clin North Am. 2002;15(2):163–5.

Chapter 7
Case 2: Linear Corneal Laceration from Broken Glass

Grayson W. Armstrong, James A. Stefater, and Yoshihiro Yonekawa

7.1 History of Present Illness

A 24-year-old woman with a history of asthma presented for evaluation and repair of a Zone I corneal laceration of the left eye with concern for retained intraocular glass foreign body.

- The patient reported that a delivery man elbowed through her glass door, resulting in an explosion of glass and a sudden foreign body sensation in her left eye with tearing.
- The patient presented directly to Massachusetts General Hospital and ophthalmology was consulted for evaluation, at which point the open globe was confirmed.
- The patient denied any visual dysfunction prior to operative repair.

7.2 Initial Trauma Evaluation

7.2.1 Visual Acuity (Without Correction)

OD: 20/25-1
OS: 20/25-1

G. W. Armstrong, M.D., M.P.H. (✉) • J. A. Stefater, M.D., Ph.D.
Department of Ophthalmology, Harvard Medical School, Massachusetts Eye and Ear, Boston, MA, USA
e-mail: grayson_armstrong@meei.harvard.edu

Y. Yonekawa, M.D.
Vitreoretinal Surgery, Harvard Medical School, Massachusetts Eye and Ear and Boston Children's Hospital, Boston, MA, USA

S. Grob, C. Kloek (eds.), *Management of Open Globe Injuries*,
https://doi.org/10.1007/978-3-319-72410-2_7

7.2.2 *Pupils*

OD: Normal, no afferent pupillary defect
OS: Normal, no afferent pupillary defect

7.2.3 *External Examination*

No other facial trauma other than a small left upper eyelid laceration.

7.2.4 *Slit Lamp Examination*

	OD	OS
Lids and lashes	Normal	Small upper eyelid non-marginal laceration
Sclera and conjunctiva	Normal	1+ injection
Cornea	Normal	Full-thickness corneal laceration extending radially from at 5 o'clock measuring 3.5 mm in length, minimally Seidel-positive
Anterior chamber	Normal	Deep, pigmented debris to wound
Iris	Normal	Normal, no peaking
Lens	Normal	Normal, no obvious violation
Vitreous	Normal	Normal

7.2.5 *Dilated Examination*

Macula/Nerve OD: Normal
Periphery OD: Normal
Macula/Nerve: OS: Normal
Periphery OS: Normal

7.2.6 *Radiographic Imaging*

Computed tomography (CT) of the orbits showed a small focus of air attenuation within the anterior chamber. No radiopaque foreign body was identified to suggest metal or glass in the eye (Fig. 7.1).

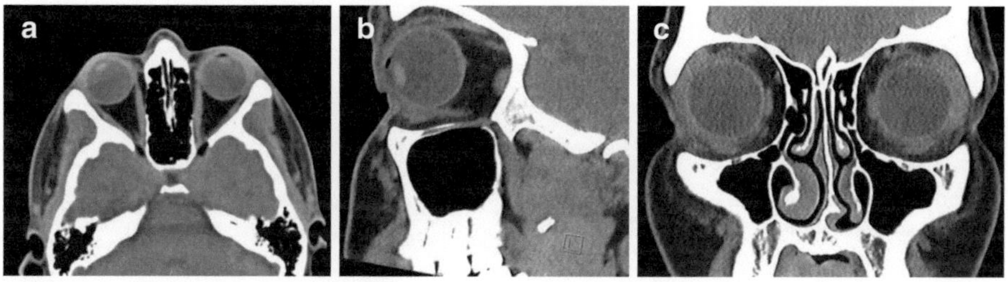

Fig. 7.1 Axial (**a**) and sagittal (**b**) CT images showing formed globes with a small amount of air attenuation within the anterior chamber. Coronal (**c**) CT image showing grossly formed globes

7.3 Surgeon's Initial Assessment and Pre-Operative Plan

The patient had a corneal Zone I globe injury of the left eye with preserved vision requiring surgical repair and no obvious intraocular foreign body on pre-operative exam and imaging.

This case illustrates the management of Zone I corneal lacerations and the potential for such wounds to result in good post-operative vision outcomes. It also demonstrates the importance of careful intra-operative exploration for potential retained foreign body material if the suspicion is present.

Corneal wound suturing is an important concept in open globe management as discussed in the prior case. The quality of the initial repair is a major determinant of the final visual outcome in corneal lacerations [1]. It is imperative to correctly approximate the corneal wound edges during suturing to avoid irregular wound healing. As mentioned in the first case, it is important to place sutures at approximately 80–90% depth in the corneal stroma. Shallow corneal suturing may result in posterior wound 'gape' and sometimes wound leaks.

Since nylon is a relatively slippery material, either a locking surgeons' knot is tied in a 3-1-1 fashion using an initial triple throw followed by two alternating single throws or a slip knot (1-1-1) can be utilized. Sufficient tension to close the wound is important to allow for some compression of the wound so the wound edges are appropriately apposed for healing. Non-shelved wounds compared to shelved wounds might require more tension for healing. Sutures that are too tight can result in unwanted astigmatism that can limit visual potential, while sutures that are too loose can result in discomfort and can collect bacteria and debris, thus risking post-operative infection and associated morbidity. In open globe injuries where the intraocular pressure may be low during surgery, it can be difficult to estimate the resulting tension of corneal sutures. As a result, it is not uncommon to replace sutures that are too tight or too loose once a water-tight seal is created and the globe is reformed. Or, if slip knot sutures were placed and the third tie not placed to secure the knot, then the tension can be adjusted on all of the sutures prior to doing the final tie. Circumstances that might require tighter sutures include: when another surgery is necessary during primary wound repair or shortly after

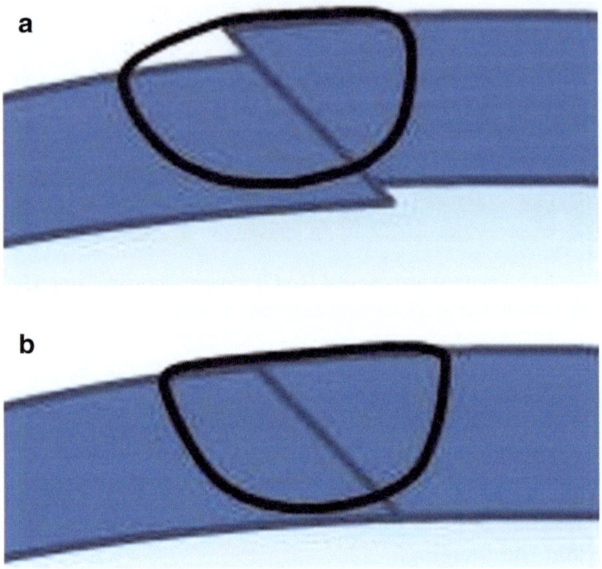

Fig. 7.2 Schematic of (**a**) shelved corneal laceration with overriding wound edge due to varied suture depth, and (**b**) well-approximated corneal wound edge resulting from uniform suture depth

(lensectomy, vitrectomy, etc.), when there is significant corneal edema, since when corneal edema resolves after repair the sutures will loosen, or often when there is a retained corneal foreign body such as a metal rod that may create the appearance of tissue loss after the foreign body is removed. Use of filtered air to inflate the anterior chamber during corneal suturing, as opposed to saline or ophthalmic viscoelastic devices, is useful to aid in reapproximation of corneal wounds.

In non-shelved corneal wounds, suture passes are placed so there is equal distance/amount of suture on both sides of the wound. However, in shelved corneal lacerations, the suture bites need to be symmetrically placed at the deeper aspect of the laceration. This is important to prevent wound override and an abnormal shape of the cornea after healing (Fig. 7.2).

The knot, once tied, is rotated within the suture tract such that the body and tail of the knot are completely embedded in the stroma. Ideally the knot is rotated away from the visual axis. Exposure of the knot or suture tail can cause irritation and pain, but may also result in unwanted corneal infection.

Careful pre-operative evaluation did not identify any obvious lenticular or intraocular foreign bodies. Intraoperatively, the surgeons planned to carefully assess for small foreign bodies that were not detected pre-operatively.

7.4 Surgical Exploration and Repair: Operative Note

The risks, benefits, and alternatives were discussed with the patient pre-operatively and the patient consented to proceed with exploration and repair of the open globe injury. The patient was brought to the operating room where the anesthesia team

proceeded with general anesthesia. A careful time-out was observed and the correct patient and the eye were identified. The left eye was prepped and draped in the usual sterile ophthalmic fashion using a Jaffe speculum to provide adequate exposure.

The patient was found to have a 3.5 mm non-shelved corneal laceration from 5 o'clock extending radially and centrally. Air was injected through a nasal paracentesis and the cornea was closed with four interrupted 10-0 nylon sutures. There was no extension of the wound past the limbus.

Upon inspection of the anterior chamber, small cream-colored foreign bodies were identified. These were aspirated from the anterior chamber with a 30-gauge cannula and sent to pathology.

A subconjunctival steroid and antibiotic injection was performed nasally away from the laceration. The speculum was removed. The patient's drape was removed under the microscope. The patient tolerated the procedure well without any complications.

7.4.1 Surgical Exploration and Repair: Pearls

- Careful intraoperative evaluation of the cornea and anterior chamber is vital in cases where retained foreign bodies may be present.
- It is important to ensure the corneal laceration does not extend beyond the limbus.
- Careful placement of corneal sutures with the appropriate amount of tension, depth, and distance on either side of the wound is important to ensure good wound closure and the best possible visual outcome.
- Use of filtered air to re-inflate the anterior chamber is useful during corneal laceration repair.

7.5 Post-Operative Course

The patient completed 48 hours of intravenous antibiotics. Post-operative day one examination revealed vision of 20/40 and a nicely repaired corneal laceration with a formed anterior chamber (Fig. 7.3).

One week later, the patient had no complaints and examination revealed a best-corrected visual acuity of 20/15-1 in the affected eye. The corneal wound was intact and Seidel negative. The posterior exam was unremarkable.

At a 6-week follow-up visit, the corneal laceration was thought to have healed and the four corneal sutures were removed after application of topical antibiotics and povidone-iodine solution in the clinic and was found to be Seidel negative.

Since removal of the corneal sutures, the vision has remained stable at 20/15. A plan for life-long polycarbonate glasses use is reinforced at each follow-up visit to prevent future eye injuries.

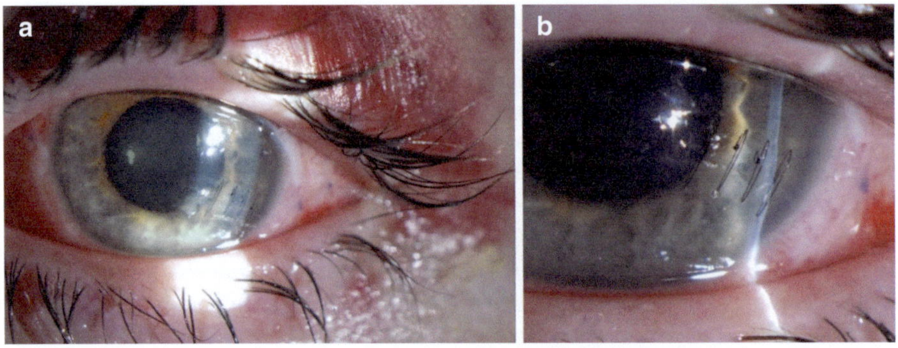

Fig. 7.3 Clinical image (**a**) showing the initial post-operative cornea with four nylon sutures in place. Higher magnification (**b**) reveals partial thickness corneal sutures with buried knots and suture tails

7.6 Final Trauma Evaluation

7.6.1 Final Visual Acuity

OD: 20/15
OS: 20/15

7.6.2 Pupils

OD: Normal, no afferent pupillary defect
OS: Normal, no afferent pupillary defect

7.6.3 Slit Lamp Examination

	OD	OS
Lids and lashes	Normal	Normal
Sclera and conjunctiva	Normal	Normal, no injection
Cornea	Normal	Inferotemporal linear scar, well healed, Seidel negative, no epithelial defect (Fig. 7.4)
Anterior chamber	Normal	Normal, no cell
Iris	Normal	Normal, no transillumination defects
Lens	Normal	Normal, clear
Vitreous	Normal	Normal

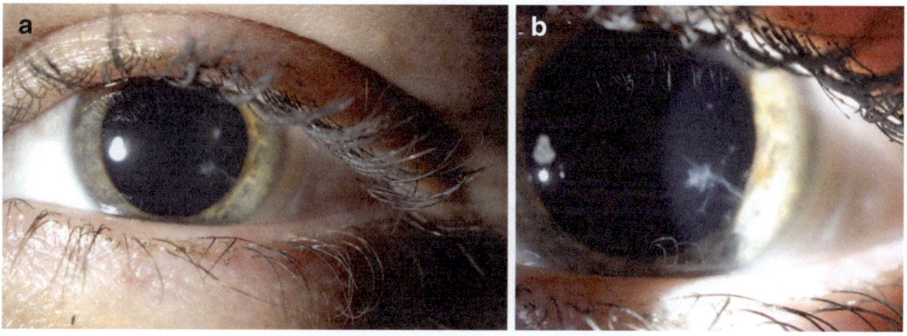

Fig. 7.4 Clinical image (**a**) showing the resulting peripheral corneal scar following suture removal. Higher magnification (**b**) reveals a linear stromal corneal scar from the initial corneal laceration in addition to scars corresponding to prior suture tracts

7.6.4 Dilated Examination

Macula/Nerve OD: Normal
Periphery OD: Normal
Macula/Nerve: OS: Normal
Periphery OS: Normal

7.7 Review and Lessons Learned

As this case illustrated, isolated corneal laceration injuries have the potential for excellent visual outcomes. The quality of the primary repair is a major determinant in the final visual outcome. Careful corneal suturing technique should be incorporated to maximize visual outcomes. This involves careful choice of suture material, suture depth and length, careful wound edge re-approximation, appropriate suture tension, use of intracameral air in the anterior chamber, and thoughtful removal of sutures at a later date. As in the first case, it is important to inform patients that their vision will likely worsen after the primary repair due to corneal edema and astigmatism from the suture placement and often the final visual outcome is not certain until follow up after the sutures are removed. Usually suture removal is considered around 6 weeks after primary repair, but can be longer depending on the length and type of corneal laceration. Fortunately, in this case, the wound appeared healed at the 6-week period and it was decided to remove all four sutures at one visit. Often a careful exam is necessary to decide whether the wound is healed and suture removal can be performed, especially all sutures in one visit. Short linear shelved or non-shelved lacerations can often have all sutures removed at once, but as will be discussed in later cases, care should be taken in limbus to limbus, stellate, complex, wounds that tend to leak, or those that present with retained corneal foreign bodies.

When in doubt, it is better to be conservative with suture removal and the sutures can be removed over several visits.

In cases of Zone I corneal lacerations, careful examination of the entire globe is paramount. Retained intraocular foreign bodies may not be seen on initial ophthalmic exam and may only be identified as a result of careful intraoperative evaluation. Retained foreign bodies may result in significant morbidity, such as cataract, glaucoma, endophthalmitis, chalcosis, siderosis bulbi, varying degrees of uveitic reaction, or decreased visual acuity [2]. Glass can often be difficult to identify, so it is important to look closely.

7.8 Key Learning Points

- Zone I corneal lacerations can result in excellent visual outcomes, as in this case with resulting 20/15 vision in the affected eye. Care should be taken to ensure the appropriate placement and tension of corneal sutures depending on the type and shape of the wound.
- Careful evaluation of the cornea and anterior chamber for potential retained intraocular foreign bodies should be performed, as pre-operative examination may not allow for adequate assessment of retained material.

References

1. Sullivan P. The open globe: surgical techniques for the closure of ocular wounds. London: Eyelearning; 2013.
2. Loporchio D, Mukkamala L, Gorukanti K, et al. Intraocular foreign bodies: a review. Surv Ophthalmol. 2016;61(5):582–96.

Chapter 8
Case 3: Stellate Corneal Laceration from a Motor Vehicle Accident

Yvonne Wang, Natalie Wolkow, and Seanna Grob

8.1 History of Present Illness

An 18-year-old man with no significant past medical history was transferred to the Massachusetts Eye and Ear (MEE) emergency room with an open globe injury of the right eye.

- The patient was a passenger in a car when the vehicle swerved off the road and hit a side-rail. The car windshield was broken and a piece of glass hit his right eye. Immediately after the accident his vision in the right eye became blurry. He reported that he could only see shapes and colors. He did not have any loss of consciousness and the airbag in the vehicle did not deploy.
- He was seen at another hospital and was found to have an open globe of the right eye, but no other injuries from the accident. A computed tomography (CT) scan of the orbits showed a flattened anterior chamber in the right eye compared to the left (Fig. 8.1). He was transferred to MEE for further management.

8.2 Initial Trauma Evaluation

8.2.1 Visual Acuity (Without Correction)

OD: Counting fingers at 6 inches. There was no improvement with pinhole.
With near card: 20/400 pinhole 20/200
OS: 20/20-1

Y. Wang, M.D. (✉) • N. Wolkow, M.D., Ph.D. • S. Grob, M.D., M.A.S.
Department of Ophthalmology, Harvard Medical School, Massachusetts Eye and Ear, Boston, MA, USA
e-mail: Yvonne_wang@meei.harvard.edu

S. Grob, C. Kloek (eds.), *Management of Open Globe Injuries*,
https://doi.org/10.1007/978-3-319-72410-2_8

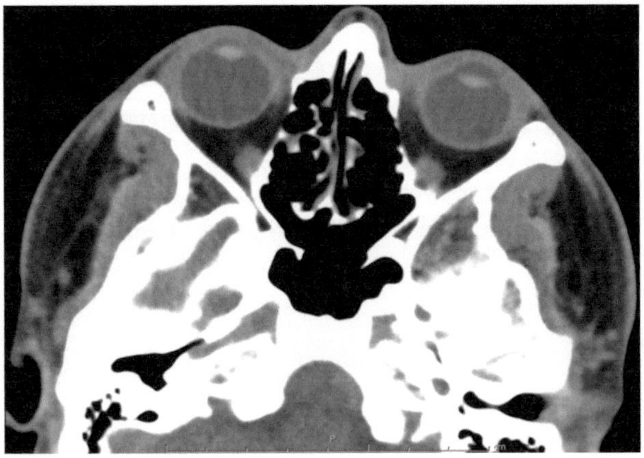

Fig. 8.1 The CT scan showed no intraocular foreign body and a shallow anterior chamber on the right, which was concerning for an open globe injury

8.2.2 *Pupils*

OD: Irregular, no afferent pupillary defect by reverse
OS: Round, briskly reactive

8.2.3 *External Examination*

Mild periorbital swelling on the right

8.2.4 *Slit Lamp Examination*

	OD	OS
Lids and lashes	Periorbital swelling	Normal
Sclera and conjunctiva	1+ diffuse injection	Normal
Cornea	Complex full-thickness corneal laceration extending superiorly through the visual axis. Seidel positive. Superior iris strands protruding anteriorly into the cornea, with pigment over the endothelium centrally. Large triangular-shaped laceration beginning at 12 o'clock, with the apex in the visual axis, that extends nasally with multiple other associated triangular components (Fig. 8.2)	Normal
Anterior chamber	Shallow, 3–4+ cell and fibrin, hazy view, with small amount of hemorrhage	Normal
Iris	Debris over the iris with a few spots of hemorrhage. Iridocorneal touch superiorly with some incarceration of the iris in the wound.	Normal
Lens	Fibrin debris over the lens. Difficult to determine the integrity of the lens capsule given corneal edema, corneal laceration and fibrin.	Normal
Vitreous	Poor view	Normal

8.2.5 Dilated Examination

Macula/Nerve OD: No view
Periphery OD: No view
Macula/Nerve OS: Normal
Periphery OS: Normal

8.2.6 Radiography Imaging

The CT scan showed no intraocular foreign body, but a shallow anterior chamber on the right, which was concerning for an open globe injury (Fig. 8.1).

8.3 Surgeon's Initial Assessment and Pre-Operative Plan

This patient was found to have a Zone I open globe injury of the right eye from glass hitting the eye during a motor vehicle accident. The patient was taken to the nearest local hospital for a full trauma evaluation to rule out any other bodily injuries and then was transferred to MEE for further management of his ocular injury.

The initial assessment of this case is similar to a standard Zone I injury as seen in Case 1 and 2 (Chapters 6 and 7). However, this patient had a complex stellate laceration, which can be more difficult or time-consuming to close. Given the stellate nature of the wound, the view of the lens was too hazy to rule out lens capsular involvement, and this was discussed with the patient. Even in cases where the lens can be clearly evaluated on the initial exam the view into the anterior chamber to the lens is quite poor after a stellate corneal wound repair which may hinder the ability to complete a lens removal during the primary surgery. It can be helpful to draw out the shape of the corneal laceration seen on initial examination because if there is a delay

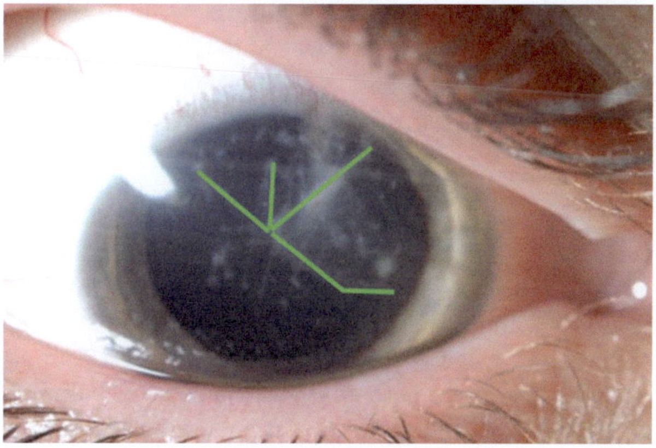

Fig. 8.2 Schematic of the stellate corneal laceration of the right eye which was formed by four lacerations extending from a central location, forming three separate triangular components (The schematic is overlaid on a post-operative month four photograph of the eye, at which point all sutures had been removed)

to the operating room, corneal edema can obscure the view of the shape of the laceration. Often on initial examination in the operating room, tracing out the shape of the corneal laceration with a 30-gauge cannula on syringe (something that will not further traumatize corneal tissue) can also help determine the shape of the laceration and full extent of the wound. There may be more apices involved in these stellate wounds than can be clearly seen in the emergency department. Once the shape of the wound is determined, it is important to align the apices of the wound primarily. It is also important to release one's grasp of corneal tissue as soon as possible to avoid macerating the apices of the wound or other parts of the wound, which could make closure of the wound without leaks more challenging.

This case highlights the challenges of repairing a complex corneal wound with a stellate pattern, and the importance of a step-wise suture removal in a complex stellate corneal wound. Additionally, management of post-operative persistent photophobia is discussed.

8.4 Surgical Exploration and Repair: Operative Note

In the pre-operative area, the patient was identified and the right eye was marked. He was brought into the operating room where general anesthesia was induced. His right eye was prepped with povidone iodine (5% on the ocular surface and 10% on the skin) and draped in the usual sterile ophthalmic fashion. Jaffe lid speculae were used to retract the eyelids to minimize pressure on the globe. Under the operative microscope the wound was examined. It was almost a limbus to limbus Zone I complex stellate, full-thickness laceration affecting the superior half of the cornea, extending from approximately 9:30 to 3 o'clock, consisting of four triangular shelved components (see Fig. 8.2). The conjunctiva was noted to be injected, the pupil was poorly dilated, and a small amount of iris tissue was caught in the superonasal lacerations. The conjunctiva appeared intact and there was no chemosis or signs of extension of the wounds posteriorly past the limbus.

A paracentesis was made temporally with a 15° blade. This was used to inject filtered air intracamerally in order to reform the anterior chamber. The intracameral air injection dislodged the trapped iris tissue from the corneal wound. At this point the anterior chamber was noted to flatten rapidly as the air would leak through the corneal wounds. Initially, 10-0 nylon sutures were used in an interrupted fashion to unite and join the apices of the triangular pieces of the stellate wound. Additional sutures were placed to join the sides of these triangular pieces to help form the globe. Some of the initial sutures had to be removed and replaced with new ones as the globe took shape, either because they were loose or needed to be repositioned to make the wound water-tight. Filtered air was injected as needed to reform the anterior chamber. As sutures were placed, the filtered air remained in the anterior chamber without leaking. Once the globe appeared intact and reformed, the corneal wound was tested with a fluorescein strip and found to still have a small area of leakage centrally where all of the apices were joining. Additional corneal sutures were then placed to reinforce this junction site. Sutures were placed to direct force towards the apex of the triangular components to prevent leaking in this area. A total of sixteen 10-0 nylon sutures were placed and the knots were buried. Additional testing with fluorescein was performed and the globe was found to be Seidel negative. Greater than 50% of the intracameral air was removed with a cannula, and the globe was re-formed with balanced salt solution. The globe was found to be water-tight. The paracentesis wound was hydrated. An 18-mm Kontour bandage contact lens was placed over the cornea in case of future small areas of leakage due to the complexity of the corneal laceration and for patient comfort. Subconjunctival cefazolin-dexamethasone was injected temporally, taking care not to displace the contact lens. The Jaffe speculae were removed. Tobramycin-dexamethasone ophthalmic drops and atropine 1% drops were placed in the right eye. The eyelids were taped lightly with a steri-strip, and a patch and Fox shield were placed over the eye. The patient tolerated the procedure well without complications.

8.4.1 Surgical Exploration and Repair: Pearls

- Alignment of the apices is an important initial step when repairing a stellate laceration. Take time to determine the exact shape of the corneal laceration and ensure that all triangular components are properly positioned before suturing.
- Sutures may need to be replaced and repositioned as the triangular components start to come together in order to ensure the wound is watertight.
- Direct sutures towards the apex (instead of perpendicular to the wound) in order to ensure there are no gaps that may cause leaks at the apex junction.
- Placing a bandage contact lens at the end of the case may be helpful in cases with complex corneal lacerations or lacerations that are prone to leaking during the case. If there is a brisk leak at the end of the case though, likely sutures need to be adjusted. The bandage contact lens can also be helpful with patient comfort if any corneal epithelium is missing at the conclusion of the repair.

8.5 Post-Operative Course

The patient was seen on post-operative day 1 and the contact lens was not removed. His vision was counting fingers at 2 feet. He completed the standard post-operative intravenous antibiotics and was discharged on the standard post-operative topical medications (gatifloxacin, prednisolone, and atropine). At post-operative week 1, he had a visual acuity of 20/200 with pinhole. The contact lens was removed on post-operative week 2 and the wound was Seidel negative. His visual acuity was 20/125.

The first sutures were removed at post-operative week 7. Suture removal was approached in a step-wise fashion. Only 4 of the 16 sutures were removed initially (Fig. 8.3a, b). Then on post-operative week 10 an additional 5 sutures were removed. and the remaining 7 sutures were removed on post-operative week 12 (Fig. 8.4). At

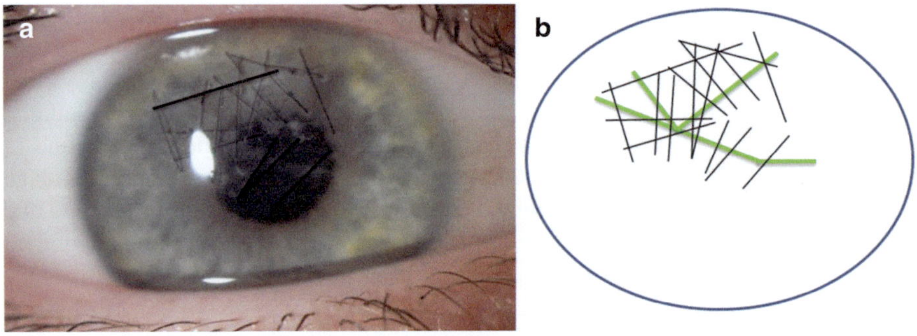

Fig. 8.3 The stellate laceration was closed with 16 overlapping sutures. Four sutures were removed at post-operative week 7. (**a**) An external photograph of the right eye at post-operative week 10, with 12 remaining sutures visible, and the 4 previously removed sutures are drawn in. (**b**) A schematic of the laceration and initial suture placement

Fig. 8.4 Post-operative week 12. There are seven remaining sutures

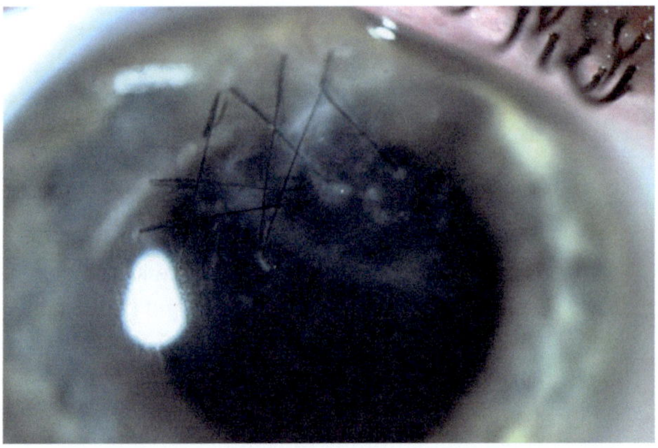

week 12, after all of the sutures had been removed (Fig. 8.5), a small focal cataract in the far supero-temporal periphery of the lens with an overlying iris transillumination defect was noted as well as a trace central posterior subcapsular cataract.

Despite improving visual acuity after removal of all sutures, the patient started to report significantly bothersome photophobia and ocular discomfort. Initially, it was thought that there may be trace residual inflammation, and a trial of prednisolone 1% once daily was prescribed for 2 weeks. There was no improvement in symptoms, so it was discontinued. Gonioscopy and ultrasound biomicroscopy confirmed that there was no sign of retained foreign body and no obvious violation of the posterior capsule of the lens. The small focal anterior cataract was seen on biomicroscopy, but

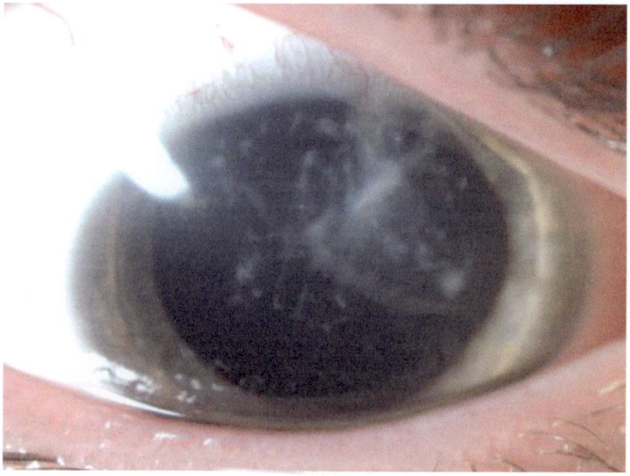

Fig. 8.5 Post-operative week 14. All sutures have been removed

no sign of an intralenticular foreign body was noted. The patient was evaluated by a cornea specialist who thought the persistent photophobia was likely related to the ocular surface and recommended continued artificial tears. An evaluation by the contact lens specialist was recommended to see if a contact lens would improve his vision and his symptoms of photophobia/irritation. Although the patient was evaluated by a contact lens specialist, he was not interested in using contacts. At his 6-month post-operative examination, his photophobia had resolved with use of artificial tears several times per day. Cataract extraction for the posterior subcapsular cataract was also recommended, but the patient deferred.

8.6 Final Trauma Evaluation

8.6.1 Final Visual Acuity Without Correction

OD: 20/70 pinhole 20/40-2
OS: 20/20

8.6.2 Manifest refraction

	Sphere	Cylinder	Axis	Dist
Right	+1.00	−2.50	070	20/40 + 2
Left	+0.50	−0.50	045	20/20

8.6.3 *Pupils*

OD: Round and briskly reactive, no afferent pupillary defect
OS: Round and briskly reactive, equal, no afferent pupillary defect

8.6.4 *Slit Lamp Examination*

	OD	OS
Lids and lashes	Normal	Normal
Sclera and conjunctiva	Normal	Normal
Cornea	Superior corneal scarring, small narrow superior pannus	Normal
Anterior chamber	Normal, no cell	Normal
Iris	Round, temporal/superotemporal arc of concentric transillumination defect (TID) no significant hippus	Normal
Lens	Focal cataract at 10:30 o'clock with associated pigment clump peripherally, 2+ central posterior subcapsular cataract	Normal
Vitreous	Normal	Normal

8.6.5 *Dilated Examination*

Macula/Nerve OD: Normal
Periphery OD: Normal
Macula/Nerve OS: Normal
Periphery OS: Normal

8.7 Review and Lessons Learned

Stellate lacerations are challenging to close due to their complex structure and suture placement and the fragility of the corneal tissue apices and flaps. Aligning the apices is an important first step. If this is not done properly, there may be a gap at the apex that will leak at the end of the case. In cases such as this one where there are multiple apices, a surgeon must take his or her time to carefully align all of the apices before suturing to avoid having to reposition flaps and remove sutures later in the case. Excessive repositioning of sutures can tear or macerate the already friable corneal tissue, making the wound even more difficult to seal. Thus, careful planning of suture placement at the beginning of the case is essential. Drawing out

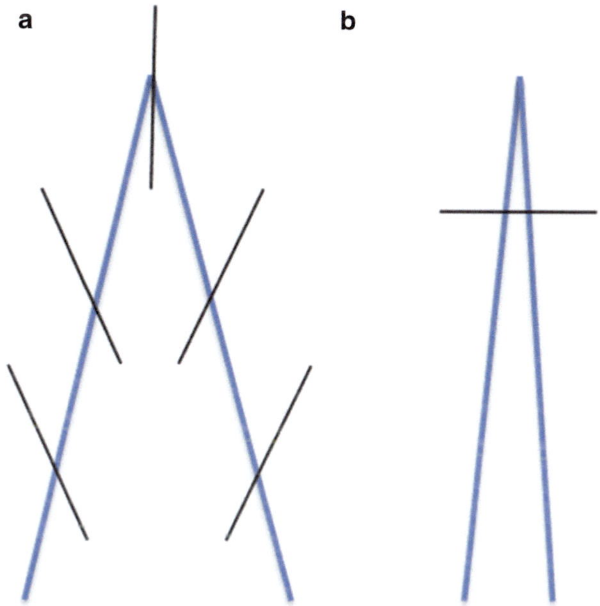

Fig. 8.6 Techniques for suturing apical flaps. (**a**) Sutures are angled towards the apex to direct their forces towards the points of leakage. (**b**) If the flap is too thin or friable, a suture can be placed across the apex to hold it in place

a picture or mentally reviewing a picture of suture placement can be helpful at the beginning of the case.

The usual teaching for suturing corneal lacerations is that the suture should be placed perpendicular to the wound to avoid slippage of the wound edges [1]. However, in V-shaped lacerations, sometimes it is helpful if the sutures are placed at an angle to direct the forces towards the apex (Fig. 8.6a). This allows for tighter apposition of the wound edges. In cases where the apex is too fragile or too thin to pass a suture, one or more sutures can be placed across the apex to hold it down (Fig. 8.6b). Other techniques for closing stellate lacerations include adjustable sutures, purse-string sutures and corneal glue.

Adjustable sutures are useful in situations where multiple sutures are being placed (either with a stellate or limbus to limbus corneal wound), as tension may be adjusted prior to locking them. The advantages of adjustable sutures include the ability to loosen or tighten the sutures to distribute the tension more evenly across a wound, minimizing the chances of a wound leak and need for removing and replacing sutures that become too loose or tight once others are placed. Additionally, adjustable sutures require fewer throws and have a slimmer profile, allowing them to be rotated more easily into the cornea. There are multiple techniques to tying adjustable corneal sutures such as the adjustable slide knot [2], or the adjustable square knot [3]. The main disadvantage to adjustable corneal sutures is that it may be difficult to keep track of all the suture tails in a complex wound.

One of the challenges of stellate lacerations is that closing one flap can open up adjacent wounds. This leads to repeated adjustment and repositioning of sutures to close all the flaps. Purse-string sutures (Fig. 8.7a) and butterfly sutures

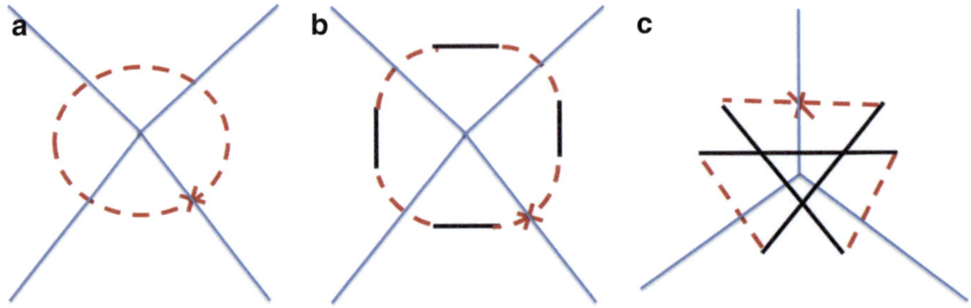

Fig. 8.7 Continuous sutures for stellate wounds. (**a**) The classic purse-string suture is completely buried. (**b**) Eisner purse-string modification. (**c**) Akkins star-shaped suture

are useful for bringing together multiple apices with a single suture, and are effective at distributing equal force across all the flaps [4]. These sutures direct all of the forces towards the center of the stellate wound. The Eisner purse-string [5] (Fig. 8.7b) and the Akkin star-shaped suture [6] (Fig. 8.7c) are examples of modified purse-string and butterfly suture techniques. The disadvantage to these techniques is that they are technically difficult. The surgeon must be careful to avoid excessive manipulation of the apices. Furthermore, because these techniques use a continuous suture, step-wise suture removal is not possible, possibly compromising the integrity of the wound if this single suture breaks.

Testing for wound leakage using fluorescein should be performed at the end of the case. The anterior chamber should be reformed with balanced salt solution, and a drop of concentrated fluorescein should be applied directly to the wound with a fluorescein strip. If there is a brisk leak, additional sutures are often needed. A bandage contact lens can be placed at the end of the case for patient comfort after a complex wound repair or if there is concern that the wound might leak minimally as the corneal edema resolves.

In this case, the contact lens was kept in the eye, even during examination, until post-operative week 2 to prevent disruption of corneal healing. Since it is not possible to test for Seidel positivity with a contact lens in place, it is important to note that the anterior chamber is well formed. If the anterior chamber is flat on post-operative examination despite a contact lens, then the patient likely needs to be taken back to the operating room for repair of a wound leak.

The standard timing of corneal suture removal in open globe repair is 6 weeks. Removing sutures too early may result in wound leak or dehiscence, while removing sutures too late increases corneal scarring. A step-wise approach to removing sutures is recommended for a stellate wound or limbus to limbus laceration (see Case 5, Chapter 10) due to the higher risk of wound leak or dehiscence. In this case, the sutures were removed over a course of three visits, each 2–3 weeks apart. The apical sutures should be removed last.

This patient's post-operative course was complicated by persistent photophobia which significantly compromised his vision despite improving acuity. The differential for post-operative photophobia includes irregular astigmatism, anterior chamber inflammation, elevated intraocular pressure, corneal scarring, ocular surface disease, iris defects, and cataract. In open globe injuries, it is also important to consider retained foreign bodies in the lens or the angle which can be very small and missed on initial imaging. Contact lenses are a good option for treating ocular surface irregularities [8]. A rigid contact lens can be used to correct for astigmatism. Colored contact lenses can be used to minimize glare from mydriasis or transillumination defects. In this case, it was likely ocular surface irritation which improved with time with frequent artificial tears.

8.8 Key Learning Points

- In complex stellate lacerations, it is helpful to evaluate the exact shape and structure of the wound before starting to place sutures. Aligning the apices of the triangular components of the wound should be the initial step in repair.
- When repairing apical lacerations, angle the sutures towards the apex to prevent gaping of the wound at these junctions.
- For very narrow or friable flaps, place a suture across the apex to hold it down instead of through the apex.
- Adjustable sutures can be used to avoid repeated removal and repositioning of sutures in complex lacerations.
- Corneal adhesives or a bandage contact lens can be used at the end of the case to prevent post-operative wound leaks.
- Remove sutures in a step-wise fashion over several visits to avoid wound leaks.

References

1. Lin DT, Webster RG Jr, Abbott RL. Repair of corneal lacerations and perforations. Int Ophthalmol Clin. 1988;28:69–75.
2. Dangel ME, Keates RH. The adjustable slide knot—an alternate technique. Ophthalmic Surg. 1980;11:843–6.
3. Narváez J, Jones J, Zumwalt M, Mahdavi P. Reversed needle pass clear-corneal or limbal incision suturing technique using the 3-throw (1-1-1) adjustable square knot. J Cataract Refract Surg. 2012;38:929–32.
4. Sullivan P. The Open Globe. Surgical techniques for the closure of ocular wounds. London: Eyelearning; 2013. iBook.
5. Eisner G. Eye surgery: an introduction to operative technique, 2nd, fully rev. and expanded ed. Berlin: Springer; 1990:xiv, 317. p. 26.
6. Akkin C, Kayikcioglu O, Erakgun T. A novel suture technique in stellate corneal lacerations. Ophthalmic Surg Lasers. 2001;32:436–7.
7. Mascai M. Ophthalmic microsurgical suturing techniques. Berlin: Springer; 2007. p. 57.
8. Titiyal JS, Sinha R, Sharma N, Sreenivas V, Vajpayee RB. Contact lens rehabilitation following repaired corneal perforations. BMC Ophthalmol. 2006;6:11.

Chapter 9
Case 4: Zone I Pediatric Open Globe Management

James A. Stefater, Ankoor S. Shah, and Seanna Grob

9.1 History of Present Illness

A 4-year-old boy presented with a Zone I open globe injury of the left eye after being poked with a wooden stick.

- The child was playing in a campground when he was accidently hit directly in the left eye with a wooden stick.
- The child's mother noted a small amount of blood initially from the left eye, but the child had only mild symptoms such as tearing and irritation.
- He was seen by a local ophthalmologist who was concerned for an open globe injury of the left eye and referred the patient to Massachusetts Eye and Ear (MEE) for further evaluation.

Electronic Supplementary Material The online version of this chapter (https://doi.org/10.1007/978-3-319-72410-2_9) contains supplementary material, which is available to authorized users.

J. A. Stefater, M.D., Ph.D. (✉) • S. Grob, M.D., M.A.S.
Department of Ophthalmology, Harvard Medical School, Massachusetts Eye and Ear, Boston, MA, USA
e-mail: james_stefater@meei.harvard.edu

A. S. Shah, M.D., Ph.D.
Department of Ophthalmology, Harvard Medical School, Boston Children's Hospital and Massachusetts Eye and Ear, Boston, MA, USA

S. Grob, C. Kloek (eds.), *Management of Open Globe Injuries*,
https://doi.org/10.1007/978-3-319-72410-2_9

9.2 Initial Trauma Evaluation

9.2.1 Visual Acuity (Without Correction)

OD: 20/20
OS: Light perception

9.2.2 Pupils

OD: Round, no afferent pupillary defect by reverse
OS: Irregular

9.2.3 External Examination

Normal

9.2.4 Slit Lamp Examination

	OD	OS
Lids and lashes	Normal	Normal
Sclera and conjunctiva	Normal	Trace injection
Cornea	Normal	Large, curvilinear, vertical laceration extending from 12:00 to 6:30 o'clock through the pupillary axis, nasal iris to wound
Anterior chamber	Normal	Shallow with fluffy white material extending from lens capsule through pupil to the cornea – possible fibrin versus lens material
Iris	Normal	Nasal iris entrapped in corneal wound
Lens	Normal	Difficult view, unable to confidently examine the integrity of the lens
Vitreous	Normal	No view

9.2.5 Dilated Examination

Macula/Nerve OD: Normal
Periphery OD: Normal
Macula/Nerve: OS: No view
Periphery OS: No view

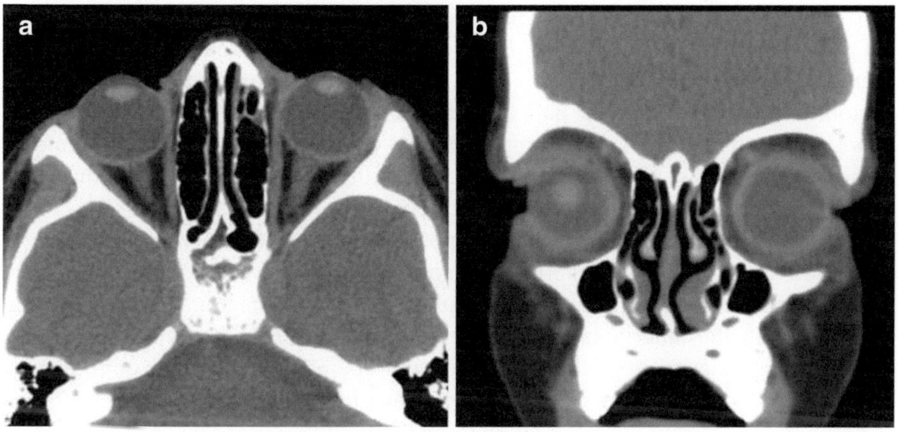

Fig. 9.1 Axial (**a**) and coronal (**b**) computed tomography (CT) images showing a normal globe on the right and a deformed globe on the left with concern for lens violation

9.2.6 Radiographic Imaging

Computed tomogrpahy (CT) of the orbits showed an irregular globe contour suggestive of a lacerated globe of the left eye (Fig. 9.1) without evidence of an intraocular foreign body. The anterior surface of the lens was noted to be mildly distorted raising concern for lens capsule violation and possible traumatic cataract.

9.3 Surgeon's Initial Assessment and Pre-Operative Plan

This case raises four important points beyond repair of a standard Zone I laceration (see Case 1):

1. Extreme caution should always be used when relying on a child's complaints or symptoms as a component of clinical decision making;
2. Pre-operative approach to possible lens involvement;
3. Amblyopia treatment is a key component of the post-operative management of young children; and
4. Timing and strategy of suture removal that requires a return trip to the operating room (discussed in Case 1).

In cases of pediatric eye injury, a clinical exam should be attempted. Many children will allow a thorough examination to be performed, which can inform pre-operative planning. Patients may be relatively asymptomatic on presentation. The absence of symptoms should not lower the suspicion that a patient has an open globe injury. If a clinical exam cannot be achieved to rule out an open globe injury, an examination under sedation or anesthesia is critical (as discussed in Case 1). A CT scan should be done pre-operatively to rule-out an intraocular foreign body if there is concern for an open globe injury and can also give clues to the presence of a globe injury in children or patients that are not cooperate with a pre-operative exam. Moreover, historical elements provided by a child may not be accurate or available. Imaging studies can identify occult injuries or mechanisms of injury that may guide the initial approach in these patients.

Second, this patient had concern for possible lens violation on presentation. A collection of white fluffy material was noted posterior to the corneal laceration, representing exuberant fibrin or lens material. The CT imaging report suggested irregularity to the anterior aspect of the lens and possible lens violation. These findings were discussed with the parents pre-operatively. Surgical consent was obtained for lensectomy if there was clear lens involvement and significant lens material in the anterior chamber noted intraoperatively.

9.4 Surgical Exploration and Repair: Operative Note

Informed consent was obtained, and the operative left eye was verified and marked. A comprehensive examination was initiated under anesthesia. A dilated examination of the right eye was completed and was normal. Examination of the anterior segment of the left eye revealed no new findings beyond what was found during presentation. There was a poor view on dilated funduscopic examination of the left eye due to the corneal laceration and the resulting poor dilation due to the uveal prolapse. The right eyelids were taped closed, and the eye was shielded. The left eye was prepared with Betadine 10% solution in the periocular region and 5% solution in the fornices. A sterile eye drape exposed the left eye, and a Jaffe eyelid speculum was used to provide adequate exposure. The patient was found to have a curvilinear vertical corneal laceration extending from 12:00 to 6:30 o'clock, at least two-thirds of the diameter of the cornea. This laceration tracked through the visual axis. There was no extension past the limbus. There was white material surrounding the inferior area of iris prolapse, and it was unclear if this was fibrin that had accumulated in the anterior chamber or lens material. The view to the lens in this area was compromised by the corneal laceration, corneal edema, and iris. A temporal paracentesis was made directed towards the wound and filtered air was injected to reform the anterior chamber. A cyclodialysis spatula was inserted through this incision, and several gentle sweeps were used to "pull" the iris back into the eye. During these sweeps, it was clear that the iris had adhered to the cornea in the location of the prolpase. The corneal wound was closed with multiple interrupted 10-0 nylon sutures. Filtered air was injected periodically to reform the anterior chamber. The filtered air from the anterior chamber was removed once the entire wound had been closed, and the anterior chamber was filled with balanced salt solution. The suture knots were rotated such that they were buried in the corneal stroma. Fluorescein staining was applied to the wound, and it was confirmed to be free of leaks. Given the poor view of the anterior chamber and lens after repair of the corneal laceration due to corneal edema and given the uncertain lens status, it was decided not to proceed with primary lensectomy.

At the conclusion of surgery, a subconjunctival injection of Cefazolin and Dexamethasone was given inferonasally away from the laceration. Atropine 1% ophthalmic drops were used to retract the iris away from the wound and rotate the lens-iris diaphragm posteriorly to prevent re-prolapse of uveal tissue through the repaired laceration in case it began to leak as the edema cleared. Neomycin sulfatepolymixin b sulfate and dexamethasone ophthalmic ointment was instilled on the eye to help with prevention of infection and to decrease inflammation. The drape was removed, and a sterile eye patch and shield were placed over the left eye.

9.4.1 Surgical Exploration and Repair: Pearls

- Surgical repair of pediatric open globe injuries should start with a careful exam under anesthesia of both eyes as even the best bedside exam is limited. Make sure to look for eyelid lacerations and lacerations with canalicular involvement, as well as injuries of both eyes by completing thorough anterior and posterior segment examinations.
- If lens violation cannot be adequately assessed pre- or intraoperatively, the best course is to leave the lens at the time of initial globe repair. The patient can be followed closely post-operatively as the cornea clears and the view improves, which can also allow for a safer subsequent surgery if a lensectomy is required. One can also look for other signs of lens disruption including increasing inflammation and elevated intraocular pressure post-operatively. Moreover, violated lens capsules that do not self-seal will become evident over 3–7 days after the injury. The gradual hydration of the lens material with aqueous will lead to prolapse of a white, fluffy material into the anterior chamber originating from the lens.
- A lensectomy is best avoided if possible in young children due to concerns of amblyopia and loss of accommodation.

9.4.2 Surgical Video

See Video 9.1 of surgical repair

9.5 Post-Operative Course

The patient was admitted to MEE to complete a 48 hour course of intravenous antibiotics. See Case 1 or Chap. 2 for pediatric antibiotic dosing. On post-operative day one, he had hand motions vision in the left eye. The exam of the lens and posterior pole was still limited due to corneal edema. A B-scan ultrasound showed a normal-appearing, posterior lens capsule, unremarkable vitreous, and attached retina. The patient was discharged home on topical prednisolone acetate 1% 6 times daily, gatifloxacin 0.3% four times daily, and atropine sulfate 1% twice daily all to the left eye. They were also instructed to avoid vigorous activity and to keep a shield over the eye at all times.

The patient followed up with pediatric ophthalmology at 1 week post-operatively, at which time the cornea had significantly cleared. The white material seen at presentation was likely exuberant fibrin as it had resolved with post-operative steroids and time allowing a clear view of the lens. The lens was found to be clear without evidence of any anterior capsule disruption. There was a faint posterior capsule haze centrally representing an early posterior subcapsular cataract, likely due to the decompression of the globe causing transient dysfunction of the lens epithelial cells maintaining the anterior-posterior ionic gradient. A view to the posterior pole showed mild optic disc edema and dilation and tortuosity to the retinal vasculature likely from decompression of the globe while it was open. There were no abnormalities noted of the macula or peripheral retina.

The patient was subsequently followed weekly by a pediatric and cornea specialist closer to his home and was noted to be doing well. He returned to MEE one month after the injury at which time his vision was 20/125 with pinhole improvement to 20/100. At that time, the patient was booked for suture removal in the operating room. (See Case 1 for discussion of suture removal in pediatric patients or uncooperative adults). The patient then underwent corneal suture removal in the operating room. Half of the sutures were removed in an alternating fashion, and the wound was tested and found to be secure and water-tight; so, the remaining sutures were also removed. At the conclusion of suture removal, the wound was again tested with fluorescein application and found to be devoid of leak. The patient then continued to follow with the pediatric and cornea specialist closer to home, so the final trauma clinic evaluation in this case is the day after suture removal and does not include a visual acuity after a trial contact lens or prescription glasses. Outside records show current visual acuity with glasses to be 20/60 in the left eye.

9.6 Final Trauma Evaluation

9.6.1 Final Visual Acuity

OD: 20/20
OS: 20/125 pinhole 20/100

9.6.2 Pupils

OD: Round, no afferent pupillary defect by reverse
OS: Irregular

9.6.3 Slit Lamp Examination

	OD	OS
Lids and lashes	Normal	Normal
Sclera and conjunctiva	Normal	White and quiet
Cornea	Normal	Vertical corneal scar (Fig. 9.2)
Anterior chamber	Normal	Formed, quiet
Iris	Normal	Irregular
Lens	Normal	Faint central posterior capsular haze, clear centrally with intact anterior capsule
Vitreous	Normal	Normal

9.6.4 Dilated Examination

Macula/Nerve OD: Normal
Periphery OD: Normal
Macula/Nerve: OS: Normal
Periphery OS: Normal

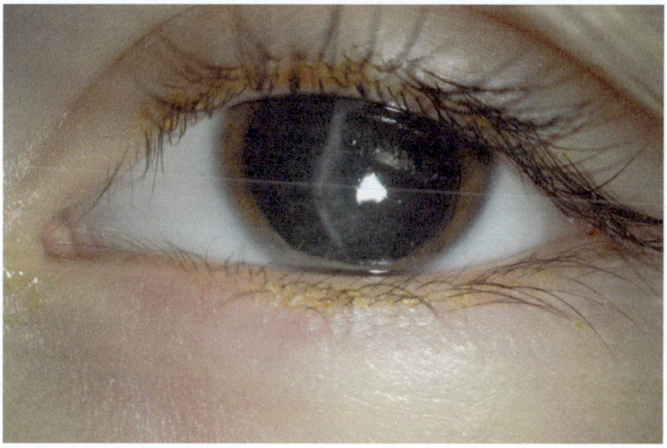

Fig. 9.2 Slit lamp photograph of the left eye showing vertical linear corneal scar after suture removal

9.7 Review and Lessons Learned

This child had a severe ocular injury with light perception vision on presentation. At the time of presentation to the Emergency Department, he was calm and unperturbed by the vision loss or any eye pain.

A clinical examination should always be attempted on presentation. If there is any question about the presence of significant ocular trauma, the child should be taken to the operating room for an exam under anesthesia with possible repair of injuries. When there is concern for possible lens capsule violation pre-operatively, it is important to discuss the possibility of lensectomy as part of the surgical consent. If there is clear lens violation and a clear view after repair of the open globe injury, primary lensectomy may be an option to limit the number of trips to the operating room and exposures to general anesthesia for a child. If the initial assessment of lens damage is questionable, as in this case, where exuberant fibrin may appear like lens material and the lens may actually be intact, it is best to wait on surgical removal and reevaluate the situation when the view has improved.

Especially with children of amblyogenic age, it is best to avoid lensectomy if the lens capsule is not clearly violated. Amblyopia therapy should be started as early as possible post-operatively. Some children can start this therapy at 1 week after surgical repair if they are comfortable and cooperative. This therapy is typically patching of the non-injured or normal eye. If amblyopia is confirmed, the patching therapy should be increased to be therapeutic for amblyopia treatment. Optimizing refractive correction is of paramount importance as well. However, refraction and dispensing of the final prescription is typically left until 2 weeks after suture removal as the refractive error will fluctuate and the time and cost of prescription lenses can be prohibitive in obtaining glasses every few weeks.

When considering initiation of amblyopia therapy, the social situation must be considered. Some families and parents may be able to process the injury, all of the appointments, the eye drops, and the patching. However, some may be overwhelmed with too many tasks; in these cases, initial follow up visits and eye drop compliance are essential and patching should be deferred until a later date. It is important to work with each family individually to make sure the patient is getting the necessary care. Amblyopia can develop within days of vision deprivation depending on the age of the child and his or her own host response to an acute perturbation to visual development. Thus, it is critical for the eye trauma specialist to manage amblyopia or involve pediatric ophthalmology colleagues immediately to obtain the best possible outcome.

As discussed in Case 1, suture removal should be considered starting at around 4 weeks after the initial repair. Sutures will often need to be removed in the operating room under general anesthesia. Ideally, one can remove all the sutures with only one trip to the operating room to limit the child's exposure to anesthesia.

9.8 Key Learning Points

- A patient might have minimal pain or symptoms on presentation and still have an open globe injury. A careful clinical examination in the clinic or operating room is necessary to rule out severe ocular trauma.
- If lens involvement is questionable on initial examination, it is best to defer lens removal until the cornea clears and the view improves. This will allow for a detailed evaluation of the lens to determine if lens removal is required.
- Consider initiating amblyopia management around post-operative week one with patching of the non-injured or normal eye. Correction of induced ametropia with glasses is typically reserved for 2 weeks after suture removal.

Chapter 10
Case 5: Limbus to Limbus Corneal Laceration from Nail Gun Injury

Rohini Rao, John B. Miller, and Seanna Grob

10.1 History of Present Illness

23-year-old-man with history of bipolar disorder and substance abuse presents with concern for open globe of the left eye.

- The patient reports using a nail gun earlier in the day of presentation. The nail gun was spring-loaded and sprung back and hit his left eye. He immediately felt pain and fluid run down his face.
- He was seen at another hospital where a CT scan confirmed an open globe and showed no evidence of an intraocular foreign body.
- On presentation at Massachusetts Eye and Ear (MEE), he reported significant pain and decreased vision in his left eye.

10.2 Initial Trauma Evaluation

10.2.1 Visual Acuity (Without Correction)

OD: 20/20
OS: Hand Motion

R. Rao, M.D. (✉) • S. Grob, M.D., M.A.S.
Department of Ophthalmology, Harvard Medical School, Massachusetts Eye and Ear, Boston, MA, USA
e-mail: rohini_rao@meei.harvard.edu

J. B. Miller, M.D.
Vitreoretinal Surgery, Department of Ophthalmology, Harvard Medical School, Massachusetts Eye and Ear, Boston, MA, USA

S. Grob, C. Kloek (eds.), *Management of Open Globe Injuries*,
https://doi.org/10.1007/978-3-319-72410-2_10

10.2.2 Pupils

OD: Round and reactive
OS: Irregular, minimally reactive, no afferent pupillary defect by reverse

10.2.3 External Examination

Periorbital swelling on the left side.

10.2.4 Slit Lamp Examination

	OD	OS
Lids and lashes	Normal	Normal
Sclera and conjunctiva	Normal	Corneal laceration approaching limbus bilaterally
Cornea	Normal	Limbus to limbus full-thickness laceration
Anterior chamber	Normal	Layered hyphema inferiorly, flat
Iris	Normal	Peaked at 4 o'clock
Lens	Normal	Displaced anteriorly, likely lens capsule violation and traumatic cataract
Vitreous	Normal	Vitreous in anterior chamber

10.2.5 Dilated Examination

Macula/Nerve OD: Normal, cup to disc ratio of 0.4
Periphery OD: Normal
Macula/Nerve: OS: No view
Periphery OS: No view

10.2.6 Radiographic Imaging

Computed tomography (CT) of the orbits showed open globe of the left eye with no evidence of intraocular foreign body.

10.3 Surgeon's Initial Assessment and Pre-Operative Plan

This patient presented with significant pain. He had a history of substance abuse and therefore, may have had a lower pain tolerance. The patient had also been evaluated by multiple physicians at an outside hospital before transfer to MEE. Due to his significant pain and fatigue from visits to multiple hospitals and multiple examinations, it was difficult to complete a thorough pre-operative examination. The majority of adults understand the importance of a complete exam and will do their best to cooperate, but they are often worried about the prospect of losing vision and are exhausted from the hospital experience and multiple examinations. If this overlies a history of psychiatric illness, especially anxiety disorders, it can make a complete pre-operative examination difficult. Similar to pediatric cases, it is ideal if a complete exam is done prior to going to the operating room, however sometimes it is not possible due to patient cooperation, despite a calm and encouraging approach. Although this patient's pre-operative exam was challenging, it was clear that he had a limbus to limbus corneal laceration and likely lens involvement.

The placement and length of corneal sutures is important in repair of corneal lacerations. Tight central corneal sutures can induce central corneal flattening and astigmatism. Astigmatism can be reduced by placing shorter, spaced out, suture passes centrally and then progressively longer passes towards the corneal periphery, which is called the Rowsey-Hays technique (Fig. 10.1) [1, 2]. Longer compressive sutures in the periphery creates flattening in the periphery with compensatory steepening in the center, creating a more spherical cornea. Shorter suture passes centrally can also allow for improved view if retinal surgery is needed subsequently; however, the shorter the

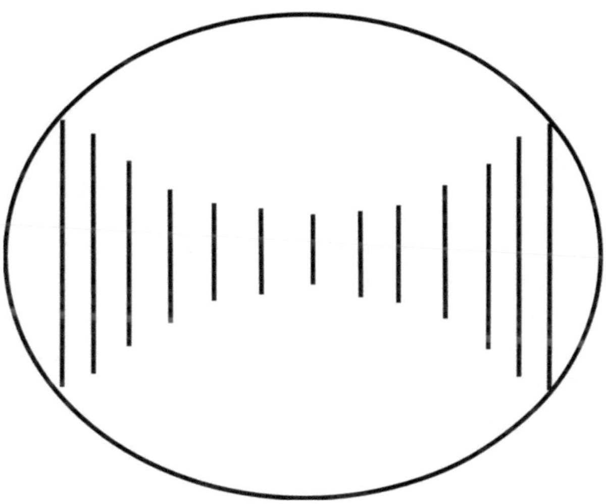

Fig. 10.1 Demonstration of the Rowsey-Hays surgical closure for corneal wound

suture pass, the more difficult it is to rotate the suture and bury the knot at the end of the case. Often astigmatism induced by tight sutures disappears after suture removal, so the primary goal of wound closure is to close the eye.

If corneal tissue is not aligned properly or there is wound override, corneal astigmatism may be permanent. This is important in long and shelved corneal wounds. Aligning the wound can be done by ensuring the limbus is aligned first. Then, you can use the 50/50 rule with corneal suture placement. Place a suture in the center of the wound and keep cutting each part of the wound in half by placing additional sutures until an adequate number of sutures are placed. Wound override can be prevented by ensuring the suture bites are symmetrically placed at the deeper aspect of the wound or cornea (compared to symmetric placement of bites with respect to the surface of the wound) (Chap. 7, Fig. 7.2).

After repairing a long corneal wound similar to this case, it is often necessary to replace sutures. If the usual 3-1-1 knot is tied with the 10-0 nylon suture, then it is important to make sure the eye is at physiologic pressure before tying it down and that it is adjusted to the appropriate tightness. Tying one suture more tightly, may loosen an adjacent suture. After all the sutures are placed, then it will be clear which sutures are too loose or too tight and need to be removed and replaced. In addition, if the suture knots cannot be buried, then they might need to be replaced. As this can be time consuming, it can be useful to use adjustable sutures in these limbus to limbus cases, as discussed in Case 3 (Chap. 8). Then, once all of the sutures are placed, the tightness of each suture can be adjusted before permanently tying each one down. These are often a 1-1-1 knot specifically tied to form a slip knot after the second tie. The 1-1-1 knot at times seems to be less bulky and may rotate more easily as well.

Knot rotation is a very important step at the conclusion of the repair. If knots and suture tails are left exposed, the patient will have foreign body sensation or discomfort. The knots can also be a conduit for mucous collection and potentially a suture abscess or corneal infection.

10.4 Surgical Exploration and Repair: Operative Note

The risks, benefits, and alternatives were discussed with the patient pre-operatively and the patient consented to proceed with exploration and repair of the open globe injury. The patient was brought to the operating room where the anesthesia team proceeded with general anesthesia. A careful time-out was observed and the correct patient and the eye were identified. The left eye was prepped and draped in the usual sterile ophthalmic fashion using a Jaffe speculum to provide adequate exposure. On initial examination, the patient was found to have a limbus to limbus corneal laceration extending from approximately 10 to 4 o'clock with extension past the limbus at both ends approximately 1–2 mm. The anterior chamber was shallow and lens capsule violation was noted. The lens also appeared to be cut in half along a similar course to the corneal laceration. Lens material was in the anterior chamber, especially superiorly. There was vitreous prolapsing from the corneal wound. A Weck-Cel (Beaver-Visitec, Waltham, MA) vitrectomy was completed to clear the vitreous from the wound in order to allow for closure. Two 9-0 nylon sutures were used to align the limbus at either end of the laceration. 10-0 nylon suture was used to place 12 interrupted sutures across the limbus to limbus corneal laceration. A supersharp blade was used to create a paracentesis at 1:30 o'clock and balanced saline solution followed by filtered air was used to form the anterior chamber and move the lens material away from the corneal endothelium. A lensectomy could not be safely performed after complete repair of the corneal laceration since the view to the lens was significantly obscured due to corneal edema and the newly placed sutures and there was known vitreous in the anterior chamber suggesting posterior capsule involvement.

A peritomy was performed temporally. Gentle exploration with blunt dissection was performed with Westcott scissors. No further scleral extension of the wound was identified other than the 1–2 mm that was noted initially. The conjunctiva was closed with an 8-0 Vicryl suture in an interrupted fashion. A subconjunctival steroid and antibiotic injection was performed nasally and inferiorly away from the laceration. The speculum was removed. The patient's drape was removed under the microscope. Atropine and neomycin sulfate polymixin b sulfate and dexamethasone ophthalmic ointment were placed in the eye. A sterile eye patch and shield were placed. The patient tolerated the procedure well without any complications.

10.4.1 Surgical Exploration and Repair: Pearls

- A Weck-cel vitrectomy can be helpful to clear vitreous from corneal wound before beginning wound closure.
- Make sure to align the limbus and the corneal wound to prevent unwanted corneal astigmatism.
- Keep dividing the wound in half with suture placement to allow for even placement of sutures and good alignment of the wound.
- Consider the Rowsey-Hays technique when closing limbus to limbus corneal lacerations.
- Resist removal of the lens if the view is significantly compromised after corneal repair. The situation can be more clearly assessed after corneal edema improves and then the decision can be made whether to remove the lens with an anterior approach or to refer to a retina specialist.

10.5 Post-Operative Course

The patient was admitted to MEE to complete a 48 hour course of intravenous antibiotics. On post-operatively day 1, his vision was slightly improved to counting fingers vision in the left eye with a Seidel negative corneal wound (Fig. 10.2a).

B-scan ultrasound was obtained that revealed mild vitreous debris with an attached retina, but with an irregular posterior lens capsule, suggesting posterior lens capsule violation. He was discharged home on the usual regimen of eye drops.

He followed up with the retina service 1 week later where his vision remained counting fingers at 1 foot with an IOP of 15 mmHg. Exam at that time more clearly revealed a traumatic cataract with the lens practically cut into two halves and no clear view posteriorly (Fig. 10.2b). He subsequently underwent a pars plana vitrectomy and lensectomy 2 weeks after initial open globe repair. Intraoperatively a nasal choroidal rupture was identified.

By two months after this lensectomy and vitrectomy, his vision improved to 20/60 pinhole 20/40 with a + 10 diopter lens (Fig. 10.3). At this point, suture removal was initiated. Five sutures within the limbus to limbus laceration repair were removed initially. One month later, the final nine sutures were removed without complication, leaving a central corneal scar (Fig. 10.4). The patient followed up

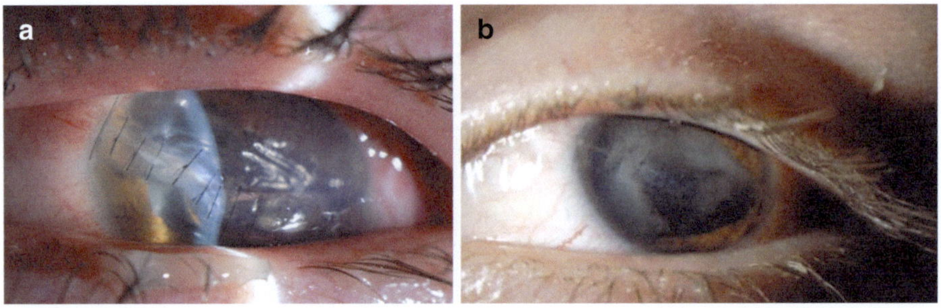

Fig. 10.2 Clinical image of the patient. (**a**) 1 day after open globe repair showing multiple vertical nylon corneal sutures across the limbus to limbus laceration with a swollen cornea and poor view into the anterior chamber. (**b**) 1 week after open globe repair showing improved cornea edema and a lens that has been cut almost in half from the nail gun and a traumatic cataract

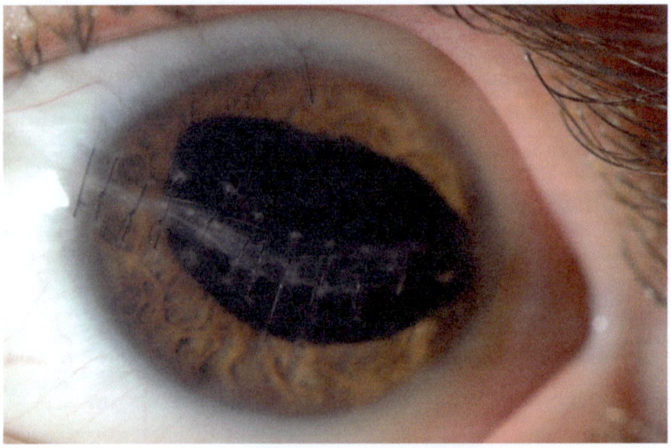

Fig. 10.3 Clinical image of the patient 2 months after initial open globe repair and 6 weeks after vitrectomy showing intact corneal sutures, irregular pupil with some iris tissue loss and aphakia

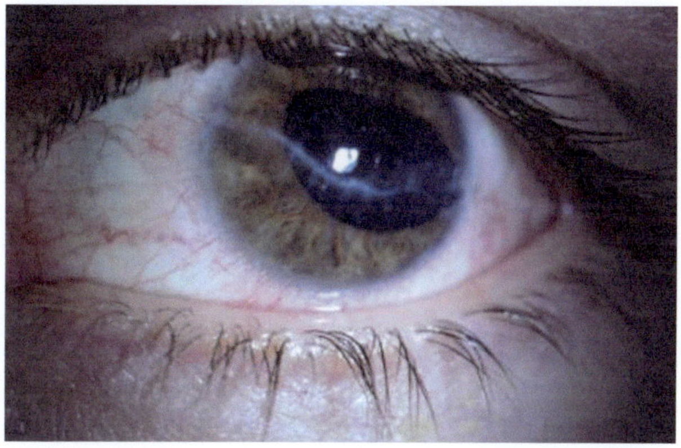

Fig. 10.4 Clinical image of the patient 6 months after initial open globe repair showing central curvilinear corneal scar and associated faint suture scars after all sutures had been removed

with the contact lens service approximately six weeks after final suture removal and was able to achieve 20/25 vision with a rigid contact lens.

10.6 Final Trauma Evaluation

10.6.1 Final Visual Acuity

OD: 20/25
OS: 20/25 with contact lens

10.6.2 Pupils

OD: Round, no afferent pupillary defect by reverse
OS: Irregular, with loss of iris tissue superotemporally

10.6.3 Slit Lamp Examination

	OD	OS
Lids and lashes	Normal	Normal
Sclera and conjunctiva	Normal	Normal
Cornea	Normal	Healing limbus-limbus laceration
Anterior chamber	Normal	Normal
Iris	Normal	Atrophy and tissue loss superotemporally
Lens	Normal	Aphakic
Vitreous	Normal	Status post pars plana vitrectomy

10.6.4 Dilated Examination

Macula/Nerve OD: flat, cup to disc ratio 0.4
Periphery OD: Normal
Macula/Nerve: OS: Flat and attached, cup to disc ratio 0.4
Periphery OS: Attached retina, nasal choroidal rupture, poor peripheral view

10.7 Review and Lessons Learned

Nail gun injuries can result in devastating ocular injury and visual compromise (see Case 34 (Chap. 39) as well) [3, 4]. Often, these types of injuries occur in patients who use nail guns at work [4–6]. A discussion about the use of protective eye wear at work is an important part of the care for any patient who works as an electrician, carpenter, constructor, plumber, or in any capacity where there is potential for eye injury at work. It is important to encourage them to use the same eye protection at home as they do at work when using these tools. Nail gun injuries can also be associated with intraocular, intraorbital or facial, or intracranial foreign bodies, so it is crucial to rule out foreign bodies with CT imaging pre-operatively [6].

Lens capsule violation with traumatic cataract is a frequent finding in nail-gun related penetrating injuries [5, 6]. Sometimes, lens material can clearly be seen in the anterior chamber on pre-operative or intraoperative examination. However, subtle areas of lens capsule violation can be obscured by an injured, swollen cornea. It is also difficult to confidently assess the integrity of the posterior lens capsule in such situations. The view into the eye worsens after repair of the corneal laceration due to corneal edema as well. If there is concern for posterior capsule violation, it is important to refer to a retina specialist for a more detailed posterior segment examination and possible lensectomy and vitrectomy. Primary lensectomy at time of globe repair or shortly thereafter with a swollen cornea can lead to incomplete lens removal while also exposing the patient to unnecessary risk due to poor visualization. It is often most prudent to wait several days after the initial repair for the cornea to deturgesce. By allowing time for the corneal edema to improve, cataract removal with or without pars plana surgical techniques can be more safely completed. (See Cases 17–20 (Chaps. 22–25) for other examples of lens involvement.)

Slow suture removal is important in the limbus to limbus corneal lacerations. Removing too many sutures too quickly can lead to wound destabilization and wound dehiscence, as can happen after other types of corneal surgery [7]. We recommend removing the corneal sutures in a staged fashion, similar to that discussed in Case 3 (Chap. 8) with stellate corneal wounds. Remove a portion of the sutures and have the patient return 2–3 weeks later (or longer) for additional suture removal. Often, we recommend waiting longer than the usual 6 weeks to even initiate suture removal in these patients. For this patient, we started suture removal around 10 weeks. He had issues with attending his follow up visits which accounts for the 4 week follow up in between suture removal dates. Since this is a significant amount of time, patients often have to be encouraged and counseled through this time period before they can get fitted for a contact lens.

10.8 Key Learning Points

- In limbus to limbus lacerations, make sure to align the limbus and the corneal wound to prevent unwanted post-operative corneal astigmatism.
- Keep dividing the wound in half with suture placement to allow for even placement of sutures and good alignment of the wound.
- Consider the Rowsey-Hays technique when closing limbus to limbus corneal lacerations—shorter suture lengths centrally with progressively longer sutures peripherally—to prevent central corneal flattening and astigmatism.
- Delay removal of the lens if the view is significantly compromised after corneal repair.
- Slow and staged suture removal is key in preventing wound dehiscence in limbus to limbus corneal lacerations. Go slow and prevent a headache of a situation later!

References

1. Hamill MB. Corneal and scleral trauma. Ophthalmol Clin N Am. 2002;15:185–94.
2. John B, Raghavan C. Open globe injuries-primary repair of corneoscleral injuries. Kerala J Ophthalmol. 2010;22:225–34.
3. Lee BL, Sternberg PJ. Ocular nail gun injuries. Ophthalmology. 1996;103:1453–7.
4. Burger BM, Kelty PJ, Bowie EM. Ocular nail gun injuries: epidemiology and visual outcomes. J Trauma. 2009;67:1320–2.
5. Kolomeyer AM, et al. Nail gun-induced open-globe injuries: a 10-year retrospective review. Retina. 2014;34:254–61.
6. Bauza AM, et al. Work-related open-globe injuries: demographics and clinical characteristics. Eur J Ophthalmol. 2013;23:242–8.
7. Mannan R, Jhanji V, Sharma N, Pruthi A, Vajpayee RB. Spontaneous wound dehiscence after early suture removal after deep anterior lamellar keratoplasty. Eye Contact Lens. 2011;37:109–11.

Chapter 11
Case 6: Dehiscence of Penetrating Keratoplasty from Blunt Trauma

Emma Davies and Yoshihiro Yonekawa

11.1 History of Present Illness

A 43-year-old woman with past ocular history of keratoconus in both eyes with previous penetrating keratoplasty 20 years ago in the right eye presents with pain and vision loss after blunt trauma to the right eye.

- She reports that she was opening a closet door when something fell and hit her right eye.
- She noticed immediate decrease in vision and flashes of light in the right eye.
- She denies any other trauma or loss of consciousness.
- She presents immediately to emergency room for an evaluation.

11.2 Initial Trauma Evaluation

11.2.1 Visual Acuity (Without Correction)

OD: Light perception
OS: 20/125-1

E. Davies, M.D. (✉)
Department of Ophthalmology, Harvard Medical School, Massachusetts Eye and Ear, Boston, MA, USA
e-mail: Emma_Davies@meei.harvard.edu

Y. Yonekawa, M.D.
Vitreoretinal Surgery, Harvard Medical School, Massachusetts Eye and Ear and Boston Children's Hospital, Boston, MA, USA

S. Grob, C. Kloek (eds.), *Management of Open Globe Injuries*,
https://doi.org/10.1007/978-3-319-72410-2_11

11.2.2 Pupils

OD: Distorted, no relative afferent pupillary defect by reverse
OS: Round and reactive

11.2.3 External Examination

No significant facial ecchymoses or lacerations noted on examination.

11.2.4 Slit Lamp Examination

	OD	OS
Lids and lashes	Normal	Normal
Sclera and Conjunctiva	Subconjunctival hemorrhage inferiorly, trace diffuse injection	Normal
Cornea	Status-post penetrating keratoplasty, no sutures remaining, dehisced wound from 1 o'clock to 8 o'clock with prolapsed vitreous and uvea (Fig. 11.1a, b)	Apical cone with Vogt's striae but no scarring, Fleischer ring
Anterior chamber	Flat	Formed
Iris	Distorted contour with iris prolapse through the wound inferiorly	Normal
Lens	Aphakia	1+ Nuclear sclerosis
Vitreous	Vitreous prolapse through the wound inferiorly	Clear

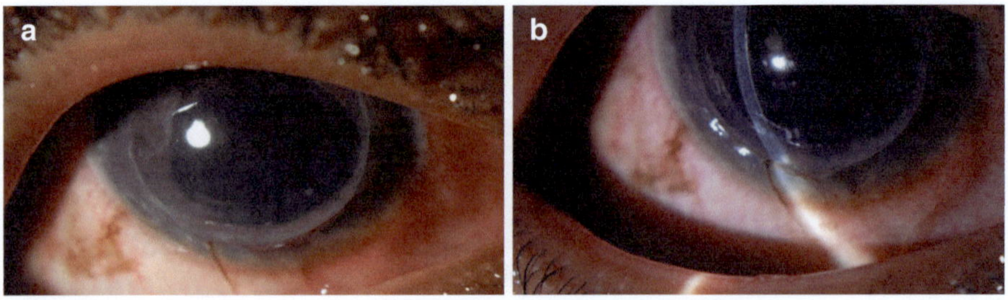

Fig. 11.1 Pre-operative slit lamp photograph of the right eye demonstrating dehiscence of the previous penetrating keratoplasty wound inferiorly with extrusion of uveal tissue and vitreous (**a**). Corneal graft tissue over-riding the host corneal tissue is demonstrated by the slit beam step-off inferiorly (**b**)

11.2.5 Dilated Examination

Macula/Nerve OD: Multiple lobules of posterior choroidal detachment
Periphery OD: Retina attached, no breaks appreciated
Macula/Nerve: OS: Macula flat, disc sharp
Periphery OS: Normal, no retinal hole, tear, or detachment

11.2.6 Radiographic Imaging

CT of the orbits shows loss of the globe contour consistent with a ruptured globe of the right eye without evidence of intraocular foreign bodies and intact globe contour of the left eye. There are no orbital fractures or intracranial injuries.

11.3 Surgeon's Initial Assessment and Pre-Operative Plan

The patient presented with inferior traumatic wound dehiscence 20 years after her prior penetrating keratoplasty for keratoconus. She had traumatic extrusion of her crystalline lens, some uveal tissue, and vitreous through the wound. This case highlights several important features of open globe injury in the setting of penetrating keratoplasty.

Open globe injury occurs in 1–5.8% of patients with a previous penetrating keratoplasty [1]. The site of rupture after blunt trauma in these cases typically occurs at the graft-host junction, indicating weakness at the incision despite wound healing. This wound dehiscence occurs most commonly in the inferonasal quadrant in keratoconus patients but otherwise most commonly in the superonasal quadrant [1, 2]. Nasal dehiscence is likely related to distribution of force from a common temporal site of impact, given less protection from orbital bones temporally, and inferior dehiscence in keratoconus is likely related to the thinner stroma in the inferior cornea in this entity. The wound dehiscence in cases with sutures still in place in the graft are significantly smaller, indicating that limiting wound gape is an important factor in preventing large dehiscences as in this current case [2].

The associated anterior segment injuries with dehisced penetrating keratoplasty wounds include iris prolapse (85% of cases), hyphema (60% of cases), and lens extrusion (60% of cases) while the posterior segment injuries include vitreous prolapse (60% of cases), vitreous hemorrhage (55% of cases), and retinal detachment within the first 6 months after trauma (20% of cases) [2]. The most predictive pre-operative factors for worse final visual outcome are lens extrusion and vitreous prolapse [3]. The worse outcome in these settings is likely related to larger size of wound dehiscence and damage to posterior structures. Retinal detachment and choroidal hemorrhage at the time of presentation obviously portend an even worse prognosis.

Further surgical intervention after initial wound repair is needed in approximately 50% of dehisced penetrating keratoplasty cases. The subsequent surgeries are typically replacement of the corneal transplant due to graft failure from endothelial cell loss and vitreoretinal intervention for retinal detachment or non-resolving vitreous hemorrhage [1].

In the current case, immediate repair of the wound dehiscence with reposition of the extruded uveal tissue was performed. The patient was counseled regarding the guarded visual outcome given the extrusion of her crystalline lens and vitreous to the wound. She was aware of the risk for possibly needing a second eye procedure to treat any posterior segment pathology. She understood that the goal of the initial repair was to reapproximate the wound and close the eye to minimize the risk of infection and inflammation.

Since globe irregularity, corneal transplant over-ride, and extensive corneal edema is common in the setting of transplant dehiscence, these types of wounds are often best repaired by continually placing sutures half-way along the opening to gain adequate closure (Fig. 11.2). Appropriate length of sutures should be ensured by keeping the distance from the graft-host junction to the entrance point in the transplant tissue equal to the distance from the graft-host junction to the exit point in the host tissue. The adjustment of suture tightness may be difficult in trauma cases but sutures that are slightly tight are more optimal than loose sutures given that corneal edema at the time of repair will likely detergence over time and correspondingly loosen sutures. It is recommended that sutures be placed for closure of the wound and then replaced as needed to ensure appropriate tightness.

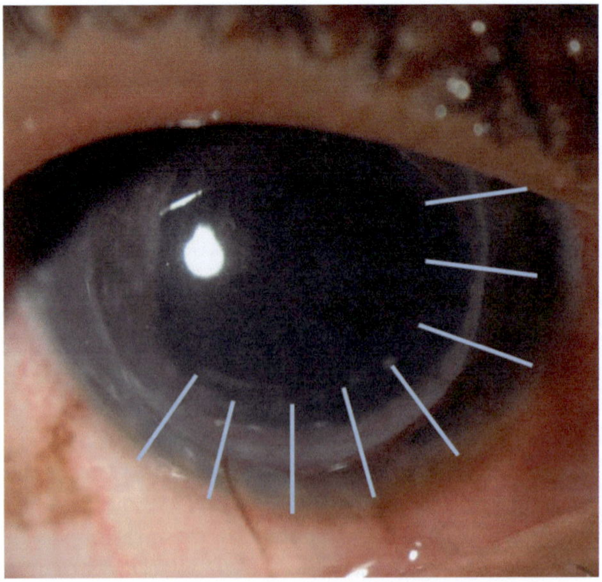

Fig. 11.2 Image demonstrating appropriate location for sutures (marked with lines) in closure of dehisced corneal transplantation wound

11.4 Surgical Exploration and Repair: Operative Note

Informed consent was obtained for repair of the traumatic wound dehiscence in the right eye. The operative eye was verified and marked. The uninjured left eye was taped and shielded for protection. The right eye was then prepped and draped in the usual sterile ophthalmic fashion. A Jaffe lid speculum was placed to gain adequate exposure with minimal pressure on the globe. Eight interrupted 10-0 nylon sutures were placed, each bisecting the region of wound dehiscence radial to the wound, until the wound was completely closed. A cyclodialysis spatula was used throughout the closure of the wound to ensure complete repositioning of the uveal tissue and vitreous inside the eye. An anterior vitrectomy was deemed unnecessary at the time of closure as all vitreous was able to be swept into the eye with uveal tissue. All sutures were tied and the knots buried at the side of host corneal tissue. The wound was ensured to be watertight with a fluorescein strip. A subconjunctival injection of cefazolin and dexamethasone was placed superotemporally away from the site of previous dehiscence. The Jaffe lid speculum and sterile drape were carefully removed. Several drops of gatifloxacin and an application of maxitrol ointment were placed in the right eye. The eyelids were closed and an eye patch and eye shield were placed over the eye for protection.

11.4.1 Surgical Exploration and Repair: Pearls

- Close the corneal wound by continuing to bisect the region of wound gape with interrupted sutures radial to the wound
- Slightly longer suture passes and tighter sutures are preferred when closing traumatic wound dehiscence to ensure adequate wound closure in the setting of possible tissue maceration.
- Perform anterior vitrectomy and reposition of uveal tissue as needed at the time of initial repair, but delay any necessary iris repair, secondary intraocular lens placement, and retinal detachment repair.

11.5 Post-Operative Course

On post-operative day 1, the patient had visual acuity of count fingers at one foot in the right eye. The wound dehiscence was completely closed with interrupted 10-0 nylon sutures with no uveal tissue or vitreous to the wound. Dilated eye examination continued to show a choroidal detachment in the right eye. The patient was evaluated by the retina service one week after the repair and found to have resolution of the choroidal detachment and no retinal detachment. Given the expulsion of vitreous at the time of the initial injury, she was informed of the risks for delayed retinal detachment and possible need for vitrectomy in the future. Follow-up retina examinations showed no evidence of retinal tear or detachment, and so no further vitreoretinal intervention was required.

Two months after wound repair, she was noted to have all sutures intact at the graft-host junction, but evidence of early graft rejection that was treated with increased topical steroid eye drops. Starting at the post-operative 6-month visit, the majority of the interrupted sutures were removed using topography and the manifest refraction as a guide to reduce astigmatism. One year after her traumatic wound dehiscence, she was noted to have development of microcystic edema in the inferonasal periphery of the transplant, believed to be related to vitreous touch at this site. Given overall stability of the graft, however, repeat transplantation procedure was deferred.

The patient was initially fitted for a hybrid contact lens for treatment of her aphakia, as she had a prior history of rigid gas permeable contact lens intolerance used to treat keratoconus. She had problems removing the hybrid lens from her eye and several episodes of corneal abrasions related to lens wear. She was thus fit with a scleral lens and subsequently a BostonSight® PROSE device. She found maintenance of these lenses difficult and reported still being able to notice anisometropia despite lens usage (given the necessary high plus power needed for treatment of the aphakia in the right eye and the high negative power needed for treatment of the keratoconus in the left eye). Given her problems with a variety of lenses, surgical treatment for her aphakia was discussed as secondary intraocular lens placement (likely intrascleral fixation of an intraocular lens) in the right eye. The patient is currently considering this surgical option for management of her aphakia.

11.6 Final Trauma Evaluation

11.6.1 Final Visual Acuity

OD: 20/70 with scleral lens in place
OS: 20/40+2 with scleral lens in place

11.6.2 Pupils

OD: 6 mm, surgical pupil, no afferent pupillary defect by reverse
OS: 4 mm

11.6.3 Slit Lamp Examination

	OD	OS
Lids and lashes	Normal	Normal
Sclera and Conjunctiva	Normal	Normal
Cornea	Status post keratoplasty, graft clear centrally but with thickening and microcystic edema inferonasal periphery, two interrupted sutures intact, peripheral anterior synechiae from 1 to 7:30 o'clock, vitreous to graft-host margin inferiorly	Apical cone with Vogt's striae but no scarring, Fleischer ring
Anterior chamber	Vitreous in the anterior chamber	Normal
Iris	Surgical pupil	Normal
Lens	Aphakia	Normal
Vitreous	Pigment in the anterior vitreous face	Normal

11.6.4 Dilated Examination

Macula/Nerve OD: Epiretinal membrane
Periphery OD: Normal, no retinal hole, tear, or detachment
Macula/Nerve: OS: Macula flat, disc sharp
Periphery OS: Normal, no retinal hole, tear, or detachment

11.7 Review and Lessons Learned

This case demonstrates how blunt trauma after penetrating keratoplasty commonly results in wound dehiscence along the graft-host junction often associated with hyphema, iris prolapse, vitreous prolapse, and even lens extrusion. The wound should be closed with interrupted sutures and all clean uveal tissue repositioned inside the eye as soon as possible. Despite pre-operative appearance of the globe, adequate closure of a dehisced penetrating keratoplasty is possible as rupture occurs at the graft-host junction without loss of tissue (Fig. 11.3a, b). Other surgical procedures, such vitreoretinal procedures and secondary intraocular lens placement should be delayed until after primary closure. The risk for corneal transplantation rejection and failure after trauma are high and the patient should be educated about warning signs for each, including eye pain, photosensitivity, decreased vision, and

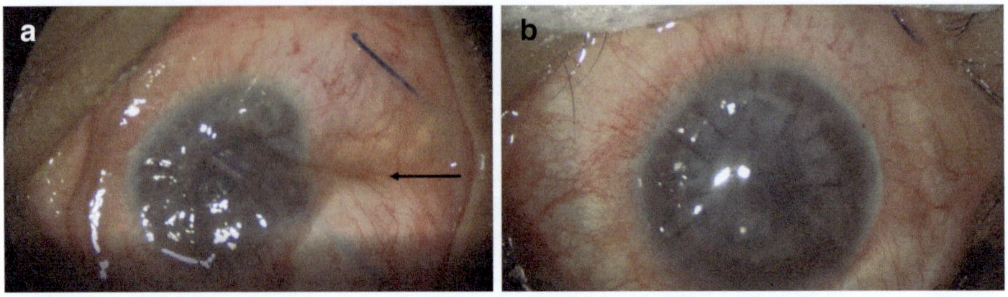

Fig. 11.3 Intra-operative photographs from a different case of dehisced penetrating keratoplasty. Note the severely deflated globe with indentation of the sclera (black arrow) and corneal edema of the penetrating keratoplasty margins (**a**). At the end of the repair surgery, note the return of the globe contour and appropriate closure of the wound with ten interrupted sutures (**b**)

cloudy vision. Treatment for graft rejection includes topical and potentially systemic steroids and ultimately may require repeat corneal transplantation surgery for definitive treatment.

Given that an open globe injury may occur with even mild blunt trauma at any time after penetrating keratoplasty, it is important to educate patients that wound dehiscence is a life-long risk after this surgery [4]. During the consent process for a full-thickness corneal transplantation, patients should be counseled regarding the need to wear daily protective eyewear after penetrating keratoplasty.

Treatment for aphakia can be difficult, particularly in patients with contact lens intolerance or persistent anisometropia symptoms but should include a discussion regarding secondary intraocular lens placement. In the current patient, the secondary intraocular lens placement surgery would be challenging due to the vitreous in the anterior chamber and peripheral anterior synechiae and thus should be combined with an anterior vitrectomy and iris synechiolysis.

11.7.1 Key Learning Points

- Blunt trauma in an eye with previous penetrating keratoplasty often results in wound dehiscence along the graft-host junction.
- Associated anterior segment complications include hyphema, iris prolapse, and lens extrusion, while associated posterior segment complications include vitreous prolapse, vitreous hemorrhage, and retinal detachment.
- Immediate repair of wound dehiscence should be performed; however, any necessary vitreoretinal procedures or secondary intraocular lens procedures should usually be delayed with timing of reoperation depending on the pathology.
- The risk of transplant rejection and transplant failure after blunt trauma should be discussed with the patient.

References

1. Goweida M, Helaly H, Ghaith A. Traumatic wound dehiscence after keratoplasty: characteristics, risk factors, and visual outcome. J Ophthalmol. 2015;2015:1–5.
2. Steinberg J, Eddy MT, Katz T, Fricke O, Richard G, Linke S. Eur J Ophthalmol. 2012;22(3):335–41.
3. Lam F, Rahman M, Ramaesh K. Traumatic wound dehiscence after penetrating keratoplasty-a cause for concern. Eye. 2007;21:1146–50.
4. Ma J, Rapuano C, Hammersmith K, Nagra P, Dai Y, Azari A. Outcomes of wound dehiscence post penetrating keratoplasty. Cornea. 2016;35(6):778–83.

Chapter 12
Case 7: Zone II Open Globe Injury from Cell Phone

K. Matthew McKay, Eric D. Gaier, Seanna Grob, and John B. Miller

12.1 History of Present Illness

A 72-year-old man with history of chronic contact lens use and overwear presents with concern for open globe of the right eye.

- The patient reports accidental blunt trauma from the corner of a cell phone with subsequent vision loss.
- He was standing next to someone holding a cellphone and turned suddenly, hitting his right eye on the corner of the cell phone.
- Computed tomography (CT) imaging was performed at the referring facility where a tetanus vaccine was administered and intravenous antibiotics were started.

12.2 Initial Trauma Evaluation

12.2.1 Visual Acuity (with Correction, Contact Lenses)

OD: Hand motion
OS: 20/20-1

K. Matthew McKay, M.D. (✉) • E. D. Gaier, M.D., Ph.D. • S. Grob, M.D., M.A.S.
Department of Ophthalmology, Harvard Medical School, Massachusetts Eye and Ear, Boston, MA, USA
e-mail: matthew_mckay@meei.harvard.edu

J. B. Miller, M.D.
Vitreoretinal Surgery, Department of Ophthalmology, Harvard Medical School, Massachusetts Eye and Ear, Boston, MA, USA

S. Grob, C. Kloek (eds.), *Management of Open Globe Injuries*,
https://doi.org/10.1007/978-3-319-72410-2_12

12.2.2 *Pupils*

OD: Poor view due to hyphema, no relative afferent pupillary defect by reverse
OS: 3 to 2 mm, no relative afferent pupillary defect

12.2.3 *External Examination*

Normal

12.2.4 *Slit Lamp Examination*

	OD	OS
Lids and lashes	Normal	Normal
Sclera and conjunctiva	Nasal, inferior, and superior bullous subconjunctival hemorrhage with nasal area of subconjunctival pigment concerning for uveal prolapse	Normal
Cornea	Significant peripheral neovascularization	Significant peripheral neovascularization
Anterior chamber	4+ red blood cells with a 2.5 mm layered hyphema	Normal
Iris	Limited view	Normal
Lens	No view	Normal
Vitreous	No view	Normal

12.2.5 *Dilated Examination*

Macula/Nerve OD: No view
Periphery OD: No view
Macula/Nerve: OS: Normal
Periphery OS: Normal

12.2.6 *Radiographic Imaging*

CT imaging showed no evidence of an intraocular foreign body and preserved globe contour bilaterally (Fig. 12.1).

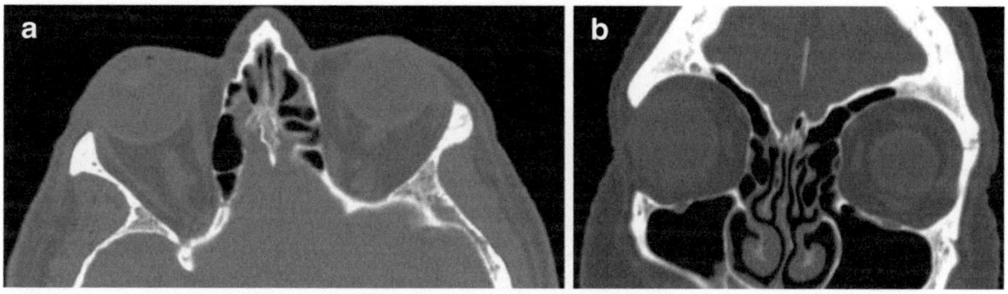

Fig. 12.1 CT imaging. (**a**) Axial and (**b**) coronal sections of the orbits showing no evidence of an intraocular foreign body and preserved globe contour of both eyes

12.3 Surgeon's Initial Assessment and Pre-Operative Plan

This patient had a Zone II open globe injury of the right eye due to blunt trauma.

This case serves to illustrate the basics of Zone II injury evaluation and repair, focusing on two important clinical points: (1) The signs that should raise suspicion for an open globe injury in ambiguous cases. (2) A technique for avoiding uveal incarceration during repair. We also discuss the mechanism of injury specific to this patient's case.

Due to the blunt nature of this injury, the conjunctiva was intact on presentation. It can be difficult to definitively diagnose an open globe injury under these circumstances, especially when CT imaging shows a normal globe contour (Fig. 12.1). Any case of blunt globe trauma resulting in a region of bullous subconjunctiva on the external globe and impaired review to the retina underlying that region of subconjunctival hemorrhage should undergo globe exploration. If there is an area for which there is high suspicion, a very careful clinical examination at the slit lamp is a reasonable first step. Sometimes conjunctiva can be gently moved to explore an area of concern, but we do not recommend putting any pressure on the globe that could worsen uveal prolapse. This patient had an area nasally with some pigmented tissue beneath the intact conjunctiva that was concerning for an area of scleral rupture. In these cases, we advise a low threshold for taking patients to the operating room.

The mechanism of injury is also an important factor in judging the likelihood of an open globe injury, and therefore, in determining the necessity of exploration in the operating room. The low velocity and blunt nature of our patient's injury did not suggest a high likelihood of open globe injury, but the presence of extensive subconjunctival hemorrhage, subconjunctival pigment and limited view to the posterior pole drove our decision to proceed to the operating room (Fig. 12.2). Blunt trauma generally causes open globe injuries by the deformation of the wall of the globe. Anterior-posterior compression and distension at the equator splits the globe, usually circumferentially either at or close to the limbus or behind the muscle insertions. Our patient's past ocular history is remarkable for chronic contact lens

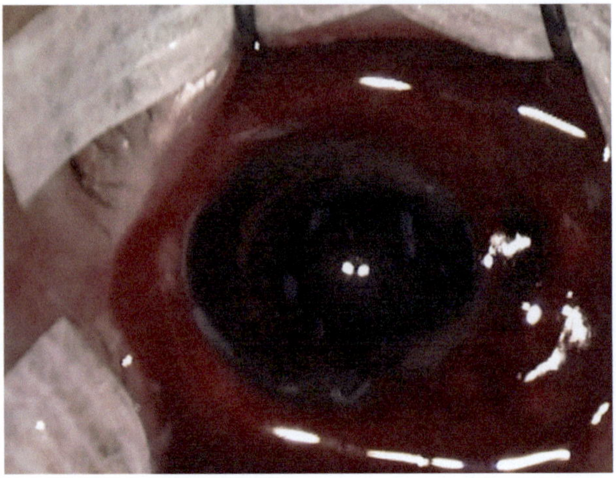

Fig. 12.2 Pre-operative photograph prior to initiation of repair showing dense, bullous, subconjunctival hemorrhage and layering hyphema

use and significant overwear and the corneal examination was notable for significant peripheral neovascularization in both eyes and thinned scleral tissue. Chronic inflammation related to contact lens abuse may have led to scleral thinning and a susceptibility to globe rupture in this case. We found no previous reports of open globe injuries related to chronic contact lens use in the literature.

At the age of 72, our patient is significantly older than the average patient to present with an open globe injury (41.5 years) based on a review of 848 open globe injuries. However, globe rupture is the most common mechanism of open globe injury in the geriatric population (88% versus only 29% of younger patients). Older patients were also significantly more likely to present with Zone II and Zone III injuries ($P < 0.0001$) and to have undergone previous intraocular surgery ($P < 0.0001$) [1].

The initial step to exploration of suspected open globe injuries is a conjunctival peritomy. Special attention should be paid to the quadrant(s) in question, but it is important to initiate the peritomy in the 180° meridian tangential to, and never directly over that area. The peritomy is typically limbal-based with small radial incisions extending posteriorly either at 3 and 9 o'clock or 6 and 12 o'clock depending on the location of the injury. Blunt Wescott scissors or curved Stevens scissors can be used for blunt dissection. Usually we start with blunt Wescotts and then proceed to using curved Stevens to achieve a more posterior view of the globe when searching for a more posterior rupture site. Curving the Steven's scissors along the globe in the 4 oblique meridians allows for efficient exploration while avoiding the extraocular muscle insertions. It is important to dissect down to bare sclera and expose the scleral edges of the wound. It can be easy to dissect between Tenon's and conjunctiva, but this may lead to difficulty finding more posterior wounds. At the site of suspected rupture, it is important to dissect gently so as not to worsen uveal prolapse. The scleral wound should be cleaned so the wound edges can be clearly seen for suturing.

In our patient's case, a vertical, full-thickness, perilimbal scleral defect was noted. We recommend interrupted 8-0 nylon sutures on a spatulated needle to repair

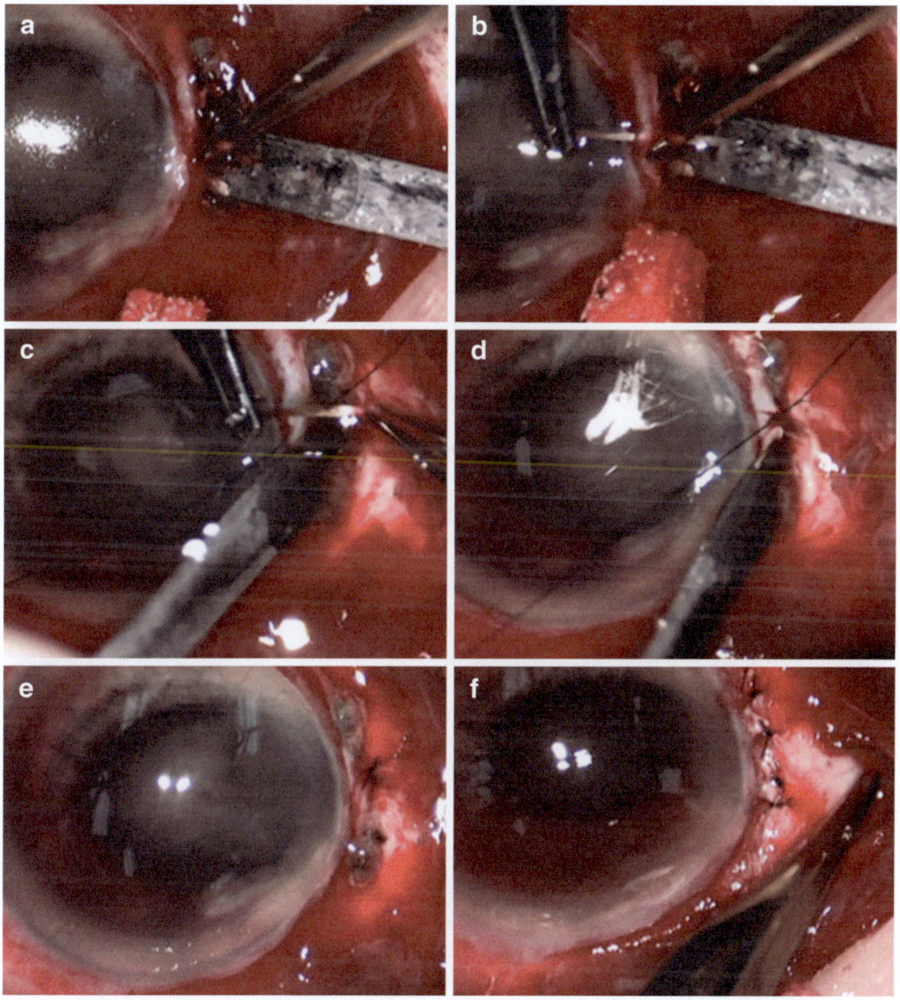

Fig. 12.3 Intraoperative photographs for scleral laceration repair. (A-D) The iris spatula technique. (**a**) The iris spatula is used to depress/reinsert the iris to expose the margin of the scleral laceration in which the first suture pass will enter and exit. (**b**) Using toothed forceps, to control the scleral margin, the suture is passed partial thickness to exit over the iris spatula and pulled through. (**c**) The needle is then re-loaded and the iris spatula is placed to expose the opposing margin of the scleral laceration. Again, the needle is passed partial thickness through the scleral margin and pulled through (**d**). The iris spatula can assist to ensure complete deposition of uveal tissue as the sclera is closed. (**e**) The laceration after the first scleral suture has been tied. (**f**) The laceration after all sutures have been tied

scleral ruptures or lacerations. The prolapsed uveal tissue can be carefully reposited into the globe or held out of the way of the suture passes with an iris spatula. Sometimes it is necessary to hold the uveal tissue out of the wound with the iris spatula and sew over the uveal tissue. Once enough sutures have been placed, uveal tissue will no longer prolapse from the eye. This is a very important step to prevent uveal or retinal incarceration in the wound (Fig. 12.3).

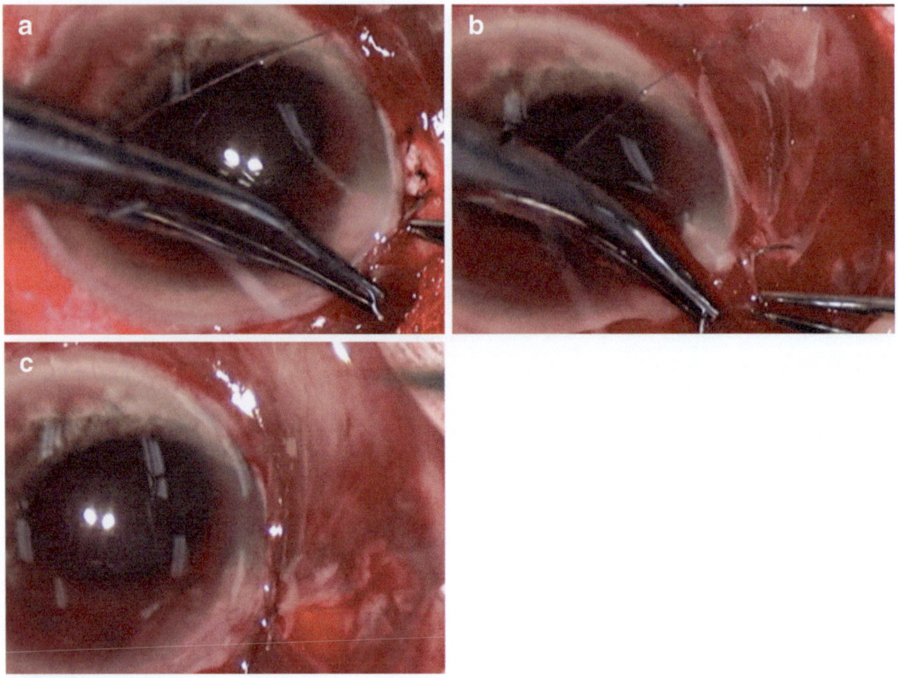

Fig. 12.4 Intraoperative photographs for conjunctival peritomy closure. (**a**) 8-0 Vicryl suture needle passing through the inferior conjunctival peritomy border and inferonasal episclera. Countertraction is applied with smooth-tip forceps to facilitate exit of the needle tip. (**b**) The other edge of the conjunctival peritomy is placed over the needle tip to completely cover the sclera. (**c**) The suture is tied

After the sclera is fully repaired and the globe is water-tight, the conjunctival peritomy can be closed. We use 8-0 Vicryl suture with anchoring to the perilimbal episclera using superficial partial thickness episcleral bites at the locations of the radial incisions and sometimes at 12 o'clock to prevent conjunctival override onto the superior cornea (Fig. 12.4).

12.4 Surgical Exploration and Repair: Operative Note

Informed consent was obtained and the operative eye was verified and marked. The right eye was prepped and draped in the usual sterile ophthalmic fashion using a Jaffe speculum to provide adequate exposure.

A 180° nasal peritomy was initiated from 12 to 6 o'clock in the location of concern for globe rupture. Gentle exploration with blunt dissection was performed with Westcott scissors to expose the rupture site.

The patient was found to have a 7 mm perilimbal full-thickness laceration of the sclera with iris prolapse following the limbal contour nasally. The iris was gently placed in the eye using the iris spatula and the laceration was sutured with interrupted 8-0 nylon sutures. An iris spatula was used to prevent uveal incarceration.

The conjunctiva was then closed with interrupted 8-0 Vicryl sutures with episcleral bites. A subconjunctival steroid and antibiotic injection was performed temporally away from the laceration. The speculum was removed. The patient's drape was removed under the microscope. The patient tolerated the procedure well without any complications.

12.4.1 Surgical Exploration and Repair: Pearls

- A conjunctival peritomy should be initiated tangential to the area of high suspicion and should allow full exposure of the area of concern when exploring potential open globe injuries.
- An iris spatula can be a useful tool for repositing uveal tissue or holding uveal tissue out of the wound during repair in order to prevent uveal incarceration within the wound.
- 8-0 nylon interrupted sutures are the suture of choice for scleral laceration repair.
- 8-0 Vicryl suture can be used to close the conjunctival peritomy at the conclusion of the case.

12.5 Post-Operative Course

The patient was admitted to complete a 48 hour course of intravenous antibiotics. On post-operative day 1, the patient's vision had improved to counting fingers at 3 feet, and then 20/200 as his hyphema cleared over the next several days. The intraocular pressure was noted to be elevated at 32 mmHg and topical medical therapy brought the intraocular pressure to 15 mmHg within the next 2 days. Though the view to the posterior chamber was still limited by hyphema, a traumatic cataract was noted without evidence of capsular violation. View to the posterior segment was limited by vitreous hemorrhage and a B scan ultrasound revealed dome shaped membranous elevations in the superior and inferior temporal periphery, representing small choroidal detachments. The patient was referred to a retina specialist and was seen 5 days after globe repair.

On follow up in retina clinic, the patient had improved visual acuity of 20/63 (best corrected), but was still bothered by the decreased vision from his traumatic cataract and the persistent vitreous hemorrhage. At post op week 3, the patient underwent cataract extraction and intraocular lens placement along with pars plana vitrectomy for persistent vitreous hemorrhage and concern for a retinal tear noted on B-scan ultrasound.

12.6 Surgeon's Secondary Assessment and Pre-Operative Plan

This patient has undergone a repair of a Zone II open globe injury after blunt trauma, and has been referred for evaluation by a retina surgeon for concern of a possible retinal tear and choroidal hemorrhage noted on B-scan ultrasound in the post-operative course. Additionally, the patient was noted to have a progressive traumatic cataract and persistent vitreous hemorrhage.

This case serves to illustrate the possibility of posterior structure involvement in open globe injuries. In cases such as this, complications from the initial injury such as hyphema or vitreous hemorrhage may limit view on dilated fundus examination, requiring reliance on ultrasound to guide clinical management. Our patient continued to have persistent vitreous hemorrhage with possible additional posterior pathology, like a retinal tear, prompting a secondary surgery by vitrectomy.

The presence of a progressive cataract after trauma raises the possibility of capsular violation even in the absence of clear evidence on exam. Zonular dialysis is a frequent occurrence in the setting of traumatic cataracts which greatly increases the difficulty of traditional phacoemulsification. Given the presence of vitreoretinal pathology as well as a visually significant cataract, we elected to proceed with cataract removal in combination with vitreoretinal surgery. With concurrent pars plana vitrectomy (PPV), cataract extraction and intraocular lens placement can be completed safely and effectively to achieve a good visual outcome [2].

Patients with open globe injuries, especially in the presence of vitreous hemorrhage are at high risk for the development of fibrovascular proliferation and tractional retinal detachment. Experimental evidence and clinical practice have indicated that pars plana vitrectomy may serve to minimize this risk. In their 1979 rhesus monkey study, Cleary and Ryan demonstrated the detrimental effect of blood in the vitreous after a full-thickness injury. Only monkeys that received autologous blood injection at the time of injury developed tractional retinal detachment [3]. Early pars plana vitrectomy should be considered in any case considered high risk for developing these complications though the timing of surgery is still controversial. Various groups recommend a range of timing for vitrectomy from 3 days to 1 month after injury [4].

12.6.1 Second Surgical Repair: Operative Note

After the operative eye was identified and marked in the pre-operative area, the patient was wheeled to the operating room. The right eye was prepped and draped in the usual ophthalmic sterile fashion. Three ports were made inferotemporal, superotemporal and superonasally 3.5 mm posterior to the limbus with a 23-gauge valve trocar system. The infusion was inserted into the inferotemporal port. The

Supersharp blade was used to create a superonasal paracentesis, viscoelastic was injected into the anterior chamber and then the superior clear cornea incision was made using the keratome. A cystotome was used to initiate the capsulorrhexis and Utrata forceps were used to complete it. There was an area of zonular dialysis nasally measuring about 3–4 o'clock hours and the lens was noted to be unstable. The lens was phacoemulsified in a chop fashion. A small anterior capsular tear was noted superotemporally as well as a posterior capsular tear. One half of the nucleus had not been emulsified. At that point, we decided to perform a pars plana lensectomy. The cutter was used to remove any remaining lens material and then a core vitrectomy was completed. Dissection of the vitreous base was performed 360°. No breaks were found. Then, viscoelastic was injected into the sulcus space in order to create an adequate plane for lens placement. The clear corneal incision was then enlarged in order to accommodate the MA60AC lens, 23.5 diopters. This lens was injected into the sulcus space, centered, and haptics rotated well into the sulcus. The viscoelastic was removed from the anterior chamber and then the incision was closed with a 10-0 nylon suture. The paracentesis was hydrated and all ports were removed and the sclerotomies were closed with 7-0 Vicryl sutures. Subconjunctival cefazolin and dexamethasone were injected at the end of the case. The eye was dressed with neomycin, polymixin B, and dexamethasone ointment. The eye was patched and the patient was wheeled to the post-operative care unit in stable condition.

12.6.2 Second Surgical Repair: Pearls

- A poor view and/or an inability to rule out retinal injury due to media opacities, such as progressive traumatic cataract, vitreous hemorrhage or hyphema may prompt a secondary surgery to properly assess the posterior segment for additional traumatic injuries.
- Ocular trauma can often lead to zonular dialysis or weakness, increasing the chances for dropped lens material with a standard cataract extraction approach.
- Concurrent pars plana vitrectomy and cataract extraction with intraocular lens placement can be successful in achieving good visual outcome in patients with visually significant cataract and vitreous hemorrhage while minimizing complications and the need for additional surgery.

12.7 Final Trauma Evaluation

12.7.1 Final Visual Acuity (Without Correction OD, with Correction OS)

OD: 20/20-1
OS: 20/20

12.7.2 *Pupils:*

OD: Irregular, non-reactive
OS: 4 to 3 mm, no afferent pupillary defect

12.7.3 *Slit Lamp Examination* (Fig. 12.5)

	OD	OS
Lids and lashes	Normal	Normal
Sclera and conjunctiva	4 limbal nylon sutures nasally under conjunctiva	Normal
Cornea	Significant peripheral neovascularization	Significant peripheral neovascularization
Anterior chamber	Normal	Normal
Iris	Irregular pupil margin, nasal tear	Normal
Lens	Sulcus intraocular lens, open posterior capsule	Normal
Vitreous	s/p PPV	Normal

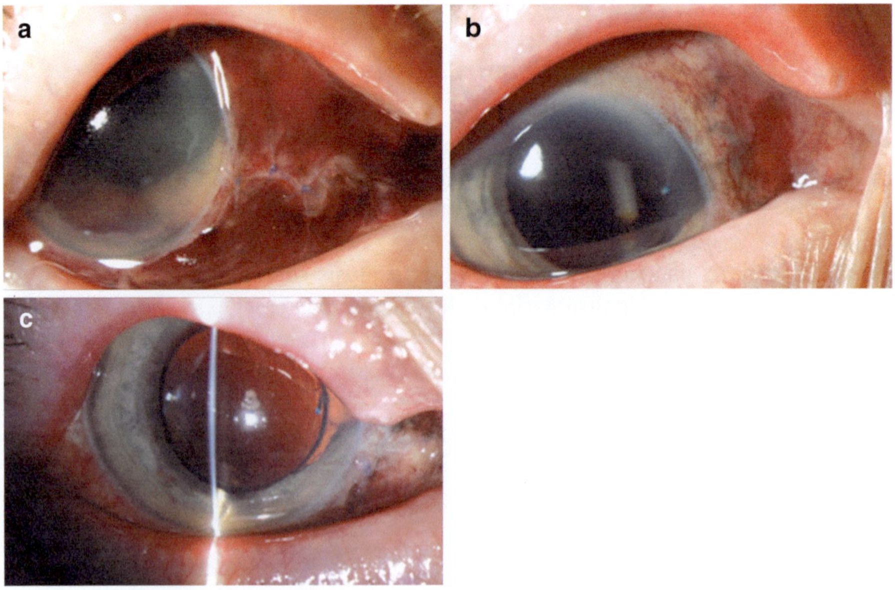

Fig. 12.5 External post-operative photographs taken (**a**) the day following primary surgery and (**b**, **c**) the day following pars plana vitrectomy and lensectomy

12.7.4 Dilated Examination

Macula/Nerve OD: Mild epiretinal membrane. 0.2 cup to disc ratio
Periphery OD: Normal
Macula/Nerve: OS: Normal, 0.2 cup to disc ratio
Periphery OS: Normal

12.8 Review and Lessons Learned

Signs of underlying Zone II globe rupture resulting from blunt injury can be subtle. Bullous subconjunctival hemorrhage, areas of subconjunctival pigment, low intraocular pressure and obscuration of the posterior segment should alert the clinician to the possibility of an underlying ruptured globe regardless of the injury mechanism. Advanced age, high myopia, prior ocular surgery, chronic topical medication use (especially corticosteroids), and long-standing inflammation (as was likely a contributing factor in our case related to contact lens abuse) may further increase susceptibility due to mechanical weakening of the eye wall.

Uveal tissue can become incarcerated within a full-thickness injury to the eye as the pressure differential from within the eye forces intraocular contents outward. The prolapsed uveal tissue can plug the wound and thus, the patient can present with a normal globe contour on imaging and even intraocular pressures within the normal range. It is important to maintain a high index of suspicion in these cases. A detailed clinical examination at the slit lamp is key to diagnosis, as findings on the CT scan may be subtle or may show a normal globe contour. The clinician should have a low threshold for exploration when any high risk factors or signs are present.

Exploration, beginning with a conjunctival peritomy, can be focused on areas of particular concern. If the location of the rupture site is unknown, a 360° peritomy must be initiated and all quadrants explored, including the sclera posterior to muscle insertions. An iris spatula can be a useful tool to reposit uveal tissue or hold uveal tissue out of wound while ensuring proper placement of sutures and minimizing the risk for uveal incarceration. The suture of choice for most scleral lacerations is an 8-0 nylon suture on a spatulated needle and interrupted sutures should be placed to align and repair the scleral wound.

12.8.1 Key Learning Points

- Suspicion for open globe injury should be maintained when any risk factors or clinical signs are present.

- A small area of pigmented tissue beneath the conjunctiva can be a sign of potential rupture in that location.
- Maintain a low threshold for surgical exploration to rule out an open globe in cases concerning for possible rupture.
- 8-0 nylon suture on a spatulated needle is used for repair of scleral lacerations.
- Ensure no uveal tissue is incarcerated in the scleral wound.

References

1. Andreoli MT, Andreoli CM. Geriatric traumatic open globe injuries. Ophthalmology. 2011;118(1):156–9.
2. Assi A, Chacra CB, Cherfan G. Combined lensectomy, vitrectomy, and primary intraocular lens implantation in patients with traumatic eye injury. Int Ophthalmol. 2008;28(6):387–94.
3. Cleary PE, Ryan SJ. Histology of wound, vitreous, and retina in experimental posterior penetrating eye injury in the rhesus monkey. Am J Ophthalmol. 1979;88(2):221–31.
4. Mittra RA, Mieler WF. Controversies in the management of open-globe injuries involving the posterior segment. Surv Ophthalmol. 1999;44(3):215–25.

Chapter 13
Case 8: Extracapsular Cataract Extraction Wound Rupture

Mohammad Dahrouj, Tavé van Zyl, Lucy H. Young, and Seanna Grob

13.1 History of Present Illness

An 84-year old man with history of hypertension and extracapsular cataract extraction (ECCE) in both eyes 30 years prior was transferred to our facility with concern for an open globe of the left eye.

- The patient reports that he was punched with a fist to the left eye 5 hours prior to arrival and suffered complete loss of vision directly following the attack.

13.2 Initial Trauma Evaluation

13.2.1 Visual Acuity (Without Correction)

OD: 20/20
OS: Hand motion

13.2.2 Pupils

OD: Round, reactive
OS: Dilated, irregular

M. Dahrouj, M.D., Ph.D. (✉) • T. van Zyl, M.D., • L. H. Young, M.D., Ph.D.
S. Grob, M.D., M.A.S.
Department of Ophthalmology, Harvard Medical School, Massachusetts Eye and Ear, Boston, MA, USA
e-mail: mohammad_dahrouj@meei.harvard.edu

S. Grob, C. Kloek (eds.), *Management of Open Globe Injuries*,
https://doi.org/10.1007/978-3-319-72410-2_13

13.2.3 External Examination

No lacerations or bony step-offs (Fig. 13.2).

13.2.4 Slit Lamp Examination

	OD	OS
Lids and lashes	Normal	Periorbital ecchymosis, mild edema
Sclera and conjunctiva	Normal	Bullous subconjunctival hemorrhage 360°, 3 piece intraocular lens extruded and visible beneath conjunctiva superiorly
Cornea	ECCE incision well healed	No epithelial defect
Anterior chamber	Anterior chamber intraocular lens, deep, quiet	Well formed with 1.8 mm layering hyphema; fibrinous and possible vitreous debris at pupil plane
Iris	Transillumination defects, superotemporal peripheral iridectomy, round	Irregular pupil, iris tissue not visible superiorly
Lens	Anterior chamber intraocular lens	No lens visible
Vitreous	Posterior vitreous detachment	No view behind fibrinous debris and heme

13.2.5 Dilated Examination

Macula/Nerve OD: Normal
Periphery OD: Normal
Macula/Nerve: OS: No view
Periphery OS: No view

13.2.6 Radiographic Imaging

Computed tomography (CT) of the orbits showed no fractures (Fig. 13.1). Significant findings included left-sided bullous subconjunctival hemorrhage, large choroidal hemorrhages, and relatively preserved globe contour. There was no intraocular foreign body; an intraocular lens could not be identified. There was no intracranial injury.

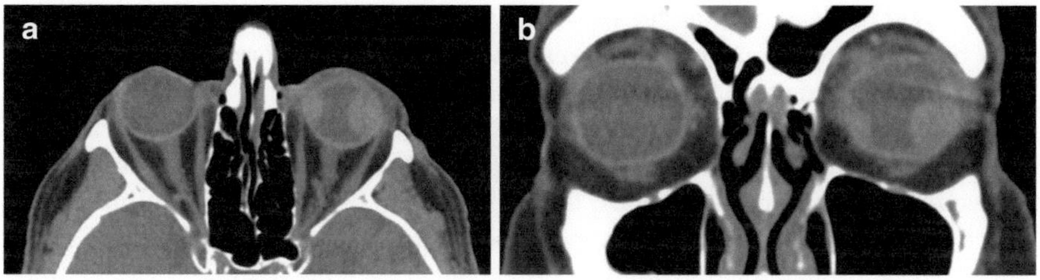

Fig. 13.1 Non-contrast CT images of the orbits. (**a**) Axial and (**b**) coronal images show normal globe on the right and a choroidal hemorrhages with irregular globe contour on the left

13.3 Surgeon's Initial Assessment and Pre-operative Plan

The patient had a Zone II open globe injury of the left eye secondary to traumatic extracapsular cataract extraction (ECCE) wound dehiscence following blunt trauma with extrusion of his intraocular lens beneath the conjunctiva.

Exam showed 360° bullous subconjunctival hemorrhage, an extruded 3-piece intraocular lens beneath the conjunctiva, loss of iris tissue superiorly, hyphema, and no view to the posterior pole. Exam of the fellow eye showed a well-healed ECCE wound superiorly with an anterior chamber intraocular lens (ACIOL).

This case illustrates the importance of obtaining a good history from the patient regarding prior intraocular surgeries. It is helpful to know when the patient had cataract surgery and by whom. Because the patient often does not remember the details of their cataract surgery, the ophthalmologist must often do some investigative work when evaluating an ocular trauma. It can be very helpful to examine the fellow eye to identify the type of cataract surgery the patient might have had in the past. Having the patient look down and examining the conjunctiva and sclera along the superior limbus might reveal a previous extracapsular cataract surgery scar (compared to a clear corneal incision scar). Seeing that this patient had an ECCE surgery on the right with the clinical history and clinical exam on the left, increased our suspicion of an ECCE wound rupture. The patient does not have to be elderly to have had ECCE. If the patient had cataract surgery from an ophthalmologist who was trained to do cataract surgery by ECCE or if there was a complication during a cataract surgery that required conversion to a larger wound, the patient can have a similar presentation after trauma.

Similar to the Zone II rupture discussed in case 7 (Chap. 12), it is important to expose the scleral edges of the wound in order to carefully re-approximate the wound. Open globe injury following ECCE usually occurs at the prior surgical incision site, which is not usually difficult to identify.

However, it is important to proceed with gentle intraoperative exploration with blunt dissection using blunt Westcott scissors to preserve any undamaged tissue or prolapsed uveal tissue. If the incision is mostly scleral, then an 8-0 nylon suture on a spatulated needle can be used to place interrupted sutures and the knots can be rotated away from the limbus and buried under the conjunctiva. If the wound is just along the limbus, then a 9-0 nylon or even a 10-0 nylon may be better since a portion of the suture pass will be in corneal tissue. Then the knots can either be rotated away from the cornea and covered by conjunctiva or can be rotated and buried. Since the initial cataract surgery wound followed the limbus, the traumatic wound is in the same orientation and can be closed by placing sutures radial to the limbus, similar to how an ECCE wound would be closed after a cataract surgery.

13.4 Surgical Exploration and Repair: Operative Note

The risks, benefits, and alternatives were discussed with the patient pre-operatively and the patient consented to proceed with exploration and repair of the open globe injury. The patient was brought to the operating room where the anesthesia team proceeded with general anesthesia. A careful time-out was observed and the correct patient and eye were identified. The left eye was prepped and draped in the usual sterile ophthalmic fashion using a Jaffe speculum to provide adequate exposure.

A 180° peritomy was initiated superiorly. Gentle exploration with blunt dissection immediately revealed the patient's 3-piece intraocular lens in the subconjunctival space superiorly (Fig. 13.2c, d). The lens was removed from the field in its entirety and sent to pathology. The superior quadrants were then gently explored via blunt dissection with Westcott scissors.

The patient was found to have a rupture of his prior extracapsular cataract wound extending from 11 o'clock to 2:30 o'clock just posterior and parallel to the limbus. Prolapsed iris and ciliary body tissue were evident as was a small amount of vitreous. A limited Weck-Cel® (Beaver-Visitec, Waltham, MA) vitrectomy was performed taking care to remove vitreous from the wound, but not to pull on vitreous. The wound was then closed with eight interrupted sutures using 9-0 nylon placed radial to the limbus.

The conjunctiva was then closed with interrupted 8-0 Vicryl sutures. A subconjunctival steroid and antibiotic injection was performed inferiorly away from the wound. The speculum was removed. The patient's drape was removed under the microscope. The patient tolerated the procedure well without any complications.

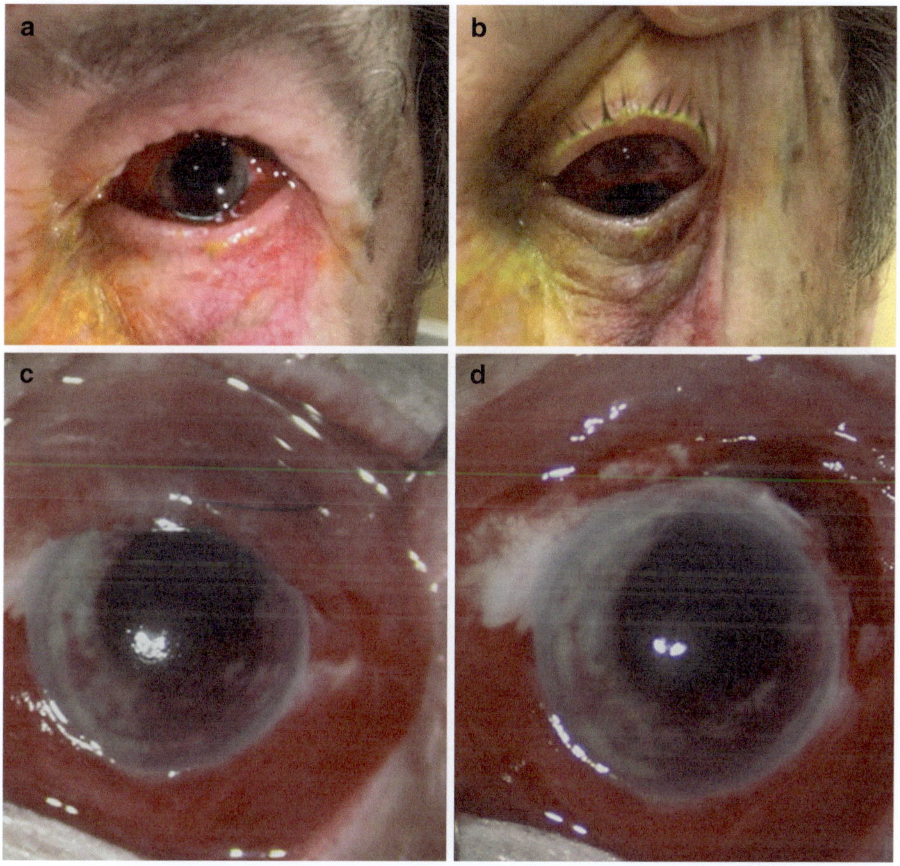

Fig. 13.2 External photographs (**a** and **b**) of patient on presentation showing 360 subconjunctival hemorrhage and irregular dilated pupil. Intraoperative photographs (C and D) showing 360 subconjunctival hemorrhage with extruded 3-piece intraocular lens superiorly with blue haptics visible subconjunctivally (**c**), and uveal tissue prolapsing through the dehisced wound seen following 180° peritomy (**d**)

13.4.1 Surgical Exploration and Repair: Pearls

- For surgical planning, it can be helpful to know about a history of ECCE surgery. Traumatic dehiscence of an ECCE wound should always be considered in older patients with a history of cataract surgery performed at a time when ECCE was more prevalent, who present with an open globe injury following blunt trauma to the eye. Evaluating the fellow eye for an ECCE scar can be helpful.

- Careful blunt dissection along the limbus can help exposed the ruptured ECCE wound. An iris spatula can be helpful to keep prolapsed uveal tissue out of the wound when suturing.
- Take time to look for a prolapsed intraocular lens; often the lens is under the conjunctiva.

13.5 Post-operative Course

The patient was admitted to MEE to complete a 48 hour course of intravenous antibiotics. On post-operative day 1 he still had hand motion vision, with no view to the posterior pole due to dense vitreous hemorrhage. A B scan ultrasound showed vitreous hemorrhage with peripheral choroidal effusions, attached retina and subretinal hemorrhage (Fig. 13.3).

The patient returned 6 days after initial repair for evaluation by a retina specialist. Visual acuity was hand motion with minimal view posteriorly. Following the initial visit, the patient returned twice to the retina clinic at 3-week intervals to assess the vitreous hemorrhage and the size of his choroidal effusion. Vision remained count fingers at 3 feet with minimal view posteriorly secondary to persistent vitreous hemorrhage, however the size of the choroidal effusion improved.

At this point, it was safe to proceed with pars plana vitrectomy (PPV). The options were discussed with the patient who agreed to proceed with surgery to clear the visual axis and maximize visual potential. This took place 10 weeks following the initial injury. Intraoperatively, as the vitreous hemorrhage was cleared, the patient was found to have low lying temporal and nasal choroidal effusions, and a dense epiretinal membrane over the posterior pole. The retina was attached and there were no retinal breaks.

The patient was followed closely by the retina and trauma service. On post op week 1 after PPV, the vision was count fingers at 3 feet, 20/300 with +11 D lens and

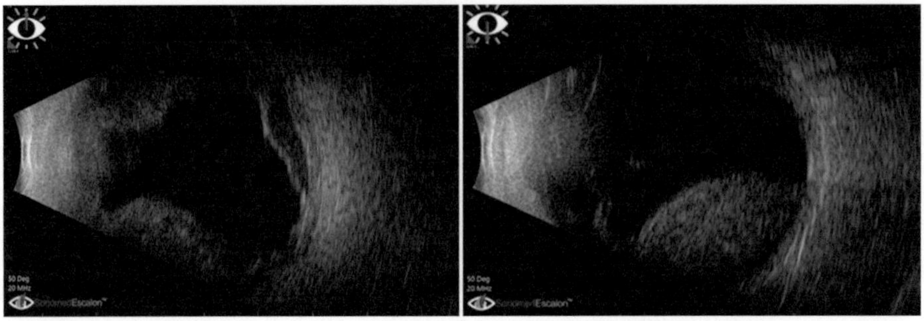

Fig. 13.3 B scan ultrasonography following initial repair demonstrated vitreous debris, peripheral choroidal and subretinal hemorrhages and an attached retina

pinhole 20/125. The patient was scheduled to see the optometry service for a rigid gas permeable contact lens fitting.

13.6 Final Trauma Evaluation

Prior to seeing the optometry service, the patient noticed decreased vision in the left eye. Exam showed total retinal detachment with inferior proliferative vitreoretinopathy. The options were discussed with the patient, who agreed to proceed with pars plana vitrectomy, membrane peel and silicone oil insertion. At the time of publication of this chapter, the patient was awaiting surgery.

13.6.1 Final Visual Acuity

OD: 20/20
OS: Count fingers at face

13.6.2 Pupils

OD: Round and reactive
OS: Dilated and irregular

13.6.3 Slit Lamp Examination

	OD	OS
Lids and lashes	Normal	Normal
Sclera and conjunctiva	Normal	Superior nylon sutures intact with no surrounding injection
Cornea	ECCE incision well healed	Ruptured ECCE wound closed with eight interrupted sutures (Fig. 13.4)
Anterior chamber	Anterior chamber intraocular lens, deep and quiet	Trace remaining vitreous near the wound superiorly
Iris	Transillumination defects, peripheral iridotomy	Dilated and irregular pupil, with loss of tissue from 11 to 1 o'clock and inferior pigment
Lens	Anterior chamber intraocular lens	Aphakia
Vitreous	Posterior vitreous detachment	Clear, status post pars plana vitrectomy

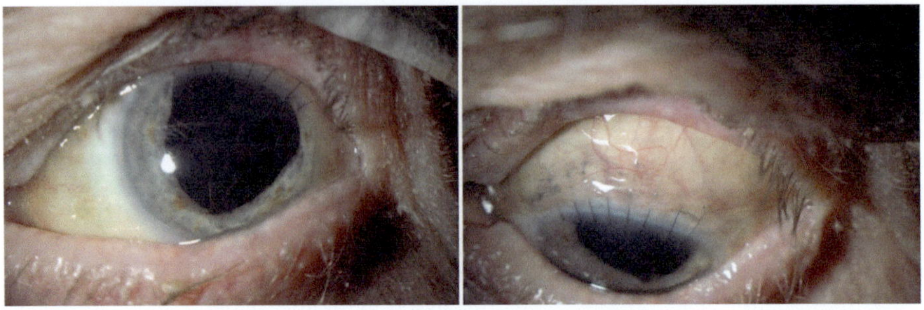

Fig. 13.4 Anterior segment slit lamp photographs showing eight nylon limbal sutures superiorly, with loss of iris tissue superiorly

13.6.4 Dilated Examination

Macula/Nerve OD: Normal
Periphery OD: Normal
Macula/Nerve: OS: Normal nerve with detached macula
Periphery OS: Total retinal detachment with proliferative vitreoretinopathy inferiorly

13.7 Review and Lessons Learned

In cases of open globe injury in older patients, it is important to determine if there is any history of eye surgery. As in this case, a history of extracapsular cataract extraction constitutes a higher risk for open globe injury secondary to wound dehiscence even with minor blunt trauma. However, many patients are not familiar with the cataract extraction technique that was used during their surgery. In this situation, examining the fellow eye and finding an ECCE scar is very helpful and suggestive of a possible ECCE surgery in the injured eye. This can increase the suspicion of an ECCE wound rupture and can help with surgical planning.

Open globe injury due to traumatic pseudophakic (ECCE) wound dehiscence has been associated with poor final visual outcome. In a retrospective chart review of 848 open globe injuries repaired at our institution [1], Kloek et al. found that 63 (7.4%) of open globe injuries were due to traumatic dehiscence of a cataract surgery wound. The majority of these ruptures (56/63, or 89%) occurred among patients with prior extracapsular cataract extractions, and the majority occurred after falls. Furthermore, visual outcomes in the ECCE wound dehiscence group were significantly worse compared to patients presenting without wound dehiscence (hand motion compared to 20/40, respectively; $P = 0.0002$).

Traumatic pseudophakic (ECCE) wound dehiscence has also been associated with increased risk of posterior pathology such as choroidal hemorrhage (attributed to a rapid drop in intraocular pressure due to large wound gape) and retinal detachment, which contributes to their particularly poor prognosis. Our patient had significant vitreous hemorrhage on presentation and choroidals noted on B scan. Although he did not have a retinal detachment noted during the initial vitrectomy, he later developed proliferative vitreoretinopathy that lead to retinal detachment and a decrease in his vision.

Proliferative vitreoretinopathy (PVR) is a common complication following ocular injury and is usually associated with poor visual outcome [2]. In a large retrospective chart review study, PVR occurred in 71 (4%) of 1654 injured eyes. This study also found that the time from injury to onset of PVR was associated with the type of trauma: the shorter interval (median 1.3 months) was observed in perforated globe, followed by rupture (median 2.1 months). Moreover, it was found that vitreous hemorrhage was the strongest independent predictive factor for the development of PVR with an odds ratio of 31. For this reason, it is usually recommended to proceed with pars plana vitrectomy early within 2–3 weeks following initial injury in order to clear the visual axis, maximize visual potential and prevent the development of PVR. This was not the case here as our patient had large choroidal effusion which makes it unsafe to proceed with surgery and resulted in delaying the surgery for 10 weeks.

13.8 Key Learning Points

- Always consider ECCE wound dehiscence as a mechanism for open globe injury in patients with a history of cataract surgery, especially among elderly patients presenting with open globe injury following a fall or other blunt trauma to the eye.
- Careful history-taking and examination of the fellow eye is essential in determining the intraocular surgical history and the risks for wound dehiscence following blunt trauma.
- Open globe injury with ECCE wound dehiscence has a particularly poor prognosis and requires multiple surgeries in attempt at visual rehabilitation; this should be discussed early on with the patient to aid in management of their expectations.

References

1. Kloek CE, Andreoli MT, Andreoli CM. Characteristics of traumatic cataract wound dehiscence. Am J Ophthalmol. 2011;152(2):229–33.
2. Cardillo JA, et al. Post-traumatic proliferative vitreoretinopathy. The epidemiologic profile, onset, risk factors, and visual outcome. Ophthalmology. 1997;104(7):1166–73.

Chapter 14
Case 9: Zone I/II Open Globe Injury from Metal Bearing

Eric D. Gaier, Yoshihiro Yonekawa, and Seanna Grob

14.1 History of Present Illness

A 56-year-old healthy male marine mechanic presented by referral for concern of open globe injury of the left eye.

- The patient was removing a bearing from a spindle on a boat trailer using a hand tool and it flew into his eye, under the safety goggles he was wearing.
- The patient reported immediate onset of severe pain and "greying" of vision in the left eye.
- Computed tomography (CT) imaging performed at the referring hospital revealed deformed globe contour on the left with no intraocular or intraorbital foreign bodies and no orbital fractures (Fig. 14.1).

14.2 Initial Trauma Evaluation

14.2.1 Visual Acuity (Without Correction)

OD: 20/60 pinhole 20/30
OS: Counting fingers at 1 foot

E. D. Gaier, M.D., Ph.D. (✉) • S. Grob, M.D., M.A.S.
Department of Ophthalmology, Harvard Medical School, Massachusetts Eye and Ear, Boston, MA, USA
e-mail: eric_gaier@meei.harvard.edu

Y. Yonekawa, M.D.
Vitreoretinal Surgery, Harvard Medical School, Massachusetts Eye and Ear and Boston Children's Hospital, Boston, MA, USA

S. Grob, C. Kloek (eds.), *Management of Open Globe Injuries*,
https://doi.org/10.1007/978-3-319-72410-2_14

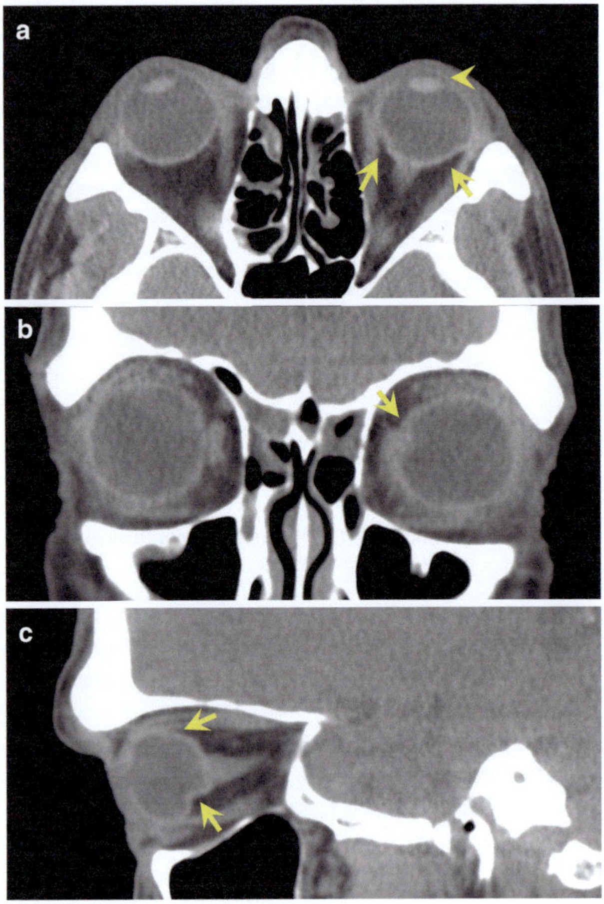

Fig. 14.1 Non-contrast CT images performed by the referring hospital and reviewed at the time of presentation. Axial (**a**), coronal (**b**), and sagittal (**c**) cuts are displayed and demonstrate irregular globe contour (arrows) suggestive of an open globe injury. The anterior chamber is shallow on the left compared to the right (**a**; arrow head). There are no evident facial fractures or foreign bodies

14.2.2 Pupils

OD: Round
OS: Irregular, no relative afferent pupillary defect by reverse

14.2.3 External Examination

Within normal limits; upper and lower eyelid marginal lacerations.

14.2.4 Slit Lamp Examination

	OD	OS
Lids and lashes	Normal	Upper and lower eyelid marginal lacerations
Sclera and conjunctiva	Normal	Nasal subconjunctival hemorrhage and conjunctival laceration
Cornea	Normal	Arcuate nasal full-thickness defect extending from the limbus at 7:30 o'clock to the limbus at 10:30 o'clock with uveal prolapse; Decemet's membrane folds evident temporally
Anterior chamber	Normal	3 mm hyphema; shallow
Iris	Normal	Irregular; iris protrusion from 7:30 to 10:30 o'clock
Lens	Normal	Pigment deposition on the anterior lens capsule; no apparent lenticular violation
Vitreous	Normal	Vitreous hemorrhage

14.2.5 Dilated Examination

Macula/Nerve OD: Normal
Periphery OD: Normal
Macula/Nerve: OS: Optic nerve sharp and pink, macula attached (poor view)
Periphery OS: Poor view

14.2.6 Radiographic Imaging

Non-contrast CT of the orbits showed deformation of globe contour on the left without intraocular or orbital foreign body (Fig. 14.1).

14.3 Surgeon's Initial Assessment and Pre-operative Plan

The patient had a Zone I/II open globe injury of the left eye with uveal prolapse from a projectile that required surgical repair. This case serves to demonstrate two key principles in Zone I/II open globe repair: (1) a useful technique to reposit anteriorly prolapsed uveal tissue and (2) the importance of aligning the corneal limbus.

Anteriorly prolapsed uveal tissue, much like iris prolapsing through the main phacoemulsification wound during cataract surgery, can be difficult to directly reposit. The surgeon should make every effort to minimize further trauma to the iris by avoid pinching or grasping the tissue with forceps. The anterior chamber may be collapsed at the beginning of surgical repair, and expansion of this space is necessary for uveal repositioning. With an open and leaking wound, injection of balanced salt solution is unlikely to adequately maintain this space. Injection of filtered air helps to better stabilize the anterior chamber due to capillary surface tension of the bubble [1]. Injected air also serves to stabilize the anterior chamber during subsequent suturing of large corneal rupture sites and/or lacerations. A cyclodialysis spatula inserted through a contrapositioned paracentesis can then be gently used to sweep the uveal tissue back through the defect, minimizing secondary uveal trauma (Fig. 14.2a). Necrotic, devascularized, or contaminated uveal tissue should be truncated rather than reposited. Even if uveal tissue is truncated, the sweeping method described above should be employed prior to closure because no uveal tissue should ever be left within the wound. This motion can also be completed at the conclusion of the repair to ensure there was no iris or other tissue incorporated into suture passes.

Alignment of the corneal limbus is a critical initial step of Zone I/II open globe repairs. Reconstruction of this landmark helps to orient and guide the remainder of the operation, and is especially helpful in complex or extensive injuries (Fig. 14.2b, c). Proper alignment of the corneal limbus helps to achieve

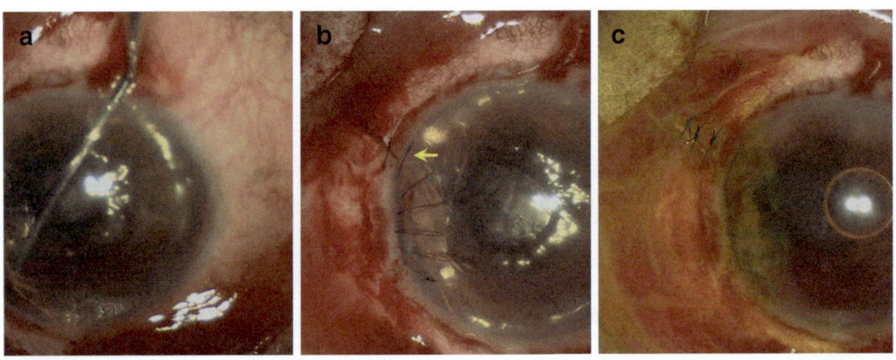

Fig. 14.2 Intraoperative images showing repair of the corneal and scleral rupture. (**a**) Sweeping of prolapsed uveal tissue using a cyclodialysis spatula under injected filtered air. The nasal defect is out of view. (**b**) Corneal rupture site repair using 10-0 nylon suture. Yellow arrow indicates the limbal 9-0 nylon suture, which was the first suture placed in this repair. (**c**) Scleral rupture site repair using 8-0 nylon suture

an optimal anatomic and refractive outcome. From this point, the corneal defect is typically closed to help stabilize the anterior chamber, followed by the scleral component.

14.4 Surgical Exploration and Repair: Operative Note

The risks, benefits, and alternatives were discussed with the patient pre-operatively and the patient consented to proceed with exploration and repair of the open globe injury. The patient was brought to the operating room where the anesthesia team proceeded with general anesthesia. A careful time-out was observed and the correct patient and the eye were identified. The left eye was prepped and draped in the usual sterile ophthalmic fashion using a Jaffe speculum to provide adequate exposure. A 180° peritomy was initiated from 12:00 to 6.00 o'clock. Gentle exploration with blunt dissection into the superonasal and inferonasal quadrants was performed with Westcott scissors followed by Stevens tenotomy scissors to evaluate for posterior eye trauma. The patient was found to have a 5 mm nasal shelved corneal full-thickness defect from the limbus at 7:30–10:30 o'clock, which extended an additional 5 mm radially (superonasally) past the limbus. There was uveal and vitreous prolapse through the corneal wound, and a ~3 clock-hour iridodialysis was appreciated in the nasal quadrant. There was not an obvious break in the anterior lens capsule, but the capsule posterior to the corneal rupture site was difficult to assess.

A paracentesis was made with a supersharp blade at the 1:00 o'clock position. The anterior chamber was reformed using filtered air. Uveal tissue was carefully reposited into the eye with a cyclodialysis spatula (Fig. 14.2a). The corneal limbus was reapproximated superonasally with a single 9-0 nylon suture (Fig. 14.2b; yellow arrow). The shelved corneal rupture site was closed with 10-0 nylon sutures. The shelved component of the corneal defect was very thin at the edge of the wound, so longer suture passes were placed in order to incorporate enough tissue to hold the suture. The scleral component of the defect was closed with 8-0 nylon sutures (Fig. 14.2c). Care was taken to ensure no uveal tissue or vitreous was incorporated into the wound repair. The defect was tested for integrity with a fluorescein strip and was determined to be watertight. The paracentesis was hydrated and was found to be watertight.

The conjunctiva was then closed with interrupted 8-0 Vicryl sutures. A subconjunctival steroid and antibiotic injection was performed inferonasally away from the injury site. The speculum was removed. The patient's drape was removed under the microscope. An atropine drop and maxitrol ointment were placed in the left eye and a sterile patch and shield were applied. The patient tolerated the procedure well without any complications.

14.4.1 Surgical Exploration and Repair: Pearls

- A useful approach to repositing prolapsed uveal tissue is sweeping from a contrapositioned paracentesis using a cyclodialysis spatula under injected filtered air.
- Repair of Zone I/II open globe injuries that cross the limbus should begin by approximating the corneal limbus, typically using 9-0 nylon suture.

14.5 Post-operative Course

The patient was admitted and completed a 48 hour course of intravenous antibiotics.

At the post-operative day 1 evaluation, the patient demonstrated hand motion vision with no view to the posterior pole in the affected left eye primarily secondary to corneal edema and vitreous hemorrhage. A B-scan ultrasound showed hyper-reflective debris in the inferior vitreous and an attached retina.

Subsequent follow up revealed steady improvement in visual acuity to 20/200 without correction and 20/60 with a manifest refraction on post-operative day 10. As his vitreous hemorrhage was clearing, observation was recommended by the retina team, who followed the patient closely over the ensuing weeks. Polycarbonate lenses were prescribed. The patient's visual acuity with spectacle correction improved to 20/40 with staged suture removal that was complete at the post-operative month 2 visit (Fig. 14.3a–c). His retina remained attached (Fig. 14.4a, b).

Along this course, the patient had continued ocular pain and developed a habit of frequently rubbing the eye despite strong recommendation and reminders to avoid touching the eye. Artificial tears helped minimally. This discomfort continued after all corneal sutures had been removed. Based on the focal nature of injection and some follow up visits, it was postulated that the scleral suture tails were irritating his bulbar and palpebral conjunctiva. Trimming of the most prominent suture tails improved his ocular symptoms.

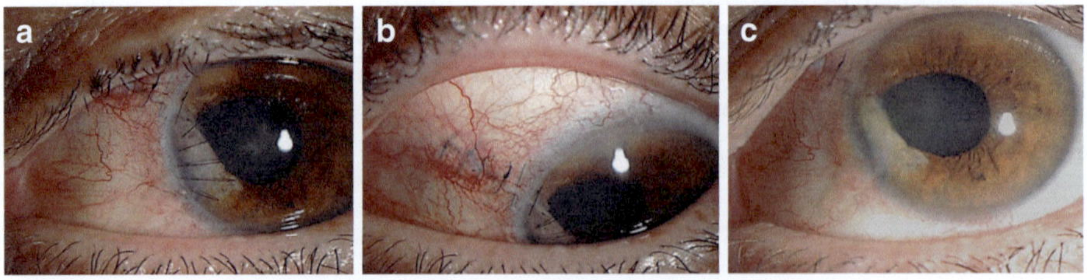

Fig. 14.3 Post-operative images. (**a**, **b**) Post-operative month 2 photographs showing the corneal (**a**) and scleral (**b**) components of the rupture. (**c**) Post-operative month 4 photographs after corneal suture removal

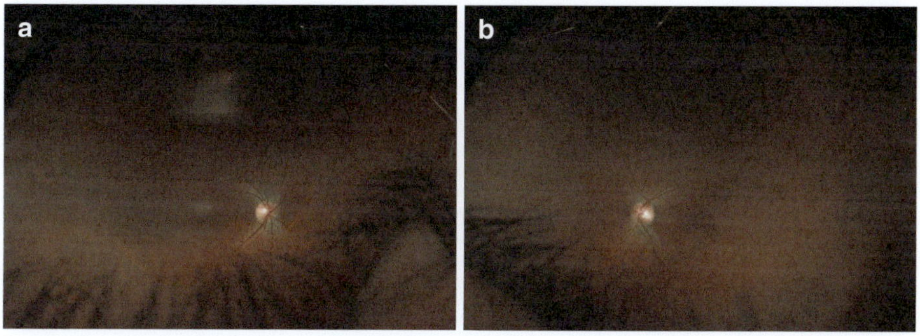

Fig. 14.4 Widefield fundus images taken at post-operative month 3 of the right (unaffected) eye (**a**) and the left (affected) eye (**b**) with resolving vitreous hemorrhage and debris

The patient also described glare that interfered with his vision and ability to drive. He did not have a significant/causative cataract, and his symptoms were not improved with artificial tears. Therefore, his glare was attributed to his traumatic mydriasis secondary to pupillary sphincter tear (Fig. 14.3c). A soft contact lens with a painted light brown iris and 4 mm pupil helped with his glare. He was referred to a cornea specialist for evaluation and is considering a pupilloplasty, iridoplasty, and synechiolysis procedure.

14.6 Final Trauma Evaluation (9 Months After Injury)

14.6.1 Final Visual Acuity

OD: 20/80 pinhole 20/20
OS: 20/40−1 with plano soft contact lens

14.6.2 Manifest Refraction (4 Months After Injury)

OD:	−1.75	−1.00	178	20/20
OS:	−0.50	−1.00	005	20/80

14.6.3 Pupils

OD: Round
OS: Irregular, peaked nasally, no relative afferent pupillary defect by reverse

14.6.4 Slit Lamp Examination

	OD	OS
Lids and lashes	Normal	Normal
Sclera and conjunctiva	Normal	Nylon scleral sutures buried superonasally with trace overlying injection
Cornea	Normal	Corneal scar nasally with associated neovascularization inferiorly
Anterior chamber	Normal	Formed, quiet
Iris	Normal	Iris sphincter tear nasally with associated transillumination defect and peaked pupil nasally, 3 clock hours of iridodialysis nasally
Lens	Normal	1+ nuclear sclerosis with nasal focal opacity outside the visual axis
Vitreous	Normal	Minimal debris with inferior hemorrhage resolving

14.6.5 Dilated Examination

Macula/Nerve OD: Normal
Periphery OD: Normal
Macula/Nerve: OS: Normal
Periphery OS: Attached, no retinal breaks

14.7 Review and Lessons Learned

A key objective of primary open globe injury repair is to close the laceration in the eye in a watertight fashion. Prolapsed uveal tissue should be reposited if viable, and truncated if not viable, but most importantly the defect must be free of tissue so that the margins can be closed. Inclusion of material or ectopic tissue in the defect leads to leaks and increased risk of infection in the short term. In the long term, contraction and fibrosis of the tissue can distort the ocular surface and intraocular contents that compromise the final visual and cosmetic outcome, and epithelial ingrowth may also occur.

The iris can be easily damaged in open globe injuries. This can occur directly during the injury; for example, the iris could be torn/cut by penetrating injuries/projectiles or ruptured/denervated by blunt trauma. Alternatively or in addition, the iris can be secondarily damaged. Prolapsed iris is stretched and can become ischemic when its vascular supply is compromised as it protrudes through a tight, edematous corneal defect. Manipulation of the iris during open globe repair can further damage the iris sphincter. Care should be taken during the surgery to minimize further damage to the iris. In the case of prolapsed uveal tissue, the above described method of sweeping internally helps to reposit prolapsed tissue while minimizing damage. Although this technique was used in our patient, the iris sphincter was torn, possibly a direct result of the injury. As a result, the patient was left with symptomatic glare, which can be addressed with a painted soft contact lens or subsequent pupilloplasty.

Full-thickness ocular defects that cross the corneal limbus should always be approached by aligning the limbal margin as an initial step. An analogous application of this principle is alignment of tarsus as a primary step in repairing eyelid lacerations that span the eyelid margin, and the importance of the second suture in penetrating keratoplasties. Failure to reconstruct alignment in these cases can lead to significant anatomic and functional defects that are nearly impossible to correct after completion of the initial healing stages. Most notably, proper alignment of the corneal limbus is critical to obtaining a reasonable refractive outcome.

Ocular trauma patients with Zone I-involving injuries require special refractive considerations. Significant, irregular corneal cylinder can be corrected using rigid gas-permeable contact lenses if they can be tolerated (unfortunately not in our patient's case) [2, 3]. Colored iris lenses, more commonly available as soft contact lenses, can help address photophobia or glare induced by iris defects, which are common in penetrating Zone-I injuries. Patients are often left aphakic after a penetrating Zone I or II injury that violates the lens capsule and the resulting cataract must be removed (rationale discussed elsewhere), so prescription of an aphakic contact lens is often necessary with some adjustments to address other symptoms or refractive sequelae of the injury. Contact lens prescription and management is often best handled by an optometrist with experience in treating trauma patients.

14.8 Key Learning Points

- Gentle repositioning of the iris using a sweeping technique helps to clear the wound of prolapsed tissue and minimizes secondary iris trauma, which can have long-term sequelae.
- Alignment of the corneal limbus is a critical initial step of Zone I/II open globe repairs.
- Zone I-involving open globe injury patients have much to gain from optometric consultation and contact lens fitting.

References

1. Vora GK, Haddadin R, Chodosh J. Management of corneal lacerations and perforations. Int Ophthalmol Clin. 2013;53(4):1–10.
2. Zheng B, Shen L, Walker MK, et al. Clinical evaluation of rigid gas permeable contact lenses and visual outcome after repaired corneal laceration. Eye Contact Lens. 2015;41(1):34–9.
3. Kanpolat A, Ciftci OU. The use of rigid gas permeable contact lenses in scarred corneas. CLAO J. 1995;21(1):64–6.

Chapter 15
Case 10: Zone I/II Open Globe Injury from Blunt Trauma with a Wrench

Huy V. Nguyen, Durga S. Borkar, John B. Miller, and Seanna Grob

15.1 History of Present Illness

A 24-year-old man with history of substance abuse presents with concern for open globe of the left eye.

- The patient reports he was pulling a staple out of some wood with a wrench with significant force when the wrench snapped back and hit him in his left eye.
- He was seen at an outside hospital and CT imaging was consistent with an open globe injury so he was transferred to Massachusetts Eye and Ear (MEE).
- He reports decreased vision and pain in the left eye.

15.2 Initial Trauma Evaluation

15.2.1 Visual Acuity (Without Correction)

OD: 20/25
OS: 20/60 pinhole 20/50

H. V. Nguyen, M.D. (✉) • D. S. Borkar, M.D. • S. Grob, M.D., M.A.S.
Department of Ophthalmology, Harvard Medical School, Massachusetts Eye and Ear, Boston, MA, USA
e-mail: huy_nguyen@meei.harvard.edu

J. B. Miller, M.D.
Vitreoretinal Surgery, Department of Ophthalmology, Harvard Medical School, Massachusetts Eye and Ear, Boston, MA, USA

S. Grob, C. Kloek (eds.), *Management of Open Globe Injuries*,
https://doi.org/10.1007/978-3-319-72410-2_15

15.2.2 Pupils

OD: Round, brisk reaction, no afferent pupillary defect
OS: Irregular, sluggish reaction, no afferent pupillary defect

15.2.3 External Examination

No facial lacerations

15.2.4 Slit Lamp Examination

	OD	OS
Lids and lashes	Normal	Normal
Sclera and conjunctiva	Normal	4.7 mm laceration involving the cornea at 2 o'clock and extending inferotemporally, crossing the limbus at 3 o'clock and extending into the sclera, with vitreous prolapse through the wound
Cornea	Normal	4.7 mm laceration involving the cornea at 2 o'clock and extending inferotemporally, crossing the limbus at 3 o'clock and extending into the sclera with a large epithelial defect centrally
Anterior chamber	Normal	1.8 mm layered hyphema
Iris	Normal	Transillumination defect at 3 o'clock
Lens	Normal	No cataract
Vitreous	Normal	Normal

15.2.5 Dilated Examination

Macula/Nerve OD: Enlarged cup to disc ratio
Periphery OD: Normal
Macula/Nerve: OS: Enlarged cup to disc ratio
Periphery OS: Vitreous hemorrhage inferiorly, with choroidal rupture at 5 o'clock

15.2.6 Radiographic Imaging

Computed tomography (CT) of the orbits showed a ruptured globe of the left eye without evidence of an intraocular foreign body. There were no orbital fractures. No intracranial injury identified.

15.3 Surgeon's Initial Assessment and Pre-operative Plan

The patient had a Zone I/II open globe injury involving the limbus of the left eye requiring surgical repair.

This case is notable for a single full-thickness laceration involving both the cornea and sclera. In Zone I/II injuries involving the limbus, it is essential to carefully align the limbus first during repair. A choroidal rupture was identified on dilated fundus exam (Fig. 15.1), although this does not change the operative strategy for globe repair.

As always in trauma patients, a thorough physical exam must be performed to rule out any associated facial or eyelid lacerations. This patient did not have any associated external injuries.

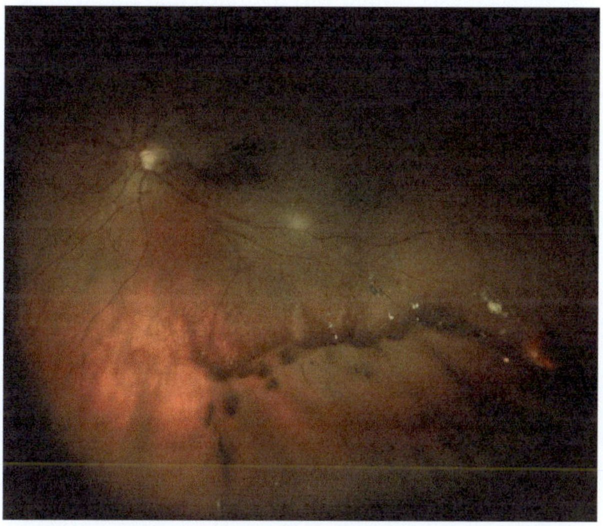

Fig. 15.1 Fundus photo with choroidal rupture OS

15.4 Surgical Exploration and Repair: Operative Note

The risks, benefits, and alternatives were discussed with the patient pre-operatively and the patient consented to proceed with exploration and repair of the open globe injury. The patient was brought to the operating room where the anesthesia team proceeded with general anesthesia. A careful time-out was observed and the correct patient and the eye were identified. The left eye was prepped and draped in the usual sterile ophthalmic fashion using a Jaffe speculum to provide adequate exposure.

A superonasal paracentesis was made using a 15° blade and 0.12 forceps. Filtered air was injected through the paracentesis to reform the anterior chamber. The patient was found to have an approximately 5 mm Zone I/II laceration originating supero-temporally (approximately 2 o'clock) on the cornea and crossing the limbus. Vitreous prolapse was noted through the wound and a Wek-cel vitrectomy was performed to remove the incarcerated vitreous from the wound. A small amount of iris prolapse was noted and was gently reposited in the anterior chamber with an iris spatula. The laceration was then closed using five simple interrupted 10-0 nylon sutures. Additional filtered air was injected through the paracentesis as needed while suturing. Then the filtered air was removed from the anterior chamber and was replaced with balanced salt solution. A fluorescein strip was used to check the integrity of the sutured laceration. The laceration was found to be Seidel negative. The paracentesis wound was hydrated and found to be watertight.

A subconjunctival steroid and antibiotic injection was performed inferotemporally away from the laceration. The speculum was removed. The patient's drape was removed under the microscope. Atropine and maxitrol ointment were placed in the left eye and then a sterile patch and shield were applied. The patient tolerated the procedure well without any complications.

15.4.1 Surgical Exploration and Repair: Pearls

- In cases with Zone I/II injury involving the limbus, it is important to carefully align the limbus with interrupted sutures.
- Make sure to carefully examine any laceration for presence of prolapsed vitreous, as this needs to be addressed prior to wound closure.

15.5 Post-operative Course

The patient was admitted to MEE to complete a 48 hour course of intravenous antibiotics. On post-operative day one his vision in the left eye was 20/150 pinhole 20/100. His corneo-scleral stitches were in good position (Fig. 15.2). A B-scan ultrasound was performed given the presence of vitreous hemorrhage which did not

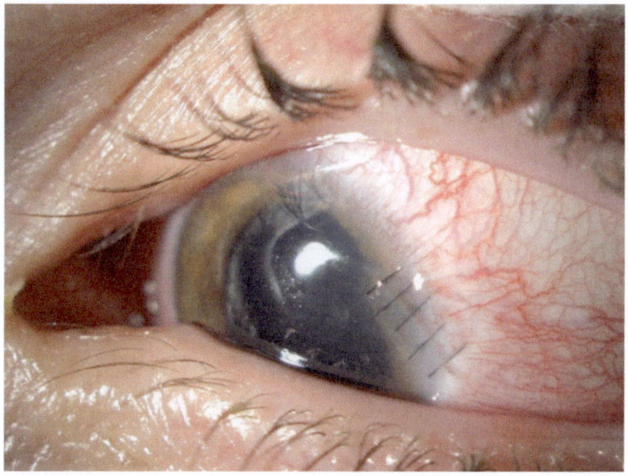

Fig. 15.2 Anterior segment slit lamp photograph of the left eye showing the laceration immediately after repair

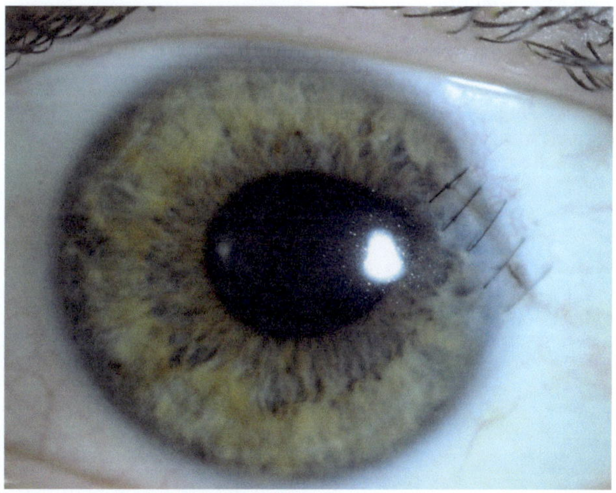

Fig. 15.3 Anterior segment slit lamp photograph of the left eye 2 months after globe repair showing the five nylon sutures in place

show any evidence of retinal tears, detachment, or dialysis. The retina service was consulted for evaluation of the patient's choroidal rupture.

The patient followed up 5 days after repair with a retina specialist and visual acuity in the left eye was 20/63 pinhole 20/32. The choroidal rupture was better visualized and there were still no signs of retinal tears, detachments, or dialysis. The lifetime risk for choroidal neovascular membrane and the subsequent need for annual dilated fundus exams were carefully reviewed with the patient. The patient's vision improved to 20/40 pinhole 20/25 by the post-op week 1 visit.

Eight weeks after his injury, the corneal sutures were removed in the trauma clinic, per standard practice and the wound appeared well healed (Fig. 15.3). His choroidal rupture was found to be resolving and there were no signs of any developing choroidal neovascular membrane (Fig. 15.4). On 3 month followup, the

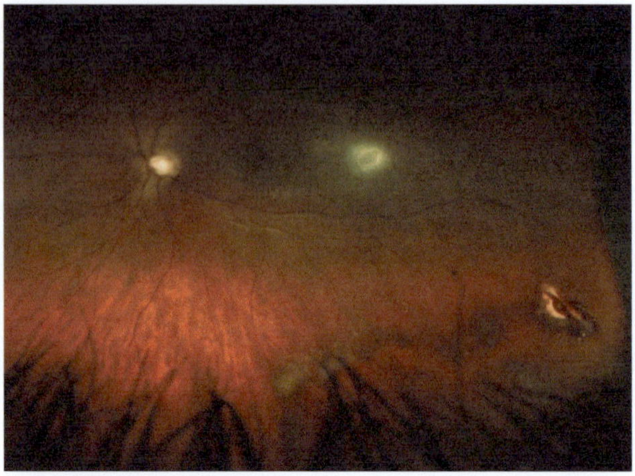

Fig. 15.4 Fundus photograph of the left eye 3 months after globe repair. Note the resolving choroidal rupture

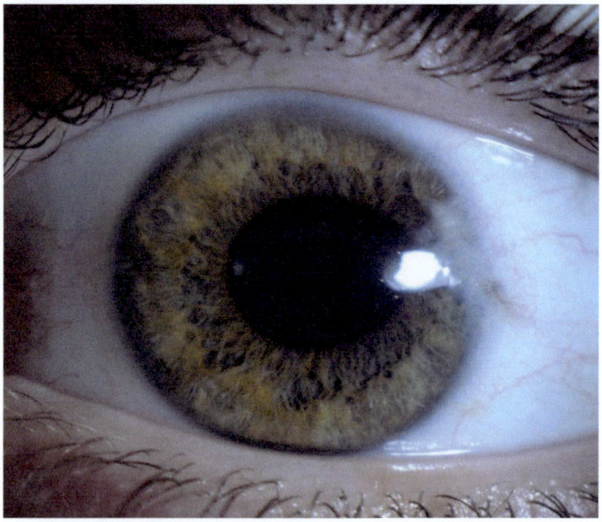

Fig. 15.5 Anterior segment slit lamp photograph 3 months after globe repair, with well-healing scar on the corneal surface

patient was found to have a well-healed wound (Seidel negative) (Fig. 15.5). He was referred to the glaucoma service for initial evaluation given his enlarged cup-to-disc ratios and family history of glaucoma.

15.6 Final Trauma Evaluation

15.6.1 Final Visual Acuity

OD: 20/20
OS: 20/20

15.6.2 *Pupils*

OD: Round, no afferent pupillary defect
OS: Round, no afferent pupillary defect by reverse

15.6.3 *Slit Lamp Examination*

	OD	OS
Lids and lashes	Normal	Normal
Sclera and conjunctiva	Normal	Normal
Cornea	Normal	Well-healed 4.7 mm Zone I/II laceration starting at 2 o'clock and extending inferotemporally, no sutures
Anterior chamber	Normal	No cell
Iris	Normal	Peaking towards wound, iris defect with transillumination at 3 o'clcok
Lens	Normal	Normal
Vitreous	Normal	Normal

15.6.4 *Dilated Examination*

Macula/Nerve OD: Enlarged cup to disc ratio
Periphery OD: Normal
Macula/Nerve: OS: Enlarged cup to disc ratio
Periphery OS: Resolving choroidal rupture at 5 o'clock, no heme

15.7 Review and Lessons Learned

This patient had a large laceration through the limbus involving nearly equal parts cornea and sclera. In order for optimal repair, the wound should be apposed. Prolapsed vitreous or iris can be subtle and may prevent good alignment, so a careful examination at the slit lamp is essential. In this case there was prolapsed vitreous which was removed with a Weck-cel vitrectomy, and a small segment of prolapsed iris was gently reposited into the anterior chamber with an iris spatula.

For wounds involving the limbus, it is important to align the limbus first before completing the rest of the laceration repair. Sutures should be made longer near the limbus and shorter towards the central cornea, and care should be taken to ensure that entry and exit points are equidistant from the wound edge. As with other standard open globe repairs, corneal sutures should be passed through 90% corneal depth and scleral sutures should be 75–90% deep, with entry and exit at least 1 mm from the wound edge.

As with all traumatic open globe injuries, a careful and thorough dilated fundus exam is crucial for identifying retinal pathology. This patient was found to have a small choroidal rupture on initial examination, which was partially hidden by the vitreous hemorrhage. Choroidal ruptures are breaks in the choroid, Bruch's membrane, and retinal pigment epithelium occurring in up to 5–10% of blunt ocular injuries. With blunt trauma, the globe undergoes mechanical compression and sudden hyperextension. The sclera may resist these forces and the retina is protected due to its elasticity, but the middle layers have neither this tensile strength nor elasticity and thus are prone to rupture. The traditional teaching is that choroidal rupture occurs in closed globe injuries, but in a review of 111 cases at MEE from 1993 to 2011, 28% of choroidal ruptures occurred in open globe injuries [1]. The choroidal rupture will typically heal within 2–3 weeks after the initial injury, although hemorrhages might persist for 2–3 months. Foveal involvement, presence of dense subfoveal hemorrhage, and development of extensive pigmentary changes in the macula portend a worse prognosis. A major complication of choroidal rupture is choroidal neovascularization, which may occur in up to 10–20% of patients, usually in their first year after injury. There is an increased risk of developing CNV with longer ruptures (50% in ruptures >2.35 mm in length), and treatment includes anti-VEGF, laser photocoagulation, or photodynamic therapy [1].

The patient was evaluated by the Retina service immediately after globe repair and followed up in clinic at 1 week, 3 weeks, and 3 months after injury to monitor for complications of choroidal rupture.

15.8 Key Learning Points

- In cases that involve the limbus, it is important to carefully realign the limbus first before suturing the rest of the laceration.
- In patients with choroidal rupture, it is important to have close followup with the retina service to assess for other retinal injuries.
- Patients with choroidal rupture will need lifetime monitoring with a dilated fundus exam and occasional fluorescein angiogram to detect any choroidal neovascular membrane that might grow through the choroidal rupture.

Reference

1. Patel MM, Chee YE, Eliott D. Choroidal rupture: a review. Int Ophthalmol Clin. 2013;53(4): 69–78. https://doi.org/10.1097/IIO.0b013e31829ced74.

Chapter 16
Case 11: Zone III Open Globe Injury from Fall

Jay Wang, Seanna Grob, and Dean Eliott

16.1 History of Present Illness

An 80-year-old woman presents with concern for open globe of the right eye.

- The patient reports tripping on a curb and falling forward, hitting the right side of her face on the pavement. The patient denied any other trauma or loss of consciousness.
- She was seen at another hospital where an initial trauma survey was negative, except computed tomography (CT) imaging showed a right orbital floor fracture and bedside examination was concerning for open globe injury. She was transferred to Massachusetts Eye and Ear (MEE) for further management of her ocular injury.
- She reports one flash of light at the time of injury and only being able to discern shadows in the right eye.

Electronic Supplementary Material The online version of this chapter (https://doi.org/10.1007/978-3-319-72410-2_16) contains supplementary material, which is available to authorized users.

J. Wang, M.D. (✉) • S. Grob, M.D., M.A.S.
Department of Ophthalmology, Harvard Medical School, Massachusetts Eye and Ear, Boston, MA, USA
e-mail: jay_wang@meei.harvard.edu

D. Eliott, M.D.
Vitreoretinal Surgery, Department of Ophthalmology, Harvard Medical School, Massachusetts Eye and Ear, Boston, MA, USA

S. Grob, C. Kloek (eds.), *Management of Open Globe Injuries*,
https://doi.org/10.1007/978-3-319-72410-2_16

16.2 Initial Trauma Evaluation

16.2.1 Visual Acuity (Without Correction)

OD: Hand Motion at 3 feet
OS: 20/25

16.2.2 Pupils

OD: Round, no afferent pupillary defect
OS: Round, no afferent pupillary defect

16.2.3 External Examination

Two facial lacerations of right eyebrow and forehead

16.2.4 Slit Lamp Examination

	OD	OS
Lids and lashes	Periorbital ecchymosis	Normal
Sclera and conjunctiva	Bullous 360° subconjunctival hemorrhage, lids not able to close over bullous hemorrhage	Normal
Cornea	Descemet membrane folds	Normal
Anterior chamber	4+ cell and pigment, non-layering hyphema	Normal
Iris	Normal, regular	Normal
Lens	Posterior chamber intraocular lens	Posterior chamber intraocular lens
Vitreous	Dense vitreous hemorrhage	Normal

16.2.5 Dilated Examination

Macula/Nerve OD: Hazy view secondary to vitreous hemorrhage
Periphery OD: Hazy view secondary to vitreous hemorrhage
Macula/Nerve: OS: Normal
Periphery OS: Normal

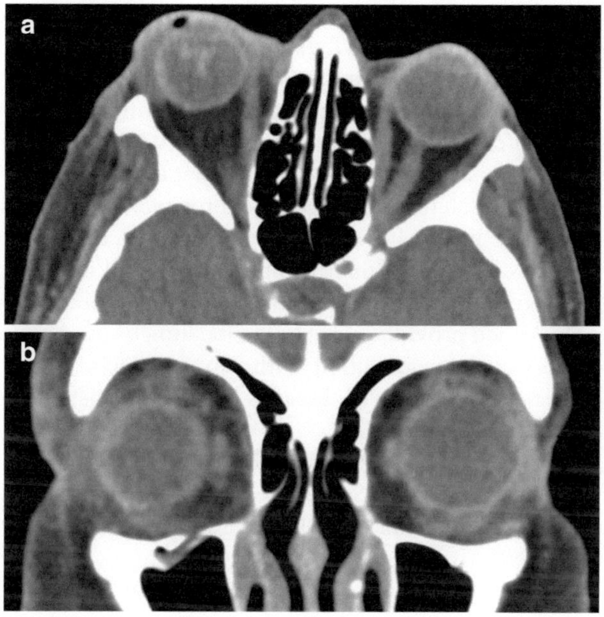

Fig. 16.1 Axial (**a**) and coronal (**b**) CT images showing a normal globe on the left and irregular scleral borders on the right with a hyperdensity within the right globe suggesting intraocular hemorrhage concerning for open globe injury. The orbital floor fracture can also be seen on the coronal image

16.2.6 Radiographic Imaging

CT of the orbits (Fig. 16.1) showed a right inferior orbital floor fracture, irregular scleral borders, and hyperdensity within the right globe likely representing hemorrhage without evidence of intraocular foreign body. No intracranial injury identified.

16.3 Surgeon's Initial Assessment and Pre-operative Plan

This patient presented with ocular trauma resulting in 360° subconjunctival hemorrhage, hyphema, and dense vitreous hemorrhage. The CT scan demonstrated a right globe with an irregular scleral border, decreased volume, and intraocular hemorrhage all concerning for an open globe injury, in addition to an inferior orbital floor fracture on the right.

There must be a high clinical suspicion for open globe injury in cases with bullous subconjunctival hemorrhage and no view to the fundus. One should proceed with the presumption of globe rupture until exploration in the operating room can be done to rule out globe injury. A globe can appear formed on CT imaging and still have a large posterior rupture. However, if there is 360° subconjunctival hemorrhage and clear view to the fundus underlying the region of subconjunctival hemorrhage that shows no evidence of trauma, then exploration is not needed.

There was a high level of concern for a posterior Zone III rupture in this case. Careful review of the CT may show an irregularity in globe contour indicating the location of the defect in the sclera. For posterior ruptures, globe exploration starts with a 360° conjunctival peritomy at the limbus with small relaxing incisions at 3 and 9 o'clock. Then gentle dissection with blunt Westcott scissors into all four quadrants is completed. It is important to take care to ensure the dissection plane is on bare sclera. If dissection is propagated with Tenon's still in place over the sclera, it can be very difficult to locate and expose the rupture site. This is similar to exposure of the Zone II injuries discussed in previous cases. While dissecting in the four quadrants, some dark choroidal blood or pigment or vitreous might be seen, which provides clues to the location of the rupture site. If the wound is more posterior, then dissection with blunt Westcott scissors should be followed by dissection with curved Stevens tenotomy scissors to allow for more posterior dissection and exposure.

In the majority of posterior Zone III injuries, it is necessary to isolate extraocular muscles. Sometimes it is necessary to hook muscles in order to find a rupture site that can often be found just posterior to the muscle insertions where the scleral tissue is the thinnest. Other times it is necessary to hook muscles in order to better expose the rupture site with gentle rotation of the eye taking care not to prolapse uveal contents, or to isolate and remove the muscle for better exposure to close the rupture, or to identify the muscles so they are not injured during dissection and to examine the muscles to ensure they were not injured in the trauma. Isolating muscles can be done with a Gass muscle hook that has a small hole in the hook where a 2-0 silk suture can be threaded. After hooking the muscle with the muscle hook, the 2-0 silk can be pulled through and kept looped around each muscle. Make sure to remove the silk sutures at the conclusion of the case.

Exposure of posterior ruptures can be difficult. In addition to using the extraocular muscles for gentle ocular rotation, there are several other techniques that can be helpful. After clearing with anesthesia, sometimes the patient's head can be slightly rotated to help expose the side of the rupture. Retractors are also great for exposure. The Schepens orbital retractor can be used, however, at times this retractor can seem large during posterior globe repair. Thin malleable retractors can be especially helpful and do not take up too much space, allowing room to get a suture needle into position.

Once the leading edge of a posterior globe rupture site has been identified it can be helpful to initiate wound closure at one end of the laceration and march suture by suture back along the wound. Posterior ruptures often involve uveal prolapse and it may be difficult to identify the posterior scleral edge with all of the uveal tissue in the way. By identifying one end of the wound, sutures can be placed and uveal tissue slowly and carefully reposited with each suture. As each suture is placed, there is less uveal prolapse and eventually it gets easier to suture and visualize the wound. It is important to identify each end of the wound in order to ensure the entire rupture site has been repaired.

16.4 Surgical Exploration and Repair: Operative Note

The risks, benefits, and alternatives were discussed with the patient pre-operatively and the patient consented to proceed with exploration and repair of the open globe injury. The patient was brought to the operating room where the anesthesia team proceeded with general anesthesia. A careful time-out was observed and the correct patient and the eye were identified. The right eye was prepped and draped in the usual sterile ophthalmic fashion using a Jaffe speculum to provide adequate exposure. A 360° peritomy was initiated with relaxing incisions nasally and temporally. Gentle exploration with blunt dissection into the four quadrants was performed with Westcott scissors followed by Stevens tenotomy scissors to evaluate for posterior eye trauma. While dissecting into the superotemporal quadrant dark blood was noted concerning for posterior rupture in this area. The lateral and superior rectus were isolated with a Gass muscle hook followed by a 2-0 silk suture.

The patient was found to have an 11-mm full-thickness scleral rupture 11-mm posterior to the limbus superotemporally in the right eye with vitreous and uveal tissue prolapse. The inferior extent of the rupture site was located just superior to the superior edge of the lateral rectus. The most superior extent of the rupture site was found to be just posterior to the insertion of the superior rectus muscle. The lateral muscle fibers of the superior rectus appeared to be disrupted from the trauma as the rupture site extended just below these fibers. A Weck-Cel vitrectomy was completed. This rupture site was closed with multiple interrupted 8-0 nylon sutures. A malleable retractor was used for exposure of the site and an iris spatula was used to prevent uveal incarceration in the wound. After the scleral rupture site was closed, the silk muscle sutures were removed. Subconjunctival blood was evacuated due to the significant bullous subconjunctival hemorrhage that was noted pre-operatively and was causing poor eyelid closure and exposure. The conjunctiva was then closed with interrupted 8-0 Vicryl sutures. A subconjunctival steroid and antibiotic injection was performed away from the laceration. The speculum was removed.

Attention was then directed to the two facial lacerations of the right brow and forehead. One was closed with two interrupted 5-0 plain gut sutures and another was closed with a single 5-0 plain gut suture.

16.4.1 Surgical Exploration and Repair: Pearls

- Before proceeding to the operating room, it is helpful to review the CT scan for clues as to the location of possible posterior rupture(s).
- Exploration for globe injury typically begins with a 360° conjunctival peritomy with blunt dissection into the four oblique quadrants looking for any bleeding or prolapse of uvea.
- It can be helpful to isolate the extraocular muscles when looking for a rupture site and also to assist with exposure of the injury once found.

- Once the rupture site has been identified, it is important to achieve adequate exposure and to identify both ends of the wound.
- An iris spatula is useful for repositing the uvea and holding it out of the way while suturing the rupture.

16.4.2 Surgical Video

Please see Video 16.1

16.5 Post-operative Course

The patient was admitted to MEE to complete a 48 hour course of intravenous antibiotics. On post-operative day one she remained hand motion vision with no view to the posterior pole. A B-scan ultrasound showed multiple membranous interfaces, some with attachment to the optic nerve.

She was also evaluated by the MEE oculoplastics service for management of the orbital fracture. There was no indication for surgical repair given its small size, minimal herniation of orbital contents, full motility, and recent ruptured globe repair.

She then followed up 8 days after open globe repair with a retina specialist and visual acuity was light perception with no view posteriorly. A repeat B-scan ultrasound showed evidence of 360° large appositional choroidal hemorrhage with a retinal detachment in a tight configuration (Fig. 16.2). Dense membranous tissue

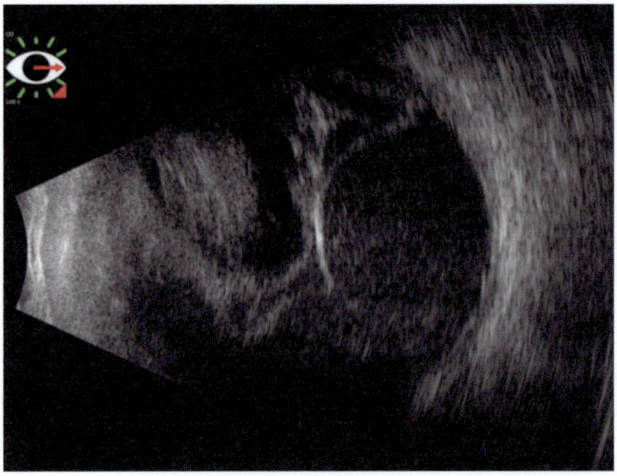

Fig. 16.2 B-scan ultrasound of the right eye showing appositional choroidals, retinal detachment, and vitreous hemorrhage

was also noted just posterior to the intraocular lens. The severity of the clinical findings and the likelihood of a poor prognosis was discussed with the patient. In elderly patients with evidence of severe vitreoretinal trauma and very limited prognosis, surgical intervention is not always pursued. In this case, there was dense choroidal hemorrhage, and in eyes with this finding there can sometimes be remarkable visual recovery after vitreoretinal surgery. Thus, in this patient, we decided to proceed with surgical intervention. The options were discussed with the patient who agreed to proceed with a pars plana vitrectomy, membrane peel, probable relaxing retinectomy, endolaser, and silicone oil placement with drainage of choroidal hemorrhage. This surgery took place about 15 days after globe repair.

16.6 Vitreoretinal Surgical Repair: Operative Note

The right eye was prepped and draped in routine sterile fashion. A wire lid speculum was placed. A 23-gauge surgery was performed. An anterior chamber infusion was first placed in anticipation of draining the choroidal hemorrhage. A peritomy was performed, and the inferior and lateral rectus muscles were isolated on 2-0 silk suture. Cautery was used to expose sclera in the inferotemporal quadrant. A cutdown was performed with a 69 Beaver blade. The choroidal hemorrhage drained freely.

The chamber deepened and then it was safe to put in the instruments. Cannulas and trocars were placed 3.0 mm posterior to the limbus in the usual locations. The tip of the infusion was visualized before it was turned on. Pars plana vitrectomy was then carried out with the vitreous cutter.

There was an intraocular lens in the bag. A temporal paracentesis was created to remove blood from the surface of the lens. The same paracentesis site was used as the anterior chamber infusion. The case was extremely difficult as there was dense hemorrhage. Eventually the vitreous cutter and the fiberoptic light source were able to remove the vitreous so that the retina could be visualized. The retina was incarcerated in the scleral wound from 9 o'clock to 12 o'clock. There was a total retinal detachment present. There was blood under the retina, as well as a significant amount of membranes. The retina was cut free from the incarceration site after diathermy was performed. Then membranes were extensively peeled on the surface of the retina. There also was a large hole inferonasally and two small holes surrounding it. After complete membrane peeling on the surface of the retina, subretinal membranes were peeled. This was extremely difficult as well and required considerable time and effort. The final retinectomy extended from 7:30 clockwise to 1 o'clock and was present on the temporal edge of the macula. After complete relief of traction, perfluorocarbon liquid was placed over the posterior pole. The retina flattened nicely with no traction remaining anywhere. Endolaser was then applied confluently along the retinectomy edge and to any other areas of pathology, which were quite extensive. A good endolaser pattern was achieved. A fluid-air exchange was then performed using the soft-tipped cannula and the fiberoptic light source. The retina stayed nicely attached with no traction remaining anywhere. Perfluorocarbon liquid was washed free from the posterior pole with balanced salt solution. Each of the three sclerotomies were sutured with 7-0 Vicryl after small incisions were made in the overlying conjunctiva. Silicone oil was placed up to the pupil plane and intraocular lens as demonstrated with a chimney. Endolaser had been performed 360°. No peripheral iridectomy was needed because the intraocular lens was in the bag. Conjunctiva was closed with multiple interrupted sutures. During this procedure, it was necessary to remove the central corneal epithelium with a Beaver blade. Pressure was checked at the conclusion of the procedure and was normal. The eye was flushed with Betadine, then dressed with Maxitrol ointment and a patch and shield, and the patient was extubated and transferred to the recovery room in good condition, having tolerated this procedure well. There were no complications.

16.6.1 Vitreoretinal Surgical Repair: Pearls

- Indications to drain a suprachoroidal hemorrhage include choroidal apposition, the simultaneous presence of a retinal detachment and/or vitreous hemorrhage [1], all of which were present in this case.
- A posterior draining sclerotomy is the most commonly used technique to drain suprachoroidal hemorrhages.
- The infusion port may be placed in the anterior chamber through a paracentesis to reform a shallow or collapsed anterior chamber.
- All traction must be relieved on the retina in order to achieve flattening. This includes pre-retinal and sub-retinal membranes, as well as sites of incarceration. Relaxing retinectomies may be necessary to relieve traction.
- Perfluorocarbon is often needed to flatten the retina in complex cases with significant traction, and silicone oil to ensure adequate tamponade.

16.7 Post-operative Course

On post-operative day one, the vision had improved to 20/300 and the retina was noted to be attached (Fig. 16.3a). The silicone oil was subsequently removed 6 months later, and the vision improved further to 20/125 (Fig. 16.3b). The retina remained attached without any signs of proliferative vitreoretinopathy.

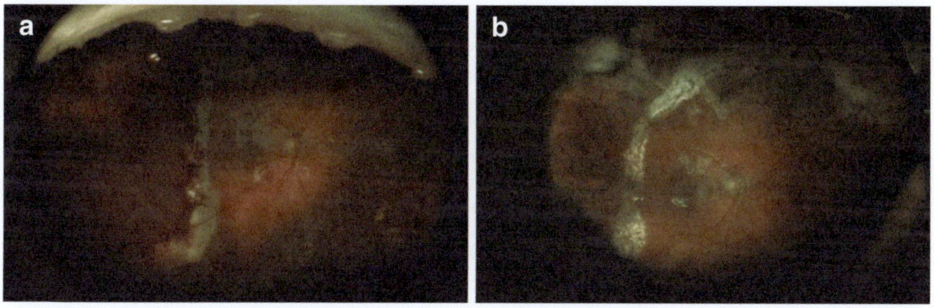

Fig. 16.3 Fundus photos of the right eye 1 day post-operatively (**a**), and 6 months post-operatively (**b**) showing the temporal retinectomy edge and an otherwise attached retina

16.8 Final Trauma Evaluation

16.8.1 Final Visual Acuity

OD: 20/200 pinhole 20/125
OS: 20/30 pinhole 20/20

16.8.2 Pupils

OD: Round, no afferent pupillary defect
OS: Round, no afferent pupillary defect

16.8.3 Slit Lamp Examination

	OD	OS
Lids and lashes	Normal	Normal
Sclera and conjunctiva	Mild subconjunctival hemorrhage	Normal
Cornea	Peripheral neovascularization, multiple pigmented keratic precipitates on endothelium	Normal
Anterior chamber	Normal	Normal
Iris	Normal	Normal
Lens	Posterior chamber intraocular lens	Posterior chamber intraocular lens
Vitreous	Normal	Normal

16.8.4 Dilated Examination

Macula/Nerve OD: Pink and sharp, macula flat with pigmentary changes
Periphery OD: Retina attached, relaxing retinectomy from 6 to 2 o'clock, fibrosis superotemporally without traction
Macula/Nerve: OS: Normal
Periphery OS: Normal

16.9 Review and Lessons Learned

It is important to maintain a high level of suspicion for occult posterior globe rupture in cases of significant ocular trauma with 360° bullous subconjunctival hemorrhage and no view to the posterior pole. On CT imaging, the globe contour may be irregular, and may provide clues as to the location of an occult rupture. Vitreous hemorrhage and hemorrhagic choroidals, or other signs of trauma, can also be demonstrated on CT imaging. However, a regular globe contour does not eliminate the possibility of a globe rupture. A dilated fundus examination is necessary to evaluate for evidence of vitreous hemorrhage or localized full-thickness scleral injury.

Surgical exploration for possible occult Zone III open globe injury begins with a 360 conjunctival peritomy, followed by blunt dissection into the four oblique quadrants and isolation of the four rectus muscles. It is important to look behind the rectus muscles, as the sclera is thinnest just posterior to the muscle insertions. Prolapse of uvea or dark choroidal blood may indicate the location of the full-thickness scleral wound. Once the site of rupture has been identified, ideally it should be followed posteriorly to locate the posterior most extent of the rupture. There may be cases, however, where it may not be possible to achieve complete closure if the rupture extends too far posteriorly. At some point, more harm than good may be done in trying to close very posterior ruptures, as exposing the wound might result in worsening uveal prolapse (Chap. 5.6.1). Use of an iris spatula can keep uvea out of the wound while it is being sutured, but even with careful closure, often some retinal or uveal incarceration is noted intraoperatively during subsequent retina surgery.

Zone III injuries are more commonly associated with retinal detachment so prompt retina consultation after primary closure is important [2]. Traumatic retinal detachments are difficult to repair because they are often extensive and are complicated by vitreous hemorrhage, retinal incarceration, and fibrotic membranes. The risk for developing proliferative vitreoretinopathy is high [3]. Care must be taken to relieve all traction on the retina, performing relaxing retinectomies as necessary. Perflurocarbon liquid is often needed to flatten the retina, and silicone oil may be used as the tamponade agent. Large appositional suprachoroidal hemorrhages should be drained, especially with a concurrent retinal detachment and vitreous hemorrhage, as in this case. The visual prognosis in such cases is guarded and should be communicated clearly to the patient. Occasionally, the visual outcome is better than expected, like in this patient with a final visual acuity of 20/125.

16.10 Key Learning Points

- The presence of 360° bullous subconjunctival hemorrhage and no view to the posterior pole in the setting of blunt ocular trauma should raise suspicion for occult posterior globe rupture.
- Evaluation by a retina specialist should be obtained promptly after primary closure to assess for the need for further retina surgery.
- Traumatic retinal detachment can be difficult to repair even in the hands of experienced vitreoretinal surgeons.
- Zone III globe injuries have a poor visual prognosis and it is extremely important to properly manage the patient's expectations.

References

1. Meier P, Wiedemann P. Massive suprachoroidal hemorrhage: secondary treatment and outcome. Graefes Arch Clin Exp Ophthalmol. 2000;238:28–32. http://www.ncbi.nlm.nih.gov/pubmed/10664049. Accessed 13 June 2017.
2. Stryjewski TP, Andreoli CM, Eliott D. Retinal detachment after open globe injury. Ophthalmology. 2014;121:327–33. http://www.ncbi.nlm.nih.gov/pubmed/24011994. Accessed 13 June 2017.
3. Eliott D, Stryjewski TP, Andreoli MT, Andreoli CM. Smoking is a risk factor for proliferative vitreoretinopathy after traumatic retinal detachment. Retina. 2017;37(7):1229–35. http://www.ncbi.nlm.nih.gov/pubmed/27787448. Accessed 13 June 2017.

Chapter 17
Case 12: Zone III Rupture Requiring Muscle Take-Down After Hockey Stick Injury

Tavé van Zyl and Seanna Grob

17.1 History of Present Illness

A 31-year-old otherwise healthy male presented with concern for an open globe injury of the left eye.

- He was playing hockey and was exiting the arena to secure his protective face shield, which had come loose, when another player's hockey stick struck his left eye.
- He noted blurry vision en route to the locker room, which progressed to almost complete loss of vision.

17.2 Initial Trauma Evaluation

17.2.1 Visual Acuity (Without Correction)

OD: 20/20-2
OS: Hand Motion

T. van Zyl, M.D. (✉) • S. Grob, M.D., M.A.S.
Department of Ophthalmology, Harvard Medical School, Massachusetts Eye and Ear, Boston, MA, USA
e-mail: tave_vanzyl@meei.harvard.edu

S. Grob, C. Kloek (eds.), *Management of Open Globe Injuries*,
https://doi.org/10.1007/978-3-319-72410-2_17

17.2.2 Pupils

OD: 4 mm, round, briskly reactive
OS: 5 mm, minimally reactive, afferent pupillary defect (APD) by reverse

17.2.3 Intraocular Pressure

OD: 21
OS: Deferred

17.2.4 External Examination

Left-sided periorbital edema and ecchymosis. No facial lacerations.

17.2.5 Slit Lamp Examination

	OD	OS
Lids and lashes	Normal	Upper and lower eyelid edema, periorbital ecchymosis
Sclera and conjunctiva	Normal	360° bullous subconjunctival hemorrhage with darker tissue (possibly uveal tissue or blood clot) noted superotemporally
Cornea	Normal	1+ descemet folds
Anterior chamber	Normal	Deep, 3–4+ red blood cells
Iris	Normal	Normal
Lens	Normal	In normal position, obscured by anterior chamber hemorrhage
Vitreous	Normal	Dense vitreous hemorrhage

17.2.6 Dilated Examination

Macula/Nerve OD: Normal
Periphery OD: Attached, unremarkable
Macula/Nerve: OS: No view due to dense vitreous hemorrhage
Periphery OS: No view due to dense vitreous hemorrhage

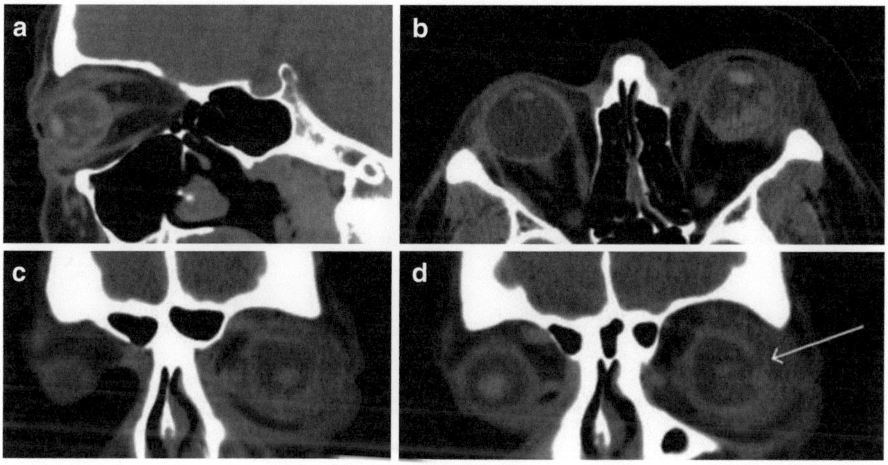

Fig. 17.1 Pre-operative CT scan of the orbits. Saggital view demonstrates irregular globe contour with heterogeneous intraocular hyperdensities. The crystalline lens appears in normal position (**a**). Axial view demonstrates similar findings highlighting the majority of hyperdense material laterally and posteriorly within the globe and scleral discontinuity temporally (**b**). Coronal images demonstrate the irregular globe contour, extensive subconjunctival hemorrhage (**c**) and a clear area of scleral discontinuity superotemporally (**d**)

17.2.7 Radiographic Imaging

Computed tomography (CT) of the orbits showed no orbital fractures. There was a minimally displaced nasal bone fracture. The left globe was small and abnormal in contour, consistent with ruptured globe, and there was a heterogeneous density in the posterior globe likely consistent with vitreous hemorrhage. There was adjacent hyperdense soft tissue likely representing the combination of intraocular content extrusion and adjacent soft tissue injury. The lens was intact and in normal position. The extraocular muscles were unremarkable. No radiodense foreign body was identified (Fig. 17.1).

17.3 Surgeon's Initial Assessment and Pre-operative Plan

This patient almost certainly has an open globe injury following blunt trauma and likely has a posterior rupture site in the superotemporal region. Supporting findings include the 360° bullous subconjunctival hemorrhage with pigmented tissue underneath, dense vitreous hemorrhage without a view to the posterior pole, and CT evidence of abnormal globe contour with visible discontinuity of the scleral wall superotemporally.

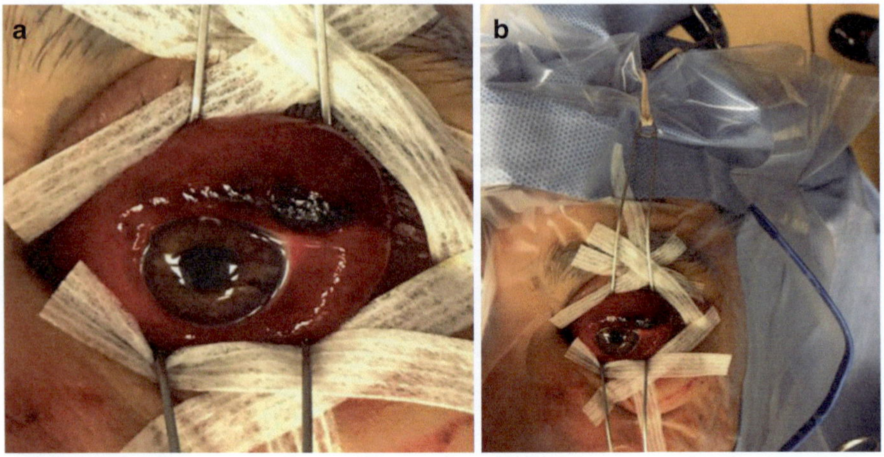

Fig. 17.2 Pre-operative external photo shows a soft globe, with bullous 360 subconjunctival hemorrhage with pigmented subconjunctival tissue superiorly, round pupil, deep anterior chamber with scattered heme on the iris and anterior lens capsule. There was no view posteriorly (**a**). Demonstration of surgical draping features use of the Jaffe-style lid speculum, which avoids undue pressure on the globe by lifting the palpebral circle off the globe via the force of the elastic rubber bands. The Steri-strip placement keeps eyelashes and the lid margin retracted and out of the wounds (**b**)

As mentioned in a prior case, CT imaging can be very helpful in determining the location of a posterior rupture. It is helpful to carefully analyze the scan prior to repair, not only to rule out intraocular or orbital foreign bodies and/or other trauma, but also for surgical planning. Sometimes you can see the distortion of the sclera on CT imaging. Coronal images can often be helpful to look for these areas of scleral distortion or discontinuity (depending on the location of the rupture). The location of intraocular hemorrhage on the CT scan may also help direct you to the location of the rupture. For example, in this case, there is a large collection of likely intraocular hemorrhage temporally on the axial CT scan (Fig. 17.2b). You can also see deepening of the anterior chamber in the traumatized eye as a possible sign of posterior rupture on CT imaging.

The lack of pupil distortion (peaking) can suggest that the rupture is further posterior than Zone II. However, sometimes you can see even mild corectopia or mild lens dislocation in a posterior rupture slightly towards the location of the posterior rupture. For example, if the rupture was temporally, you may see mild displacement of the pupil or lens temporally and this may provide a clue to the location of the posterior rupture.

As discussed in a prior chapter, it is often necessary in posterior ruptures to isolate the extraocular muscles. This is important in order to identify the muscles so they are not injured during exploration and repair, to examine the muscles for trauma, and for evaluation and exposure of the sclera posterior to the muscle insertion sites for any trauma. Hooking muscles in the trauma setting can be challenging. Passing a Gass muscle hook, with a 2-0 silk suture pre-threaded through the hole in the toe, between the sclera and the rectus muscle, and then removing the hook while holding one end of the silk suture, is often the simplest approach. Special care must be taken to gently guide the toe of the hook underneath the entirety of the muscle and away from the sclera, as there may be a rupture site posterior to the muscle you are trying to isolate. The muscle may also have been injured making it difficult to know if you have the entire muscle or not. Taking pause and ensuring that all muscle fibers have been hooked at this step is crucial, as it may become necessary later on to disinsert the muscles in order to better expose the rupture site. Therefore, in addition to the 2-0 silk suture on a wheel to isolate muscles, we often have a double-armed, 6-0 Vicryl on an S-29 spatulated needle ready, in case a muscle needs to be isolated and disinserted during globe repair. It is best to try and complete the repair without having to disinsert a muscle, but if the wound cannot be visualized, there is too much uveal extrusion to visualize the posterior edge of the sclera without better exposure, or it is just posterior to the muscle insertion and cannot be repaired, then you can consider disinserting a muscle in order to appropriately repair the globe.

Disinserting a muscle from the sclera is similar to strabismus surgery. Make sure to isolate the muscle in its entirety, checking that there are no additional muscle fibers on either side of your hook, and mark the center of the muscle insertion for re-insertion subsequently in the case. You can use the double-armed, 6-0 Vicryl on an S-29 spatulated needle to place a full-thickness central one-third bite and tie it with a 3-1-1 knot. Then, with each arm you can place imbricating bites on either end of the central one-third bite. This is best done by entering the muscle near your central knot, and passing the needle at a partial thickness depth through the lateral one-third of the muscle and then returning back towards the center with a locking, full-thickness bite. This would also be performed on the medial one-third with the other arm of the double-armed suture. Once you know the muscle is secure with your Vicryl suture, you can use blunt Westcott scissors to disinsert the muscle. Make sure you note which arm of the suture is on either side of the muscle, so when you reinsert the muscle it is not twisted or distorted.

Prior to going to the OR for globe repair, the patient was also examined by Head and Neck Surgery (ENT) due to his nasal fractures to ensure there was no septal hematoma and that the fracture did not require immediate surgical repair. Given that there was minimal displacement of the nasal bone and there was no hematoma, observation was recommended.

17.4 Surgical Exploration and Repair: Operative Note

The risks, benefits, and alternatives were discussed with the patient pre-operatively and the patient consented to proceed with exploration and repair of the open globe injury. The patient was brought to the operating room where the anesthesia team proceeded with general anesthesia. A careful time-out was observed and the correct patient and eye were identified. The left eye was prepped and draped in the usual sterile ophthalmic fashion using a Jaffe speculum to provide adequate exposure.

The upper and lower eyelids were noted to be edematous with ecchymosis. There was significant 360° bullous subconjunctival hemorrhage, especially superotemporally (Fig. 17.2). There was corneal edema and hemorrhage in the anterior chamber. The view of the lens was obscured by heme and there was no view posteriorly.

A 360° peritomy was initiated with radial relaxing incisions at 3 o'clock and 9 o'clock. The eye was noted to be soft during gentle blunt dissection. Gentle exploration with blunt dissection into the four quadrants was performed with Westcott scissors followed by Stevens tenotomy scissors to evaluate for posterior eye trauma. There was extensive bullous subconjunctival hemorrhage. While exploring in the inferotemporal and superotemporal quadrants, uveal pigment and dark choroidal heme were visualized concerning for a posterior rupture in these areas. The superior, inferior, and lateral rectus muscles were then isolated with a Gass muscle hook followed by 2-0 silk sutures.

The patient was found to have an approximately 16 mm, curvilinear scleral rupture approximately 15–16 mm posterior and parallel to the limbus extending from 2 o'clock to 5 o'clock (Fig. 17.3). There was extensive uveal prolapse. The distal ends of the rupture site were identified and the wound edges were reapproximated with interrupted 8-0 nylon sutures.

The rupture ran underneath and posterior to the lateral rectus muscle. Closure of the wound was attempted without removing the lateral rectus muscle, but there was a difficult view due to the posterior location of the rupture and the degree of uveal prolapse. Therefore, it was necessary to disinsert the lateral rectus from the globe in order to achieve adequate exposure to explore the extent of the wound and repair the rupture. After isolating the muscle, a pole test was performed and it was felt that the entire muscle was hooked. A 6-0 Vicryl double-armed suture on an S-29 needle was used to place a full-thickness central bite followed by a partial-thickness pass and a full-thickness locking bite on either side of the muscle. The center of the muscle

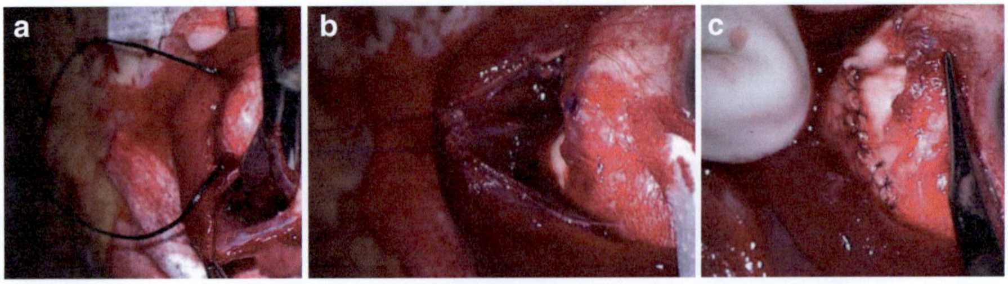

Fig. 17.3 Surgeon's view during open globe repair. After 360 peritomy and gentle exploration there was no rupture identified in Zone II. After the lateral rectus muscle was identified, hooked, and isolated with a 2-0 silk, Westcott scissors were used to gently dissect further posteriorly (**a**). The scleral rupture was identified 15 mm posterior to the limbus from 2 o'clock to 5 o'clock and ran posterior to the insertion of the lateral rectus, which was disinserted to provide adequate exposure for complete closure (**b**). Demonstration of the aspect of the scleral wound that extended under the lateral rectus. The lateral rectus insertion site is identified by the tip of the closed Westcott scissors (**c**)

was marked at its insertion site on the sclera. The muscle was then carefully dissected from the globe. The remainder of the rupture site was then better exposed. The uveal tissue was carefully and gently reposited into the eye. The wound edges were reapproximated with multiple interrupted 8-0 nylon sutures. An iris spatula was used and care was taken to avoid incarceration of intraocular contents in the wound. Upon satisfactory closure of the wound, the lateral rectus muscle was sutured back to its original insertion site via partial thickness scleral passes.

The four quadrants were gently explored once again to ensure no other full-thickness ruptures and none were noted. The conjunctiva was then closed with interrupted 8-0 Vicryl sutures. A subconjunctival steroid and antibiotic injection was performed nasally away from the laceration. The speculum was removed under the microscope. The patient's drape was removed under the microscope. The patient tolerated the procedure well without any complications.

17.4.1 Surgical Exploration and Repair: Pearls

- Closing the most proximal or accessible portion of a large scleral rupture before proceeding with further exploration can enhance stability and integrity of the globe during subsequent manipulations.
- If the scleral wound extends under the insertion of a rectus muscle, the involved muscle may be temporarily disinserted to improve exposure of the wound for repair.
- Wounds extending posterior to the equator should be closed very carefully with diligent avoidance of torqueing the globe and causing more extraocular prolapse of intraocular tissues as this will inevitably lead to incarceration.
- If the full extent of the wound cannot be safely visualized without torqueing the globe and causing uveal extrusion, the best treatment may be to leave the most posterior portion of a rupture unsutured (however, this is debated). If you feel you are doing more harm than good in closing a very posterior rupture, then that is a good time to stop.

17.5 Post-operative Course

The patient was admitted to MEE to complete a 48 hour course of intravenous antibiotics. On post-operative day one, he had light perception vision, with no view to the posterior pole. A B-scan ultrasound showed membranous elevations extending from the nerve consistent with a total retinal detachment, in addition to vitreous hemorrhage and thickened choroid.

He followed up 5 days after repair with a retina specialist and visual acuity remained light perception and there was still minimal view posteriorly. In the setting of a total retinal detachment, the poor visual prognosis was discussed at length with the patient, but surgical repair in attempt at visual rehabilitation was offered. The retina specialist additionally suggested a second opinion with another retina specialist due to the complexity and severity of the injury prior to proceeding with repair, and this was pursued the following day and yielded the same recommendation.

The patient agreed to proceed with complex retinal detachment repair involving a 23-gauge endoscopic pars plana vitrectomy, lensectomy, retinectomy, endolaser, perfluorocarbon and silicone oil tamponade and associated procedures. This took place 10 days following the initial open globe repair under monitored anesthesia care with subtenon's block. Intraoperatively, the patient was found to have significant vitreous hemorrhage and fibrin, which was removed until the underlying retina could be visualized. Upon visualization, the retina was found to be incarcerated into the temporal scleral wound. There was also significant foreshortening of the retina with funnel formation. After further exploration, a 360° retinotomy was completed to relax the retina. Then, perfluorocarbon was introduced into the eye and used to flatten the retina. Endolaser was applied at all the edges of the retina. Perfluorocarbon was removed and a complete air-fluid exchange was performed. An inferior peripheral iridectomy was created and the eye was filled with silicone oil.

On post-operative day one following complex retinal detachment repair, the patient had light perception vision and the intraocular pressure (IOP) was 6 mmHg. There was still an APD by reverse, as noted on initial exam. The retina was attached under oil. On post-operative week one, his vision remained light perception but his IOP was symptomatically elevated at 41 mmHg, felt to be a steroid response. He was started on topical dorzolamide 2%/timolol 0.5% and brimonidine 0.15%, which improved his IOP to the mid-teens. At post-operative week 2, he was noted to have developed a new total hyphema/vitreous hemorrhage, impairing view to the retina. The silicone oil fill precluded adequate visualization of the retina via B-scan. Given that his IOP remained in the mid-teens and there was no corneal blood staining, observation was recommended (Fig. 17.4).

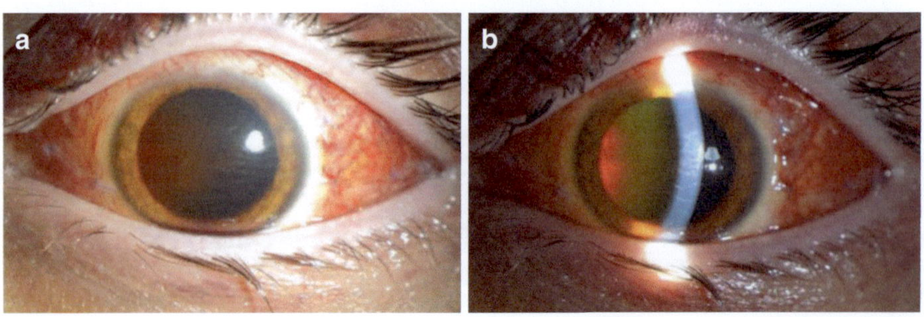

Fig. 17.4 External photographs of left eye post-operative week one status post Zone III open globe repair with lateral rectus take-down. Conjunctival peritomy with radial relaxing incisions at 3 and 9 o'clock are well apposed with 8-0 Vicryl sutures (**a**). Slit beam photograph highlights Descemet folds in the setting of post-op inflammation and relative hypotony (IOP 7). The anterior chamber is formed; there is a mild cataract, and vitreous hemorrhage is evident posterior to the lens (**b**)

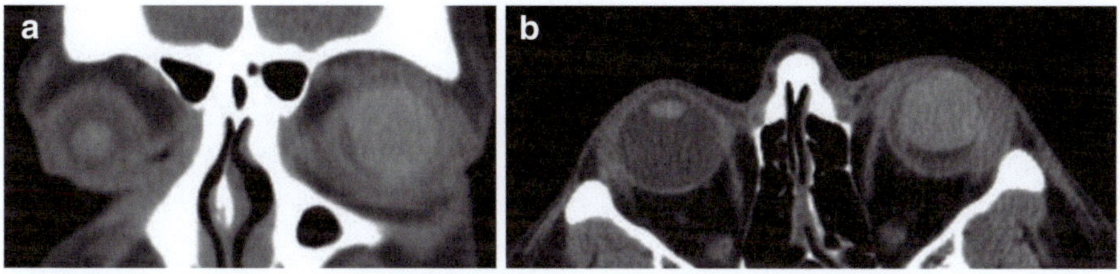

Fig. 17.5 CT face was obtained at post-operative week one s/p retinal detachment repair for evaluation of the nasal bone fracture. The left globe demonstrates improved contour and decreased periocular soft tissue swelling. The silicone oil is evident as homogeneous hyperdense material within the globe. Coronal view (**a**). Axial view (**b**)

Fig. 17.6 Wide-field color fundus photo of left eye following 23-gauge complex retinal detachment repair with silicone oil. The retina is attached superiorly with a funnel detachment at the optic nerve. The scarred site of injury with traction and associated PVR is noted temporally

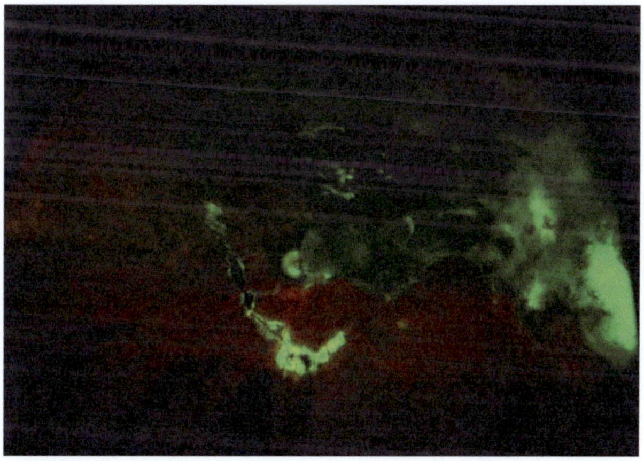

The patient continued to follow-up on a weekly basis, alternating with the retina and eye trauma services. His hyphema cleared approximately 2 months after it was first noted, at which point the follow-ups were extended to a monthly basis.

Eight months following the injury, the patient continued to have light perception vision and the IOP was 14. He remained on prednisolone four times daily, atropine twice daily, and brimonidine twice daily. Posterior examination revealed a stable exam with the retina attached under oil superiorly, and folded under traction around the optic nerve and inferiorly, with proliferative vitreoretinopathy (PVR) in the central macula (Figs. 17.5 and 17.6). Observation was recommended by the retina service and the topical eye drop regimen was unchanged.

17.6 Final Trauma Evaluation

8 months post open globe repair

17.6.1 Final Visual Acuity

OD: 20/20
OS: Light Perception

17.6.2 Pupils

OD: 4 mm, round, brisk reaction
OS: 5 mm minimally reactive, + afferent pupillary defect by reverse

17.6.3 Intraocular Pressure

OD: 18
OS: 14

17.6.4 Slit Lamp Examination

	OD	OS
Lids and lashes	Normal	Normal
Sclera and conjunctiva	Normal	Normal
Cornea	Normal	Normal
Anterior chamber	Normal	Normal, 2–3+ silicone oil droplets
Iris	Normal	Normal
Lens	Normal	Aphakia
Vitreous	Normal	Silicone oil

17.6.5 Dilated Examination

Macula/Nerve OD: Normal
Periphery OD: Attached, unremarkable
Macula/Nerve: OS: Slight pallor, extensive traction around optic nerve head, submacular choroidal scarring, PVR over central macula
Periphery OS: Attached superiorly, dense fibrosis with funnel centrally

17.7 Review and Lessons Learned

High velocity blunt trauma to the globe often results in large ocular ruptures with devastating anatomic and visual consequences. The sites most likely to result in ocular rupture in these scenarios are as follows:

- Corneoscleral limbus
- Immediately posterior to the rectus insertions where the sclera is thinnest (0.3 mm). The medial rectus inserts 5.5 mm posterior to limbus, inferior rectus at 6.6–6.9 mm, lateral rectus at 6.9 mm, and superior rectus at 7.0–7.7 mm
- The equator (approx. 14 mm posterior to limbus depending on axial length), where it is 0.4–0.5 mm thick
- Insertion of the optic nerve; and
- Site of previous intraocular surgery or trauma

In addition to exploration and identification of the site of scleral rupture, goals of initial repair include restoration of the integrity of the globe and, importantly, avoidance of further injury to ocular tissues. If the scleral rupture is long or runs posteriorly, the most accessible portion should be reapproximated first as this will provide structural support that allows for further manipulation in the safest possible manner.

If the rupture runs beneath a rectus muscle, the muscle can be temporarily disinserted utilizing the same technique as is used in strabismus surgery, after careful isolation with a Gass hook followed by 2-0 silk suture (see op note above for more details). Disinserting the muscle provides the needed exposure to safely close the wound without putting undue pressure on the globe or damaging the muscle, which may happen if suturing is attempted while the muscle remains in its natural position.

As discussed previously (see Chap. 5.6.1), controversy remains as to whether ruptures extending posterior to the equator should be surgically repaired. Surgeons who recommend abstaining from attempted repair posterior to the equator assert that the torque and manipulation required to access the posterior-most aspect of the wound is excessive and would likely lead to further extrusion of intraocular contents and increase the likelihood of retinal incarceration in the wound. Instead, if the posterior aspect of a wound extending beyond the equator is left unsutured, the wound is expected to granulate and become sealed by Tenon's fascia. Those in favor of suturing the wound in its entirety assert that complete closure allows for more timely restoration of pressure in the eye, improved overall integrity and reduced risk of recurrent rupture, and reduced risk of sympathetic ophthalmia and infection. Our practice is to assess on a case-by-case basis intraoperatively; we aim for complete closure in all cases but will forego doing so in situations of an extremely posterior wound that would require extensive pressure on the globe to access or so posterior that a suture needle cannot be mobilized into the location for repair.

17.8 Key Learning Points

- 360 bullous subconjunctival hemorrhage after blunt trauma is highly suspicious for posterior globe rupture, especially if pigmented tissue is visualized beneath the conjunctiva.
- Long ruptures that run beneath rectus muscles may require disinsertion of the muscles to provide adequate exposure.
- Repair of posterior ruptures should be attempted with extreme caution to avoid excessive pressure on the globe, which will lead to further extraocular prolapse of intraocular tissues.

Suggested Reading

Basic and clinical science course, AAO 2014-2015, Section 2, Chapter 2. p. 37–81.

Chapter 18
Case 13: Zone II/III Laceration from a Cat Claw

Natalie Wolkow, Seanna Grob, and John B. Miller

18.1 History of Present Illness

A 52-year-old woman with history of diabetes mellitus, depression, hypertension, hypothyroidism and lupus, presents with concern for open globe of the left eye.

- Her cat was sitting on her lap and reached up and scratched her left eye and left face with its claw.
- The patient noticed a sudden decrease in vision and was brought to Massachusetts Eye and Ear for evaluation.

18.2 Initial Trauma Evaluation

18.2.1 Visual Acuity (Without Correction)

OD: 20/60 pinhole 20/25
OS: Hand Motion

Electronic Supplementary Material The online version of this chapter (https://doi.org/10.1007/978-3-319-72410-2_18) contains supplementary material, which is available to authorized users.

N. Wolkow, M.D., Ph.D. (✉) • S. Grob, M.D., M.A.S.
Department of Ophthalmology, Harvard Medical School, Massachusetts Eye and Ear, Boston, MA, USA
e-mail: natalie_wolkow@meei.harvard.edu

J. B. Miller, M.D.
Vitreoretinal Surgery, Department of Ophthalmology, Harvard Medical School, Massachusetts Eye and Ear, Boston, MA, USA

S. Grob, C. Kloek (eds.), *Management of Open Globe Injuries*,
https://doi.org/10.1007/978-3-319-72410-2_18

18.2.2 Pupils

OD: No afferent pupillary defect
OS: No afferent pupillary defect by reverse

18.2.3 External Examination

Small scratch on left side of face

18.2.4 Slit Lamp Examination

	OD	OS
Lids and lashes	Normal	Few small ecchymoses
Sclera and conjunctiva	Normal	Superior conjunctival laceration. A visible scleral laceration noted beneath the conjunctival laceration, slowly Seidel positive with possible vitreous prolapse
Cornea	Normal	Normal
Anterior chamber	Normal	1-mm layering hyphema, 4+ cell (red blood cells)
Iris	Normal	Peaked superiorly prior to dilation
Lens	Normal	Poor view due to anterior chamber heme
Vitreous	Normal	Poor view due to heme

18.2.5 Dilated Examination

Macula/Nerve OD: Normal
Periphery OD: Normal
Macula/Nerve: OS: No view due to vitreous hemorrhage
Periphery OS: No view due to vitreous hemorrhage

18.2.6 Radiographic Imaging

Computed tomography (CT) of the orbits showed two intraocular hemorrhages of the left eye, likely choroidal hemorrhages. No foreign bodies or fractures were seen (Fig. 18.1).

18.3 Surgeon's Initial Assessment and Pre-operative Plan

The patient had a Zone II and possibly III open globe injury (Fig. 18.2) with vitreous hemorrhage. Choroidal hemorrhages were also noted on CT imaging (Fig. 18.1). Our first priority was to close the open globe injury.

The globe should be handled gently prior to and during surgery to minimize any further prolapse of intraocular contents. Patients with more anterior scleral lacerations can do well if there is minimal disruption of the intraocular contents and the wound is repaired carefully. Given the vitreous and choroidal hemorrhages, it is important to inform the patient of the potential need for additional surgeries after the initial open globe repair. A B-scan ultrasound should be completed the day after

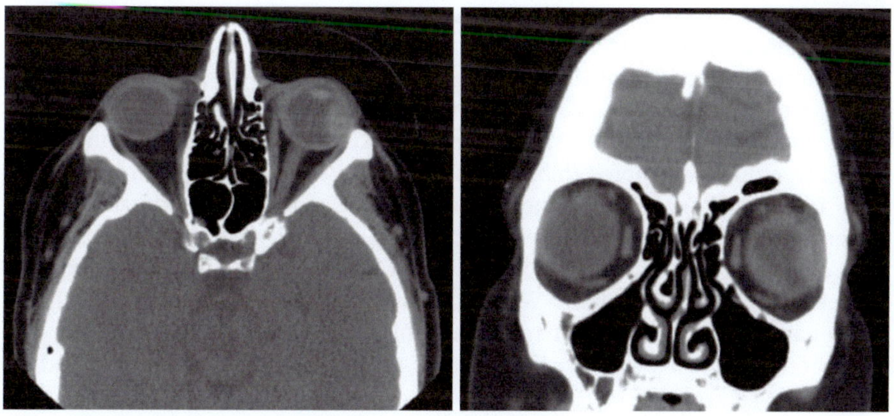

Fig. 18.1 Axial (left) and coronal (right) CT images without contrast demonstrating choroidal hemorrhages in the left eye

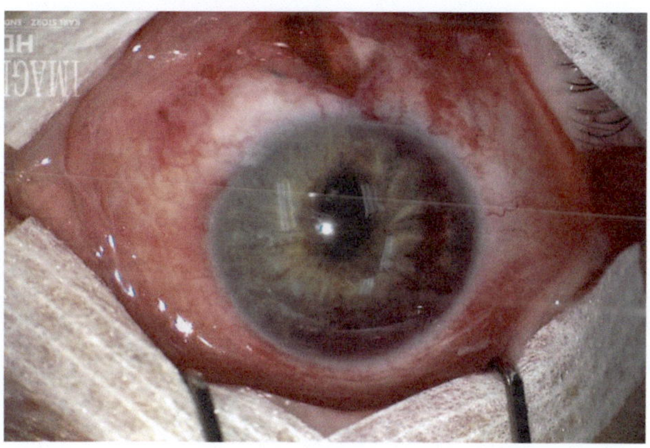

Fig. 18.2 Pre-operative photograph of the left eye showing the superior conjunctival and scleral laceration with a slightly peaked pupil superiorly and intraocular hemorrhage

open globe repair to further assess the status of the retina and posterior segment. Precise placement of the partial thickness interrupted 8-0 nylon sutures to close the laceration with care to prevent uveal incarceration in the wound is important.

18.4 Surgical Exploration and Repair: Operative Note

The risks, benefits, and alternatives were discussed with the patient pre-operatively and the patient consented to proceed with exploration and repair of the open globe injury. The patient was brought to the operating room where the anesthesia team proceeded with general anesthesia. A careful time-out was observed and the correct patient and eye were identified. The left eye was prepped and draped in the usual sterile ophthalmic fashion using Jaffe specula to provide adequate exposure.

The patient was found to have a superior conjunctival laceration (Fig. 18.2) and a vertical superior full-thickness scleral laceration. A superior peritomy was created from 10 o'clock to 2 o'clock to aid in visualization of the scleral laceration. Gentle blunt dissection with Wescott scissors exposed the scleral laceration. The scleral laceration was noted to begin 1 mm posterior to the limbus and continued for 7 mm to the insertion of the superior rectus muscle, approximately 8 mm posterior to the limbus. The edges of the scleral wound were approximated with interrupted partial thickness 8-0 nylon sutures (Fig. 18.3). Gentle exploration and further blunt dissection with Westcott scissors into the superotemporal and superonasal quadrants did not reveal any further extension of the wound. The superior rectus muscle was hooked with a 2-0 silk suture on a Gass hook, and the

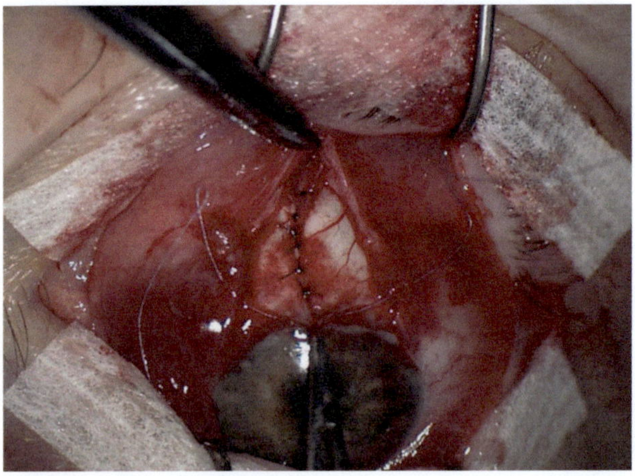

Fig. 18.3 Intraoperative photograph demonstrating the extent of the scleral laceration. Please see surgical video for more details of the repair

sclera behind the muscle insertion was carefully examined. The laceration was noted to stop at the insertion of the muscle and did not extend beyond the muscle insertion. The conjunctiva was then closed with interrupted 8-0 Vicryl sutures. A subconjunctival steroid and antibiotic injection was performed temporally away from the laceration. The speculum was removed. The patient's drape was removed under the microscope. The patient tolerated the procedure well without any complications. Atropine and neomycin sulfate, polymyxin b sulfate and dexamethasone ointment were placed in the eye and a sterile patch and shield were placed.

18.4.1 Surgical Exploration and Repair: Pearls

- To expose the laceration site, gentle blunt dissection with blunt Wescott scissors is necessary. Care must be taken to avoid pressure on the globe to prevent further prolapse of intraocular contents.
- The assistant surgeon may find an iris spatula useful to hold prolapsed uveal tissue and/or vitreous out of the wound while the surgeon sutures the wound closed. Prolapsed vitreous can be excised with Vannas scissors, but one should not pull on the vitreous when excising it from the wound.
- When a laceration reaches the border of an extraocular muscle, the muscle should be hooked and the sclera posterior to the muscle must be visualized to ensure that there is no continuation of the wound.

18.4.2 Surgical Video

Please see Video 18.1.

18.5 Post-operative Course

Post-operatively the patient had a B-scan ultrasound given the poor view due to vitreous hemorrhage, which confirmed the choroidal hemorrhages and absence of retinal detachments (Fig. 18.4). The week after open globe repair she was seen by a retina specialist. Her vision had improved significantly from hand motions to pinhole 20/30 as the vitreous hemorrhage settled. She was also found to have 360° of shallow choroidal hemorrhages, the greatest inferotemporally, and no retinal

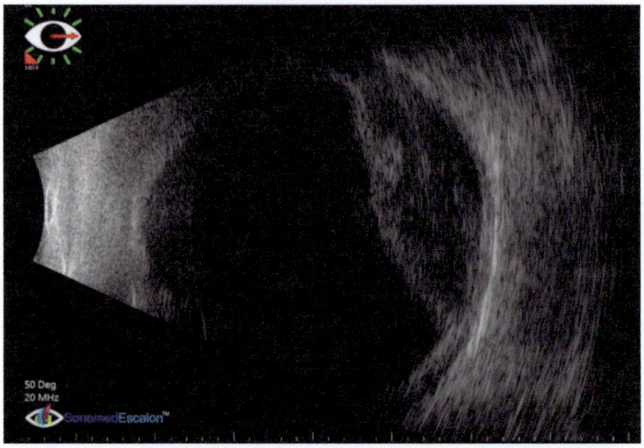

Fig. 18.4 B-scan ultrasound of the left eye on post-operative day 1, confirming the choroidal hemorrhages first seen on CT scan. The retina is attached

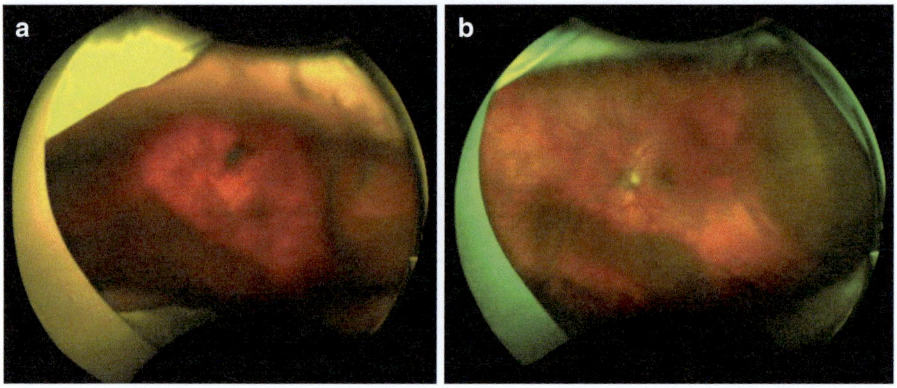

Fig. 18.5 (**a**) Optos fundus photograph of the left eye on post-operative week 1 demonstrating the 360° shallow peripheral choroidal hemorrhages. (**b**) Optos fundus photograph of the left eye on post-operative week 5 demonstrating significant improvement of choroidal hemorrhages with conservative management

breaks or detachments (Fig. 18.5). Given the significant improvement in vision and the peripheral location of the choroidal hemorrhages, close monitoring was recommended. Over the subsequent months, the choroidal hemorrhages slowly resolved without need for surgical intervention.

18.6 Final Trauma Evaluation

18.6.1 Final Visual Acuity

OD: 20/100, pinhole 20/20-1 sc
OS: 20/50-2 pinhole 20/25-2

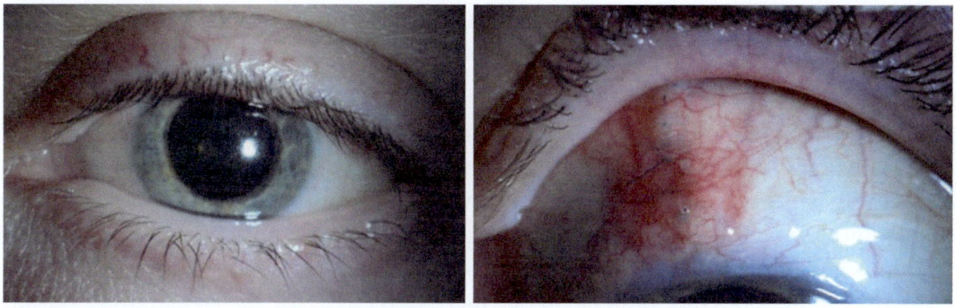

Fig. 18.6 Follow up slit lamp photographs demonstrating a well-healed scleral laceration with mild injection in the area due to exposed nylon sutures tails that required trimming

18.6.2 Pupils

OD: No afferent pupillary defect
OS: No afferent pupillary defect by reverse

18.6.3 Slit Lamp Examination

	OD	OS
Lids and lashes	Normal	Normal
Sclera and conjunctiva	Normal	Conjunctival laceration healed. Nylon sutures noted below the healed corneal laceration superiorly. A suture tail was exposed requiring trimming (Fig. 18.6)
Cornea	Normal	Normal
Anterior chamber	Normal	Normal
Iris	Normal	Normal
Lens	Normal	Cortical spokes
Vitreous	Normal	Old vitreous hemorrhage

18.6.5 Dilated Examination

Macula/Nerve OD: Normal
Periphery OD: Normal
Macula/Nerve: OS: Normal
Periphery OS: Small residual temporal peripheral choroidal hemorrhage

18.7 Review and Lessons Learned

Zone II/III open globe injuries often have poor final visual outcomes, largely because many of them are the result of blunt ocular injury with significant extrusion of intraocular contents and retinal detachment; however, anterior scleral lacerations from sharp objects, such as a sharp cat claw, may have a very good visual outcome, as seen in our patient. Sharp scleral lacerations may have minimal uveal or vitreous prolapse and if closed carefully, can lead to minimal disruption of the intraocular contents. However, the patient is at increased risk for post-operative retinal detachment and has a high likelihood of needing additional surgeries, so it is important to inform the patient of these risks.

Like many patients with Zone II/II open globe injuries, this patient had choroidal hemorrhages. In her case they were present 360° and were shallow. The management of choroidal hemorrhages is a subject of debate [1], without clearly defined guidelines as to when to intervene. In general the approach is conservative, especially for small choroidal hemorrhages, with observation recommended initially, as choroidal hemorrhages often slowly spontaneously resolve. Fortunately, our patient's choroidal hemorrhages resolved without need for surgical intervention and with a great final visual acuity.

At times, choroidal hemorrhages may need to be evacuated because of their effects on visual acuity or because of the development of retinal traction and detachments. When choroidal hemorrhages resorb, the vitreous may remain in a contracted state, predisposing to vitreous traction on the retina and retinal detachment. In such situations, pars plana vitrectomy is needed to release traction [1]. Blood from choroidal hemorrhages may be drained through the same incisions that are made to insert the trochars for vitrectomy avoiding the need for separate sclerotomies. Choroidal hemorrhages are usually evacuated after 2–3 weeks, because the clotted blood needs to liquify somewhat before it can be removed.

There are a limited number of studies in the literature pertaining to suprachoroidal hemorrhages. One study in 1993 from Bascom Palmer reviewed all suprachoroidal hemorrhages that presented within a 10 year period and were followed for at least 3 months [2]. In total, 106 cases were identified, of which the largest number, 35 (33%), were in the setting of trauma. Of the patients with trauma, the majority, 33 cases, were in the setting of sharp trauma, while only 2 were in the setting of blunt trauma. Overall features in this series that correlated with poor visual outcome were co-existence of a retinal detachment on presentation and 360° (or four quadrant) hemorrhages [2]. There was no difference in outcomes among patients with and without "kissing" choroidal hemorrhages, although patients with "kissing" suprachoroidal hemorrhages underwent secondary drainage of hemorrhages at a much higher rate (65%) than those without "kissing" hemorrhages (33%). Of patients with hemorrhages presenting secondary to trauma, the majority (25 out of 35) had surgical closure of their traumatic wound and observation of the hemorrhages, no patients had a primary sclerotomy for drainage at the time of presentation, only one patient underwent sclerotomy for drainage at a later time, while nine patients underwent a later pars plana vitrectomy with or without a scleral buckle.

A more recent retrospective study was performed at Mass Eye and Ear in 2014 examining the accuracy of B-scan ultrasonography in patients with open globe injury [3]. Of 965 open globes over a 10 year period, 210 underwent B-scan ultrasonography. Of these 210 open globes, 37 (18%) had hemorrhagic choroidal detachments, and 7 (3%) had kissing choroidals on the initial B-scan study [3]. Of the 37 patients with hemorrhagic choroidal detachments, 19 (51%) underwent some type of retinal surgery at a later point. In those 19 cases, the hemorrhagic choroidal detachment was confirmed intraoperatively in 8 cases, but not in the other 11. This discrepancy in clinical and B-scan diagnosis may in part be due to resolution of choroidal detachment between the time of B-scan and the time of surgery, particularly since B-scan ultrasonography was extremely accurate in diagnosing other pathology, such as retinal detachment (100%) and intraocular foreign bodies (100%). Although this study does not focus on the management of choroidal hemorrhages in patients with open globe injuries, it does conclude that choroidal hemorrhages and kissing choroidals are both significant predictors of poor final visual outcome [3].

18.8 Key Learning Points

- B-scan ultrasound should be performed on post-operative day one on all patients without an adequate view of the posterior segment to assess for retinal detachment and choroidal hemorrhages.
- Shallow choroidal hemorrhages may be monitored, very large choroidal hemorrhages may need to be drained.
- Zone II/III laceration-type injuries may have better final visual outcome than blunt ruptures where there is a greater chance of expulsion of intraocular contents.

References

1. Charles S, Calzada J, Wood B. Chapter 30: Management of suprachoroidal hemorrhage. In: Vitreous microsurgery. 5th ed. Philadelphia: Lippincott Williams and Wilkins; 2011. p. 241–24.
2. Reynolds MG, Haimovici R, Flynn HW Jr, DiBernardo C, Byrne SF, Feuer W. Suprachoroidal hemorrhage. Clinical features and results of secondary surgical management. Ophthalmology. 1993;100(4):460–5.
3. Andreoli MT, Yiu G, Hart L, Andreoli CM. B-scan ultrasonography following open globe repair. Eye (Lond). 2014;28(4):381–5.

Chapter 19
Case 14: Penetrating Zone II/III Open Globe Injury from a Knife

Durga S. Borkar, Dean Eliott, and Seanna Grob

19.1 History of Present Illness

A 31-year-old man with no past ocular history presents with an open globe injury of the left eye.

- The patient reports he was on a fishing trip with his friends and struck his left eye with a fishing knife while trying to cut a zip tie.
- He was seen at an outside hospital and computed tomography (CT) imaging was consistent with an open globe injury of the left eye. After receiving intravenous vancomycin and ceftazidime as well as a tetanus booster, he was transferred to Massachusetts Eye and Ear (MEE) for further evaluation.

19.2 Initial Trauma Evaluation

19.2.1 Visual Acuity (Without Correction)

OD: 20/20
OS: 20/100

Electronic Supplementary Material The online version of this chapter (https://doi.org/10.1007/978-3-319-72410-2_19) contains supplementary material, which is available to authorized users.

D. S. Borkar, M.D. (✉) • S. Grob, M.D., M.A.S.
Department of Ophthalmology, Harvard Medical School, Massachusetts Eye and Ear, Boston, MA, USA
e-mail: durga_borkar@meei.harvard.edu

D. Eliott, M.D.
Vitreoretinal Surgery, Department of Ophthalmology, Harvard Medical School, Massachusetts Eye and Ear, Boston, MA, USA

S. Grob, C. Kloek (eds.), *Management of Open Globe Injuries*,
https://doi.org/10.1007/978-3-319-72410-2_19

19.2.2 Pupils

OD: No afferent pupillary defect
OS: No afferent pupillary defect

19.2.3 External Examination

Within normal limits bilaterally

19.2.4 Slit Lamp Examination (Left Eye)

	OD	OS
Lids and lashes	Normal	Periorbital dried sanguinous secretions; no lid lacerations
Sclera and conjunctiva	Normal	Curvilinear Zone II/III laceration starting near 6 o'clock at the limbus and extending inferiorly with uveal and vitreous prolapse
Cornea	Normal	Edema and inferior Descemet's folds
Anterior chamber	Normal	Shallow
Iris	Normal	Inferior iris defect prolapsing to laceration
Lens	Normal	Normal
Vitreous	Normal	Vitreous hemorrhage

19.2.5 Dilated Examination

Macula/Nerve OD: Normal
Periphery OD: Normal
Macula/Nerve: OS: Hazy view
Periphery OS: Poor view, grossly attached

19.2.6 Radiographic Imaging

Noncontrast CT of the orbits (Fig. 19.1) showed abnormal contour of the left globe without intraocular foreign body. No orbital fractures were noted.

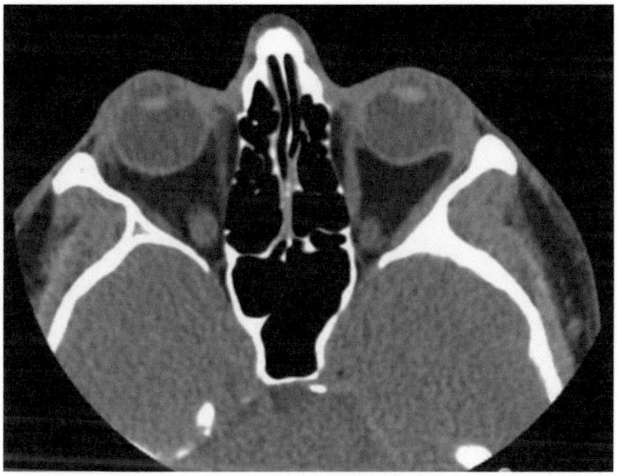

Fig. 19.1 Axial CT image showing a normal globe on the right and a deformed globe on the left with no evidence of intraocular foreign body

19.3 Surgeon's Initial Assessment and Pre-operative Plan

The patient had a Zone II/III open globe injury of the left eye requiring surgical repair.

This case illustrates a few important areas of discussion beyond the standard repair of a Zone II/III laceration. These are: the importance of a thorough posterior segment exam on presentation to evaluate for a posterior strike site, exit wound, or choroidal rupture in the case of a penetrating injury and additional planning to prevent uveal or vitreous incarceration in penetrating injuries with significant uveal or vitreous prolapse.

In this case, a thorough posterior exam was performed but the view was slightly limited by vitreous hemorrhage. This may often be the case and illustrates the need for careful serial exams post-operatively in conjunction with a retina specialist as needed to evaluate for retinal pathology. Additionally, a CT scan is imperative to rule out an intraocular foreign body in the case of a penetrating injury with limited view posteriorly on presentation.

For many Zone II/III injuries, significant vitreous and uveal prolapse may be present. Performing a limited Wek-cel vitrectomy early in the case prior to wound closure can be helpful to prevent vitreous incarceration in the wound. Furthermore, the use of a surgical assistant to reposit prolapsed uveal tissure with an iris spatula can be helpful while suturing the wound closed to prevent uveal incarceration.

19.4 Surgical Exploration and Repair: Operative Note

The risks, benefits, and alternatives were discussed with the patient pre-operatively and the patient consented to proceed with exploration and repair of the open globe injury. The patient was brought to the operating room where the anesthesia team

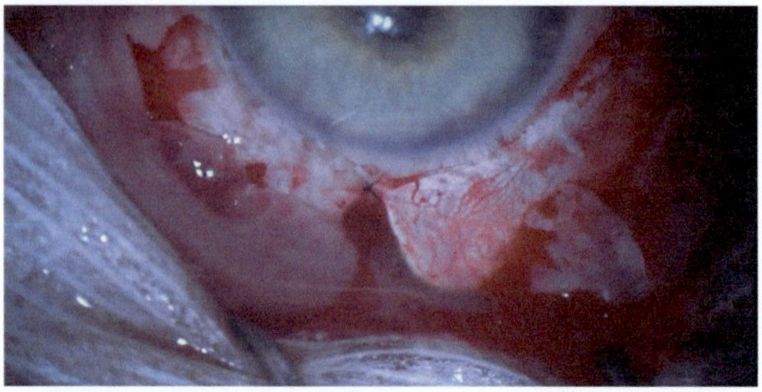

Fig. 19.2 An intraoperative photo after an initial inferior 180° peritomy was performed showing an approximately 11–12 mm full-thickness curvilinear scleral laceration with vitreous and uveal prolapse starting just below the limbus inferiorly at 6 o'clock and extending temporally and inferiorly into the inferotemporal quadrant

proceeded with general anesthesia. A careful time-out was observed, and the correct patient and eye were identified. The left eye was prepped and draped in the usual sterile ophthalmic fashion using a Jaffe speculum to provide adequate exposure.

An inferior 180° peritomy was initiated with relaxing incisions at 3 and 9 o'clock. Gentle exploration with blunt dissection into the inferior quadrants was performed with blunt Westcott scissors. The patient was found to have an approximately 11–12 mm full-thickness curvilinear scleral laceration with vitreous and uveal prolapse starting just below the limbus inferiorly at 6 o'clock and extending temporally and inferiorly into the inferotemporal quadrant (Fig. 19.2). A gentle Wek-Cel vitrectomy was performed prior to wound closure due to the presence of significant vitreous prolapse. An iris spatula was used during closure of the laceration to prevent incarceration of uvea into the scleral laceration. The laceration was closed with 11 interrupted 8-0 nylon sutures. Further exploration was then completed to ensure the full extent of the laceration was identified and closed.

The conjunctiva was then closed with multiple interrupted 8-0 Vicryl sutures. A subconjunctival steroid and antibiotic injection was performed superotemporally away from the laceration. The speculum and patient's drape were removed under the microscope. Atropine and neomycin and polymyxin B sulfates and dexamethasone ophthalmic ointment were placed in the left eye. A sterile pad and shield were placed over the left eye. The patient tolerated the procedure well without any complications.

19.4.1 Surgical Exploration and Repair: Pearls

- In Zone II/III lacerations with significant vitreous prolapse, a Wek-Cel vitrectomy performed prior to wound closure is useful to prevent vitreous incarceration. Take care to not pull on vitreous.

- For lacerations with significant uveal prolapse, an assistant can use an iris spatula during closure of the scleral laceration to prevent uveal incarceration.
- Place partial thickness sutures, typically 8-0 nylon, approximately 1 mm apart for closure of a scleral laceration.

19.4.2 Surgical Video

Please see Video 19.1

19.5 Post-operative Course

The patient was admitted to MEE to complete a 48 hour course of intravenous antibiotics. On post-operative day one, his vision was 20/100 pinholing to 20/40 in the left eye with a 1 mm hyphema. On fundus exam, there was concern for possible retinal detachment or retinal incarceration inferotemporally in the area of the Zone II/III laceration. However, the view was limited secondary to vitreous hemorrhage.

A retina consultation was performed on post-operative day one. Fundus examination revealed a likely peripheral choroidal rupture inferiorly, and B scan confirmed an attached retina. Close observation was recommended. The patient was discharged on atropine twice a day, prednisolone acetate six times a day, and gatifloxacin four times a day in the operative eye.

The patient was seen in follow up on post-operative day three and week two by the retina service and confirmed to have a likely choroidal rupture in the inferior periphery (Fig. 19.3) with improved vitreous hemorrhage. By post-operative week two, his vision had improved to 20/40 pinholing to 20/25 in the operative eye. The

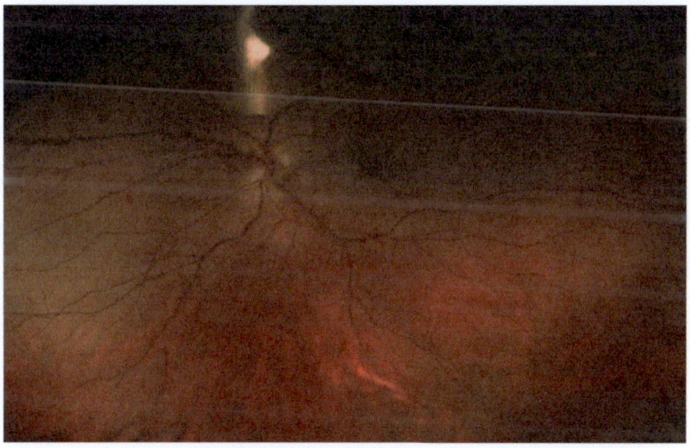

Fig. 19.3 A wide field fundus photo of the left eye at post-operative week two showing two curvilinear areas in the inferior periphery concerning for a peripheral choroidal rupture

patient was counseled on the need for regular monitoring by a retina specialist to monitor for possible development of choroidal neovascularization or retinal detachment.

A final trauma service examination was performed at post-operative month one. At this time, his vision was stable at 20/40 pinholing to 20/25 in the operative eye. Slit lamp examination revealed resolution of the hyphema noted on post-operative day one. There was some irregularity of the conjunctiva inferiorly. The fundus exam remained stable. The patient had been visiting from out of town at the time of his injury and further follow up arrangements were made for him closer to home.

19.6 Final Trauma Evaluation

19.6.1 Final Visual Acuity

OD: 20/20
OS: 20/40 pinhole 20/25

19.6.2 Pupils

OD: Round, no afferent pupillary defect
OS: Round, no afferent pupillary defect

19.6.3 Slit Lamp Examination

	OD	OS
Lids and lashes	Normal	Normal
Sclera and conjunctiva	Normal	Vicryl sutures nasally, inferiorly, and temporally. Trace chemosis in these areas with some irregularity of the conjunctiva inferiorly
Cornea	Normal	Clear
Anterior chamber	Normal	No cell
Iris	Normal	Normal
Lens	Normal	Possible area of opacification inferiorly posterior to iris
Vitreous	Normal	Normal

19.6.4 Dilated Examination

Macula/Nerve OD: Normal
Periphery OD: Not dilated, previously normal
Macula/Nerve: OS: Normal
Peripheral OS: Two inferior arcuate white lines, no retinal tear or detachment

19.7 Review and Lessons Learned

In penetrating injuries, there is often vitreous hemorrhage present. However, it is important to perform a thorough posterior exam on presentation whenever possible to look for a posterior strike site or exit wound. Additionally, the use of CT imaging is especially imperative in these cases to rule out the presence of an intraocular foreign body.

In cases that present with a Zone II/III laceration, there can be significant vitreous and uveal prolapse. Wek-cel vitrectomy can be helpful to ensure there is no vitreous incarceration in the wound. Additionally, the use of an iris spatula by the surgical assistant to reposit prolapsed uvea while the surgeon is suturing can be helpful to prevent uveal incarceration in the wound.

While Zone II/III penetrating lacerations present with significant pathology, these cases can often have good visual outcomes if the laceration remains peripheral without significant damage to the retina or a subsequent retinal detachment. Studies have shown that penetrating Zone III injuries can often have better visual outcomes than posterior injuries due to blunt trauma [1, 2].

In this case, the patient was noted to also have an associated peripheral choroidal rupture. Although the choroidal rupture did not have a significant impact on the patient's visual outcome because of the peripheral location of the rupture, he was advised to have close follow up to monitor for complications including choroidal neovascularization and retinal detachment. In a series of patients with choroidal rupture from either closed or open globe trauma, the incidence of choroidal neovascularization was 11% and the incidence of retinal detachment was 14% [3].

19.8 Key Learning Points

- Penetrating injuries and lacerations can often have better visual outcomes than injuries from blunt trauma.

- Although many cases of penetrating trauma may be complicated by vitreous hemorrhage, it is important to do a thorough posterior exam when possible to evaluate for a strike site or exit wound.
- Associated choroidal rupture may occur in patients with significant penetrating injuries; however, choroidal rupture may not have a significant impact on the final visual acuity if it is peripheral.

References

1. Agrawal R, Ho SW, Teoh S. Pre-operative variables affecting final vision outcome with a critical review of ocular trauma classification for posterior open globe (Zone III) injury. Indian J Ophthalmol. 2013;61(10):541–5.
2. Rahman I, Maino A, Devadason D, Leatherbarrow B. Open globe injuries: factors predictive of poor outcome. Eye (Lond). 2006;20(12):1336–41.
3. Ament CS, Zacks DN, Lane AM, et al. Predictors of visual outcome and choroidal neovascular membrane formation after traumatic choroidal rupture. Arch Ophthalmol. 2006;124(7):957–66.

Chapter 20
Case 15: Zone II/III Open Globe due to Stab Wound from Knife Assault During Intimate Partner Violence

Tavé van Zyl, Demetrios Vavvas, and Seanna Grob

20.1 History of Present Illness

A healthy woman in her 40s with no prior ocular history was transported by ambulance to Massachusetts General Hospital after a domestic partner assault with a knife, during which she sustained multiple facial, chest, and back lacerations.

- The patient reported blurry vision and pain in the left eye.
- Computed tomography (CT) imaging of the orbits raised concern for an open globe injury of the left eye with associated vitreous hemorrhage.
- Ophthalmology service was consulted.

20.2 Initial Trauma Evaluation

20.2.1 Visual Acuity (Without Correction)

OD: 20/20
OS: Count Fingers at 2 feet

T. van Zyl, M.D. (✉) • D. Vavvas, M.D., Ph.D. • S. Grob, M.D., M.A.S.
Department of Ophthalmology, Harvard Medical School, Massachusetts Eye and Ear, Boston, MA, USA
e-mail: tave_vanzyl@meei.harvard.edu

S. Grob, C. Kloek (eds.), *Management of Open Globe Injuries*,
https://doi.org/10.1007/978-3-319-72410-2_20

20.2.2 Pupils

OD: 3 mm
OS: 3.5 mm irregular, peaked and displaced superonasally, poorly reactive
No afferent pupillary defect by reverse

20.2.3 Intraocular Pressure (Tonopen)

OD: 22 mmHg
OS: Deferred

20.2.4 External Examination

4.5 cm laceration above left brow, 1 cm laceration on chin sutured by primary trauma team

20.2.5 Slit Lamp Examination

	OD	OS
Lids and lashes	Normal	Periorbital ecchymosis and edema
Sclera and conjunctiva	Normal	Patchy slightly raised subconjunctival hemorrhage almost 360°
Cornea	Normal	Normal, no epithelial defects or lacerations
Anterior chamber	Normal	Deep compared to fellow eye Small amount of heme resting on iris, no layering hyphema (patient supine)
Iris	Normal	As above, peaked superonasally
Lens	Normal	Normal
Vitreous	Normal	1+ vitreous heme

20.2.6 Dilated Examination

Macula/Nerve OD: Flat, normal
Periphery OD: Attached, normal
Macula/Nerve: OS: Hazy view due to vitreous hemorrhage, macula possibly detached
Periphery OS: Hazy view, bullous elevation temporally, superiorly and nasally suspicious for retinal detachment

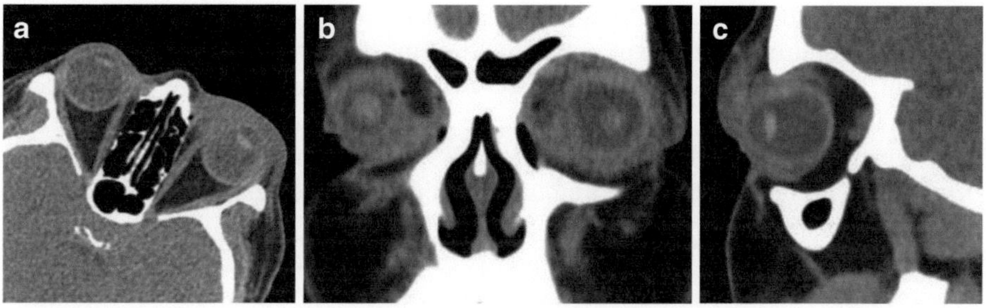

Fig. 20.1 Pre-operative CT orbits. Axial CT images showed deepening of the left anterior chamber relative to the right (**a**); coronal CT images showed irregular globe contour nasally with preseptal soft tissue swelling (**b**); sagittal CT images showed flattening of the left globe superiorly (**c**)

20.2.7 Radiographic Imaging

CT of the orbits showed intact orbital rims without evidence of fracture. The left anterior chamber was deepened, with layering hyperdense material along the temporal and posterior aspects of the left vitreous body. On sagittal CT images, the left globe had a somewhat flattened appearance relative to the right. There was extensive soft tissue swelling along the left prefrontal scalp extending to the left preseptal region. There was no intraocular foreign body (Fig. 20.1).

20.3 Surgeon's Initial Assessment and Pre-operative Plan

The patient had acutely decreased vision in the left eye, patchy flat subconjunctival hemorrhage extending 360°, a deepened anterior chamber, a peaked pupil, vitreous hemorrhage and a deep laceration above the brow on the ipsilateral side. She denied any blunt trauma to the eye. Together with CT imaging revealing an irregular globe contour, these historical and physical exam findings raised concern for a posterior penetrating open globe injury requiring exploration.

20.4 Surgical Exploration and Repair: Operative Note

The risks, benefits, and alternatives were discussed with the patient pre-operatively and the patient consented to proceed with exploration and repair of the open globe injury and repair of the brow laceration. The patient was brought to the operating room where the anesthesia team proceeded with general anesthesia. A careful timeout was observed and the correct patient and eye were identified. The left eye was prepped and draped in the usual sterile ophthalmic fashion using a Jaffe speculum to provide adequate exposure.

A limited 120° peritomy was initiated nasally and superiorly in the area of suspected rupture. Gentle exploration with blunt dissection into the superonasal quadrant was performed with Westcott scissors followed by Stevens tenotomy scissors to assess the injury and evaluate the extent of posterior eye trauma.

The patient was found to have an oblique, 15 mm full-thickness scleral laceration beginning 3 mm posterior to the limbus at 10 o'clock and extending posteriorly and nasally (Fig. 20.2). The posterior two-thirds of the wound was found to run adjacent to the superior border of the medial rectus muscle. There was vitreous and uveal tissue prolapse notable more anteriorly and superiorly in the wound, but minimal prolapse was noted posteriorly. The medial rectus muscle was isolated with a muscle hook, inspected and confirmed to be uninjured. The scleral laceration was carefully closed with multiple 8-0 nylon sutures placed in an interrupted fashion. An iris spatula was used to keep vitreous and uveal tissue out of the wound edges during closure. Care was also taken to avoid damage to the medial rectus muscle.

The conjunctiva was then closed with interrupted 8-0 Vicryl sutures. A subconjunctival steroid and antibiotic injection was performed nasally away from the laceration. The speculum was removed.

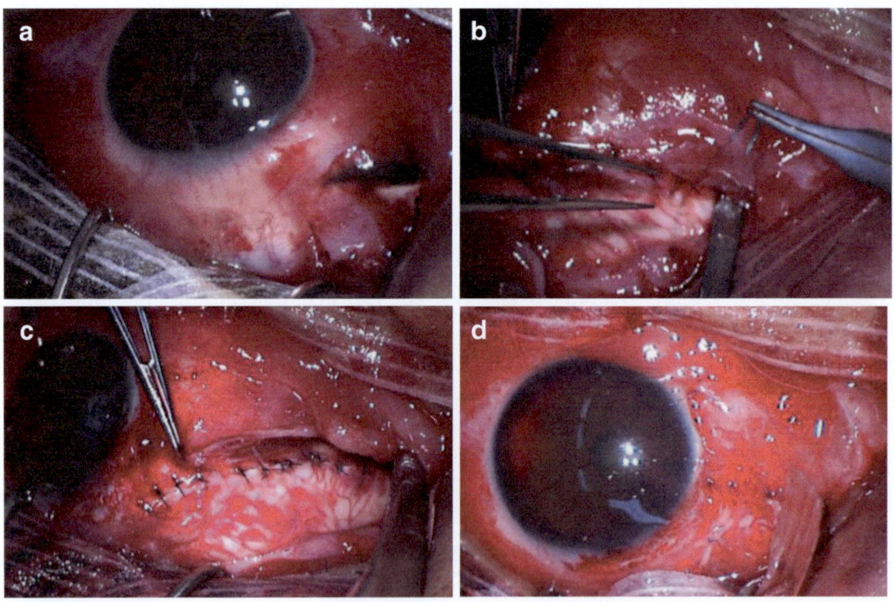

Fig. 20.2 Intraoperative photos of open globe repair. Gentle infraduction with a 0.12 forceps revealed the full-thickness scleral laceration with vitreous and uveal tissue prolapse superonasally (**a**). An iris spatula prevented incarceration of uveal tissue in the wound while suturing; the medial rectus muscle ran parallel to the wound and was carefully avoided (**b**). The wound measured approximately 15 mm (**c**). Once the scleral wound was repaired, the conjunctiva was closed with interrupted 8-0 Vicryl sutures (**d**)

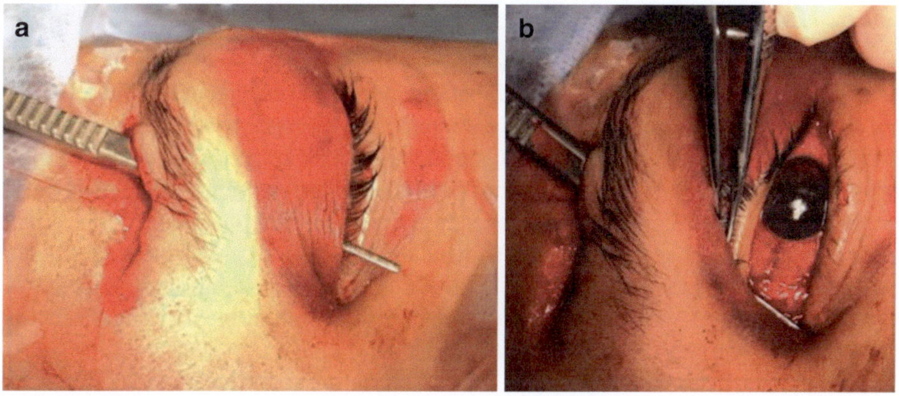

Fig. 20.3 Intraoperative examination revealed that the supra-brow stab wound communicated with the periocular space and likely represented the initial entry site (**a**, **b**). There was no injury to the lid margin or canalicular system

Attention was then turned to the left brow laceration. It was inspected and found to communicate with the left periocular space and likely represented the entrance wound to the scleral laceration (Fig. 20.3). The wound was closed with three interrupted 5-0 Vicryl deep sutures followed by multiple interrupted 5-0 nylon sutures to approximate the skin edges.

The patient's drape was removed under the microscope. A steroid-antibiotic ophthalmic ointment and atropine drops were applied to the eye followed by a sterile soft patch and protective shield. Bacitracin ointment was applied to the brow laceration. The patient was extubated in the operating room and tolerated the procedure well without any complications.

20.4.1 Surgical Exploration and Repair: Pearls

- Eyes with signs of posterior rupture should be gently but thoroughly explored in the operating room.
- Cautious mobilization of the globe using 0.12 forceps by an assistant can allow for improved exposure of the wound. Care must be taken to avoid undue pressure on the globe, which may lead to further extrusion of intraocular contents and increased risk of uveal tissue incarceration.
- Extraocular muscles residing in the vicinity of the wound should be identified, inspected for injury, and avoided during surgical repair of the sclera.

20.5 Post-operative Course

The patient remained admitted as an inpatient at MGH to complete a 48 hour course of intravenous antibiotics and receive support and referrals to social services and Intimate Partner Violence resources. On post-operative day one she had hand motion vision, with a hazy view to the posterior pole due to vitreous hemorrhage. Binocular indirect ophthalmoscopy revealed elevations in the retina suspicious for retinal detachment and a B-scan ultrasound showed multiple membranous interfaces noted within the vitreous cavity with points of attachment to the posterior pole (Fig. 20.4). Noted superonasal was a shallow elevation of a membrane extending from the peripapillary region to the posterior pole.

The patient was evaluated by the retina service on post-operative day 4 and on post-operative day 7 she underwent 23-gauge pars plana vitrectomy. Intraoperatively, upon clearance of the vitreous hemorrhage, the retina was found to be attached. Thorough scleral depressed examination confirmed that there were no retinal breaks besides the injury-related chorioretinal scar in the superonasal quadrant and a nearby area of subretinal hemorrhage extending inferiorly.

The patient was followed closely by the retina and trauma services over the following weeks. The subretinal hemorrhage slowly resolved revealing a choroidal rupture site superonasally (Fig. 20.5). The retina remained attached. At her most recent follow-up visit, 7 months after the injury, her best-corrected visual acuity was 20/25+ and her retina was attached without signs of overt proliferative

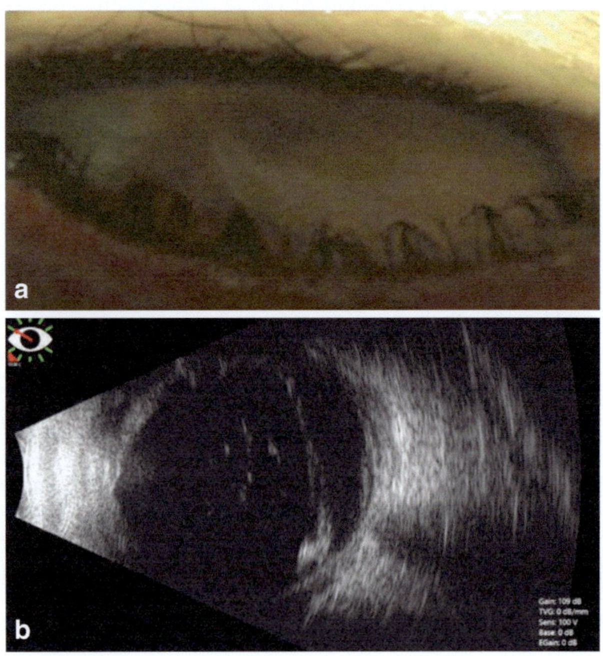

Fig. 20.4 Post-op day 3 after open globe repair. Dilated exam was hazy due to vitreous hemorrhage but showed membranous elevations supero-nasally and super-temporally suspicious for macula-involving retinal detachment (**a**). B-scan showed multiple membranous interfaces within the vitreous cavity with points of attachment to the posterior pole (**b**)

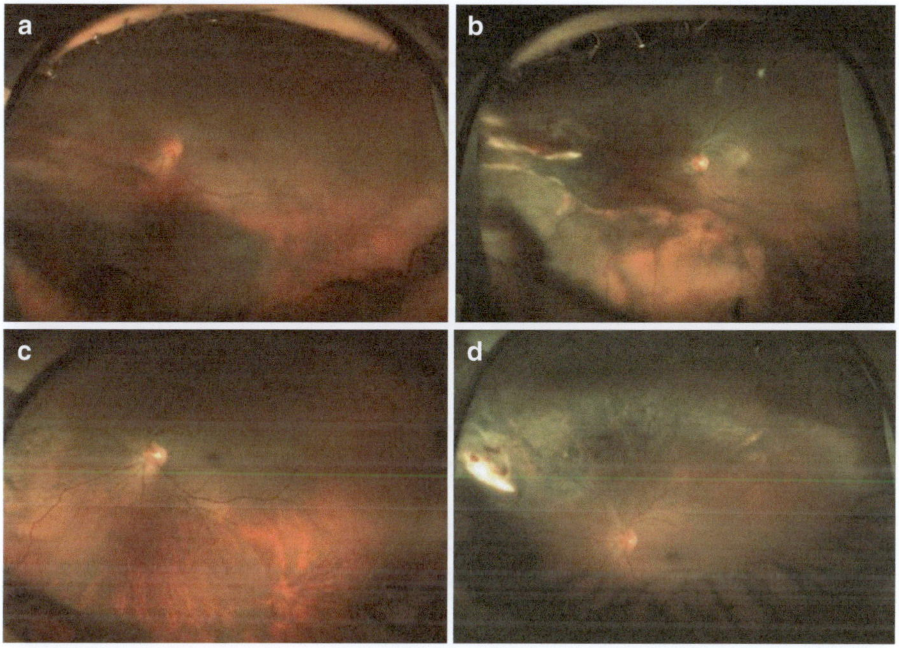

Fig. 20.5 Post-operative resolution of subretinal hemorrhage. Following clearance of vitreous hemorrhage after 23-gauge pars plana vitrectomy, a large subretinal hemorrhage was monitored. Widefield fundus photo on post-operative day 1 (**a**); post-operative week 6 (**b**); and post-operative week 9 (**c**, **d**)

vitreoretinopathy (PVR). She will continue to be followed closely by the retina service as she remains at high risk for retinal detachment [1].

20.6 Final Trauma Evaluation

20.6.1 Final Visual Acuity

OD: 20/20
OS: 20/30 pinhole 20/25

20.6.2 Refraction

OD	−0.25 − 0.25 × 105	20/20
OS	Plano − 1.25 × 145	20/25+

20.6.3 Pupils

OD: 4 mm, round
OS: 4 mm, round, slightly irregular, reactive, no afferent pupillary defect

20.6.4 Slit Lamp Examination

	OD	OS
Lids and lashes	Normal	Normal
Sclera and conjunctiva	Normal	Superonasal scleral nylon sutures in place; covered by conjunctiva
Cornea	Normal	Normal
Anterior chamber	Normal	Normal
Iris	Normal	Normal
Lens	Normal	1+ nuclear sclerosis with diffuse 2+ posterior subcapsular cataract
Vitreous	Normal	Status post pars plana vitrectomy

20.6.5 Dilated Examination

Macula/Nerve OD: Flat, normal
Periphery OD: Attached, normal
Macula/Nerve: OS: Flat, normal
Periphery OS: Choroidal rupture site nasally with scarring, resolved subretinal heme

20.7 Review and Lessons Learned

This case demonstrates several important aspects of the clinical exam that must be considered when evaluating for presence of an open globe injury (OGI). Even if no lacerations or ruptures are immediately visible on clinical examination, suspect a posterior OGI if the eye in question has a markedly deeper anterior chamber compared to the fellow eye (taking into account the lens status), or a peaked pupil, as was noted in this case. Intraocular pressure should not be used as an indicator of OGI as eyes with posterior OGI may have a normal (even raised) intraocular pressure. Vitreous hemorrhage, although not sufficient evidence in itself, can serve as another clue that the globe has been penetrated. Finally, nearby lacerations in the setting of a knife attack should also raise concern for penetrating ocular injury.

This case also demonstrates that incomplete detachment of the posterior hyaloid interface in the setting of vitreous hemorrhage can give the appearance of retinal detachment both ultrasonographically and clinically. During the vitrectomy, care was taken not to disturb the injured retina at the site of the scleral laceration. Most of the success in this case should be attributed to the careful closure without much traction during the primary repair. Subsequent to the vitrectomy, careful frequent monitoring should be employed because patients are high risk for PVR and retinal detachment. If visualization is difficult, B-scans should be utilized; however, they should be interpreted cautiously. Repeat examinations in short term intervals to reveal changes may be a preferred first option instead of surgery.

Studies have demonstrated that penetrating OGI are generally associated with more favorable outcomes as compared to blunt ruptures and this case is aligned with these findings [2]. This patient will require close follow-up nonetheless, as she remains at high risk for retinal detachment [1].

Intimate partner violence (IPV) is a major public health issue. Several studies have identified the head, neck, and face (including the eyes) as the most common sites of IPV-associated injury and ophthalmologists should therefore maintain a high degree of suspicion for IPV when caring for patients presenting with ocular injuries without a well-defined mechanism (e.g. motor vehicle collision) [3, 4]. If IPV is suspected or confirmed, referral to appropriate services prior to discharge from the medical facility is essential, as is careful documentation often including photographic evidence. Services to consider include social work, psychiatry, psychology, counseling services, law enforcement, local agencies (e.g., women's shelters), and the National Domestic Abuse Hotline (1-800-799-SAFE).

20.8 Key Learning Points

- A deepened anterior chamber on slit lamp exam and/or CT imaging when compared with fellow eye can suggest a posterior (Zone II or III) open globe injury.
  - *Caveat: account for the lens status of each eye.*
- A peaked or corectopic pupil will often "point" to the location of an occult scleral defect.
- Sharp, penetrating OGI (e.g. knife wounds) without IOFB often carry a more favorable prognosis compared to blunt ruptures, even if posterior in location.
  - *These patients still require careful, frequent monitoring as they remain at high risk for PVR and retinal detachment.*
- Victims of IPV require not only management of their immediate injuries but also support and referral to intimate partner violence resources prior to discharge from the medical facility.

References

1. Brodowska K, Stryjewski TP, Papavasileiou E, Chee YE, Eliott D. Validation of the retinal detachment after open globe injury (RD-OGI) score as an effective tool for predicting retinal detachment. Ophthalmology. 2017;124(5):674–8. https://doi.org/10.1016/j.ophtha.2016.12.032.
2. Rahman I, Maino A, Devadason D, Leatherbarrow B. Open globe injuries: factors predictive of poor outcome. Eye (Lond). 2005;20(12):1336–41. https://doi.org/10.1038/sj.eye.6702099.
3. Beck SR, Freitag SK, Singer N. Ocular injuries in battered women. Ophthalmology. 1996; 103(1):148–51. https://doi.org/10.1016/S0161-6420(96)30748-3.
4. Clark TJ, Renner LM, Sobel RK, et al. Intimate partner violence: an underappreciated etiology of orbital floor fractures. Ophthalmic Plast Reconstr Surg. 2014;30(6):508–11. https://doi.org/10.1097/IOP.0000000000000165.

Chapter 21
Case 16: Zone I/II/III Open Globe Injury with Retinal Strike Site and Post-operative Strabismus

Benjamin Jastrzembski, Katherine E. Talcott, Seanna Grob, Dean Eliott, and Ankoor S. Shah

21.1 History of Present Illness

An otherwise healthy 13-year-old boy presents with concern for an open globe injury of the left eye.

- The patient reported he was at camp and was using a pocket knife to cut zip ties. The knife slipped and penetrated his left eye with immediate pain and decreased vision.
- He was seen at an outside hospital, where intravenous (IV) antibiotics were started and computed tomography (CT) imaging of the orbits was obtained. He was then transferred to Massachusetts Eye & Ear (MEE) for further care.

21.2 Initial Trauma Evaluation

21.2.1 Visual Acuity (Without Correction)

OD: 20/30
OS: Hand motion

B. Jastrzembski, M.D. (✉) • S. Grob, M.D., M.A.S.
Department of Ophthalmology, Harvard Medical School, Massachusetts Eye and Ear, Boston, MA, USA
e-mail: Benjamin_jastrzembski@meei.harvard.edu

K. E. Talcott, M.D.
Vitreoretinal Surgery, Wills Eye Hospital, Philadelphia, PA, USA

D. Eliott, M.D.
Vitreoretinal Surgery, Department of Ophthalmology, Harvard Medical School, Massachusetts Eye and Ear, Boston, MA, USA

A. S. Shah, M.D., Ph.D.
Department of Ophthalmology, Harvard Medical School, Boston Children's Hospital and Massachusetts Eye and Ear, Boston, MA, USA

S. Grob, C. Kloek (eds.), *Management of Open Globe Injuries*,
https://doi.org/10.1007/978-3-319-72410-2_21

21.2.2 Pupils

OD: Round and reactive
OS: Inferior peaking, no afferent pupillary defect by reverse testing

21.2.3 External Examination

Normal, no lacerations

21.2.4 Slit Lamp Examination

	OD	OS
Lids and lashes	Normal	Normal
Sclera and conjunctiva	Normal	2+ injection
Cornea	Normal	8 mm, inferior nasal, linear laceration starting at 9 o'clock and extending 3 mm onto the inferior sclera at 6 o'clock with uveal prolapse from wound
Anterior chamber	Normal	Shallow with small layered hyphema
Iris	Normal	Iris prolapse from wound inferiorly
Lens	Normal	Anterior displacement of the lens with difficult view secondary to hyphema
Vitreous	Normal	No view

21.2.5 Dilated Examination

Macula/Nerve OD: Normal
Periphery OD: Normal
Macula/Nerve: OS: No view
Periphery OS: No view

21.2.6 Radiographic Imaging

CT of the orbits showed a deformity of the left globe contour with a small amount of vitreous hemorrhage. There was mild asymmetric soft tissue attenuation in the region of the left inferior rectus muscle that was thought to represent a small amount of hemorrhage. No fracture or foreign body was seen (Fig. 21.1).

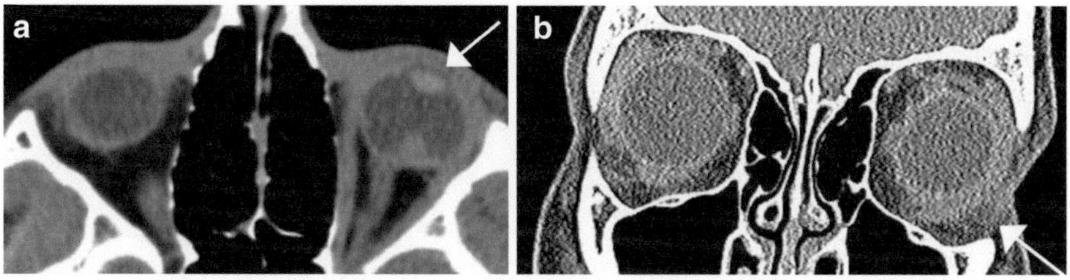

Fig. 21.1 Axial (**a**) and coronal (**b**) CT images showing a normal globe on the right and signs concerning for an open globe injury on the left side. There is intraocular hemorrhage and irregularity of the scleral contour with mild soft tissue attenuation in the region of the left inferior rectus that may represent hemorrhage or the prolapsed uvea

21.3 Surgeon's Initial Assessment and Pre-operative Plan

This child had a Zone I/II/III open globe injury of the left eye caused by a pocketknife requiring surgical repair.

This case illustrates three important areas of discussion beyond the standard repair of a Zone I/II/III laceration (see earlier cases in this book for examples) including:

1. the initial approach to a globe injury in a child;
2. management of a retinal strike site; and
3. the approach to strabismus following a globe injury.

The initial approach to a pediatric patient with open globe injury should be tailored to the child and caregivers. As with any pediatric ophthalmology visit, attention to the child's and family's psychology is key to rapport. This may facilitate a less traumatic experience for the patient and family and a better pre-operative examination. Nonetheless, depending on the child's age, maturity, and pain, the pre-operative examination may be extremely limited. When the child is uncooperative, it is best to be conservative and wait to perform an examination under anesthesia rather than risk (further) expulsion of intraocular contents. The treating ophthalmologist should emphasize this point directly to any primary trauma, emergency department or surgery team to prevent repeated exams and manipulation of the eye.

As with any open globe injury surgery, it is important to emphasize to the caregivers or the parents and patient, if age appropriate, that the goal of the initial surgery is to close the eye to prevent further damage or infection. Restoration of vision is the second goal after initial repair, and this may involve additional surgeries and close follow up post-operatively. Although an adult caregiver gives consent on behalf of a child for surgery, it is best practice to discuss the surgery with the pediatric patient and obtain consent from the patient as well as the guardian at a level appropriate to their maturity and cognition.

It is helpful to involve a pediatric ophthalmology specialist in the care of the patient in the early post-operative period. This way the family and patient get to know the pediatric ophthalmology specialist who will likely be caring for them in the long-term. Amblyopia prevention therapy can be started early with patching and refractive treatment to best correct the patient's vision. Pediatric ophthalmology specialists can also monitor for post-injury strabismus, which can happen even with brief periods of binocular vision disruption in children.

21.4 Surgical Exploration and Repair: Operative Note

The risks, benefits, and alternatives were discussed with the patient and his mother pre-operatively, and the patient and parents wished to proceed with open globe injury exploration and repair of the left eye. The patient was brought to the operating room where the anesthesia team proceeded with general anesthesia. A careful timeout procedure was performed, and the correct patient and eye were identified.

The left eye was prepared for surgery with Betadine 10% solution applied to the periocular region and 5% solution dropped in the fornices. Care was taken to avoid dropping Betadine solution directly into the wound of the eye and the prolapsed uveal tissue. A sterile eye drape exposed the left eye, and Jaffe eyelid speculae were used to retract the eyelids. The uvea, which had prolapsed from the eye, was gently debrided with a Beaver® blade (Beaver-Visitec International, Inc., Waltham, MA) and balanced salt solution. A limited inferior limbal peritomy was initiated with relaxing incisions at 3 and 9 o'clock with Westcott scissors. The patient was found to have a full-thickness, corneoscleral laceration extending from the 9 o'clock on the cornea just central to the limbus to the insertion of the inferior rectus muscle. The uveal contents were carefully reposited into the eye using an iris spatula and subsequent sutures were placed over the spatula to ensure that uvea was not incorporated into the wound or sutures. The limbus was re-approximated first using 9-0 nylon suture. A temporal perilimbal paracentesis incision was made at 4 o'clock and filtered air was injected as needed to maintain anterior chamber depth. The 6.5 mm corneal laceration was carefully re-approximated using 10-0 nylon interrupted sutures. The scleral laceration was re-approximated with 8-0 nylon, partial-thickness, interrupted sutures. The extent of the laceration was unable to be visualized until the inferior rectus muscle was hooked with a muscle hook followed by a 2-0 silk suture. Upon shifting the muscle with the sling suture, the full extent of the laceration was seen to terminate just posterior to the insertion of the inferior rectus muscle. The scleral laceration in total was measured at 6.5 mm. The entire laceration, including the corneal and scleral portions, was 13 mm in length. Fluorescein was then used to assure the wound did not leak with provocation after full closure. The conjunctiva was closed with interrupted 8-0 Vicryl sutures with episcleral passes to anchor the tissue appropriately at the limbus. A subconjunctival injection of steroid and antibiotics was given superotemporally away from the laceration. The speculae and drapes were removed carefully. Topical atropine 1% ophthalmic solution and dexamethasone-neomycin-polymixin B ophthalmic ointment were applied to the eye, and the eye was patched and shielded. The patient tolerated the procedure without any complications.

21.4.1 Surgical Exploration and Repair: Pearls

- When there is significant uveal prolapse, either through cornea or scleral tissue, an iris spatula may be placed over the uveal tissue, and sutures may be tied over the uveal tissue. As the sutures are secured, the iris spatula may be withdrawn, and the uveal tissue should remain in place and will not be incarcerated. After a few sutures are placed, it will be easier to prevent uveal prolapse, and it will be easier to place additional sutures.
- In cases with Zone III lacerations that extend through or near the insertion of extraocular muscles, it is important to isolate the muscle using a muscle hook with a hole such as the Gass muscle hook and a silk suture to sling the muscle. Once the muscle is hooked, the examination of the sclera posterior to the muscle insertion may be performed. If this is the case, the muscle may often be pulled aside with a muscle hook or the sling suture exposing the wound and allowing for repair without disinsertion of the muscle.

21.5 Post-operative Course

The patient was admitted to MEE to complete a 48 hour course of intravenous antibiotics. On post-operative day one, he continued to have hand motion vision, with no view to the posterior pole. There was no obvious violation of the lens, but this was difficult to assess given the hazy view from corneal edema and from hyphema. An initial B-scan ultrasound on post-operative day 1 showed vitreous hemorrhage and inferonasal tracking membranes. The choroidal layer was elevated inferotemporally.

He followed up 10 days after repair with a retina specialist. Visual acuity was hand motion, and there was still minimal view posteriorly (Fig. 21.2). A repeat B-scan ultrasound at that time showed severe traction and membranes encroaching on the macula (Fig. 21.3). The options were discussed with the patient and family,

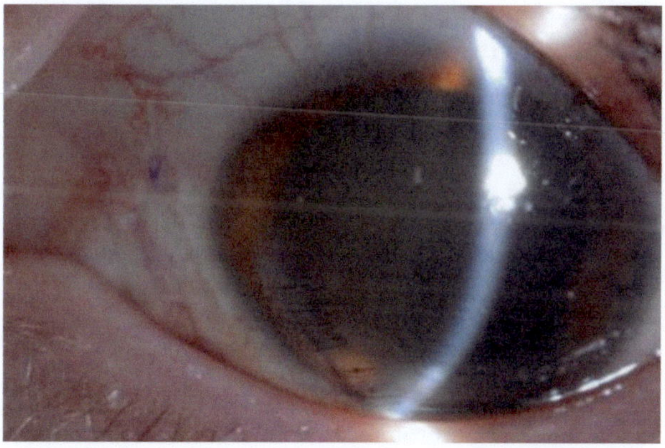

Fig. 21.2 Anterior segment, slit-lamp photograph demonstrating inferonasal corneal nylon sutures 10 days following initial repair with a dilated pupil and a hazy intraocular view

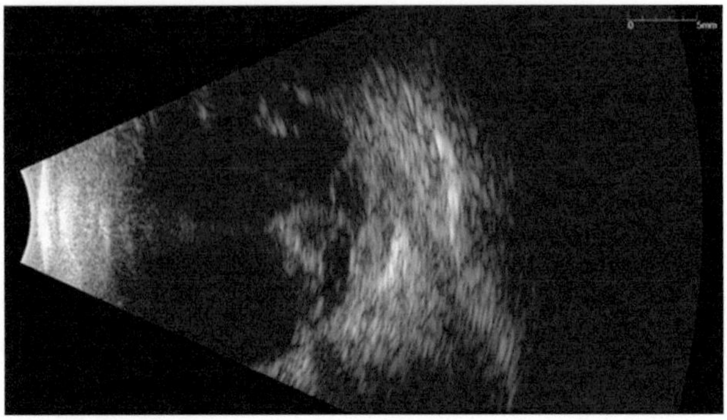

Fig. 21.3 Follow up B-scan ultrasound showing severe traction and membranes encroaching on the macula 10 days following initial repair

and they elected to proceed with a pars plana vitrectomy, lensectomy, endolaser, and membrane peel. This surgery took place 12 days after the initial repair.

Intraoperatively, the patient was found to have a scarred area inferior and temporal to the fovea through the retina and sclera suggesting an exit site of the knife injury. The scarring started in the inferior temporal macula outside of the fovea with a surrounding tractional retinal detachment. This finding established that the injury had been perforating with the knife passing through the retina and posterior sclera. A pars plana lensectomy and vitrecetomy were performed. A membrane overlying the scar was peeled, and two small retinal breaks were treated with a laser retinopexy. (See op report below.)

21.6 Second Surgical Repair: Operative Note

After informed consent was obtained, the patient was brought to the operating room and induced under general anesthesia. All risks, benefits, alternatives and complications to the procedure were fully discussed with the patient's parents pre-operatively. They understood the guarded prognosis and wished to proceed with surgery. They understood the possible progression of blindness even with surgery and they understood the possible need for additional operations. All questions were answered.

The left eye was prepped and draped in routine sterile fashion. A wire lid speculum was placed. Points were marked 3.0 mm posterior to the limbus in the usual locations. 23-gauge, valved trocars were placed transconjunctivally. Using the vitreous cutter and the fiberoptic light source, hemorrhagic axial and peripheral vitreous was removed. In addition, a pars plana lensectomy was carried out. All nucleus and cortex lens material was removed and then forceps were used to remove capsule. The vitreous hemorrhage was very dense, and it was difficult to find the retina. After considerable time and effort, it could be seen that there was a partial posterior vitreous detachment, but the vitreous was attached along the inferotemporal arcade at an exit site of the initial injury. It appeared that the knife had gone through the retina and posterior sclera. The exit site was oriented superonasal to inferotemporal in the inferior temporal macula, and there was a fibrotic scar with a localized traction retinal detachment around it. The exit site on its superonasal edge was within the macula, but not at the fovea, and its inferotemporal edge was well beyond the inferotemporal arcade. The macula and fovea were rotated inferotemporally. There was subretinal hemorrhage as well as subretinal pigment epithelial hemorrhage throughout the entire macula. There were macular striae toward the scar. In addition, there were two small tears in the inferior periphery within areas of fibrosis. The posterior hyaloid membrane was then elevated out of the fibrotic exit site and meticulous dissection was performed to release the traction. A retinectomy was not performed. Scleral depression was performed for 360° to facilitate a vitreous base dissection. As much vitreous as possible was removed and no other peripheral pathology was noted. There were significant membranes associated with the fibrotic scar, and these were peeled in their entirety. Then, when all traction was relieved, endolaser was applied to the two small breaks in the inferior periphery and around the areas of fibrosis. A fluid air exchange was performed with a soft tipped cannula using the fiberoptic light source. The small, localized tractional retinal detachment around the exit site was then reattached. No other retinal breaks were noted. The trochars were removed, and each of the three sclerotomies were sutured with 7-0 Vicryl® (polyglactin 910 suture) (Ethicon US, LLC., Somerville, NJ) after small incisions were made in the overlying conjunctiva. Air was not exchanged for gas. Conjunctiva was closed with multiple interrupted 7-0 Vicryl® sutures. A subconjunctival injection of cefazolin and dexamethasone were given. Pressure was checked, and at the conclusion of the procedure it was normal by palpation. The eye was flushed with Betadine 10% solution and dressed with dexamethaxone-neomycin-polymixin B and atropine 1% ophthalmic ointments. A patch and shield were placed, and the patient was extubated and transferred to the recovery room in stable condition having tolerated this procedure well. There were no complications.

21.6.1 Second Surgical Repair: Pearls

- Identification of an exit wound in the posterior sclera may be limited by dense vitreous hemorrhage and may not be appreciated until vitrectomy or resolution of a vitreous hemorrhage.
- Many exit wounds require retinectomy to remove the retina that is typically incarcerated in the wound. In this case, there was minimal traction and no retinal incarceration so a retinectomy around the exit site was not necessary.
- Some perforating injuries have extensive submacular hemorrhage that can be removed. In this case, there was thin submacular hemorrhage that did not require removal.

21.7 Post-operative Course

The patient was followed closely by the retina and trauma service over the following weeks. Eight weeks after his injury, the wound appeared well-healed, and the corneal sutures were removed in the trauma clinic. He was 20/300 without correction of his aphakia. Due to the patient being hesitant about trying a contact lens, he was not referred to the contact lens service until approximately 6 months after the injury. At that time, he was fitted with a tinted Orion soft contact lens (Orion Vision Group, Marietta, GA) with best corrected visual acuity of 20/40. The patient later switched to an Alden HP Toric soft contact lens (Alden Optical Laboratories, Inc., Lancaster, NY) 2 months later, which was better tolerated. With the improvement in his visual acuity with the contact lens, the patient developed binocular, constant horizontal diplopia.

He was referred to a pediatric ophthalmology specialist, and he was found to have a moderate-angle left exotropia, similar at distance and at near, likely related to sensory deprivation. However, his vision had dropped to 20/125 with the contact lens, and he was referred back to the contact lens optometry service to insure his vision had been optimized with a refitting and refraction of his aphakic contact lenses. Often, the angle of deviation is altered by suboptimal vision, and the angle of misalignment is critical to the surgical dosing of strabismus surgery. In addition, ideal refraction facilitates neurologically-based, fine-tuning of the post-operative eye alignment following strabismus surgery thereby allowing fusion of disparate images and resolution of diplopia.

His sensorimotor examination almost 16 months after his injury showed a right eye fixation preference at distance and at near, no stereopsis on Titmus fly testing, and suppression of the left eye with Worth 4-dot testing at both distance and at near. The deviations testing with ideal correction revealed an exotropia and left hypotropia with a V-pattern at distance (Fig. 21.4) and slightly larger deviation at near of an exotropia of 40–45 prism diopters and a left hypotropia of 8 prism diopters by alternate prism and cover testing. Thus, the sensorimotor evaluation impression was that of an acquired left exotropia related to sensory deprivation and disruption of binocular vision from his injury. His ocular deviation measurements were stable over 6 months (Fig. 21.5).

The patient and his mother reported that his strabismus and diplopia had decreased his self-esteem. He stated that he disliked his "lazy eye," and he was observed to avoid photographs and close one eye when chatting with peers. Upon the advice of his ophthalmologists, he had also stopped playing hockey, which was his favorite activity. He was undergoing psychotherapy to support him with these challenges, and his care-team suggested strabismus surgery as the next step in his rehabilitation. The patient and parents consented for left lateral rectus recession and left medial rectus resection on adjustable sutures for improvement in diplopia and reconstruction of ocular alignment.

Intraoperatively, the patient was found to have significant scarring around the lateral rectus muscle, making isolation of the muscle a challenge. A left lateral rectus recession of 8 mm and a left medial rectus recession of 6.5 mm using

	XT 40 LHT 6	
XT 30	XT 30 LHT 7	XT 30 LHT 8
	XT 25-30 LHT 8	

Fig. 21.4 Sensorimotor deviations tested at distance prior to strabismus surgery measured in prism diopters. *XT*=exotropia, *LHT*=left hypertropia

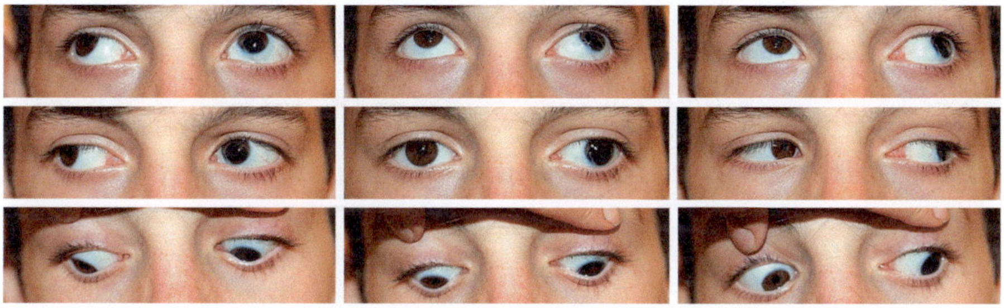

Fig. 21.5 Extraocular motility prior to strabismus surgery

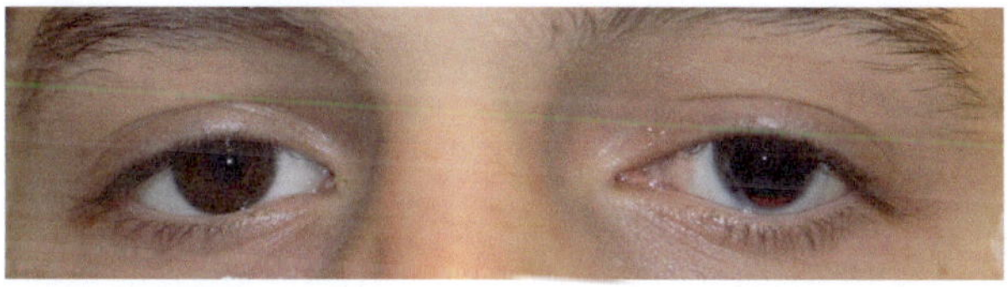

Fig. 21.6 Extraocular alignment 3 months after strabismus surgery and 31 months after his initial injury

adjustable suture technique was performed. Post-operative adjustment of alignment with the adjustable sutures was not possible, as the patient could not wear his contact lens due to chemosis, and the use of a trial frame with a high power plus lens made it too difficult to observe eye alignment. By observation, the large-angle exotropia seemed largely corrected immediately post-operatively.

The patient had significant reduction in his diplopia and the separation of the two images following strabismus surgery; but, 3 months post-operatively, he reported overlapping of two images that he simply could not fuse. He noticed that the diplopia was worse when he wore his contact lens, so he discontinued contact lens use daily. Synoptophore testing showed that he experienced metamorphopsia of the image from the left eye. This image distortion, retinal in origin from residual epiretinal membrane in the macula and from damage to the macular and foveal retina from the trauma, precluded high grade binocular vision, but placement of an obliquely oriented 3M™ Press-On™ Optics (The Fresnel Prism and Lens Co., Bloomington, MN) on his protective plano eyewear allowed resolution of diplopia when he wore his contact lens. The patient was pleased with the reconstructive appearance of the eyes and improved eye contact with others (Fig. 21.6). The parents also reported improved mood and self-esteem.

The patient will continue to follow with the contact lens optometry service, pediatric ophthalmology, and eye trauma services as it is hoped that a further improvement in his vision in the left eye might assist him in resolving his residual diplopia with time and "re-learning" of fusion.

The patient was interested in returning to play hockey. He was advised that this was reasonable as long as he wore protection for his eyes and that he and his family set guidelines on participation in sports and understood that further trauma to the eye could cause irreparable damage.

21.8 Final Pediatric Ophthalmology/Trauma Evaluation

21.8.1 Final Visual Acuity

OD: 20/15-2
OS: 20/30-2 with aphakic contact lens

21.8.2 Pupils

OD: Round, no afferent pupillary defect
OS: Round, large with loss of iris tissue inferiorly, no afferent pupillary defect by reverse

21.8.3 Alignment (as Measured by Alternate Prism and Cover Test)

Ncc (+3.00 diopters over left eye alone): Exotropia (XT) of 16 prism dioptors, left hypotropia (LHT) of 7 prism diopters
Dcc (aphakic CL): XT 8 prism diopters and LHT 7 prism diopters
Dcc:

	XT16 LHT10	
XT8 LHT5	XT8 LHT7	LHT10
	ET2 LHT6	

ET esotropia; *XT* exotropia; *LHT* left hypertropia

Right head tilt: XT6 LHT10
Left head tilt: XT10 LHT2
Double-Maddox Rod testing
OD: No torsion
OS: 8° excyclotorsion
Worth 4 Dot testing: crossed diplopia both at distance and at near

Synoptophore sensory testing: Intermittent fusion (with 12 prism diopters twisted 15° base on a plano protective glasses lens over the left eye with the aphakic contact lens inserted).

21.8.4 Slit Lamp Examination

	OD	OS
Lids and lashes	Normal	Normal
Sclera and conjunctiva	Normal	Mild conjunctival scarring inferonasally and inferotemporally at sites of strabismus surgery
Cornea	Normal	Vertical scar extending from nasal to central to inferior cornea at 6:30 o'clock at the limbus tracking inferiorly past limbus (Fig. 21.7)
Anterior chamber	Normal	Deep and quiet
Iris	Normal	Large pupil with loss of iris tissue inferior
Lens	Normal	Aphakic
Vitreous	Normal	Status post pars plana vitrectomy

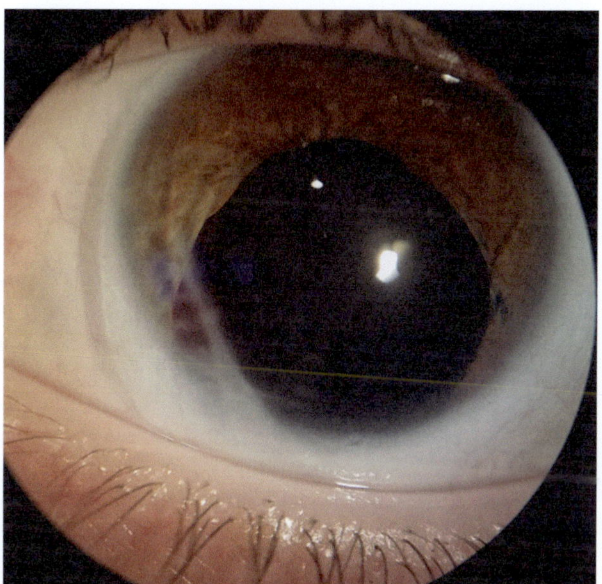

Fig. 21.7 Slit-lamp photograph of the left eye demonstrating the healed corneal-scleral laceration, iris injury, and the aphakic eye. A contact lens is noted on the eye

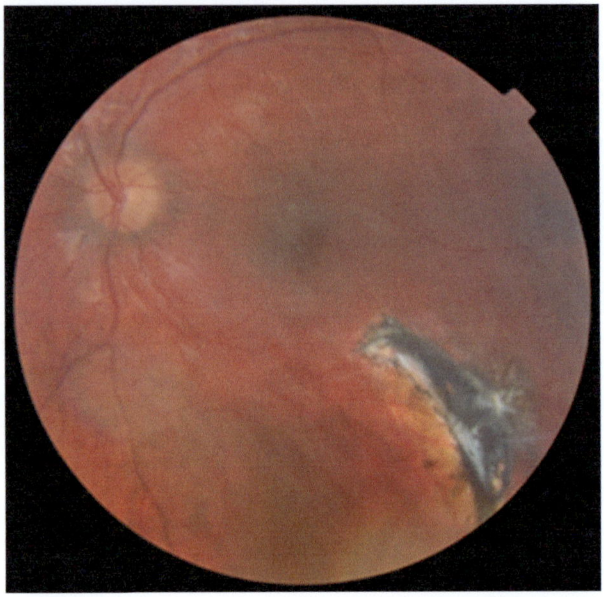

Fig. 21.8 Fundus photograph of the left eye demonstrating inferotemporal chorioretinal scar secondary to exit site from left open globe injury from a pocket knife

21.8.5 Dilated Examination

Macula/Nerve OD: Normal
Periphery OD: Normal
Macula/Nerve: OS: Normal optic nerve, slight distortion of foveal contour with epiretinal membrane, chorioretinal scar in the inferotemporal macula (Fig. 21.8)
Periphery OS: Attached, inferior laser scars and inferotemporal exit site scar

21.9 Review and Lessons Learned

In pediatric open globe injury patients, it is essential to approach the patient with developmentally appropriate care that takes into account the patient's pain, distress, and anxiety. Manipulation of the eye in an uncooperative child with a suspected open globe injury may risk expulsion of intraocular contents and in these cases it may be better to take a child to the operating room for an examination under anesthesia with globe exploration and repair than to risk further damage to the eye. If a pediatrician or pediatric ophthalmologist is available, these consultants may aide in optimizing pre-operative care for the child.

This case also demonstrates the importance of prompt evaluation by a vitreoretinal surgeon in patients with risk for posterior trauma in the open globe injury with a poor posterior view. We recommend prompt B scan ultrasound and referral to a vitreoretinal surgeon for cases with compromised views to the posterior segment.

Our patient had a non-clearing vitreous hemorrhage with concern for a tractional retinal detachment involving the macula. Intraoperatively, he was found to have a posterior exit site signifying a perforating injury. In cases with dense vitreous hemorrhage, there is no clear view for evaluation for a perforating injury. Since exit sites like this can be found very posterior towards the macula, exploring and repairing these posterior perforation exit wounds may cause more harm than good. The injured retina in these cases can be re-attached and repaired by a skilled retinal surgeon comfortable with eye trauma and may even have an excellent visual result, such as in this case.

Any patient with an open globe injury and significant vision deprivation may develop a sensory misalignment of the eyes. In young children, this is typically an esodeviation. In older children and adults, this tends to be an exodeviation, as is the case here. The development of diplopia in this case occurred because the visual rehabilitation was so good that it allowed the patient to experience two images. This is always the goal, but good vision can be frustrating for the patient in cases of image distortion due to retinal injury. The image distortion can make it very difficult to fuse images and lead to intractable diplopia.

If strabismus surgery is indicated following an open globe injury, it is important to optimize the patient's refraction prior to measuring the angle of deviation. Uncorrected refractive error will exacerbate a sensory deviation, resulting in inaccurate deviation measurements. In addition, it is advisable to ensure that the measurements are stable over at least 3–6 months prior to strabismus surgery in cases where amblyopia is not a concern.

The psychological burden of an open globe injury trauma may be especially pronounced in children. In this case, the patient was advised to refrain from hockey, a favorite athletic and social activity, and his ocular misalignment also lead to diminished self-confidence in conversations in social circles. The treating ophthalmologist is in an ideal position to query the patient and family about these issues and refer them to appropriate care.

21.10 Key Learning Points

- Avoid risking further damage to the eye with an overly ambitious pre-operative examination in an uncooperative child.
- Early involvement of pediatric ophthalmology is beneficial for evaluation of strabismus and, in patients younger than 10 years-old, for evaluation of amblyopia.
- Successful strabismus surgery in a patient following open globe injury requires stable pre-operative deviation measurements and an optimal refraction.
- Image distortion for retinal injury can lead to intractable diplopia that is frustrating and must be managed.

Chapter 22
Case 17: Zone I Open Globe Injury with Primary Lens Removal

Rohini Rao and Seanna Grob

22.1 History of Present Illness

A 47-year-old man without significant past medical history presented with pain in the right eye.

- The patient reports using a table-saw 2 days prior to presentation and being hit with a non-metallic object over the superior orbital rim of his right eye.
- He denied any pain or vision changes immediately after the incident, but subsequently experienced sharp pains, injection, progressively worsening blurry vision, and photophobia.

22.2 Initial Trauma Evaluation

22.2.1 Visual Acuity (Without Correction)

OD: Hand motion
OS: 20/25

R. Rao, M.D. (✉) • S. Grob, M.D., M.A.S.
Department of Ophthalmology, Harvard Medical School, Massachusetts Eye and Ear, Boston, MA, USA
e-mail: rohini_rao@meei.harvard.edu

S. Grob, C. Kloek (eds.), *Management of Open Globe Injuries*,
https://doi.org/10.1007/978-3-319-72410-2_22

22.2.2 Pupils

OD: Irregular
OS: Round, no afferent pupillary defect

22.2.3 External Examination

Normal.

22.2.4 Slit Lamp Examination

	OD	OS
Lids and lashes	Mild ptosis of 1 mm	Normal
Sclera and conjunctiva	1+ injection	Normal
Cornea	1.5 mm diagonal laceration superonasally, Seidel negative	Normal
Anterior chamber	Shallow, 3+ cell	Normal
Iris	Irregular pupillary margin inferotemporally	Normal
Lens	Opacified, white lens	Normal
Vitreous	No view	Normal

22.2.5 Dilated Examination

Macula/Nerve OD: No view
Periphery OD: No view
Macula/Nerve: OS: Normal
Periphery OS: Normal

22.2.6 Radiographic Imaging

Computed tomography (CT) of the orbits showed no evidence of intraocular or intraorbital foreign body or retro-orbital hematoma (Fig. 22.1).

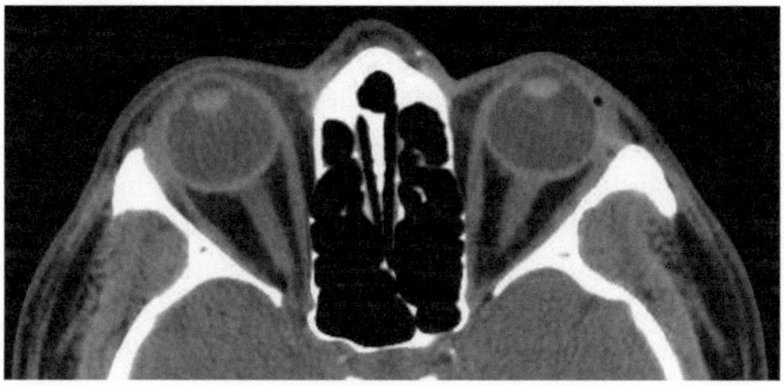

Fig. 22.1 Axial CT image showing a grossly normal appearing globe on the right with regular scleral contour, but a slightly decreased anterior chamber depth and mildly enlarged lens compared to the left

22.3 Surgeon's Initial Assessment and Pre-operative Plan

The patient has a Zone I open globe injury with a self-sealing corneal laceration. There is clear lens involvement from this trauma, as the lens was completely opacified on presentation.

Pre-operative planning in this case centers on corneal wound stability. If the corneal wound is not stable, any further surgery is more challenging. So, in general, repairing the cornea is the first step. Although the corneal wound appeared self-sealing on clinical exam, introducing a phacoemulsification probe and raising the intraocular pressure usually opens a recent corneal laceration, unless it is primarily sutured. If the cornea is clear enough after corneal wound repair, and the lens can be visualized, it can be removed during the same surgery as the open globe repair. Often with large corneal lacerations, the intraocular view diminishes significantly after corneal repair, making cataract extraction or other procedures potentially dangerous or much more challenging. So if the view is compromised, it is best to repair the cornea and control any inflammation or pressure elevation related to lens involvement and give the eye a chance to heal and the corneal view to clear before proceeding with lens removal. In this case, the corneal wound was self-sealing and small, so there was excellent visibility to the lens, allowing for safe primary lens removal.

When the lens capsule has clearly been violated, three factors need to be considered strongly: (1) capsulorrhexis construction, (2) zonular stability, (3) vitreous prolapse in cases of posterior capsular violation. When the anterior capsule has been violated, whether it be from the trauma or from simply making a paracentesis during routine cataract surgery, the site of trauma needs to be identified. Clinical examination may give clues as to the location of the anterior capsule violation. For example, there might be an area where fluffy lens material is coming forward where the violation is located. This will allow for pre-operative planning for capsulorrhexis construction. Drawing out a picture and writing out the steps can be helpful. Sometimes the anterior capsule defect is difficult to see prior to the use of trypan blue. In these cases, trypan blue can be especially helpful in identifying the remaining anterior capsule. Every attempt should be made to incorporate a small puncture site into the capsulorrhexis in order to achieve a continuous capsulorrhexis. Some anterior capsule defects are larger and might require the use of a combination of the cystotome, MST (microsurgical technology) forceps and scissors, utrata forceps, and generous use of viscoelastic to achieve the best possible capsulorrhexis.

Also, it is possible after lens trauma that zonular weakness is present, so it is important to not place too much stress on the zonules during lens removal to prevent zonular dialysis. Lastly, it is often difficult to ensure the stability and integrity of the posterior lens capsule, so there should be a low threshold to perform an anterior vitrectomy and/or use the vitrectomy for completion of the lensectomy if there is any concern for possible posterior capsule involvement. If there is a high likelihood of posterior capsule involvement, it is also an option to send the patient to a retina specialist for a pars plana lensectomy or to have them on back up if lens material does drop through posterior capsule defects.

In addition, in cases such as this one, there may be trauma to the iris sphincter and dilator muscles, leading to atonia and poor dilation, or an intraoperative situation similar to floppy iris syndrome. Iris hooks may be helpful in pupil expansion and iris stability, but care needs to be taken to avoid capturing the lens capsule within the iris hook. Iris hook placement may need to take place prior to insertion of trypan blue in order to get good stain on all parts of the remaining anterior capsule. Sometimes this can be done without placement of ophthalmic viscosurgical devices (OVD). If the anterior chamber has shallowed from lens material swelling and coming forward, then it can be helpful to place a sparing amount of cohesive viscoelastic (such as Provisc) which can more easily be rinsed out of the anterior chamber with balanced salt solution to allow for staining with trypan blue subsequently.

22.4 Surgical Exploration and Repair: Operative Note

The risks, benefits, and alternatives were discussed with the patient pre-operatively and the patient consented to proceed with exploration and repair of the open globe injury as well as cataract extraction. The patient was brought to the operating room where the anesthesia team proceeded with general anesthesia. A careful time-out was observed and the correct patient and the eye were identified. The right eye was prepped and draped in the usual sterile ophthalmic fashion using a Jaffe speculum to provide adequate exposure. Two paracentesis incisions were created with a #15 blade. The same blade was used to create five small stab incisions to insert five equally spaced iris hooks for appropriate pupil dilation due to a persistently miotic pupil. At this point, filtered air was injected into the anterior chamber followed by trypan blue to stain the anterior capsule. This was irrigated out with balanced salt solution. The anterior capsule was evaluated and it was noted that there were three anterior capsule radial tears, one superiorly and one at around 4 o'clock and one at around 8 o'clock. Viscoat was then injected into the anterior chamber. At this point, the corneal laceration was holding without evidence of leakage. A 2.4 mm keratome was utilized to enter the anterior chamber through a triplanar corneal incision. A capsulorrhexis was performed with microsurgical technology (MST) scissors followed by Utrata forceps, however, due to the already present anterior capsule tears from the trauma this was not a continuous rhexis and was completed in sections. Phacoemulsification on epinucleus setting was used to debulk the lens. Then the anterior vitrectomy handpiece was introduced as the integrity of the posterior capsule was still unknown. However, there was no visible vitreous in the anterior chamber. Then, the vitrector was used on irrigation/aspiration (I/A)—cut to remove the lens cortex. After the cortex was removed, it did not appear that there was any posterior capsule violation or that the anterior capsule tears had extended posteriorly. Viscoat was injected periodically throughout this process of lens removal to help bring the lens material forward and keep any potential vitreous back. During this process, the corneal wound was found to be leaking, so three interrupted sutures were placed using 10-0 nylon to re-approximate the wound. Then the viscoat was removed with the bimanual I/A. The iris hooks were removed. No lens was inserted due to the recent trauma and risk of infection, but sufficient capsule was noted to allow for placement of a sulcus lens in the future. Through a 30-gauge cannula, balanced salt solution was utilized to inflate the globe to normal pressure and to hydrate the main and paracentesis incisions. A 10-0 nylon was then used to close both paracenteses and the main wound. A fluorescein strip was used to check for leaks of the corneal wound and none were seen. A subconjunctival steroid and antibiotic injection was performed temporally. The speculums were removed. The patient's drape was removed under the microscope. Atropine and dexamethasone-neomycin-polymyxin B ointment was placed in the eye. A sterile ophthalmic pad and shield were applied. Having tolerated the procedure well, the patient was transferred to the recovery area in stable condition.

22.4.1 Surgical Exploration and Repair: Pearls

- Trypan blue capsular staining is especially helpful in cases of anterior capsule and lens trauma to identify the capsular tears and defects. Ideally breaks in the anterior capsule can be incorporated into a continuous capsulorrhexis. If not, multiple different instruments can be used to achieve the best possible capsulorrhexis.
- It is helpful to suture any corneal wounds prior to lens removal or as soon as the wound begins to leak. A leaking corneal wound will make lens removal challenging due to anterior chamber instability and flattening and poor quality of the surgical view with fluid constantly escaping through the corneal wound.
- Iris hooks are helpful as iris expansion devices and for iris stability. However, in cases of anterior capsular trauma, it is crucial to avoid hooking the torn capsule within the iris hook.

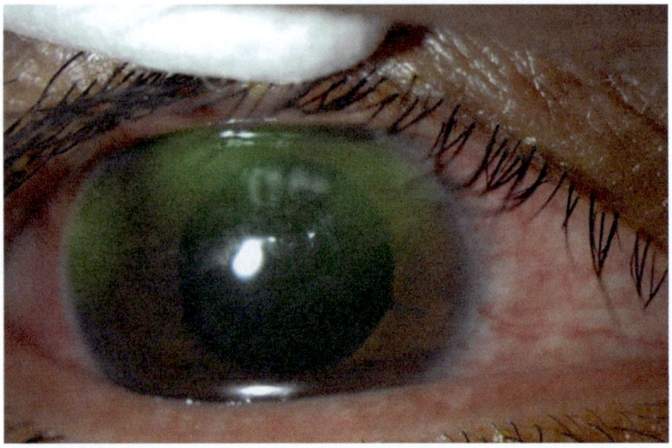

Fig. 22.2 Slit lamp clinical photo revealing a small corneal laceration with three intact nylon sutures with lingering fluorescein after exam. The eye is aphakic and pupil mid-dilated

22.5 Post-operative Course

The patient was admitted to Massachusetts Eye and Ear (MEE) to complete a 48 hour course of intravenous antibiotics. A B-scan ultrasound showed no evidence of retinal detachment or vitreous hemorrhage.

He then followed up 1 week later. With a +11.0 diopter trial lens, he was able to see 20/40 with pinhole to 20/20 in his right eye. The main wound and paracentesis sutures were removed. Five weeks later, 6 weeks after initial surgical repair, his vision was 20/30 pinhole to 20/20 with an +11.5 diopter trial lens. The three central corneal sutures were removed without complication.

He was then referred to the contact lens service at MEE for evaluation. After contact lens fitting, the patient was able to see 20/20-1 and was very happy with his vision and his contact lens. Placement of a sulcus intraocular lens was discussed with the patient, but he was so happy with his contact lens that he deferred any further surgery (Fig. 22.2).

22.6 Final Trauma Evaluation

22.6.1 Final Visual Acuity

OD: 20/25
OS: 20/20

22.6.2 Pupils

OD: Round, reactive, no afferent pupillary defect
OS: Round, reactive, no afferent pupillary defect

22.6.3 Slit Lamp Examination

	OD	OS
Lids and lashes	Normal	Normal
Sclera and conjunctiva	Normal	Normal
Cornea	1.5 mm scar from pupil superonasally, trace pigment on endothelium inferiorly	Normal
Anterior chamber	Normal	Normal
Iris	Mild posterior synechiae inferonasally 1 clock hour (iris to lens capsule)	Normal
Lens	Aphakic, posterior lens capsule appears intact with striae	Normal
Vitreous	Normal	Normal

22.6.4 Dilated Examination (Fig. 22.3)

Macula/Nerve OD: Normal, cup to disc ratio of 0.4
Periphery OD: Normal
Macula/Nerve: OS: Normal, cup to disc ratio of 0.3
Peripheral OS: Normal

22.7 Review and Lessons Learned

While the majority of patients with open globe injuries present within 24 hours of injury due to blurry vision or eye pain, not all open globe injuries manifest the same way. In fact, this patient denied a severe trauma to his eye and presented 48 hours after injury. Generally, patients with delayed presentation are less likely to have a Zone III injury and generally have good visual outcomes [1].

Upon presentation, it was clear he had suffered a penetrating injury to his eye. While the corneal wound was self-sealing and Seidel negative with provocation, there was evidence of a traumatic cataract and anterior lens capsule violation. Immediately after the injury, his vision was still good because he only had a small corneal laceration. Since the lens capsule was violated, over the subsequent 48 hours, the lens started to hydrate and opacify, affecting his visual acuity—which ultimately brought him in for evaluation. If the view to the lens is clear, the cataract should be removed to prevent lens material from coming into the anterior chamber causing inflammation and intraocular pressure elevation and to restore vision.

Infections and wound leaks are also associated with delayed presentation, secondary to poor wound healing and necrotic tissue, so it is important to monitor

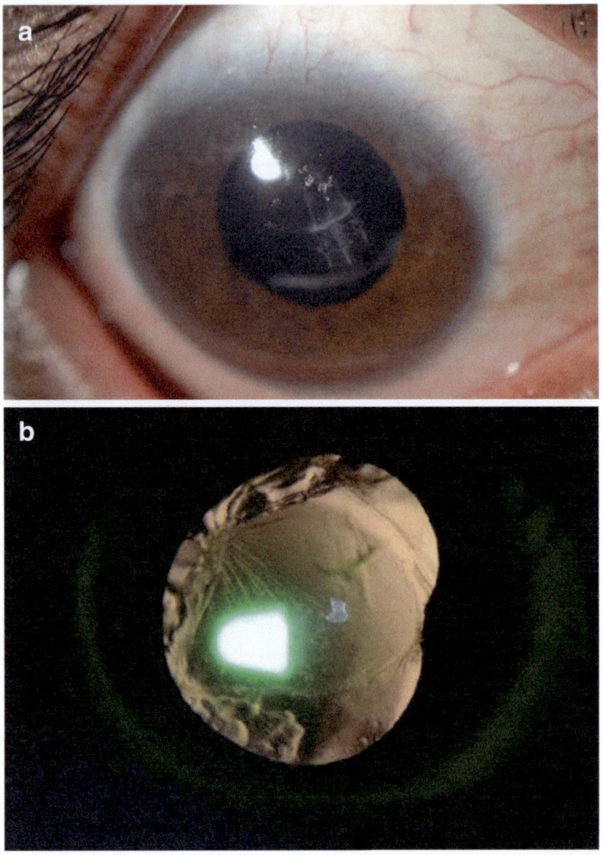

Fig. 22.3 (**a**) Slit lamp clinical photo revealing a healed corneal laceration with sutures removed. The eye is aphakic. (**b**) Slit lamp clinical photo using transillumination to reveal an intact posterior capsule with striae and an area of posterior synechiae (iris to lens capsule) from approximately 3–4 o'clock.

these injuries closely and to delay removal of sutures or removal in a staged approach (as discussed in earlier cases) so as to ensure wound stability and reduce infection risk [2]. In these cases, while a fantastic refractive outcome is always desirable, the primary concern is of globe integrity and infection prevention.

For primary traumatic cataract extraction, we often avoid the placement of an intraocular lens due to the infection risk with the placement of an implant in the setting of trauma [3]. Contact lenses can overcome a high degree of irregular astigmatism and promote vision. While training patients to wear a contact lens takes time, they are a good alternative to a second surgery for placement of a secondary intraocular lens and also can help correct the corneal astigmatism associated with the corneal laceration scar. If the patient does not tolerate a contact lens or prefers an intraocular lens, then this can be discussed after the eye has healed from the trauma and a secondary lens can be placed in a controlled, stable, non-inflammed eye several months after repair. Often patients are very happy with their contact lens, like this patient, and defer further surgery.

22.8 Key Learning Points

- When performing a removal of a traumatic cataract, utilize all the tools to help achieve a desired outcome: iris hooks for pupillary dilation and stability for improved view, trypan blue for anterior capsule staining and viewing of capsular defects, MST scissors, the cystatome, and utrata foceps for the help create a capsulorrhexis, and the bimanual I/A or vitrector for removal of the lens.
- Pre-operative planning is key for a successful surgery. It can be helpful to draw out the anterior capsule defect and think through the plan for creating a capsulorrhexis.
- Aphakic contact lenses can provide excellent vision for patients requiring a lensectomy. It is a great option for patients who do not want additional surgery and can also help correct for irregular corneal astigmatism.

References

1. Trief D, Andreoli M, Shah A, Yonekawa Y, Andreoli C. Outcomes and characteristics of open-globe injuries with delayed presentation. Invest Ophthalmol Vis Sci. 2013;54:4435.
2. Kong GYX, et al. Wound-related complications and clinical outcomes following open globe injury repair. Clin Exp Ophthalmol. 2015;43:508–13.
3. Andreoli CM, et al. Low rate of endophthalmitis in a large series of open globe injuries. Am J Ophthalmol. 2009;147:601–608.e2.

Chapter 23
Case 18: Delayed Presentation Zone I Open Globe Injury with Traumatic Cataract

Tavé van Zyl and Seanna Grob

23.1 History of Present Illness

A 63-year-old healthy man presents with concern for open globe of the right eye.

- 10 days prior to presentation, while working as a woodsman and power-sawing a tree, he felt a foreign object strike his right eye and noted decreased vision and pain.
- He initially presented to an outside urgent care clinic closer to home where he was prescribed topical gentamicin eye drops for the diagnosis of a corneal abrasion.
- Due to persistent eye pain and progressively worsening vision, he presented to Massachusetts Eye and Ear (MEE) for further evaluation.

23.2 Initial Trauma Evaluation

23.2.1 Visual Acuity (Without Correction)

OD: Hand motion at 3 feet
OS: 20/70 pinhole 20/40

Electronic Supplementary Material The online version of this chapter (https://doi.org/10.1007/978-3-319-72410-2_23) contains supplementary material, which is available to authorized users.

T. van Zyl, M.D. (✉) • S. Grob, M.D., M.A.S.
Department of Ophthalmology, Harvard Medical School, Massachusetts Eye and Ear, Boston, MA, USA
e-mail: tave_vanzyl@meei.harvard.edu

S. Grob, C. Kloek (eds.), *Management of Open Globe Injuries*,
https://doi.org/10.1007/978-3-319-72410-2_23

23.2.2 Pupils

OD: Irregular, peaked inferotemporally, minimally reactive, no afferent pupillary defect by reverse
OS: 4 mm, round, briskly reactive

23.2.3 External Examination

Normal without lacerations or ecchymosis.

23.2.4 Slit Lamp Examination

	OD	OS
Lids and lashes	Normal, deep orbit with prominent brow	Normal, deep orbit with prominent brow
Sclera and conjunctiva	2+ conjunctival injection, no scleral lacerations	Normal
Cornea	Full-thickness paracentral V-shaped laceration inferotemporally with apex pointing superotemporally measuring 3 mm on superior edge of triangle and 5 mm on inferior edge of triangle, Seidel negative without provocation, but the triangular laceration is elevated and irregular	Normal
Anterior chamber	Shallow inferotemporally with the iris bowed forward, 2+ flare, rare cell, no hypopyon	Normal
Iris	Bowed forward from lens, peaked inferotemporally, prominent iris vessels, temporal posterior synechiae	Normal
Lens	Posterior synechiae temporally, traumatic white cataract with small amount of lens material extending toward corneal wound	Normal
Vitreous	No view	Normal

23.2.5 Dilated Examination

Macula/Nerve OD: No view
Periphery OD: No view
Macula/Nerve: OS: Normal
Periphery OS: Normal

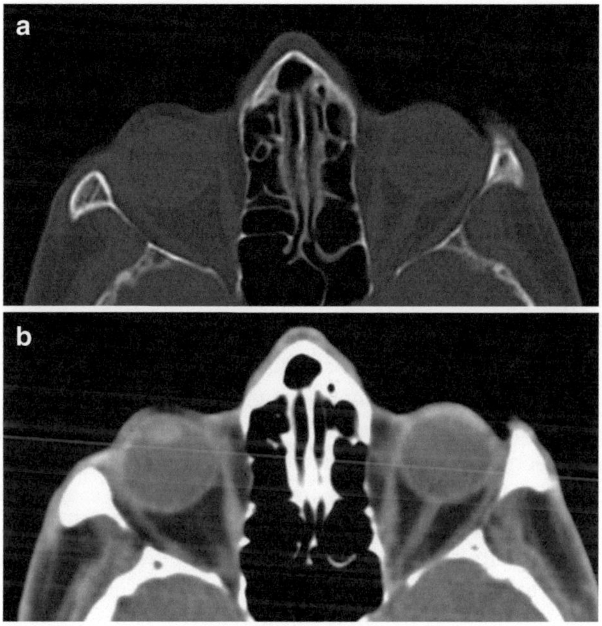

Fig. 23.1 Pre-operative CT scan of the orbits appeared unremarkable with normal, symmetric appearing globes and no fractures. Bone window (**a**), soft tissue window (**b**)

23.2.6 Radiographic Imaging

Computed tomography (CT) of the orbits showed no foreign bodies in the orbit or eye (Fig. 23.1). There was minimal preseptal soft tissue swelling. The right globe appeared formed and symmetric to the left globe with no radiologic signs of rupture or intraocular injury.

23.3 Surgeon's Initial Assessment and Pre-operative Plan

This patient presented to our institution 10 days following his eye injury. Clinical exam showed a full-thickness corneal laceration of the right eye, which was currently Seidel negative without provocation. However, even though the wound was Seidel negative, the corneal flap was elevated, poorly aligned and irregular. Given these findings, we recommended that this full-thickness laceration be taken to the operating room for repair and apposition of wound edges to promote optimal healing and visual rehabilitation. We anticipated that the wound edges may be more friable due to the delayed nature of presentation and may need gentle debridement to ensure proper healing and to prevent epithelial downgrowth. In the setting of significant corneal edema, sutures may need to be tied at higher tension—resulting in significant but short-term post-operative astigmatism—in order to ensure the wound remains Seidel negative post-operatively as the corneal edema resolves.

There was also obvious lens violation and resulting traumatic cataract, which was responsible for the patient's progressively worsening vision. Given the wound edema and corneal haze, removal of the lens at the time of globe repair may not be feasible due to poor visibility, especially in the setting of his delayed presentation. However, the patient was consented for possible removal of the traumatic cataract and anterior vitrectomy in addition to the globe repair. This was discussed at length with the patient, especially reinforcing to the patient that if the lens was not removed primarily, that the vision would likely not improve after the open globe repair due to the cataract. This discussion is important to appropriately set the patient's expectations for visual recovery.

It is important to emphasize that it is not necessary to remove a traumatic cataract primarily. There is currently no consensus regarding the optimal time of traumatic cataract extraction, and this is to some extent due to the diversity of presentations of trauma [1]. Among adults, in whom amblyopia is not an issue, the decision regarding when to proceed depends on the surgeon's preferences, the available surgical infrastructure (i.e. available instrumentation and equipment, skilled assistants and staff, etc.) at the time of open globe repair, and the extent of lens involvement and inflammation. If the view through the cornea is clear and the cataract can be safely removed, then removing the cataract initially results in one less surgery for the patient and potentially less frequent follow-ups. As mentioned briefly in the prior chapter, if the view is compromised from corneal edema after the corneal repair or due to delayed presentation, removing the cataract may be quite challenging and potentially dangerous. If the lens is not removed primarily, the patient must be watched frequently in the post-operative period to monitor for intraocular inflammation, intraocular pressure elevation, and lens material in the anterior chamber. This may be difficult for some patients with transportation issues or those who are traveling long distances. Follow up visits may need to be every 2–3 days initially in order to monitor for intraocular pressure elevation and inflammation due to exposed lens material. Patients are often started on more frequent steroid eye drops—often every 1–2 hours—when there is lens capsule violation and exposed lens material. Pressure lowering drops may also be necessary to keep intraocular pressure in the normal range.

Many patients can be well controlled with drops and closely monitored for several weeks to months prior to traumatic cataract removal. If this can be achieved, then the corneal wound is often healed and stable during traumatic cataract extraction, the eye is quiet after healing from the open globe injury, and the view through the cornea is much improved after corneal edema resolves. However, if there is an intraocular pressure spike or significant inflammation or lens material in the anterior chamber close to the endothelium that may cause worsening corneal edema, then the patient may need more urgent lens removal.

23.4 Surgical Exploration and Repair: Operative Note

The risks, benefits, and alternatives were discussed with the patient pre-operatively and the patient consented to proceed with exploration and repair of the open globe injury. The patient was brought to the operating room where the anesthesia team proceeded with general anesthesia. A careful time-out was observed and the correct patient and eye were identified. The right eye was prepped and draped in the usual sterile ophthalmic fashion using a Jaffe speculum to provide adequate exposure.

The patient was found to have a full-thickness corneal laceration in an inverted "V" configuration inferotemporally, but extending into the central visual axis with the apex pointing superiorly toward 10–11 o'clock. The superior-nasal aspect of the wound measured 3 mm and the inferotemporal aspect measured 5 mm. The cornea was edematous and the triangular flap edge was partly elevated and overriding the adjacent cornea. The anterior chamber was formed but shallow inferiorly and inferotemporally where the iris was bulging toward the wound. The iris was hyperemic with prominent vessels at the inferior margin. There was fluffy material at the pupillary plane just posterior to the corneal laceration that was consistent with lens material and was concerning for anterior capsule/lens involvement that was previously noted.

First, using a supersharp blade, a paracentesis was fashioned at 10 o'clock. Filtered air was injected into the anterior chamber. A cyclodialysis spatula was used to release the iris that was incarcerated within the inferior part of the corneal wound. After contact was made with the iris to release it from the wound, the pupil constricted significantly. The corneal wound was then closed with six 10-0 nylon sutures in an interrupted fashion. Filtered air was injected intermittently to maintain anterior chamber depth. Viscoelastic was not used. After repairing the corneal laceration, the filtered air was removed and balanced salt solution was injected into the anterior chamber to bring the intraocular pressure to a physiological level. The wound was confirmed to be watertight and Seidel negative using a fluorescein strip. A single interrupted 10-0 nylon was then placed at the paracentesis, which was also found to be watertight (Fig. 23.2).

After completion of repair of the corneal laceration, attention was turned to the lens. Due to the central location of the corneal wound, significant corneal edema, and pupillary constriction, there was a limited view to the lens and therefore, it did not seem safe to proceed with traumatic cataract extraction at that time.

A subconjunctival antibiotic and steroid injection was performed temporally. The speculum was removed. The patient's drape was removed under the microscope. Atropine and an antibiotic-steroid ointment were placed in the right eye. A sterile patch and shield were placed over the right eye. The patient tolerated the procedure well without any complications.

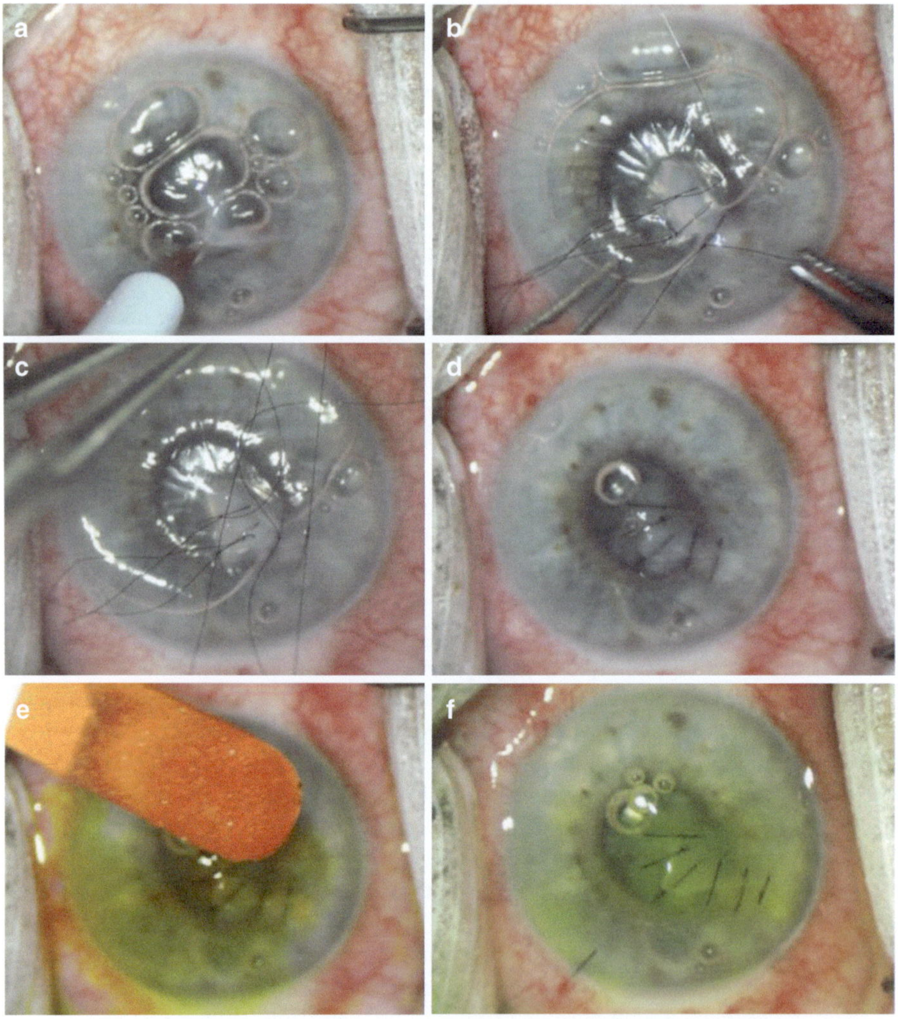

Fig. 23.2 Key steps of this delayed presentation Zone I open globe repair. After injecting filtered air into the anterior chamber through a paracentesis, the wound edges were gently debrided with a super sharp blade (**a**). The wound edges were reapproximated with granny style slipknots to allow for tension adjustment. The apex was approximated first with a long suture to ensure optimal healing (**b**, **c**). The knots were tied and buried after all sutures were adjusted to optimal tension (**d**). Wound was confirmed to be water-tight (**e**). An additional suture was placed at the wound edge to improve apposition, as well as a safety suture at the paracentesis (**f**)

23.4.1 Surgical Exploration and Repair: Pearls

- Consider repairing full-thickness corneal wounds that are healing irregularly even if Seidel negative for the best visual result.

- If significant corneal edema is present from delayed presentation, we recommend using more sutures tied at a higher tension to prevent post-operative wound leaks after the corneal edema resolves.
- In delayed presentation corneal wounds, gently debride wound edges with a blade prior to suturing, to optimize healing and prevent epithelial downgrowth.
- It is often prudent to avoid primary lens extraction at the time of globe closure if there is a poor intraocular view. Waiting several weeks and monitoring the patient may lead to an improved view and a more stable and quiet eye intraoperatively.

23.4.2 Surgical Video

Please see Video 23.1

23.5 Post-operative Course

The patient tolerated the procedure well and was discharged after he finished his 48 hour course of antibiotics. He was discharged on the standard regimen of topical drops. At the post-operative week 1 visit his visual acuity remained hand motion at 1 foot secondary to a white traumatic cataract. B-scan ultrasound confirmed no retinal detachment or significant posterior pathology. Inflammation remained well controlled with only trace cell. Risks, benefits, and alternatives regarding lens extraction were discussed and the patient was interested in proceeding with traumatic cataract extraction. The patient was scheduled for cataract extraction 1 month following primary globe closure. Due to known anterior capsule violation, delayed presentation, uncertain status of the posterior capsule, and presence of a paracentral corneal wound preventing reliable biometry, we planned to defer primary intraocular lens implantation and instead consider an aphakic contact lens fitting or secondary intraocular lens placement at a later time. The patient requested general anesthesia due to extreme anxiety about all eye-related procedures (Fig. 23.3).

23.6 Traumatic Cataract Extraction: Operative Note

A careful time out was completed and the correct patient and eye were identified. After general anesthesia was induced, a peribulbar block was performed on the right side to achieve multi-modal anesthesia and decrease the need for long acting pain medications as requested by anesthesia due to the risk associated with the patient's chronic obstructive pulmonary disease and also to provide improved exposure in a deep-set eye with a prominent brow. The patient was prepped and draped in the usual

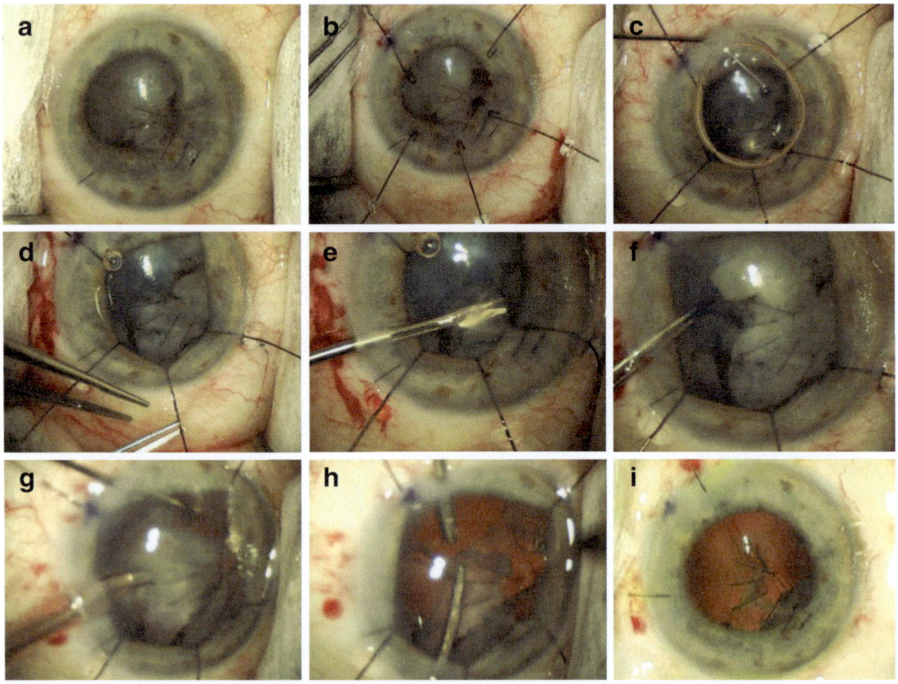

Fig. 23.3 Key steps of traumatic cataract extraction. Pre-operative photo demonstrates stable corneal wound with sutures intact (**a**). Following initial synechiolysis with a cyclodialysis spatula, iris hooks were placed (**b**). Trypan blue was used to stain the lens capsule, followed by viscoelastic (**c**). Further synechiolysis and expansion of the pupil was performed (**d**). Microscissors were required to lyse persistent synechiae at the site of penetrating injury and capsule violation inferotemporally (**e**). Capsulorrhexis of the intact anterior capsule was performed carefully with utrata forceps (**f**). Phacoemulsification using a modified stop and chop technique was performed (**g**). Residual cortex was removed with bimanual I/A (**h**). The patient was left aphakic (**i**)

sterile ophthalmic fashion. A self-retaining lid speculum was placed. A paracentesis incision was created at 2:30 o'clock and a second paracentesis was created at 9:00 o'clock. A small amount of dispersive viscoelastic was injected through the paracentesis incision into the anterior chamber and under the iris plane inferiorly in the location of the posterior synechiae. A cyclodialysis spatula was used to explore and release the inferotemporal posterior synechiae between iris and the lens in the location of the anterior lens capsule violation and posterior to the corneal laceration that was previously repaired. Microscissors were used to release areas of adhesion that could not be released with the cyclodialysis spatula. Five iris hooks were placed to achieve adequate pupillary dilation due to a persistently miotic pupil. Additional inferior posterior synechiae were noted after placement of the hooks and these were released with viscodissection and the cyclodialysis spatula. The viscoelastic was irrigated from the anterior chamber. This was followed by injection of filtered air and trypan blue to stain an otherwise obscured anterior capsule and visualize the location of the capsule defect in the setting of a white traumatic cataract. The anterior chamber was irrigated with balanced salt solution. The inferior half of the anterior lens capsule was noted to be violated with exposed lens material. Dispersive viscoelastic was injected into the anterior chamber through the paracentesis. A 2.4 mm keratome was utilized to enter the anterior chamber through a clear corneal tri-planar incision at approximately 10:30 o'clock. A cystitome was used to initiate a capsulorrhexis nasally and a utrata forceps was used to complete a curvilinear capsulorrhexis of the superior part of the intact capsule. Gentle hydrodissection was performed with balanced salt solution on a 25-gauge flat cannula in the superior quadrants. The white lens nucleus was then phacoemulsified. Residual epinuclear and cortical lens material was removed with the bimanual irrigation/aspiration instruments. The posterior capsule was noted to be intact. Residual viscoelastic was removed. The hooks were removed. Through a 30-gauge cannula, balanced salt solution was utilized to inflate the globe to normal pressure and to hydrate the main and paracentesis incisions, making them watertight. 10-0 nylon sutures were placed at the main wound as well as the paracentesis at 2:30 o'clock. The main and paracentesis incisions were noted to be watertight. A Seidel test was performed to confirm that the previously repaired corneal laceration remained watertight and no leaks were noted. A subconjunctival injection of antibiotic and dexamethasone was injected temporally. An antibiotic-steroid ointment along with a sterile ophthalmic pad and shield were applied. The patient was extubated. Having tolerated the procedure well, the patient was transferred to the recovery area in stable condition.

23.6.1 *Surgical Video*

Please see Video 23.2

23.7 Post-operative Course

The patient did well post-operatively (Fig. 23.4). He was started on typical post-operative cataract surgery eye drops and was followed closely over the subsequent weeks. Approximately 7 weeks after open globe repair and 3 weeks after traumatic cataract extraction, the patient returned to trauma clinic for corneal

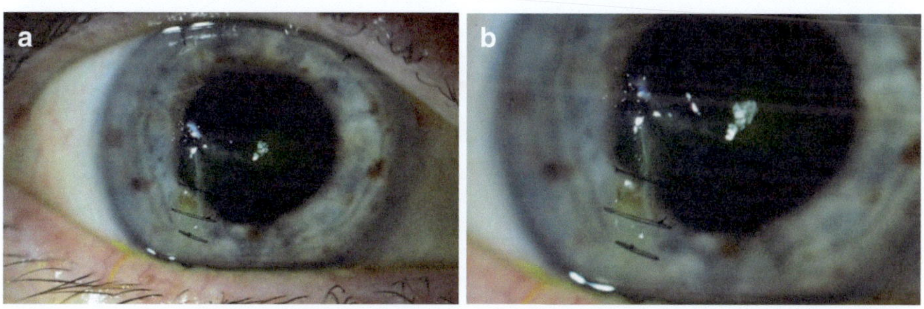

Fig. 23.4 External photo demonstrating post-operative week 1 appearance status post extraction of traumatic cataract. Corneal sutures were removed at week 2 after traumatic cataract extraction

suture removal (final exam below). Subsequent follow up was coordinated with an ophthalmologist closer to the home of the patient. We discussed the future options of evaluation for aphakic contact lens versus placement of a secondary intraocular lens.

23.8 Final Trauma Evaluation

23.8.1 Final Visual Acuity

OD: Count fingers at 1 foot (20/50 with a +11.00 lens and pinhole)
OS: 20/50 pinhole 20/30

23.8.2 Pupils

OD: 4 mm briskly reactive
OS: 3 mm briskly reactive

23.8.3 Slit Lamp Examination

	OD	OS
Lids and lashes	Normal, deep orbit	Normal, deep orbit
Sclera and conjunctiva	Normal	Normal
Cornea	Full-thickness inverted V-shaped laceration closed with six 10-0 nylon sutures in place, Seidel negative	Normal
Anterior chamber	Deep and quiet	Normal
Iris	Fairly round, some irregularity inferotemporally where there were significant synechiae	Normal
Lens	Posterior capsule appears intact	Normal
Vitreous	Normal	Normal

23.8.4 Dilated Examination

Macula/Nerve OD: Normal
Periphery OD: Normal
Macula/Nerve: OS: Normal
Periphery OS: Normal

23.9 Review and Lessons Learned

In traumatic cataract cases—unlike standard, age-related cataract cases—the pathologic changes are not limited to the lens alone and may also involve the iris, zonules, anterior or posterior capsule as well as the posterior segment. This should be discussed with the patient in advance so as to set appropriate expectations for visual outcome as well as the risk for intraoperative complications and potential need for more surgery. During surgical planning, multiple components should also be considered. The location of the traumatic injury may guide main wound placement for optimal visualization and access to problem areas. The extent of synechiae will determine whether viscosynechialysis will be sufficient or if iris hooks or a cyclodialysis spatula or microscissors are necessary to break synechiae. All of these instruments should be available intraoperatively. Zonular integrity and the presence of phacodonesis should be assessed during pre-operative exam. An attempt should be made to determine the location of the anterior capsule violation as to help with surgical planning for placement of the capsulorrhexis. The posterior capsule integrity can be assessed pre-operatively with a B-scan or ultrasound biomicroscopy (UBM). If posterior capsule is clearly involved, then it may be best to have a retina specialist on back-up on the day of cataract extraction or refer the patient to a retina specialist for pars plana lensectomy.

An anterior approach to traumatic cataract extraction can be considered if there is sufficient zonular stability and ideally an intact posterior capsule. Sometimes the posterior capsule integrity is in question pre-operatively. In these cases it is especially important to discuss with the patient the possibility of lens material falling posteriorly and needing additional surgery by a retina specialist to remove the lens. An anterior approach can still be beneficial if enough capsule can be preserved to allow for a sulcus lens to be placed at some point or even to help debulk some of the lens for the retina surgeon.

Trypan blue is often essential for visualization especially in the presence of an anterior capsule defect. A small amount can be placed and rinsed with balanced salt solution prior to placement of any ophthalmic viscosurgical devices in the eye. However, often the pupil is small before synechiolysis and placement of iris hooks, preventing good anterior capsule staining. In such circumstances, in can be helpful to use viscoat conservatively prior to staining the capsule so a good stain can still be achieved.

Synechiolysis should be attempted first with a dispersive viscoelastic; careful use of a cyclodialysis spatula can help with synechiolysis taking care to avoid damaging the anterior capsule. Often there will be tight adhesions between the iris and anterior capsule in proximity to the anterior capsular defect and these are often best lysed with intraocular microscissors to avoid undue traction and inadvertent radialization of a capsular tear. Once the iris adhesions are free, iris hooks are often helpful to provide mechanical dilation and stabilization of the pupil. Care must be taken to avoid hooking the anterior capsule tears or flaps during iris hook placement. Once the iris hooks are placed, viscoelastic can be rinsed from the anterior chamber to allow for optimal staining of the anterior capsule with trypan blue in order to better visualize the location of the anterior capsule defect.

To perform the capsulorrhexis, it is often helpful to create a flap with microscissors in the area of the defect and initiate the capsulorrhexis from there. If the anterior capsule defect can be incorporated into the capsulorrhexis, this is ideal. However, in many cases, there is a large defect in the anterior capsule and only half or a portion of a capsulorrhexis can be completed to connect it to the defect. A larger capsulorrhexis is often desirable in these situations, however should not be larger than 6 mm as this will allow for optic capture in case of posterior capsular defect. In some cases, use of the vitrector to fashion a round opening in the anterior capsule also works. Hydrodissection should be attempted only with extreme caution.

If vitreous is noted in the anterior chamber then the cataract can be removed initially via an anterior approach using the vitrector on the "cut-I/A" setting making sure to clean out all of the vitreous prior to proceeding with cataract removal. It is important to use a vitrector and not an aspirator or phacoemulsification handpiece while removing vitreous admixture in the ruptured lens matter as any traction on the vitreous can result in inadvertent retinal breaks. Pars plana vitrectomy with lensectomy performed by the retina surgeon is an alternative pathway.

The decision to place an intraocular lens (IOL) at the time of cataract removal is dependent on many factors and is also patient- and surgeon-dependent. The visual potential of the eye in question, and the visual function of the fellow eye are important factors to weigh, as well as the patient's willingness or ability to undergo another sedated procedure for secondary IOL placement. If the patient will need retina surgery in the future, the secondary lens placement can be combined at that time. Zonular integrity, remaining capsule, and the degree of residual iris tissue will also determine the ultimate strategy for lens placement, whether it is in the bag, in the sulcus, fixated to the iris or sclera. In terms of lens calculations, the fellow eye, if normal, is usually a fairly reliable resource, however refractive surprises requiring subsequent intraocular lens exchange have been reported [2]. Waiting until the corneal sutures are removed and reliable measurements can be obtained, can often lead to a more reliable lens choice, but does require another surgery for placement of the lens. Remember that an aphakic contact lens can also give some of the best results because it addresses the lens and also any corneal irregularities simultaneously.

23.10 Key Learning Points

- In adults, the timing of traumatic cataract extraction is patient- and surgeon-dependent.
- If traumatic cataract extraction is not pursued at the time of open globe repair, then the patient must be counseled in advance that the vision is unlikely to improve and that a second surgery will be required to address this.

- In traumatic cataract cases, careful pre-operative examination and surgical planning are essential for ensuring optimal visual and anatomic outcomes and reducing the risk of intraoperative complications.

References

1. Shah M, Shah S, Upadhyay P, Agrawal R. Controversies in traumatic cataract classification and management - a review. Can J Ophthalmol. 2013;48(4):251–8.
2. Cohen K. Inaccuracy of intraocular lens power calculation after traumatic corneal laceration and cataract. J Cataract Refract Surg. 2001;27(9):1519–22.

Chapter 24
Case 19: Zone I Open Globe Injury with Traumatic Cataract Requiring Secondary Lens Extraction in a Pediatric Case

Zeba A. Syed, Seanna Grob, and Ankoor S. Shah

24.1 History of Present Illness

A 10-year-old male with no past medical history presented with concern for open globe injury of the left eye.

- Earlier that morning, the patient was blending a strawberry smoothie and inadvertently placed a spoon in the blender.
- The spoon got stuck in the blender blade and shot out the side of the blender. The blender shattered and likely a plastic shard hit the patient's left eye.
- The patient visited a local eye specialist and was transferred to Massachusetts Eye and Ear with a fox shield in place for evaluation for urgent surgical repair.

24.2 Initial Trauma Evaluation

24.2.1 Visual Acuity (Without Correction)

OD: 20/20
OS: Counting fingers at 2 feet

Z. A. Syed, M.D. (✉) • S. Grob, M.D., M.A.S.
Department of Ophthalmology, Harvard Medical School, Massachusetts Eye and Ear, Boston, MA, USA
e-mail: zeba_syed@meei.harvard.edu

A. S. Shah, M.D., Ph.D.
Department of Ophthalmology, Harvard Medical School, Boston Children's Hospital and Massachusetts Eye and Ear, Boston, MA, USA

S. Grob, C. Kloek (eds.), *Management of Open Globe Injuries*,
https://doi.org/10.1007/978-3-319-72410-2_24

24.2.2 Pupils

OD: Round, reactive
OS: Fixed, peaked, no afferent pupillary defect by reverse

24.2.3 External Examination

Normal

24.2.4 Slit Lamp Examination

	OD	OS
Lids and lashes	Normal	Normal
Sclera and conjunctiva	Normal	Normal
Cornea	Normal	4.5 mm full-thickness laceration extending from 2 o'clock paracentrally towards the inferonasal periphery with perpendicular <1 mm branches (partial vs. full-thickness); Seidel positive
Anterior chamber	Normal	Collapsed
Iris	Normal	Within the cornea wound
Lens	Normal	Fibrinous material present over lens with likely lens violation
Vitreous	Normal	No view

24.2.5 Dilated Examination

Macula/Nerve OD: Normal, cup to disc ratio 0.2
Periphery OD: Attached
Macula/Nerve: OS: No view
Periphery OS: No view

24.2.6 Radiographic Imaging

Computed tomography (CT) of the orbits showed no fracture or intraocular foreign body. There was a decrease in the anterior chamber volume and irregularity of the lens concerning for an open globe on the left (Fig. 24.1).

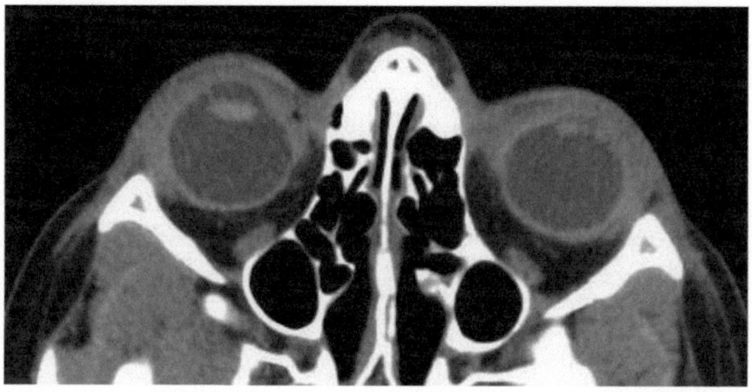

Fig. 24.1 Axial CT of the orbits showing decreased volume in the anterior chamber on the left with irregularity of the lens

24.3 Surgeon's Initial Assessment and Pre-operative Plan

This pediatric patient had a Zone I open globe injury of the left eye requiring surgical repair. The mechanism of injury was plastic from a blender shattering and hitting the left eye. There was no sign of an intraocular foreign body on clinical evaluation or on imaging. Importantly, pre-operative evaluation revealed possible lens violation. This case illustrates nuances in the management of concomitant lens violation in a pediatric open globe case.

Lens violation in pediatric open globe injuries adds another level of complexity to open globe repair. First, parents are often very anxious about the injury and adding the possibility of a traumatic cataract to the discussion can increase their concern. Second, based on age, the risk of amblyopia if the vision is blocked by a traumatic cataract or from refractive error after lens extraction is also a consideration [1, 2]. As discussed in Case 4 (Chap. 9), the pre-operative and intra-operative exams may be limited initially due to corneal edema and patient cooperation in the pediatric population. We had a high level of suspicion of traumatic cataract with lens violation in this case, but were planning to continue with primary repair of the cornea and closely follow the patient post-operatively. The patient also had a large central corneal laceration which would affect the intraocular view once the repair was complete. Postponing lens extraction would give the cornea time to heal, providing for a stable wound and therefore a stable anterior chamber during cataract extraction.

Some might elect to remove the lens primarily if there is a clear enough surgical view. The next question would then be the timing of intraocular lens placement. There have been reports of a higher rate of endophthalmitis in the setting of primary lens placement [3]. Therefore, if primary lens extraction is performed, it may be best to wait until the globe heals before placing an intraocular lens. If lens extraction takes place weeks after the globe repair and there are no signs of infection, then lens extraction with concurrent intraocular lens placement may be a good option.

The source of measurements for the choice of intraocular lens is also a consideration. If the lens is extracted primarily or prior to corneal suture removal, then measurements from the contralateral eye may be an option or the average corneal measurements can be used along with the axial length of the injured or non-injured eye.

24.4 Surgical Exploration and Repair: Operative Note

The risks, benefits, and alternatives were discussed with the patient and the patient's parents pre-operatively and they consented to proceed with exploration and repair of the open globe injury. The patient was brought to the operating room where the anesthesia team proceeded with general anesthesia. A careful time-out was observed and the correct patient and the eye were identified. The left eye was prepped and draped in the usual sterile ophthalmic fashion using a Jaffe speculum to provide adequate exposure.

The patient was found to have a vertical laceration involving two-thirds the length of the cornea and the visual axis, with stellate components at the superior and inferior ends with multiple apices. The anterior chamber was flat. There was likely lens violation with lens whitening. A temporal paracentesis was created with a supersharp blade, and filtered air was injected into the anterior chamber. The laceration was closed with multiple interrupted 10-0 nylon sutures using adjustable sutures (Fig. 24.2a, b). Filtered air was injected as needed to maintain the anterior

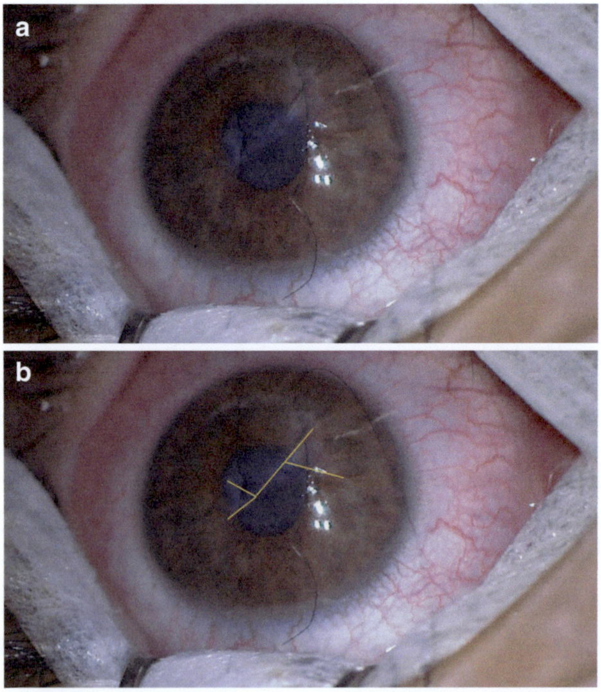

Fig. 24.2 (**a**) Early intra-operative photo showing a central corneal laceration with adjustable suture placed, a poorly dilated pupil, and hazy lens concerning for traumatic cataract. (**b**) Early intra-operative photo showing a linear representation of the structure of the corneal laceration with stellate components at both the superior and inferior aspects of the wound

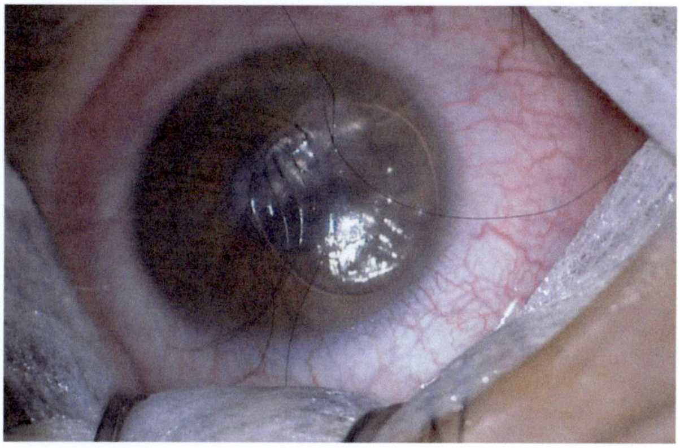

Fig. 24.3 Late intra-operative photo showing multiple adjustable sutures in position as the corneal wound is being aligned and closed. Filtered air was injected as needed into the anterior chamber to maintain anterior chamber depth during the repair

chamber depth. Sutures were removed and replaced as needed to improve alignment of the laceration edges and align the complex arrangement of apices (Fig. 24.3). All knots were buried. The air was removed and balanced salt solution was injected to fill the anterior chamber. The wound was found to be Seidel negative after the repair. The paracentesis was hydrated, and found to be watertight. A Kontur bandage contact lens was placed over the cornea due to the complex stellate corneal wound and for patient comfort.

A subconjunctival steroid and antibiotic injection was performed nasally and temporally away from the laceration. The speculum was removed. The patient's drape was removed under the microscope. The patient tolerated the procedure well without any complications.

24.4.1 Surgical Exploration and Repair: Pearls

- Adjustable corneal sutures can be helpful for stellate wounds, similar to limbus to limbus wounds.
- If the view to the lens is limited after corneal repair, then waiting until the cornea heals before performing lens extraction may be optimal to improve the view both clinically and surgically.

24.5 Post-operative Course

The patient was admitted for 48 hours of intravenous antibiotics. On post-operative day 1, the vision remained unchanged at counting fingers at 2 feet. The patient was followed closely by the pediatric ophthalmology and eye trauma services. During the first post-operative week, the cornea continued to clear, improving the view to the lens. Clinical exam clearly showed a traumatic cataract with anterior capsule

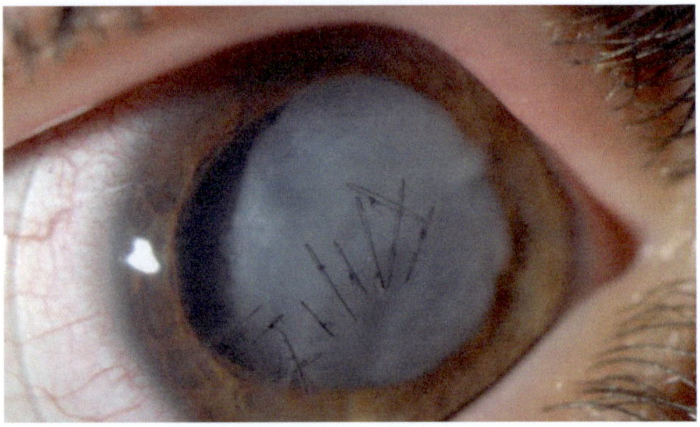

Fig. 24.4 Post-operative week 1 photo showed repaired corneal laceration with 10-0 nylon sutures in position, improved corneal edema, and a white, swollen traumatic cataract prolapsing forward into the anterior chamber

violation (Fig. 24.4). During this time, the patient's vision declined to hand motion due to progressive whitening and swelling of the lens and prolapse of the lens into the anterior chamber. Since the cornea continued to clear and the intraocular pressure remained stable, the eye was watched closely for 9 days. This allowed the corneal wound some time to heal prior to further surgical interventions. Subsequently, the patient underwent removal of the traumatic cataract with placement of an intraocular lens.

24.6 Second Surgical Repair: Operative Note

The risks, benefits, and alternatives of the procedure were discussed with the mother pre-operatively, and the mother consented to proceed with an examination under anesthesia and traumatic cataract extraction with possible intraocular lens insertion and possible vitrectomy. The patient was brought to the operating room where the anesthesia team proceeded with general anesthesia. A careful time-out was observed, and the correct patient and correct left eye were identified.

The examination under anesthesia was initiated. A cycloplegic refraction of the right eye was +0.50 + 0.50 × 90, and it was not possible to complete this on the left eye due to the traumatic cataract and corneal wound. Intraocular pressures with the Perkins tonometer were 12 mmHg in the right eye and 14 mmHg in the left with irregular mires approximately 20 minutes after induction of anesthesia. Measurements with the portable keratometer revealed K1 41.50 and K2 42.50 in the right eye. Measurements were not able to be obtained in the left eye due to the corneal irregularity from the stellate corneal laceration. Contact A-scan measurements revealed an axial length of 23.75 mm on the right and 23.50 mm on the left eye. Due to the slightly thickened appearance of the choroid on B scan of the left eye pre-operatively from the depressurization and injury to the left eye, we made a decision to proceed with biometry for intraocular lens power calculation based on the right eye keratometry and axial length, when assuming that both eyes were equivalent prior to the injury.

The left eye was prepped and draped in the usual sterile ophthalmic fashion using a speculum to provide adequate exposure. A small, localized superonasal fornix-based conjunctival flap was prepared with Westcott scissors. After achieving adequate hemostasis, a half-thickness scleral incision was made with a crescent blade, approximately 1.5 mm posterior to the limbus. It was carried anteriorly 3 mm in length with a crescent knife. A 20-gauge MVR blade was used to enter the anterior chamber through the scleral tunnel incision. Filtered air was injected into the anterior chamber. Trypan blue was then injected around the traumatic cataract in an attempt to stain an otherwise obscured view of the remaining capsule. This was washed with balanced salt solution. Viscoat was injected anterior to the traumatic cataract and lens material. A paracentesis incision was created with a 20-gauge MVR blade at 2 o'clock. The lens nucleus was then carefully removed with a 23-gauge vitrectomy cutter taking care to avoid the remaining capsule with a 23-gauge irrigating cannula in place. Residual cortical lens material was then removed carefully with aspiration and cutting as needed to remove lens material en toto and to preserve capsule. After removal of all of the lens material, the capsule was further inspected, and it was determined that the posterior capsule was intact and a large portion of the anterior capsule was also present with anterior capsule tears extending inferiorly around 5 o'clock and superiorly around 12:30 o'clock. There were some capsule-iris synechiae temporally and inferiorly that were released. Provisc was injected through the main wound to inflate the capsular bag. A 2.4 mm keratome was utilized to enter the anterior chamber through the corneoscleral incision. The intraocular lens was inserted into the capsular bag and dialed into position with the Y hook. The haptics were placed at 3 and 9 o'clock. Residual Provisc was removed with the vitrector on irrigation and aspiration mode. Through a 30-gauge cannula, balanced salt solution was utilized to inflate the globe to normal pressure. The main wound and paracentesis were closed with 10-0 nylon sutures and the knots were rotated making the incisions watertight. The conjunctiva was coapted nasally with an 8-0 Vicryl suture. The speculum was removed.

The stellate corneal laceration remained watertight throughout the procedure. It was noted during the case that the corneal laceration was slightly gaping anteriorly, but the sutures remained intact and the wound was watertight for the duration of the case. The patient's drape was removed under the microscope. A combination of neomycin, polymyxin, and dexamethasone ointment along with a sterile ophthalmic pad and shield were applied. The patient tolerated the procedure well without any complications.

24.7 Post-operative Course

Approximately 1 month later, after the eye had healed from the second surgery (Fig. 24.5), the patient was brought back to the operating room for corneal suture removal. Half of the sutures were removed initially using a #15 blade to cut and elevate the suture and then a jewelers forceps to remove them. The wound appeared stable, so the remaining half were also removed. The wound was Seidel negative after removal of all sutures.

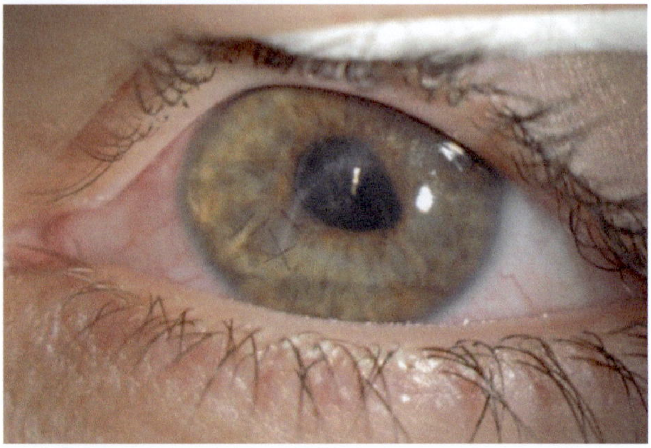

Fig. 24.5 Clinical photo after removal of the traumatic cataract with placement of an intraocular lens

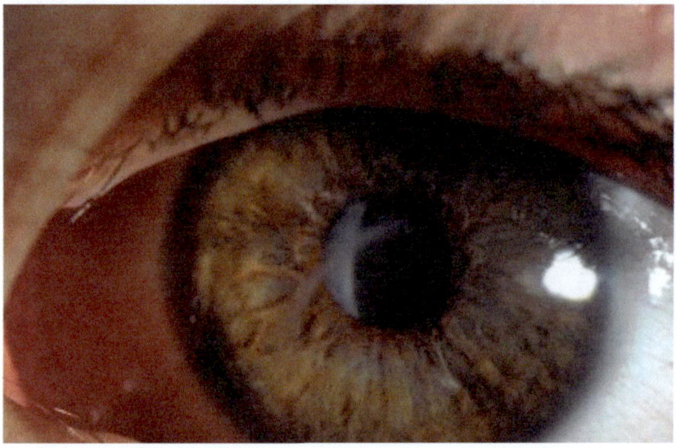

Fig. 24.6 Anterior segment photo obtained almost 6 months after the initial open globe repair showing a curvilinear scar affecting the central visual axis, a round pupil, and a clear lens implant

The patient continued to follow with the pediatric ophthalmology service. The cornea continued to heal after the sutures were removed, but it was difficult to obtain a cycloplegic refraction with retinoscopy due to an irregular and faint red reflex. After almost 5.5 months after globe repair the reflex improved, but was still irregular with two zones of reflex on either side of the laceration crossing the pupil (Fig. 24.6). The patient will be referred to the contact lens service for evaluation to see if vision can be improved with a contact.

24.8 Final Trauma Evaluation

24.8.1 Final Visual Acuity (with Correction)

OD: 20/15
OS: 20/200 pinhole 20/70-2

24.8.2 Pupils

OD: Round, reactive
OS: Round, reactive

24.8.3 Slit Lamp Examination

	OD	OS
Lids and lashes	Normal	Normal
Sclera and conjunctiva	Normal	Healed superonasal peritomy
Cornea	Normal	Stellate scar extending into visual axis
Anterior chamber	Normal	Normal
Iris	Normal	Damage to iris sphincter superiorly and temporally
Lens	Normal	Intraocular lens well-positioned in capsular bag
Vitreous	Normal	Normal

24.9 Review and Lessons Learned

Traumatic cataracts are the most common cause for severe vision decline in pediatric patients after an open globe injury, and proper management of cataract remains essential to optimize visual outcomes [1, 2]. It is necessary that traumatic cataracts be managed as soon as possible to avoid other complications, such as amblyopia, in the pediatric population.

One consideration in the management of traumatic cataracts is when to perform intraocular lens implantation with respect to closure of the primary wound and removal of the cataract. In our case, the location and extent of injury made primary lens extraction with lens implantation difficult. Although there was a high suspicion for lens capsule violation, there was not a clear view of the lens which only worsened after corneal laceration repair. For these reasons, the corneal wound was repaired primarily, and the wound was given time to heal before a second surgery involving cataract extraction with lens implantation. In other cases, the wound could be closed at the same time as cataract removal, with a choice of primary versus secondary intraocular lens implantation. Several factors should be taken into consideration, including the nature of the trauma, child's age, etc. Primary lens implantation is generally more favorable in eyes with closed globe injuries, as the risk of infection is low in the absence of a corneal laceration. Some studies advocate for simultaneous cataract extraction with lens implantation in the presence of a traumatic wound. However, with a large corneal laceration, the view could be obscured making lens extraction less safe, and there is a possible increase in risk of infection. Furthermore, the measurements used would likely be from the non-traumatized eye which could lead to inaccuracies in lens selection. Simultaneous cataract extraction with lens implantation in a separate surgery after open globe repair (as was done in this case) is also an option, and allows for some corneal healing time prior to lens extraction. This allows for a more stable anterior chamber and improved view, but could also lead to inaccuracies in lens choice depending on the measurements used (in our case we used measurements from the non-traumatized eye assuming the eyes were similar before the injury). Secondary implantation of a lens may have the benefit of allowing more accurate measurements from the injured eye for lens choice, and may have a lower risk of infection, but it would require an additional surgery and anesthesia exposure.

In cases of extensive injury to the capsule or zonules, the lens cannot be placed in the bag and should be placed in the ciliary sulcus or secured by scleral fixation. Such approaches have been shown to be successful in patients with pediatric traumatic cataract with inadequate capsular support. In this case, the lens was able to be placed in the capsular bag safely since sufficient capsule was noted during the cataract extraction.

In children, amblyopia is a major concern after open globe injury due to a lengthy period of visual rehabilitation or poor visual potential [1, 2]. Various strategies to prevent amblyopia have been studied, and patching of the uninjured eye remains the gold standard of therapy. The patient should be managed by a team including a pediatric ophthalmologist following primary repair. In our case, the patient was fortunately beyond the amblyogenic age range, which gave a little more flexibility in decision making after the open globe repair.

Recently, a pediatric ocular trauma score (POTS) was devised to predict visual prognosis after pediatric eye injury [4]. Factors indicating poorer visual prognosis include a younger age, poorer initial visual acuity, posterior eye involvement, longer wound length, globe rupture, lens involvement, and endophthalmitis. This tool may prove to be useful when counseling families of pediatric open globe injury patients, and setting practical expectations.

24.10 Key Learning Points

- In cases of pediatric globe injury with concurrent traumatic cataract, prompt management of the cataract is crucial, especially in cases when amblyopia is a risk.
- The decision on whether to perform primary wound repair with cataract extraction and lens implantation versus a staged approach depends on various factors, including the patient's age, nature of the injury, view through the cornea, and risk of infection.
- The pediatric ocular trauma score (POTS) can be very useful when counseling a patient's family about visual prognosis.

References

1. Li X, Zarbin MA, Bhagat N. Pediatric open globe injury: a review of the literature. J Emerg Trauma Shock. 2015;8(4):216–23.
2. Xu YN, Huang YS, Xie LX. Pediatric traumatic cataract and surgery outcomes in eastern China: a hospital-based study. Int J Ophthalmol. 2013;6(2):160–4.
3. Andreoli CM, Andreoli MT, Kloek CE, Ahuero AE, Vavvas D, Durand ML. Low rate of endophthalmitis in a large series of open globe injuries. Am J Ophthalmol. 2009;147(4):601–8.
4. Acar U, Tok OY, Acar DE, Burcu A, Ornek F. A new ocular trauma score in pediatric penetrating eye injuries. Eye (Lond). 2011;25(3):370–4.

Chapter 25
Case 20: Zone I Open Globe Repair with Secondary Removal of Lens Using a Pars Plana Approach

Mohammad Dahrouj, Eric D. Gaier, Seanna Grob, and Dean Eliott

25.1 History of Present Illness

A 54-year-old man with no previous medical or ocular history was transferred with concern for open globe injury of the left eye.

- The patient was prying wood planks and pulling them up towards his face when a small piece flew into his left eye. He was not wearing eye protection.
- On initial evaluation, an open globe injury was readily apparent with a large full-thickness corneal laceration.

25.2 Initial Trauma Evaluation

25.2.1 Visual Acuity (Without Correction)

OD: 20/20
OS: Hand motion

M. Dahrouj, M.D., Ph.D. (✉) • E. D. Gaier, M.D., Ph.D. • S. Grob, M.D., M.A.S.
Department of Ophthalmology, Harvard Medical School, Massachusetts Eye and Ear, Boston, MA, USA
e-mail: mohammad_dahrouj@meei.harvard.edu

D. Eliott, M.D.
Vitreoretinal Surgery, Department of Ophthalmology, Harvard Medical School, Massachusetts Eye and Ear, Boston, MA, USA

S. Grob, C. Kloek (eds.), *Management of Open Globe Injuries*,
https://doi.org/10.1007/978-3-319-72410-2_25

25.2.2 Pupils

OD: Round, reactive
OS: Irregular, non-reactive, no relative afferent pupillary defect by reverse

25.2.3 External Examination

Superficial abrasion across nasal bridge.

25.2.4 Slit Lamp Examination

	OD	OS
Lids and lashes	Normal	Normal
Sclera and conjunctiva	Normal	1+ injection with few small areas of debris buried medially
Cornea	Normal	Full-thickness 10 mm corneal laceration extending diagonally from the limbus at 8 o'clock to 2 o'clock with a stellate component nasally. Uveal material protruding through the superior portion of the laceration
Anterior chamber	Normal	Poor view, but with narrow angle with iridocorneal touch temporally
Iris	Normal	Irregular, anteriorly displaced, with iris tissue protruding from laceration
Lens	Normal	Cloudy with poor view
Vitreous	PVD	No view

25.2.5 Dilated Examination

Macula/Nerve OD: Normal
Periphery OD: Normal
Macula/Nerve: OS: No view
Periphery OS: No view

25.2.6 Radiographic Imaging

On computed tomography (CT) imaging (Fig. 25.1) the left globe was decreased in volume and irregular in shape. There was loss of volume both in the anterior and posterior segment, with decreased size of the vitreous compared to the right. No

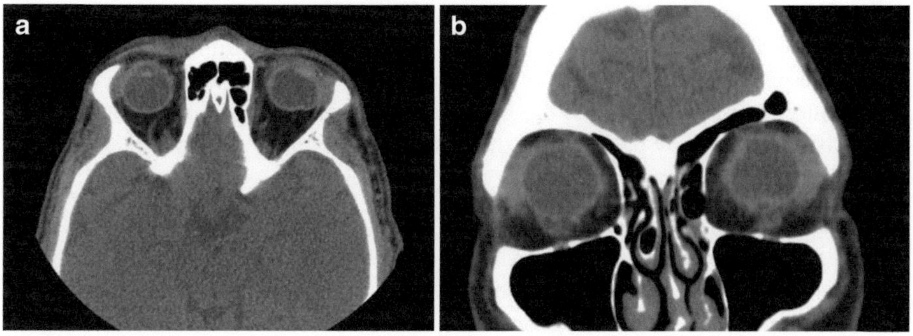

Fig. 25.1 Non-contrast CT images of the orbits. (**a**) Axial and (**b**) coronal images showing a normal globe on the right and a deformed globe on the left

radiopaque foreign body was identified in the left orbit or globe. No intracranial injury identified. No orbital fractures were noted.

25.3 Surgeon's Initial Assessment and Pre-operative Plan

The patient has a Zone I open globe injury of the left eye after a piece of wood he was pulling up on came loose and hit his eye. Examination shows an oblique, full-thickness corneal laceration with a stellate component nasally and uveal tissue prolapse.

The pre-operative plan for the Zone I laceration in this case would not differ from standard repair of stellate corneal lacerations (see earlier cases in this book for examples) despite the size of laceration. This case illustrates two important concepts beyond the standard repair of stellate Zone I laceration including: (1) the management of lens and lens capsule violation, (2) the treatment of cystoid macular edema following globe injury repair, and (3) hard contact lens fitting for irregular cylindrical refractive error.

Open globe injury with suspected lens capsule violation requires special considerations and anticipation of a staged approach. It may be intuitive to perform a primary lensectomy during the initial open globe repair (as was done in case 17 (Chap. 22)), but it is important to consider the advantages to a staged approach:

1. As discussed in an earlier case, the view through the cornea is often suboptimal immediately after the initial corneal repair due to edema, which compromises the ability to perform a lensectomy or vitrectomy or other intraocular procedures.
2. It is difficult to fully evaluate the extent of the damage to the lens and lens capsule due to the compromised view. Multiple approaches for lensectomy can be utilized, usually depending on the location and extent of trauma to the capsule and zonules. Waiting until the view to the lens clears to better assess the lens and lens capsule can allow for improved pre-operative planning.
3. Allowing the cornea to heal after repair will provide a more stable wound and will prevent leakage through the corneal wound during lens removal, which will

provide a more stable anterior chamber. Waiting can also allow the corneal edema to clear and the view to the lens to improve significantly.

4. A vitreoretinal specialist may be better equipped to remove a lens with posterior capsule violation because of the high likelihood of dropped lens material. They can also address any problems in the posterior segment noted on dilated exam or B scan during the same surgery as well.

In cases with clear posterior capsule involvement and/or obvious posterior pathology on dilated exam or B scan, it can be helpful to refer the patient to a retina specialist after globe repair. The case can either be organized as a combined case where an anterior segment surgeon removes the cataract and the retina surgeon retrieves any lost pieces, or the retina surgeon can address both the traumatic cataract and any posterior pathology. Sometimes when a retina specialist removes the lens, posterior hyaloid membrane removal is performed to decrease the risk of future retinal detachment, which may also include removal of the lens capsule. In these cases, the options for refractive correction include a contact lens, an anterior chamber lens, or an iris or scleral sutured lens. It is often helpful to wait for at least approximately 4–6 weeks after all corneal sutures are removed to get fitted for a contact lens or get measurements for placement of an intraocular lens, so corneal measurements are stable and accurate. If the patient has a corneal laceration, often the best visual acuity comes with the use of a contact lens to correct the irregular astigmatism.

25.4 Surgical Exploration and Repair: Operative Note

Informed consent was obtained and the operative eye was verified and marked. The uninjured right eye was taped and shielded for protection. The left eye was prepped and draped in the usual sterile ophthalmic fashion using a Jaffe speculum to provide adequate exposure.

The patient was found to have a ~10 mm serpentine horizontal, limbus-to-limbus corneal laceration from the 9 o'clock nasally to 2 o'clock temporally. The nasal aspect of the laceration was triangulated with a stellate focus ~3–4 mm from the limbus. There was a significant amount of diffuse corneal edema. The anterior lens capsule was violated from the trauma with lens material in the anterior chamber. There was iris protruding through the corneal laceration. A paracentesis was made at the 3 o'clock position temporally, and filtered air was injected into the anterior chamber. A cyclodialysis spatula was used to retract iris tissue out of the corneal wound. Multiple 10-0 nylon sutures were used to re-approximate the margins of the laceration, including a suture through the apex of the stellate portion of the wound nasally. The majority of the filtered air was removed. Balanced salt solution was injected through the paracentesis to bring the eye to physiologic pressure. A fluorescein strip was used to check for any wound leaks after repairing the corneal laceration and none were seen. The temporal paracentesis was sutured with a single

10-0 nylon suture. At this point, attention was turned to the anterior chamber to evaluate the lens further and, due to corneal edema, the view was difficult and it was determined it would not be safe to remove the lens at this time. There was also concern for posterior capsule involvement. A subconjunctival injection of cefazolin and dexamethasone was given inferonasally away from the laceration. The lid speculums were removed. The patient's drape was removed under the microscope. A Kontour lens (18.0 mm) was placed at the end of the case as well as atropine and tobramycin-dexamethasone eye drops.

25.4.1 Surgical Exploration and Repair: Pearls

- In cases of open globe injury with lens capsule violation, repair the corneal or scleral wound as would otherwise be done primarily. Remember the goal of the first surgery is to close the eye! Evaluating the lens and the need for primary lensectomy can be considered after the main wound is addressed. We recommend waiting to remove the lens if the view is not optimal/poor.
- Placing a bandage contact lens at the end of an open globe repair can be considered for complex corneal wounds that may be more prone to leaking or in cases where there was corneal epithelial loss from the trauma or during the repair to help with patient comfort post-operatively.

25.5 Post-operative Course

The patient was admitted and completed a 48 hour course of intravenous antibiotics. On post-operative day one, his visual acuity was still hand motion. Corneal edema and haziness improved over the following days, but the view to the posterior segment remained obscured by the opacified lens. A B-scan ultrasound showed a posteriorly tilted lens with diffusely thickened posterior capsule (concerning for posterior capsule involvement and unstable zonules), and an attached retina (Fig. 25.2a).

Six days following the initial repair, the patient was seen by a retina specialist. Visual acuity remained hand motion and on exam there were multiple lens pieces in the anterior chamber with minimal view to the posterior segment (Fig. 25.2b). Pars plana lensectomy with no lens implantation was discussed with the patient (due to concern for zonular instability and posterior capsule involvement) who elected to proceed. The surgery was performed 10 days following the initial injury and repair. In addition to the lensectomy, multiple tufts and meridional folds were noted in the superonasal quadrant intraoperatively, and endolaser was applied to this area. No retinal breaks were noted.

The patient was followed closely by the retina and trauma services. The patient's best-corrected visual acuity improved to 20/100 on the post-operative week four visit. The patient's course was later complicated by cystoid macular edema (CME)

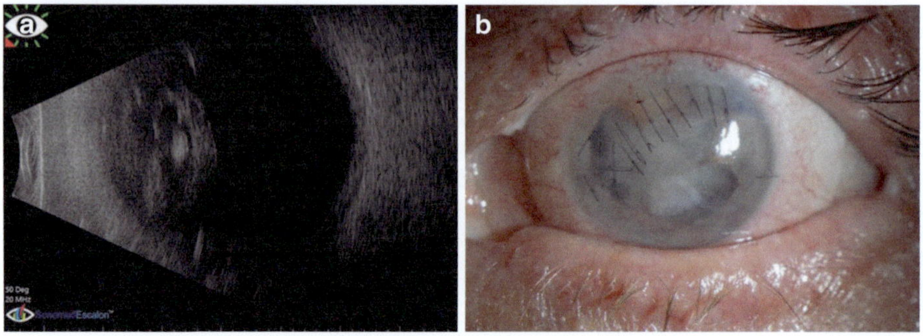

Fig. 25.2 (**a**) B scan ultrasonography following initial repair demonstrated diffusely thickened posterior lens capsule and attached retina. (**b**) Anterior segment slit lamp photograph taken 7 days following globe repair surgery showing multiple nylon sutures aligning the corneal laceration superiorly, white lens particles in the anterior chamber, and irregular pupil with loss of iris tissue

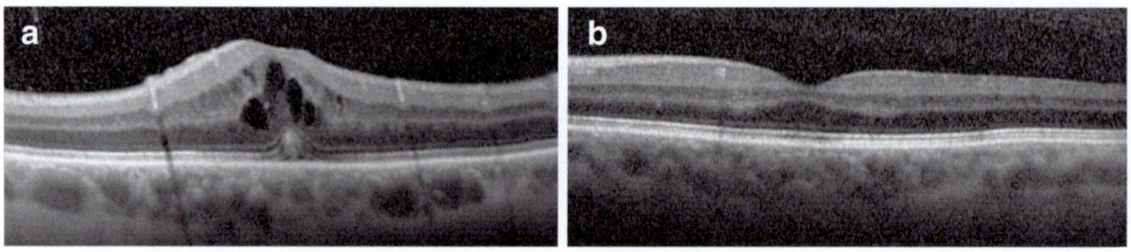

Fig. 25.3 Spectral domain optical coherence tomography (OCT) images of the left eye. (**a**) Images obtained 3 months following trauma showing cystoid macular edema (CME). (**b**) OCT images taken 4 months following treatment with ketorolac and prednisolone eye drops showing resolution of CME

3 months following the initial injury (Fig. 25.3a). Ketorolac and prednisolone eye drops four times daily were prescribed and continued for a 4-month course. Seven months following the initial injury, the patient showed resolution of his cystoid macular edema and the drops were tapered off (Fig. 25.3b).

The patient was referred to the optometry service for evaluation for a contact lens. He was fitted for a rigid gas permeable (RGP) contact lens to correct the aphakia and irregular astigmatism from his corneal wound. His visual acuity improved to 20/80+ with an RGP.

25.6 Final Trauma Evaluation

25.6.1 Final Visual Acuity

OD: 20/20
OS: 20/80 (with a rigid gas permeable contact lens)

25.6.2 *Pupils*

OD: Round, reactive
OS: Irregular, no afferent pupillary defect by reverse

25.6.3 *Slit Lamp Examination*

	OD	OS
Lids and lashes	Normal	Normal
Sclera and conjunctiva	Normal	Normal
Cornea	Normal	Limbus to limbus linear corneal scar extending from 8 to 2 o'clock (Fig. 25.4)
Anterior chamber	Normal	Trace cell
Iris	Normal	Irregular with loss of tissue superotemporally
Lens	Normal	Aphakic
Vitreous	Normal	Status post pars plana vitrectomy

25.6.4 *Dilated Examination*

Macula/Nerve OD: normal
Periphery OD: Normal
Macula/Nerve: OS: Normal
Periphery OS: Laser scars in the periphery superonasally (Fig. 25.5)

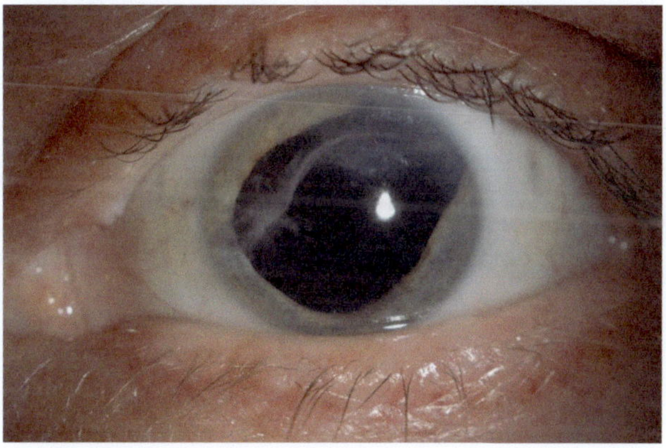

Fig. 25.4 Anterior segment slit lamp photograph taken during the last trauma evaluation (6 months following initial injury) showing corneal scar from 8 to 2 o'clock with loss of superotemporal iris tissue and a large pupil

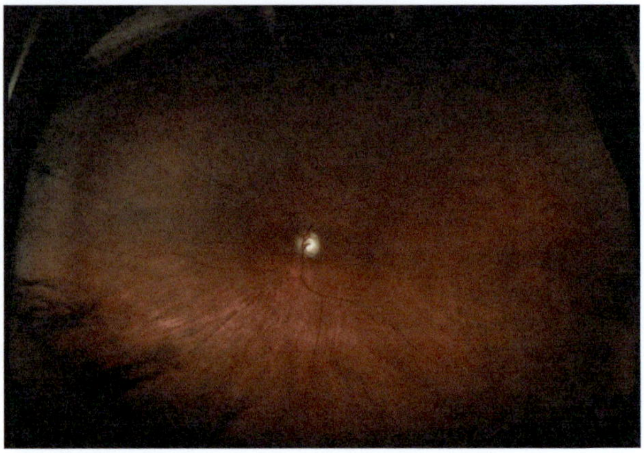

Fig. 25.5 Optos image of the left eye taken during the most recent trauma evaluation showing peripheral laser scars superonasally, but otherwise attached retina

25.7 Review and Lessons Learned

On initial repair of this 54-year-old patient's stellate, limbus-to-limbus Zone I injury, anterior lens capsule violation was evident and posterior lens capsule violation was suspected. Due to the difficult view following repair of the corneal laceration and concern for posterior lens capsule violation, we opted to take a staged approach to clear the visual axis. This is a good option even if only anterior capsule is involved, as discussed in the earlier cases. However, when there is concern for posterior capsule involvement and possibly retinal pathology, pars plana lensectomy with vitrectomy by a vitreoretinal surgeon is a good option.

Cystoid macular edema (CME) can develop following open globe injury and intraocular surgery, as occurred in our case. Management with prolonged use of topical non-steroidal anti-inflammatory and corticosteroid eye drops can lead to resolution of CME as in this case. It is important to consider CME as a reason for post-operative decreased vision in the setting of eye trauma and eye surgery (as open globe patients have many different reasons to have decreased vision, but you do not want to miss CME that can be treated). Intraocular pressure needs to be monitored carefully in patients on prolonged use of steroid eye drops.

In this case, we opted to leave the patient aphakic after traumatic cataract extraction. This decision was made for several reasons: (1) Due to the recent trauma and infection risk associated with placement of an implant in the setting of trauma, (2) Intraocular lens power calculation and keratometry measurements are more accurate after the corneal wound has healed and the corneal sutures have been removed (compared to using the fellow eye measurements) [1], and (3) The patient will likely need a contact lens anyway for best-corrected visual acuity due to the corneal astigmatism created by the corneal laceration.

Corneal scarring with irregular astigmatism and surgical aphakia present compounding visual rehabilitation challenges following open globe injury. Rigid gas permeable (RGP) contact lenses constitute a great non-surgical alternative to overcome these challenges simultaneously as they can negate irregular astigmatism and minimize anisometropia that would be caused from using glasses. In a previously published case report, 9 out of 11 patients gained 9 lines while obtaining a good contact lens tolerance [2]. Tinted RGP lenses provide additional benefit in cases of traumatic aniridia as they can improve the symptoms of photophobia as well as the cosmetic aspects of a traumatic pupil [3]. If the patient does not tolerate the lenses or has a strong interest in placing an intraocular lens, then an anterior chamber lens or an iris or scleral sutured lens can always be considered at a later date.

25.8 Key Learning Points

- A staged approach with secondary lensectomy is a good option in open globes with suspected lens capsule violation, especially if there is concern for posterior lens capsule violation and there is a poor intraocular view after corneal laceration repair.
- Pars plana vitrectomy and lensectomy should be considered when damage to the posterior capsule and zonular system is suspected.
- Cystoid macular edema following open globe injury should be considered and can be treated with a long course and slow taper of topical non-steroidal anti-inflammatory and corticosteroid.
- Rigid gas permeable contact lenses offer a useful non-surgical approach for visual rehabilitation following Zone I open globe injury with lens involvement resulting in irregular corneal astigmatism and aphakia.

References

1. Chuang LH, Lai CC. Secondary intraocular lens implantation of traumatic cataract in open-globe injury. Can J Ophthalmol. 2005;40(4):454–9.
2. Grunauer-Kloevekorn C, et al. Contact lens fitting as a possibility for visual rehabilitation in patients after open globe injuries. Klin Monbl Augenheilkd. 2004;221(8):652–7.
3. Luo WL, Tong JP, Shen Y. Rigid gas-permeable contact lens for visual rehabilitation in aphakia following trauma. Clin Exp Optom. 2012;95(5):499–505.

Chapter 26
Case 21: Zone I Open Globe Injury with Anterior Foreign Body from a Pencil Tip

Benjamin Jastrzembski, Natalie Wolkow, Seanna Grob, and Ankoor S. Shah

26.1 History of Present Illness

An otherwise healthy 11-year-old boy presented with 5.5 mm of mechanical pencil graphite penetrating the right cornea.

- The patient reported he was at school when a pencil was thrown at him and hit his right eye.
- He was seen at the school nurses' office and an outside hospital and then transferred to Massachusetts Eye and Ear (MEE) for management of his open globe injury.

26.2 Initial Trauma Evaluation

26.2.1 Visual Acuity (Without Correction)

OD: 20/50 pinhole 20/25+2
OS: 20/20-2

Electronic Supplementary Material The online version of this chapter (https://doi.org/10.1007/978-3-319-72410-2_26) contains supplementary material, which is available to authorized users.

B. Jastrzembski, M.D. (✉) • N. Wolkow, M.D., Ph.D. • S. Grob, M.D., M.A.S.
Department of Ophthalmology, Harvard Medical School, Massachusetts Eye and Ear, Boston, MA, USA
e-mail: Benjamin_jastrzembski@meei.harvard.edu

A. S. Shah, M.D., Ph.D.
Department of Ophthalmology, Harvard Medical School, Boston Children's Hospital and Massachusetts Eye and Ear, Boston, MA, USA

S. Grob, C. Kloek (eds.), *Management of Open Globe Injuries*,
https://doi.org/10.1007/978-3-319-72410-2_26

26.2.2 Pupils

OD: Round, no afferent pupillary defect
OS: Round, no afferent pupillary defect

26.2.3 External Examination

Normal, no lacerations or other trauma.

26.2.4 Slit Lamp Examination

	OD	OS
Lids and lashes	Normal	Normal
Sclera and conjunctiva	Normal	Normal
Cornea	5.5 mm-long piece of pencil graphite extending full-thickness through the cornea just central to the 8 o'clock limbus, bridging the anterior chamber and touching the anterior surface of the iris (Fig. 26.1)	Normal
Anterior chamber	+2 pigmented debris and cell, with pencil tip bridging the anterior chamber temporally and touching the anterior surface of the iris	Normal
Iris	Indented by foreign body	Normal
Lens	Normal, no cataract or lens violation seen	Normal
Vitreous	Normal	Normal

26.2.5 Dilated Examination

Macula/Nerve OD: Normal
Periphery OD: Normal
Macula/Nerve: OS: Normal
Periphery OS: Normal

26.2.6 Radiographic Imaging

Computed tomography (CT) of the orbits showed a linear foreign body in the anterior chamber of the right eye, consistent with known history of fragment of graphite (Fig. 26.2).

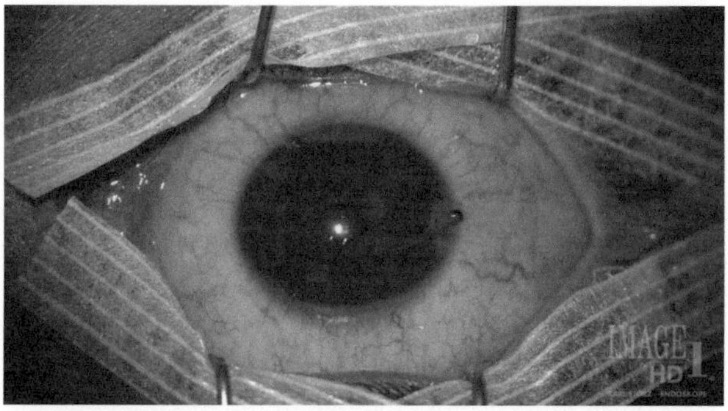

Fig. 26.1 Operating microscope photograph (surgeon view) demonstrating the pencil graphite embedded in the cornea and the anterior chamber abutting the iris

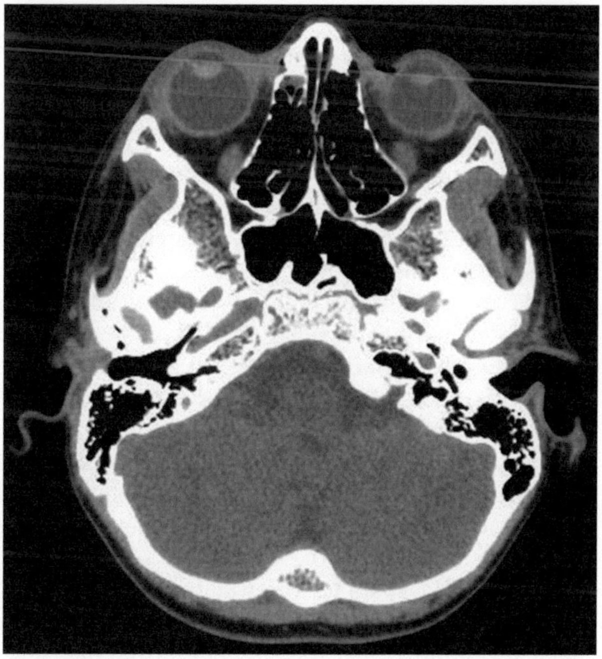

Fig. 26.2 Axial CT image showing a normal globe on the left and a fragment of pencil graphite in the cornea and anterior chamber of the right eye. The foreign body had a reading of 85 Hounsfield units

26.3 Surgeon's Initial Assessment and Pre-Operative Plan

This child had a Zone I laceration open globe injury with a retained intracorneal and anterior chamber foreign body. A classmate threw a pencil at him, and the pencil graphite became lodged in the cornea and anterior segment of the right eye. This case illustrates the basic approach to repair of an open globe injury with an intracorneal and anterior segment foreign body.

First, it is best to remove a full-thickness, intracorneal and/or anterior segment foreign body in the controlled setting of the operating room rather than in the emergency department. The foreign body may be plugging a wound leak and removing it may lead to anterior chamber collapse. It is important to communicate with all providers caring for the patient that the foreign body should not be manipulated or removed pre-operatively. The eye should be covered with a Fox shield at all times to avoid inadvertent manipulation of the eye or foreign body (as in all open globe injury cases). If a foreign body that was thought to be partial-thickness is removed and a brisk wound leak is noted, a bandage contact lens can be gently placed to slow or stop the wound leak. Alternatively, the patient may be scheduled to go to the operating room for repair quickly. Take care to not place pressure on the globe when placing a bandage contact lens.

Prior to pharmacologic dilation during the pre-operative examination, the surgeon should consider the risk of the foreign body moving with dilation, exposure of the lens to injury, or of the foreign body dropping posteriorly towards the vitreous. A dilated fundoscopic examination is almost always recommended prior to going to the operating room; however, if there is a loose foreign body in the anterior chamber, it may be best to defer dilation until the foreign body is removed in the operating room. In this case, the risk of the pencil graphite dropping was considered low as it was securely embedded in the cornea. There was a slight risk of the graphite piece injuring/touching the lens, as it was tenting the iris. Despite this risk, the patient was dilated pre-operatively without complication based on the judgment of the treating physician. Deferring dilation until after removal of the foreign body in the operating room setting would also be reasonable.

A CT scan of the orbits is always recommended pre-operatively in any open globe injury to identify intraocular foreign bodies. Although contemporary practice patterns aim to minimize exposure to iatrogenic radiation in children, the risk of an occult foreign body left in the eye or the orbit outweighs this risk as these foreign bodies may lead to significant inflammation and permanent damage to the eye from siderosis bulbi, calcosis, or endophthalmitis. Thus, CT of the orbits is routinely recommended even in children. The radiation dose for the CT orbit in this case was 3.8 millisievert (mSv). For comparison, the estimated average annual exposure to natural radiation sources is 2.4 mSv [1].

The CT scan should be reviewed by the surgeon and a radiologist and carefully scrutinized for any evidence of intraocular foreign bodies. In a case series of 74 patients with intraocular foreign bodies from the New Jersey Medical School, CT scan of the orbits was superior than clinical examination or B-scan in identifying glass and metal foreign bodies [2]. However, the utility of a CT scan is limited in identifying wood foreign bodies, as wood is hypoattenuated on CT, and may have a shifting appearance over time as the water content of the wood changes [2]. One clue on CT scan that there may be an intraocular wooden foreign body is the presence of an intraocular gas pockets.

Anterior segment foreign bodies may be removed in several different ways. If there is enough of the foreign body exposed through the cornea, forceps may be used to pull the foreign body out of the cornea. If the foreign body is fairly embedded in the cornea with minimal penetration of the anterior chamber, a 25-gauge or other size needle tip may be used to dislodge the foreign body from the cornea. If the foreign body is through the cornea and entering the anterior chamber, a paracentesis incision may be directed towards the foreign body and intraocular foreign body forceps may be used to grasp the foreign body and either push it back up through the cornea or pull it out through an enlarged corneal incision. Occasionally, docking the foreign body in a large bore needle may help with its extraction through a surgical wound, where the foreign body may get caught upon attempted removal. If the foreign body is loose in the anterior chamber or there is concern about it becoming loose and falling posteriorly, an ophthalmic viscoelastic may be injected into the anterior chamber, posterior to the foreign body, to create a barrier to it falling posteriorly during removal. Since the foreign body in this case was penetrating the cornea and the anterior chamber, the plan was to create a paracentesis, inject viscoelastic around the foreign body to secure it and protect the lens and iris, and then grasp it with forceps intraocularly and push it up through the corneal wound it created, while simultaneously grasping it extraocularly and pulling it out.

After foreign bodies are removed from the cornea, the defect that is left almost has the appearance of corneal tissue loss. For example, if a round metal rod is pulled out of the cornea, a round open defect often remains. This may often make corneal wounds with retained foreign bodies difficult to close as they are prone to leaking even with suture placement intraoperatively. Sutures may need to be tied on the tighter side to close a defect. Sometimes sutures may need to be placed and replaced adjusting wound tension several times before the wound is watertight. A cerclage suture may also occasionally be utilized to bring a round wound closed, and wound and fibrin glue are other methods that should be kept available in tough-to-close cases. A bandage contact may be placed post-operatively in wounds that are prone to leakage and left in place for several days to a week. The patient should remain on topical antibiotic drops while the contact lens is retained.

26.4 Surgical Exploration and Repair: Operative Note

The patient was brought to the operating room where the anesthesia team proceeded with general anesthesia. A careful time-out was observed, and the correct patient and eye were identified. The right eye was prepared with Betadine 10% solution in the periocular region and 5% solution in the fornices. Care was taken to avoid dropping Betadine solution directly into the wound of the eye. A sterile eye drape exposed the right eye, and Jaffe eyelid speculae were used to provide adequate exposure. A pencil lead tip of uniform diameter was noted to be lodged in the peripheral cornea just adjacent to the limbus at 8–9 o'clock, extending into the anterior chamber and pressing on the iris (Fig. 26.1). A perilimbal paracentesis incision was made at 1 o'clock with a 15° Stab Super Sharp blade directed towards the foreign body. A small pocket of Healon® (Abbott Laboratories, Abbott Park, IL) viscoelastic device was injected into the anterior chamber near the end of the pencil lead to distance the lead from the iris. Colibri forceps were used to pull on the end of the pencil lead that was extending out of the cornea from the external approach while Microsurgical Technology (MST) intraocular forceps were used to push the foreign body through the cornea from the anterior chamber/internal approach. The entire piece was easily removed and sent to pathology for cataloging. Next, the loose epithelium was scraped from the surface of the corneal wound with a #57 blade to remove residual graphite. The wound was examined and was found to be a shelved, inverted triangle. Irrigation with balanced salt solution through the paracentesis was used to remove the Healon® (Abbott Laboratories, Abbott Park, IL) from the anterior chamber and filtered air was injected to maintain the anterior chamber depth. Several 10-0 nylon sutures were placed across the corneal wound but with persistent leakage when air in the anterior chamber was exchanged for balanced salt solution. Several sutures were removed and new sutures were placed to ensure the wound was watertight, for a total of five sutures across the wound. Then, the filtered air was removed and replaced with balanced salt solution to bring the eye to physiologic pressure. The wound was tested and was found to be free of leakage. The paracentesis incision was hydrated with balanced salt solution and found to be watertight. A 16 mm diameter Kontur Precision Sphere (Kontur Kontact Lens, Co., Inc. Hercules, CA) was placed. Subconjunctival cefazolin and dexamethasone were administered away from the contact lens so as not to elevate it. The Jaffe eyelid speculae were removed, and the drape was removed. The periocular areas were cleaned, and the patient tolerated the procedure well without any complications.

26.4.1 Surgical Exploration and Repair: Pearls

- In the case of an embedded penetrating corneal foreign body, toothed forceps may be used to pull the object from outside of the eye. Alternatively, intraocular forceps can be used via the anterior chamber to push the object out through the defect it created or through an enlarged paracentesis/corneal wound.
- Viscoelastics can be used to protect intraocular structures from the foreign body and also to secure a loose foreign body from falling posteriorly while it is being retrieved.
- Corneal wounds with retained foreign bodies can be difficult to close, requiring multiple trials of sutures, and a bandage contact lens to achieve closure.

26.4.2 Surgical Video

- Please see Video 26.1.

26.5 Post-Operative Course

The patient was admitted to MEE to complete a 48 hour course of intravenous antibiotics. On post-operative day one, visual acuity in the operated eye was 20/140, and the patient had no pain. The patient was discharged after completing his intravenous antibiotics with the bandage contact lens in place. On his post-operative week one visit, visual acuity measured 20/30 and improved to 20/25 with pinhole testing. The bandage contact lens was removed, and the wound was found to be sealed. Due to the patient's age, he was scheduled for suture removal in the operating room, which was performed 4 weeks following the injury without complication.

26.6 Final Pediatric Ophthalmology/Trauma Evaluation

26.6.1 Final Visual Acuity

OD: 20/20
OS: 20/20

26.6.2 Final Manifest Refraction

OD: Plano +0.25 × 94
OS: Plano

26.6.3 Pupils

OD: Round, no afferent pupillary defect
OS: Round, no afferent pupillary defect

26.6.4 Slit Lamp Examination

Post-operative Course	OD	OS
Lids and lashes	Normal	Normal
Sclera and conjunctiva	Normal	Normal
Cornea	Trace corneal scar at temporal limbus (Fig. 26.3)	Normal
Anterior chamber	Normal	Normal
Iris	Normal	Normal
Lens	Normal, no cataract	Normal
Vitreous	Normal	Normal

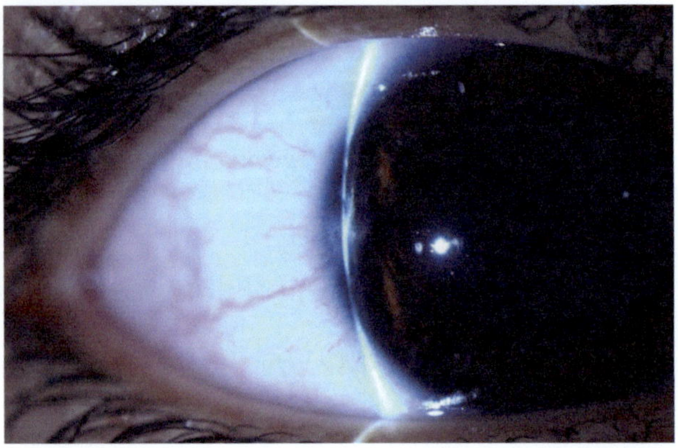

Fig. 26.3 Anterior segment, slit-lamp photograph demonstrating the temporal corneal scar 5 months following initial repair

26.6.5 Dilated Examination

Macula/Nerve OD: Normal
Periphery OD: Normal
Macula/Nerve: OS: Normal
Periphery OS: Normal

26.7 Review and Lessons Learned

In cases with an obvious full-thickness foreign body, removal should be deferred to the operating room if at all possible. Prior to dilation, a CT scan of the orbits is the modality of choice for identification of intraocular foreign bodies; research suggests that CT outperforms a pre-operative clinical examination in identifying intraocular foreign bodies [2].

An embedded corneal foreign body may be approached from the anterior chamber or externally. Viscoelastics can be helpful in securing the foreign body so it does not injure any intraocular structures and to prevent it from falling posteriorly. Closure of corneal wounds involving a penetrating foreign body may require patience and creativity as the wounds may initially keep the shape of the foreign body and be prone to leak during and after repair. Sutures may need to be replaced and adjusted. Although we try to avoid using corneal glue, it is also an option if the wound continues to leak after multiple attempts of placing sutures. A bandage contact lens is also an option with a slow leak or for wounds that tend to leak in surgery.

If the foreign body embedded in the cornea is vegetative matter, it will need to be watched carefully for infection. Fungal infection must be considered in these situations as well. Delayed presentation cases with retained intracorneal or intraocular foreign bodies may present with an infection requiring aggressive topical therapy or intracameral or intravitreal antibiotics. There are also cases of chronic uveitis caused by retained intraocular foreign bodies, so these are not to be missed. Prompt removal and repair with close follow-up may result in an excellent final visual acuity, as in this case. Chronic, retained graphite from a pencil has been reported to cause late complications such as corneal stromal edema, crystalline scars in the corneal stroma, conjunctival scarring that mimicked the appearance of conjunctival melanoma, and endophthalmitis [3–6]; thus, scraping and cleaning the wound after removal of this type of foreign body is indicated.

Visualizing the foreign body and understanding the location may be helpful for pre-operative planning. Small foreign objects might hide in the angle of the eye and gentle gonioscopy may be helpful if it cannot be visualized. This may be performed in the operating room after closure if needed. Observe for iris transillumination defects as these may also herald intraocular foreign bodies otherwise not easily visualized. An anterior segment ultrasound (ultrasound biomicroscopy) or anterior segment optical coherence tomography may be helpful in understanding the exact location and trajectory of the foreign body prior to removal as well.

26.8 Key Learning Points

- Removal of a full-thickness or intraocular foreign body should be performed in the operating room in a controlled setting.
- In cases of intraocular foreign bodies, consider the risk of the foreign body dropping to the posterior segment prior to pre-operative dilation.
- CT scan of the orbits is the ideal modality for recognizing intraocular foreign bodies, and should be performed on all open globe injury patients.

References

1. United Nations Scientific Committee on the Effects of Atomic Radiation. Sources and effects of ionizing radiation. New York: United Nations; 2010.
2. Patel SN, Langer PD, Zarbin MA, Bhagat N. Diagnostic value of clinical examination and radiographic imaging in identification of intraocular foreign bodies in open globe injury. Eur J Ophthalmol. 2012;22(2):259–68.
3. Han ER, Wee WR, Lee JH, Hyon JY. A case of retained graphite anterior chamber foreign body masquerading as stromal keratitis. Korean J Ophthalmol. 2011;25(2):128–31.
4. Jeng BH, Whitcher JP, Margolis TP. Intracorneal graphite particles. Cornea. 2004;23(3):319–20.
5. Guy JR, Rao NA. Graphite foreign body of the conjunctiva simulating melanoma. Cornea. 1985-1986;4(4):263–5.
6. Hamanaka N, Ikeda T, Inokuchi N, Shirai S, Uchihori YA. Case of an intraocular foreign body due to graphite pencil lead complicated by endophthalmitis. Ophthalmic Surg Lasers. 1999;30(3):229–31.

Chapter 27
Case 22: Zone I/II Open Globe Injury with Anterior Metallic Wire Foreign Body

Durga S. Borkar and Seanna Grob

27.1 History of Present Illness

A 21-year-old man with no past ocular history presents with an open globe injury and intraocular metallic foreign body to the left eye.

- The patient reports he works as a mechanic and was under a car when a metal spring fell and hit him in the left eye.
- He was seen at an outside hospital and was found to have a visible metallic foreign body penetrating the left globe (Fig. 27.1) and computed tomography (CT) imaging was consistent with an open globe injury and intraocular foreign body. He was transferred to Massachusetts Eye and Ear (MEE) for further management of his eye trauma.

27.2 Initial Trauma Evaluation

27.2.1 Visual Acuity (Without Correction)

OD: 20/20
OS: Count Fingers at 6 feet pinhole to 20/200

Electronic Supplementary Material The online version of this chapter (https://doi.org/10.1007/978-3-319-72410-2_27) contains supplementary material, which is available to authorized users.

D. S. Borkar, M.D. (✉) • S. Grob, M.D., M.A.S.
Department of Ophthalmology, Harvard Medical School, Massachusetts Eye and Ear, Boston, MA, USA
e-mail: durga_borkar@meei.harvard.edu

S. Grob, C. Kloek (eds.), *Management of Open Globe Injuries*,
https://doi.org/10.1007/978-3-319-72410-2_27

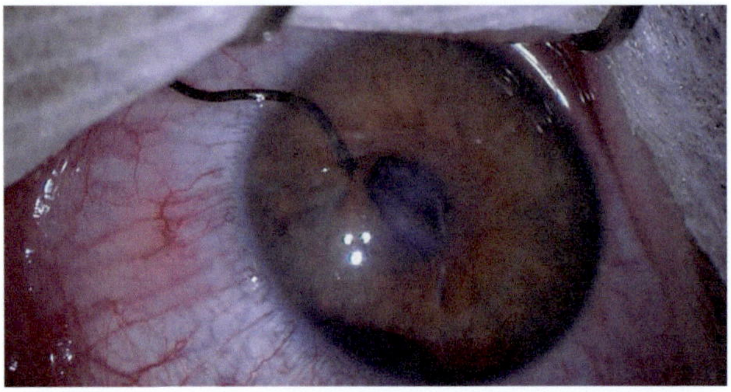

Fig. 27.1 Intraoperative clinical image of the patient's left eye prior to beginning surgery with the superonasal metal wire traveling initially superficial and then through the cornea into the anterior chamber and penetrating iris tissue at the pupillary border before coursing anteriorly to touch the posterior surface of the cornea

27.2.2 Pupils

OD: Round, no afferent pupillary defect
OS: Irregular with wire through margin of pupil, no afferent pupillary defect by reverse

27.2.3 External Examination

Normal.

27.2.4 Slit Lamp Examination

	OD	OS
Lids and lashes	Normal	Left upper eyelid edema, with wire protruding up under the left upper eyelid, conjunctival laceration on the palpebral conjunctiva of the superior eyelid
Sclera and conjunctiva	Normal	Metal wire sitting on top of conjunctiva superonasally. Unable to visualize the most nasal edge of the wire due to patient discomfort with eyelid elevation
Cornea	Normal	Entry of metal wire at limbus at 10 o'clock traveling anteriorly and intrastromally prior to entering the anterior chamber. Diffuse edema most prominent centrally where tip of wire is in contact with posterior surface of the cornea and rubbing on the endothelium
Anterior chamber	Normal	1 mm layering hyphema, blood suspended in anterior chamber at 9 o'clock, metal wire entering at 10 o'clock

	OD	OS
Iris	Normal	Wire on top of iris at 10 o'clock and traveling inferotemporally, hooking/penetrating the iris at 8 o'clock close to pupillary margin and bending anteriorly back into the anterior chamber
Lens	Normal	Possible violation of the lens capsule inferotemporally in location of where wire penetrates the iris
Vitreous	Normal	Hazy view

27.2.5 Dilated Examination

Macula/Nerve OD: Normal
Periphery OD: Normal
Macula/Nerve: OS: Hazy view
Periphery OS: Hazy view

27.2.6 Radiographic Imaging

Noncontract CT of the orbits (Fig. 27.2) showed a metallic foreign body, approximately 2–3 cm, going through the anterior segment with one end extending superonasally on top of the globe and into extraocular soft tissue. The foreign body appeared mostly preseptal. No orbital fractures were noted.

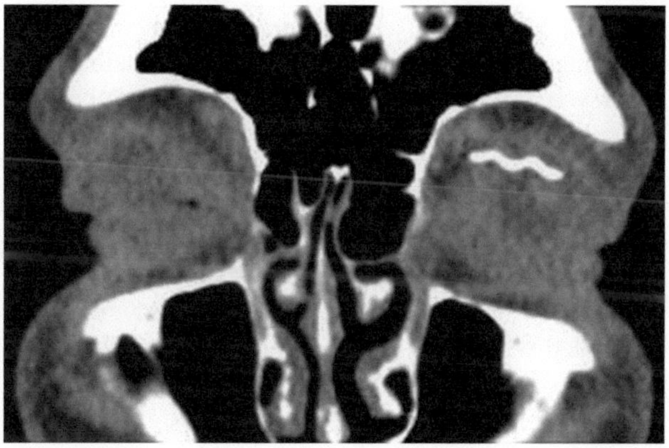

Fig. 27.2 Coronal CT image showing a normal globe on the right and a deformed globe on the left with an intraocular foreign body confined to the anterior segment

27.3 Surgeon's Initial Assessment and Pre-Operative Plan

The patient had a Zone I/II open globe injury of the left eye with an intraocular foreign body confined to the anterior segment requiring surgical repair.

This case illustrates three important areas of discussion beyond the standard repair of a Zone I/II laceration (see earlier cases in this book for examples). These are: importance of prompt surgical repair in patients with intraocular foreign bodies that may be causing continued damage to the ocular structures and further complications, and similarly to the previous case, removal of an anterior segment foreign body in the controlled setting of an operating room, and the importance of tight sutures in closing corneal lacerations from a round object causing a hole configuration after removal.

We recommend repair of all open globe injuries within 24 hours of the injury with the exception of patients who have a delayed (greater than 24 hours) presentation. However, in the case of an intraocular foreign body, additional efforts should be made to remove the foreign body and perform surgical repair as soon as possible after the diagnosis has been made. In this patient's case with an anterior segment foreign body and a round corneal entry site from the wire, prompt repair can minimize complications from rust formation as well as prevent worsening corneal edema that will only progress with time making repair and forming a watertight wound more challenging intraoperatively. Patients with foreign bodies protruding from the eye are also usually in significant discomfort and prompt repair is necessary for patients with uncontrollable pain and discomfort. In this patient, every time he blinked the wire would rub against his superior eyelid and also the posterior aspect of the cornea when the wire would rotate. Therefore, we planned to go to the operating room for removal of the foreign body and repair of the ruptured globe immediately to prevent further damage to the eyelid and orbital tissues as well as the central cornea.

As discussed previously, it is important to obtain a pre-operative CT scan for all globe patients to evaluate for a foreign body and the location and extent of the foreign body to help with surgical planning. Removal of the foreign body in the operating room is essential even if it is accessible at the slit lamp. In the operating room, you will have control of the anterior chamber depth via a paracentesis, sutures can be placed immediately in a Seidel positive wound, and the patient will also be more comfortable allowing for safer removal of the foreign body. In this case, the superonasal end of the wire was not visible at the slit lamp because it extended underneath the eyelid. A full exploration of this area was limited at the slit lamp due to patient discomfort and could be more adequately performed in the operating room to ensure the complete foreign body was removed. Removal in a more controlled setting in the operating room can also help to minimize any additional damage to the iris or lens capsule, as well as further endothelial damage in this case where the tip of the wire was touching the posterior surface of the cornea. Furthermore, removal of a foreign body that may be temporarily creating a tamponade at the corneal entry site can lead to a leaking wound, making the surgical repair in the operating room more difficult initially with a flat anterior chamber.

27.4 Surgical Exploration and Repair: Operative Note

The risks, benefits, and alternatives were discussed with the patient pre-operatively and the patient consented to proceed with exploration, removal of intraocular foreign body and repair of the open globe injury. The patient was brought to the operating room where the anesthesia team proceeded with general anesthesia. A careful time-out was observed and the correct patient and the eye were identified. The left eye was prepped and draped in the usual sterile ophthalmic fashion using a Jaffe speculum to provide adequate exposure.

The patient was found to have a 2–3 cm metallic foreign body penetrating through the cornea just anterior to the limbus at 10 o'clock passing through the iris stroma just temporal to the pupillary border and looping around to touch/scrape the corneal endothelium/posterior corneal stroma. The other end of the metallic foreign body was extending into the superonasal quadrant and hooked on the palpebral conjunctiva of the upper eyelid. A hyphema was noted in the anterior chamber. Pigment was noted on the posterior cornea, along with significant central corneal haze. The view to the lens was obscured by the corneal haze and hyphema. A temporal paracentesis was made using a 15° blade and balanced salt solution was injected into the anterior chamber. The left upper eyelid was gently lifted and the superonasal end of the metallic foreign body was exposed. Using 0.12 forceps, the metallic foreign body was gently removed from the anterior chamber taking care to avoid it rubbing on the posterior cornea or lens.

The anterior chamber was noted to be shallow after removal of the metallic foreign body and was reformed with filtered air through the paracentesis. The approximately 1 mm round penetration site was closed with 3 10-0 nylon sutures. The sutures were replaced as needed to ensure that the wound was closed appropriately and the wound was Seidel negative at the end of the case. A Kontour bandage contact lens was placed over the eye at the conclusion of the case.

A subconjunctival steroid and antibiotic injection was performed nasally and temporally away from the bandage contact lens. The speculum was removed. The patient's drape was removed under the microscope. Tobramycin-dexamethasone and timolol maleate drops were instilled in the eye. The patient tolerated the procedure well without any complications.

27.4.1 Surgical Exploration and Repair: Pearls

- In cases with an anterior segment foreign body that is accessible at the slit lamp, it is advisable to wait to remove it until the patient is in the operating room.
- Corneal lacerations from round foreign bodies that create a round hole configuration after removal can often be more difficult to close. Tight corneal sutures can be helpful to appose the wound edges and even small lacerations might require multiple sutures placed close together to seal the wound.

- For a corneal wound that seems prone to wound leaks intraoperatively, such as in the case of a round hole laceration after removal of a foreign body, placing a bandage contact lens and using a topical aqueous suppressant to decrease the chance of a wound leak in the immediate post-operative period may be helpful.

27.4.2 Surgical Video

Please see Video 27.1

27.5 Post-Operative Course

The patient was admitted to MEE to complete a 48 hour course of intravenous antibiotics. On post-operative day one he had count fingers vision with no view to the posterior pole secondary to corneal edema. A B-scan ultrasound of the left eye showed an attached retina.

He was then seen the next day and had stable count fingers vision. The anterior chamber was formed. Given the higher chance of wound leak with a round corneal laceration and presentation with a retained corneal foreign body, the bandage contact lens was left in place and aqueous suppressants were continued (timolol maleate twice a day in the left eye) along with topical antibiotic drops and atropine. Although no lens material was visible in the anterior chamber, the possibility of lens capsule violation was considered and discussed with the patient given the path of the metal wire full-thickness through the iris.

The patient was followed closely by the trauma service over the following weeks to watch for development of a cataract and also wound leaks. He was seen 1 week after surgery and the vision in the operative eye was 20/200 with improvement to 20/70 on pinhole. The bandage contact lens was removed and the aqueous suppressant discontinued since the wound was noted to be watertight. Although the corneal edema had significantly improved, there was still significant central corneal haze and pigment where the wire had abutted the posterior surface of the cornea. Fortunately, with the improvement in corneal edema, it could be determined at this point that the lens and anterior lens capsule were intact.

Two weeks post-operatively the vision continued to improve to 20/150 with pinhole to 20/30. Given that the corneal edema and haze continued to improve, the decision was made to continue to observe the patient with the understanding that the posterior corneal scar and pigment may ultimately require penetrating keratoplasty given its location in the central visual axis. Per usual practice, the three corneal sutures were removed in the trauma clinic 6 weeks post-operatively as it appeared healed and the wound remained Seidel negative (Fig. 27.3).

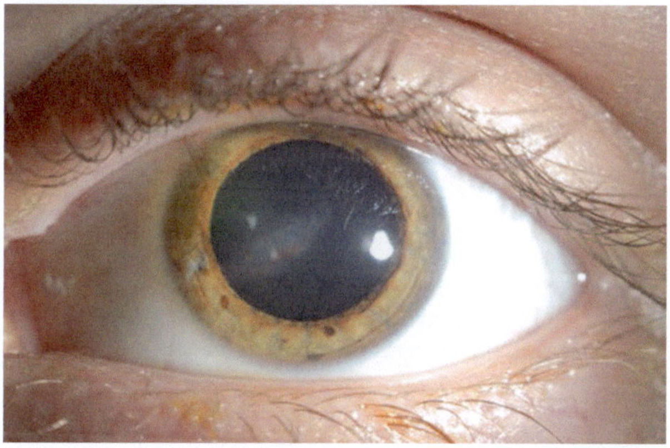

Fig. 27.3 Anterior segment slit lamp photograph at post-operative week six prior to suture removal showing three remaining nylon sutures securing the corneal entry site superonasally and a localized area of corneal scarring, pigment on the endothelium, and mild corneal heme on the posterior cornea. This area corresponds to the location of contact of the wire tip to the posterior cornea on presentation

At this point, his vision was 20/30 with pinhole improvement to 20/20. The patient was very happy with this visual outcome and deferred referral for a contact lens evaluation since his vision continued to improve. Although steroid eye drops can typically be tapered in the first month post-operatively, this patient remained on prednisolone drops once daily in the operative eye to assist in corneal healing. At this most recent visit 3 months post-operatively, his vision was 20/25 uncorrected and 20/20 with correction. The prednisolone drops were discontinued and although posterior corneal scarring and pigment remained in the visual axis, the decision was made to observe rather than proceed with further corneal evaluation and possible penetrating keratoplasty given good patient satisfaction and good visual outcome.

27.6 Final Trauma Evaluation

27.6.1 Final Visual Acuity

OD: 20/20
OS: 20/20-3 with correction

27.6.2 Pupils

OD: Round, no afferent pupillary defect
OS: Round, no afferent pupillary defect

27.6.3 Slit Lamp Examination

	OD	OS
Lids and lashes	Normal	Normal
Sclera and conjunctiva	Normal	Normal
Cornea	Normal	Corneal scar just adjacent to the limbus at 10 o'clock with central oblong corneal scar with blood staining and pigment on endothelium obliquely across visual axis (1 mm × 5 mm) in location where wire was rubbing on the back of the cornea
Anterior chamber	Normal	Normal
Iris	Normal	Small transillumination defect at 8 o'clock
Lens	Normal	Lens and anterior capsule intact, no cataract
Vitreous	Normal	Normal

27.6.4 Dilated Examination

Macula/Nerve OD: Normal
Periphery OD: Normal
Macula/Nerve: OS: Normal
Periphery OS: Normal

27.7 Review and Lessons Learned

As discussed previously, in cases that present with an anterior segment intraocular foreign body that is accessible at the slit lamp, it is important to defer removal until in the operating room. For this patient, one end of the metal wire was caught underneath the left upper eyelid and a thorough exam under anesthesia was essential to ensure that the entire wire was removed. Furthermore, a metal wire can often act as a tamponade for a round corneal wound, as in this case. Removal prior to the operating room can allow the wound to leak and the anterior chamber to flatten for a prolonged period of time, making the wound more difficult to close. Prompt surgical repair is even more imperative in these cases to decrease the chance of complications from rust formation or wound leakage and address significant patient pain or discomfort.

While all Zone I open globe injuries have the potential for wound leakage or dehiscence, corneal wounds in a round hole configuration often are more difficult to close. In these cases, multiple corneal sutures placed very close to each other may be necessary to seal the wound. It can be helpful in these small lacerations (1–2 mm) to carefully place the first corneal suture directly in the center of the corneal wound and secure it tightly. One to two sutures on either side might be necessary to address any wound leaks. Sutures sometimes need to be placed and replaced in order to perfectly place the sutures so no leaks are noted. Care must be taken to not grasp corneal tissue too tightly or any longer than necessary when passing sutures to prevent cornea tissue distortion making repair even more challenging. Rarely corneal glue is necessary to close these round corneal wounds, but it is best to try and avoid this if possible, since it can cause more corneal scarring as well as patient discomfort until it is removed.

This patient had significant posterior corneal scarring and pigment within the central visual axis, likely as a result from the tip of wire touching the posterior surface of the cornea. In this case, this improved significantly over the course of 2–3 months. Additionally, topical steroids were used for a prolonged period at a low dose to help decrease corneal scarring. Often corneal scars improve significantly with time, so options can be discussed with the patient so they are well informed, but observation may be the best option initially to monitor how much the visual acuity can improve with time. If the scarring continues to be visually significant, a penetrating keratoplasty can be considered or other surgical interventions depending on the location of the corneal scar within the cornea. These decisions will also depend on patient goals. Our patient had a great visual outcome, but did notice a blurry spot in his vision. He was not significantly bothered by this and did not want any further surgery that would keep him out of work. Other patients may have been more bothered by the scar and been interested in further interventions to try and improve vision.

27.8 Key Learning Points

- While studies have shown that most intraocular foreign bodies are posterior requiring vitrectomy for removal, between one quarter and one third of cases are anterior segment foreign bodies [1, 2]. In cases that present with an anterior segment foreign body, it is important to remove the foreign body in the operating room with immediate surgical repair of the entry site.
- Corneal lacerations in the shape of a round hole can often pose some difficulties during surgical repair and post-operatively. Multiple tight sutures can be placed adjacent to each other to decrease the chances of a wound leak as corneal edema resolves post-operatively. Placement of a bandage contact lens and use of aqueous suppressants can also be useful aids in decreasing the likelihood of a post-operative wound leak or to treat small, low flow wound leaks.
- In the case of visually significant posterior corneal scarring, it can be helpful to observe the scar for a period of time and monitor for improvement in vision. If the vision continues to be significantly affected by the scar, then a penetrating keratoplasty may be a therapeutic option.

References

1. Liu CC, Tong JM, Li PS, Li KK. Epidemiology and clinical outcome of intraocular foreign bodies in Hong Kong: a 13-year review. Int Ophthalmol. 2017;37(1):55–61.
2. Imrie FR, Cox A, Foot B, Macewen CJ. Surveillance of intraocular foreign bodies in the UK. Eye (Lond). 2008;22(9):1141–7.

Chapter 28
Case 23: Zone I Open Globe Injury with Foreign Body Extending Through the Cornea, Lens, and into Vitreous

Karen W. Jeng-Miller, Daniel Learned, and John B. Miller

28.1 History of Present Illness

A 46-year-old man with no past medical history presented with concern for open globe of the right eye.

- The patient reported he was using a metallic wire brush on a grinder and subsequently felt a projectile of one of the metal bristles in his right eye.
- He reported decreased vision, tearing and redness of the right eye.

28.2 Initial Trauma Evaluation

28.2.1 Visual Acuity (Without Correction)

OD: 20/150 pinhole 20/80-1
OS: 20/20

28.2.2 Pupils

OD: Irregular, no afferent pupillary defect by reverse
OS: Round, no afferent pupillary defect

K. W. Jeng-Miller, M.D., M.P.H. (✉) • D. Learned, M.D.
Department of Ophthalmology, Harvard Medical School, Massachusetts Eye and Ear, Boston, MA, USA
e-mail: Karen_jeng@meei.harvard.edu

J. B. Miller, M.D.
Vitreoretinal Surgery, Department of Ophthalmology, Harvard Medical School, Massachusetts Eye and Ear, Boston, MA, USA

S. Grob, C. Kloek (eds.), *Management of Open Globe Injuries*,
https://doi.org/10.1007/978-3-319-72410-2_28

28.2.3 Intraocular Pressure

OD: Deferred
OS: 20

28.2.4 External Examination

Normal

28.2.5 Slit Lamp Examination

	OD	OS
Lids and lashes	Upper lid edema	Normal
Sclera and conjunctiva	Trace injection	Normal
Cornea	1 mm × 1 mm entry wound of metal bristle at 12 o'clock in the mid periphery. Metal foreign body plugging the wound that is Seidel negative. Corneal edema noted surrounding the entry site.	Normal
Anterior chamber	Metal bristle superiorly, 2–3+ cell with fine lens particle material in the anterior chamber	Normal
Iris	Metal bristle piercing edge of the iris at 12 o'clock	Normal
Lens	Traumatic cataract, anterior lens capsule violation between 12 and 2:30 o'clock, approximately 2.5 mm high × 3.5 mm at widest extent	Normal
Vitreous	End of metal bristle going through lens into the vitreous cavity	Normal

28.2.6 Dilated Examination

Macula/Nerve OD: Normal
Periphery OD: Attached with no vitreous hemorrhage or strike site
Macula/Nerve: OS: Normal
Periphery OS: Normal

28.2.7 Radiographic Imaging

Computed tomography (CT) of the orbits showed a 1.13 cm thin curvilinear metallic foreign body extending through the anterior segment to the mid-posterior segment of the right globe consistent with an intraocular foreign body (Fig. 28.1). There was preservation of the globe contour.

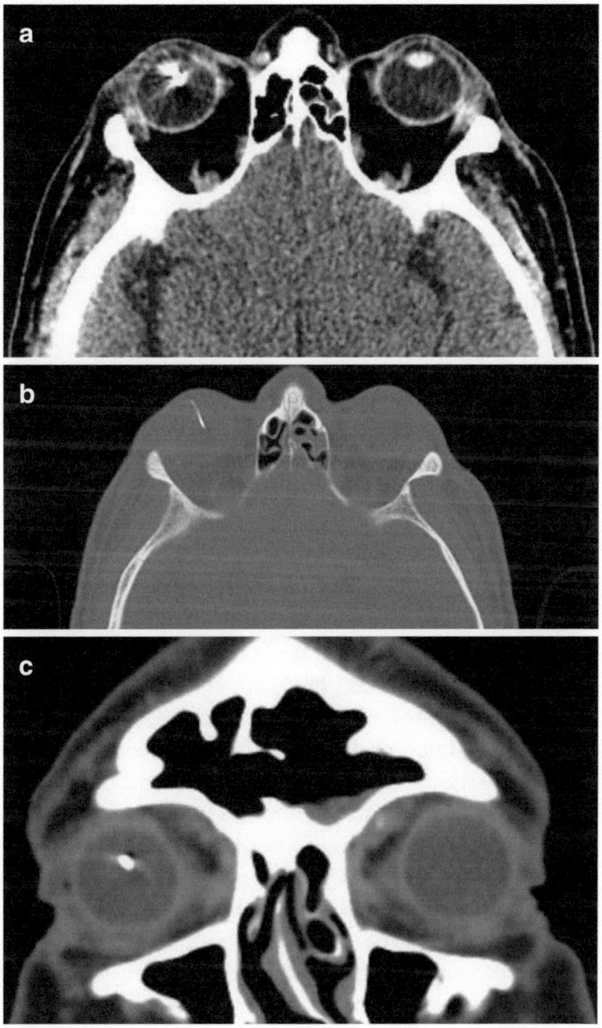

Fig. 28.1 Axial (**a**, soft tissue window and **b**, bone window) and coronal (**c**) CT images showing the presence of an intraocular foreign body on the right

28.3 Surgeon's Initial Assessment and Pre-Operative Plan

The patient had a Zone I open globe injury of the right eye with a metallic intraocular foreign body and traumatic cataract due to a metal bristle projectile requiring surgical repair.

This case illustrates removal of an intraocular foreign body via an anterior segment approach combined with a subsequent pars plana vitrectomy (PPV) and pars plana lensectomy (PPL) in addition to the standard repair of a Zone I injury. Open globes with intraocular foreign bodies spanning the anterior and posterior segment, without retina involvement, require special consideration regarding the need for a combined anterior and posterior segment repair. A fibrin capsule can develop around an intraocular metallic foreign body in the vitreous in a few hours [1] and has the possibility to result in vitreous traction/retinal tear/retinal detachment if an exclusively anterior segment repair plan is implemented. Furthermore, this patient's traumatic cataract necessitated lens removal, best accomplished via pars plana lensectomy (PPL) given the anterior and posterior capsule violation. As a result, the goal is to first extract the intraocular foreign body and stabilize the entry wound. Then attention can be directed to removal of the lens and inspection of the posterior segment for pathology if adequate visualization allows. Even in the setting of no direct injury to the retina, a pars plana vitrectomy (PPV) is likely to reduce the chance of a subsequent retinal detachment post-operatively by relieving tractional forces created by the entrance and removal of the foreign body.

The Zone I laceration pre-operative plan in this plan would not differ from standard (see earlier cases in this book for examples) after the foreign body was removed.

28.4 Surgical Exploration and Repair: Operative Note

The patient was brought to the pre-operative holding area where the correct eye was confirmed and marked. The patient then underwent intravenous sedation by the anesthesia team followed by induction of general anesthesia. In the operating room a secondary time-out was performed to identify the correct patient, eye, procedure, and any allergies. The eye was prepped and draped in the usual sterile ophthalmic fashion followed by placement of a lid speculum.

Inspection of the globe showed a linear metallic foreign body extending from the cornea into the lens and the vitreous cavity. Lens material was prolapsing into the anterior chamber from the laceration. There was no hypopyon. Trocars were used to place cannulas in the inferotemporal, superotemporal and superonasal quadrants through the pars plana in a beveled fashion. A 4 mm infusion cannula was placed through the inferonasal cannula and the infusion was confirmed in the vitreous cavity prior to turning it on.

After placement of the cannulas attention was drawn to the anterior chamber. A temporal paracentesis was made using a 15° blade. Viscoat was placed into the anterior chamber without over pressurizing the eye. Max-Grip forceps were used to enter through the paracentesis. The foreign body was grasped from the anterior chamber and then the tip was extended through the cornea giving enough room to grasp the foreign body externally with forceps. The foreign body was carefully removed following the curve of the metallic foreign body. The length of the foreign body was 15 mm in length. Viscoat was used to maintain the anterior chamber. 10-0 nylon was used to close the corneal defect. Two interrupted sutures were passed in an "x" fashion for closure. Knots were rotated into the stroma.

Next a trocar was placed through the temporal cannula to impale the lens. The vitrector was used to remove the lens. Next, the traumatic radial tear in the anterior capsule was converted into a circumferential opening with the vitrector.

Next, a standard three-port pars plana vitrectomy was performed using the light pipe, the cutter, and the RESIGHT® (Carl Zeiss Meditec, Inc., Germany) after inspection of the posterior pole. There were no areas of hemorrhage and there was no retinal strike site. A core vitreous dissection was performed. Triamcinolone acetonide injectable suspension (Triesence®) was injected on a soft tip cannula. The posterior hyaloid was not detached from the nerve. A posterior vitreous detachment was created by gentle aspiration over the optic nerve. A thorough peripheral vitreous dissection was performed with scleral depression. There were three retinal tufts noted nasally. The curved lighted laser was brought onto the field and these areas were lasered at 4, 5 and 12 o'clock. Next the corneal wound was tested and it did not leak at an intraocular pressure set at 20.

Afterwards, a partial fluid-air exchange was performed using a soft tip cannula. This was completed to a 70% gas fill. The superonasal cannula was removed and sutured using 7-0 Vicryl in an interrupted fashion. The superotemporal cannula was removed followed by the infusion cannula. These sclerotomies were then sutured with 7-0 Vicryl in interrupted fashion. The conjunctiva was closed in conjunction with the sclerotomy closure. Incisions were noted to be air tight at the end of the case. Subconjunctival injections of cefazolin and dexamethasone were administered. The lid speculum and drapes were removed. Drops of dexamethasone-neomycin-polymyxin B ointment and atropine were applied. The eye was patched and shielded.

28.4.1 Surgical Exploration and Repair: Pearls

- Removal of an intraocular foreign body and stabilization of the wound is the first step in open globe repair with foreign bodies.
- A pars plana lensectomy is indicated for lens removal with significant posterior capsular violation when adequate visualization allows.
- Careful examination of the retinal periphery is indicated for intraocular foreign bodies to rule out associated retinal breaks, detachments, or strike sites.

28.5 Post-Operative Course

The patient was admitted to complete a 48 hour course of intravenous antibiotics. On initial post-operative visits, his best-corrected visual acuity was 20/200 with pinhole. His retina remained attached during all subsequent post-operative visits. He had persistent ellipsoid zone and retinal pigment epithelium changes sub-foveally seen on optical coherence tomography (OCT) (Fig. 28.3). There were no complications relating to corneal wound dehiscence and the sutures were removed at post-operative month 4. The patient was aphakic (Fig. 28.2a) and is now 20/50-2 after secondary sulcus intraocular lens placement.

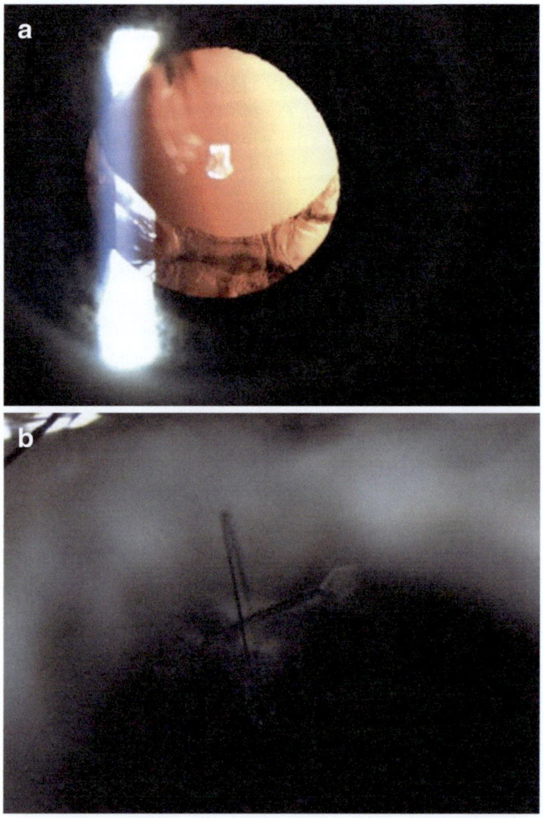

Fig. 28.2 (**a**) Anterior segment slit lamp photograph showing aphakia after trauma with a moderate remaining anterior capsule. (**b**) Corneal sutures intact at the superior corneal entry wound of the metal bristle

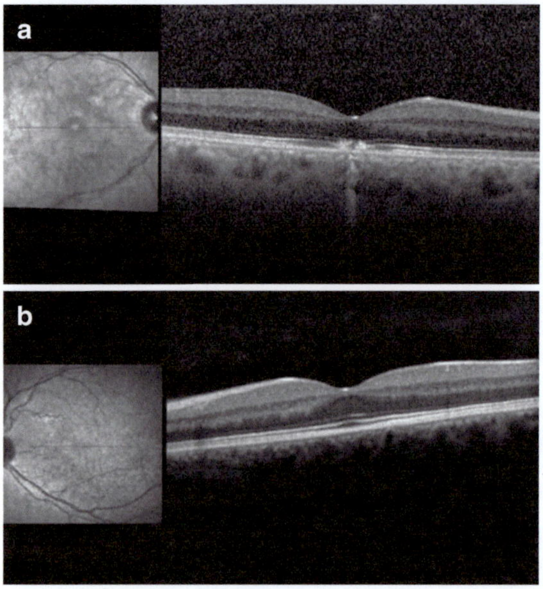

Fig. 28.3 OCT macula of the (**a**) Right eye after removal of metallic intraocular foreign body and (**b**) Normal left eye

28.6 Final Trauma Evaluation

28.6.1 Final Visual Acuity

OD: 20/60-1 pinhole 20/50-2 after secondary sulcus intraocular lens placement
OS: 20/20

28.6.2 Pupils

OD: Irregular, no afferent pupillary defect
OS: Round, no afferent pupillary defect

28.6.3 Slit Lamp Examination

	OD	OS
Lids and lashes	Normal	Normal
Sclera and conjunctiva	Normal	Normal
Cornea	Superior, mid-periphery, full-thickness corneal wound, Seidel negative	Normal
Anterior chamber	Formed	Normal
Iris	Dilated, round	Normal
Lens	Sulcus intraocular lens	Normal
Vitreous	Status post PPV	Normal

28.6.4 Dilated Examination

Macula/Nerve OD: Yellow retinal pigment epithelial changes at fovea
Periphery OD: Laser scars superonasally and nasally
Macula/Nerve: OS: Normal
Periphery OS: Normal

28.7 Review and Lessons Learned

In cases that present with intraocular foreign bodies, it is important to carefully assess the location of the intraocular foreign body, via ophthalmologic exam and CT imaging, and plan the repair accordingly. In the literature, the retina and vitreous are often cited as the most common locations of an intraocular foreign body [2, 3]. These are amenable to PPV extraction. This is supported by the thought that removal of disrupted vitreous decreases the risk for retinal detachment; furthermore, a fibrin capsule can develop around the foreign body in a few hours, necessitating PPV removal [1]. In cases where the foreign body spans the anterior segment into the posterior segment, an anterior removal of the foreign body followed by a PPV and PPL yields the most desirable result.

In cases of lens violation necessitating lens extraction, patients should be counseled on post-operative vision restoration in aphakia. The patient should understand the future need for corrective measures, including contact lenses or the potential need for future surgery for the placement of an intraocular lens.

28.8 Key Learning Points

- In cases that present with an intraocular foreign body, it is important to determine the location of the foreign body prior to repair by exam and CT imaging.
- When resources and visualization allow, ideal repair of a foreign body extending from the anterior segment into the vitreous would include both an anterior and posterior segment approach for the initial operation.
- Careful inspection of the peripheral retina is indicated when the intraocular foreign body has penetrated into the posterior segment.
- Patients may need subsequent surgeries (e.g., insertion of intraocular lens) to reach full visual potential after a pars plana lensectomy.

References

1. Nicoară SD, Irimescu I, Călinici T, Cristian C. Intraocular foreign bodies extracted by pars plana vitrectomy: clinical characteristics, management, outcomes and prognostic factors. BMC Ophthalmol. 2015;15:151.
2. Ehlers JP, Kunimoto DY, Ittoop S, Maguire JI, Ho AC, Regillo CD. Metallic intraocular foreign bodies: characteristics, interventions, and prognostic factors for visual outcome and globe survival. Am J Ophthalmol. 2008;146(3):427–33.e2.
3. Coleman DJ, Lucas BC, Rondeau MJ, Chang S. Management of intraocular foreign bodies. Ophthalmology. 1987;94(12):1647–53.

Chapter 29
Case 24: Perforating Zone I and III Open Globe Injury with Traumatic Cataract, Iris Loss, and Metallic Foreign Body Removal

J. Daniel Diaz, Miin Roh, Yoshihiro Yonekawa, Roberto Pineda, and Dean Eliott

29.1 History of Present Illness

A 47-year-old man with no prior ocular history presents with an open globe injury to the left eye.

- The patient reports he was inflating a defective car tire in the morning without eye protection when it exploded, and the subsequent blast hit him in the face. The patient denied any loss of consciousness.
- He reports immediate left eye pain and blurry vision. He was seen at an outside hospital where orbital computed tomography (CT) imaging was consistent with open globe injury of the left eye with an intraocular radioopaque foreign body. The patient was then transferred to a tertiary eye care center.
- He reports decreased vision, seeing only shadows from his left eye.

29.2 Initial Trauma Evaluation

29.2.1 Visual Acuity (Without Correction)

OD: 20/20
OS: Hand Motion at 3 feet

J. Daniel Diaz, M.D. • M. Roh, M.D., Ph.D. (✉)
Department of Ophthalmology, Harvard Medical School, Massachusetts Eye and Ear, Boston, MA, USA
e-mail: miin_roh@meei.harvard.edu

Y. Yonekawa, M.D.
Vitreoretinal Surgery, Harvard Medical School, Massachusetts Eye and Ear and Boston Children's Hospital, Boston, MA, USA

R. Pineda, M.D.
Cornea and Refractive Surgery, Department of Ophthalmology, Harvard Medical School, Massachusetts Eye and Ear, Boston, MA, USA

D. Eliott, M.D.
Vitreoretinal Surgery, Department of Ophthalmology, Harvard Medical School, Massachusetts Eye and Ear, Boston, MA, USA

S. Grob, C. Kloek (eds.), *Management of Open Globe Injuries*,
https://doi.org/10.1007/978-3-319-72410-2_29

29.2.2 *Pupils*

OD: Round and reactive
OS: Irregular and fixed, no afferent pupillary defect by reverse

29.2.3 *External Examination*

Linearly oriented punctate facial abrasions extending from lateral left lower eyelid to left lower cheek (Fig. 29.1a).

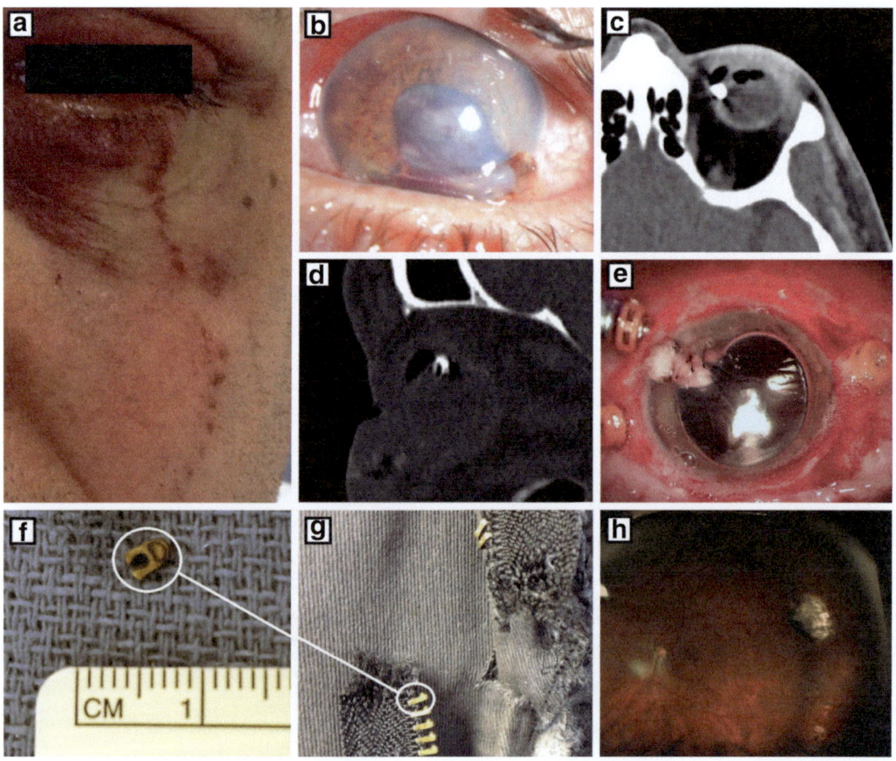

Fig. 29.1 Occult penetrating globe injury from intraocular zipper tooth. External photograph of linearly oriented punctate facial abrasions caused by jacket zipper (**a**). Slit-lamp photograph showing a Zone I penetration (**b**). Axial (**c**) and sagittal (**d**) CT scan images without contrast revealed an intraocular foreign body (IOFB) in the vitreous cavity. Pars plana vitrectomy was performed using a temporary corneal cellulose sponge to plug a corneal defect (**e**). The foreign body was identified in the extraocular space adjacent to an exit wound (**f**), which matched the zipper teeth of the patient's jacket (**g**). The retina remained attached 3 years later, and visual acuity after secondary intraocular lens implantation was 20/25 (**h**)

29.2.4 Slit Lamp Examination

	OD	OS
Lids and lashes	Normal	Punctate facial abrasion beginning at lateral left lower eyelid, no lacerations
Sclera and conjunctiva	Normal	Bullous subconjunctival hemorrhage superiorly, inferiorly, and nasally
Cornea	Normal	Full-thickness corneal laceration at 4 o'clock near limbus with iris incarceration, mild corneal edema and Descemet's membrane folds throughout (Fig. 29.1b)
Anterior chamber	Normal	2.6 mm layered hyphema inferiorly, cortical lens material extruding into anterior chamber
Iris	Normal	Irregular iris with extrusion through wound site at 4 o'clock peripherally
Lens	Normal	Anterior capsule violation with cortical material extending into the anterior chamber, remainder of lens completely opacified
Vitreous	Normal	Poor view, no vitreous prolapse appreciated

29.2.5 Dilated Examination

Macula/Nerve OD: Normal
Periphery OD: Normal, attached
Macula/Nerve: OS: No view
Periphery OS: No view

29.2.6 Radiographic Imaging

CT of the orbits showed evidence of a left globe rupture with intraocular foreign body and probable intraocular hemorrhage. There was also evidence of two preseptal foreign bodies. There was mild stranding along the left optic nerve without discrete retrobulbar hematoma. No evidence of posterior exit or intraorbital foreign bodies was noted (Fig. 29.1c, d).

29.3 Surgeon's Initial Assessment and Pre-operative Plan

At this point, the patient appeared to have suffered a Zone I open globe injury of the left eye. CT imaging showed evidence of two preseptal radio-opaque foreign bodies in the lower eyelid. The left eye also had evidence of a subluxed and disorganized crystalline lens. There was vitreous hemorrhage in the posterior segment and the radio-opaque IOFB was visualized on CT imaging. There was no evidence of a posterior exit site or further IOFBs pre-operatively.

Prompt removal of the IOFB is required to minimize the risk of traumatic endophthalmitis. Metallic IOFBs, particularly if made of iron or copper, are also toxic to the retina. The patient is otherwise healthy, without other life-threatening injuries, and could proceed with surgery. Given the need for removal of the foreign body from the posterior segment, the retina service was consulted.

A pars plana approach is considered the best approach in removal of IOFBs localized to the posterior segment. In order to obtain a better view of the posterior segment and to stabilize the eye, the corneal laceration requires repair first. Once the eye has been closed, one can proceed with the pars plana vitrectomy (PPV) and pars plana lensectomy (PPL). Pre-operative assessment to make sure there are no serous or hemorrhagic choroidal detachments are helpful in assessing whether the pars plana is available as an entry site. If the pars plana is not available, the infusion placement and other incisions can be made at the limbus. In the present case, a lensectomy was required to clear the surgeon's view to the posterior segment. A violated lens capsule with lenticular material in the anterior chamber is also very inflammatory. Once the lens has been removed, the vitreous cutter is used to clear hemorrhage and identify the IOFB.

The planned procedure therefore entails repair of Zone I open globe injury, PPV, PPL, and IOFB removal.

29.4 Surgical Exploration and Repair: Operative Note

After informed consent was obtained, the patient was brought to the operating room and induced under general anesthesia. The left eye was prepped and draped in the routine sterile fashion. A wire lid speculum was placed. First, the corneal laceration was repaired. The inferotemporal cornea had a very unusual C-shaped wound with a circular area of tissue loss at the apex of the wound and iris incarceration. The incarcerated devitalized iris tissue was excised and remnant vital tissue was irrigated and then repositioned. Next, multiple 10-0 nylon interrupted sutures were used to close the wound. Despite sutures, the area of tissue loss was left open since forceful closure of the defect at this time would result in significant corneal distortion and result in poor visualization. Therefore, the wound was plugged with a sterile cellulose sponge temporarily. (Fig. 29.1e) A dense traumatic cataract with associated iris defect was noted after repair of the corneal laceration. After a conjunctival peritomy, trocars were placed 3.0 mm posterior to the limbus in the usual locations. A complete removal of the lens nucleus and cortex was achieved by pars plana lensectomy using the vitreous cutter. Forceps were then used to remove the capsule. A pars plana vitrectomy was then carried out with the vitreous cutter and the fiberoptic light source. Vitreous hemorrhage without a posterior vitreous detachment was present. After considerable time and effort, the posterior hyaloid membrane was identified and elevated to create a posterior vitreous detachment.

After clearing the vitreous hemorrhage, whitish material indicative of sclera was noted superonasally. Further dissection from the external surface of the globe revealed an exit site at the corresponding site. The foreign body was straddling the exit site partially located within the vitreous. A gold irregularly shaped foreign body was removed through the sclera externally and sent for histopathologic examination. Interestingly, the shape of the foreign body was identical to the shape of the corneal laceration with a C configuration with a circle at the apex (Fig. 29.1f, g). The foreign body measured 4.0 × 2.0 mm with a thickness of 2.0 mm. The scleral exit site was then sutured with multiple interrupted 7-0 Vicryl sutures. After closure of the scleral laceration, inspection through the pars plana was performed which revealed retinal incarceration at the exit site. A small retinotomy was created to relieve the traction. Perfluorocarbon liquid was then used to flatten the retina. Endolaser was performed confluently around the exit site, at the area of traction, and around a small retinal hole seen at the nasal retina. A perfluorocarbon-fluid exchange was followed by fluid-air exchange using the soft tipped cannula. As an air exchange was performed, the retina remained attached with no traction remaining. Attention was then turned to the corneal wound. The cellulose sponge was removed and several additional 10-0 nylon sutures were used to close the corneal wound. After confirming complete closure of the corneal wound, air was exchanged for 14% C_3F_8 gas. The trocars were removed followed by suturing of sclerotomies with 7-0 Vicryl. The conjunctiva was also closed with multiple interrupted sutures. Subconjunctival injections of cefazolin and dexamethasone were given. The eye was flushed with povidone-iodine and dressed with dexamethasone-neomycin-polymyxin B and atropine ointment and a patch and shield. The patient was extubated and transferred to the recovery room in good condition having tolerated the procedure well.

29.4.1 Surgical Exploration and Repair: Pearls

- Cellulose sponges can be fashioned into temporary corneal plugs in cases where there is loss of corneal tissue.
- IOFBs can rest within the vitreous cavity after creating an exit wound, but may escape detection by being driven back out of the globe during vitrectomy due to the pressurized eye.

29.5 Post-Operative Course

The patient was admitted to complete a 48 hour course of intravenous antibiotics. On post-operative day one, visual acuity was light perception. The retina was grossly attached. Ten days after the initial operation, a new localized inferior retinal detachment from 3:00 o'clock to 7:30 o'clock was noted. Placement of a scleral buckle (42 band with 70 sleeve element) was performed in addition to pars plana

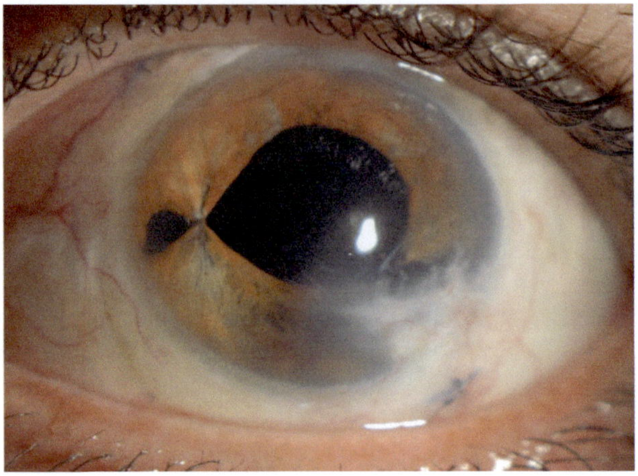

Fig. 29.2 Slit lamp photograph following anterior synechiolysis, pupilloplasty, and placement of an intrascleral fixated intraocular lens

vitrectomy followed by 14% C_3F_8 gas. The patient was followed closely by the retina service and the retina remained attached. Once the corneal sutures were completely removed, resultant irregular corneal astigmatism was corrected with rigid-gas permeable (RGP) aphakic contact lens with best corrected visual acuity of 20/80-1.

After 14 months of the retina staying attached, the focus of visual rehabilitation was then turned to the iris defect sustained during the initial open globe injury, which was causing significant photophobia. Anterior synechiolysis and pupilloplasty was performed as described below with the Cornea service (Fig. 29.2).

29.6 Surgical Exploration and Repair: Operative Note 2

After the anterior chamber was inflated using a small amount of sodium hyaluronate viscoelastic, it was also used to dissect some of the iris synechiae from the wound. A cyclodialysis spatula and microsurgical technology (MST) forceps were used to liberate all the adhesions between the iris and the cornea. Acetylcholine chloride solution was then injected intracamerally to help assess the location of the pupilloplasty sutures. 9-0 Prolene mounted on a JA255 needle was passed through the paracentesis and to both edges of the iris defect temporally. The suture was then passed through peripheral clear cornea. Kuglen hooks were used to retrieve the suture through the paracentesis and the pupilloplasty suture knot was tied using a sliding knot technique. A total of three knots using a 3-2-2 tying technique were performed. A similar procedure was performed nasally with an area of atonic dilated pupil to close the pupil and reduce its size. A suture was passed through the pupillary border at 10 o'clock, and out at 7 o'clock. The Prolene suture was tied using a similar technique as previously described, allowing the pupil aperture to obtain a more round, normal size. Following placement of the two Prolene sutures, the pupil size was approximately 4 mm in diameter.

This was followed by a secondary IOL implantation procedure (intrascleral fixated intraocular lens).

After marking the 11 o'clock and 5 o'clock positions with a marking pen on the limbus, a 5 mm peritomy was performed with Westcott scissors on each side. Hemostasis was achieved with topical brimonidine and cautery in the area of the peritomy. A supersharp blade was used to create a Y-shaped partial thickness scleral groove 2 mm posterior to the limbus, such that they are diagonally opposite to each other. A crescent blade was then used to create scleral flaps. A 20 gauge MVR blade was used to create a scleral tunnel underneath the scleral flap parallel to the limbus. The same MVR blade was then used to make a sclerotomy parallel to iris. The same procedure was performed at the 11 o'clock and 5 o'clock position. A paracentesis was made at 9 o'clock. An anterior chamber maintainer was placed through the paracentesis and a clear corneal wound was created at 1:30 o'clock with a keratome. The three-piece intraocular lens was loaded into an injector. The leading haptic and the optic of the intraocular lens was inserted into the anterior chamber and the leading haptic was grasped with MST forceps and brought through the sclerotomy at 5 o'clock. Subsequently, the trailing haptic was inserted into the eye and then was brought out through the sclerotomy at 11 o'clock. Both haptics were inserted into their respective scleral tunnel with forceps. An 8-0 nylon suture was used to fix the haptic to the scleral bed and to close the scleral flap. Conjunctiva wounds were closed with 8-0 Vicryl sutures. The pupil was round and the intraocular lens was well centered without tilting.

After the surgery, the patient reported decreased photophobia with improvement of visual acuity.

29.7 Final Trauma Evaluation

29.7.1 Final Corrected Visual Acuity

OD: 20/20
OS: 20/25

29.7.2 Pupils

OD: Round and reactive
OS: Surgical pupil, status-post pupilloplasty

29.7.3 Slit Lamp Examination

	OD	OS
Lids and lashes	Normal	Normal
Sclera and conjunctiva	Normal	Superonasal and inferotemporal sutures well covered by conjunctiva
Cornea	Normal	Inferonasal scarring with mild pannus
Anterior chamber	Normal	Normal
Iris	Normal	Status-post pupilloplasty, inferonasal and inferotemporal sutures
Lens	Normal	Scleral-fixated intraocular lens, well-positioned
Vitreous	Normal	Normal

29.7.4 Dilated Examination

Macula/Nerve OD: Retinal pigment epithelial changes at superior arcade
Periphery OD: Normal
Macula/Nerve: OS: Normal
Periphery OS: Scleral buckle elevation and chorioretinal scarring notably at 1 o'clock (site of prior retinotomy) and from 4 to 10 o'clock (Fig. 29.1h)

29.8 Review and Lessons Learned

This case covers various important topics that we often encounter during open globe repairs. Intraocular foreign bodies account for 18–41% of all open globe injuries (OGI) [1]. Most patients with OGIs with an IOFB are male, and the most common place of injury is at work, followed by home [2, 3]. IOFBs vary in composition, including glass, plastic, organic materials, and metals (zinc, aluminum, nickel, iron, copper etc.). The most common IOFB is composed of metal [4]. The IOFB is most likely to reside in the posterior segment, and visual prognosis depends on its size, zone of injury, and ensuing complications. Another factor affecting the extent of intraocular damage with IOFB is the shape of the object. A sharp object for example is more likely to enter the eye through a smaller wound, leading to less transfer of energy, however allowing for further travel into the posterior segment [5]. Metallic IOFBs, if not removed, can lead to long-term toxicity in the form of siderosis bulbi (if containing iron), and chalcosis (copper) [6, 7].

Once a thorough history and ophthalmological examination has been performed, ocular imaging is vital for the management of IOFBs. Plain film radiographs, computed tomography (CT), and ultrasonography have all been employed in assessing a patient with a concern for an IOFB [8]. While plain film X rays may miss IOFBs that are not radio-opaque, they may identify small IOFBs that were missed on thicker CT cuts. CT remains the preferred method used in cases of suspected open globes, and we recommend thin cuts. The ability to adequately examine the orbit, facial bones, and retrobulbar space is immensely helpful for surgical planning. In cases where the IOFB cannot be visualized with a CT scan (i.e., glass or plastic), ultrasonography is good alternative [9]. It is important to keep in mind that this must be performed very carefully without exerting undue pressure in open globes.

Timing of surgical IOFB removal depends on several factors, including the overall health status of the patient, whether it is associated with clinical evidence of endophthalmitis, and availability of experienced ophthalmologists. In patients with concomitant life-threatening injuries, IOFB removal may need to be delayed. The goal would then be to achieve primary globe closure. In cases of suspected infection associated with the IOFB, intravitreal and/or systemic antibiotics may be needed. Primary closure is also the goal if an experienced retina specialist is not readily available for removal of the IOFB.

Vitrectomy is employed in the removal of IOFBs from the posterior segment. Advantages include direct visualization of the IOFB, access to clearance of media opacities (traumatic cataract, hemorrhage), the collection of cultures in suspected cases of endophthalmitis, and administration of intraocular antibiotics [10]. Media opacities should be removed through core vitrectomy prior to IOFB removal. External electromagnets, forceps, and intraocular magnets have been used to extract IOFBs. Small metallic and ferromagnetic IOFBs can be removed with rare earth intraocular magnets. If there is already a scleral entry or exit site, it can be extracted through the existing site, but in general, it is better to remove IOFBs through the pars plana sclerotomies. Larger IOFBs necessitate the use of forceps and possibly the need to enlarge the sclerotomy site for extraction. External magnets are better utilized in the external surgical approach to removal of IOFBs. A study comparing the use of external magnets versus PPV and forceps in the removal of IOFB resulted in better anatomical and functional outcomes with better post-operative visual acuity in the group that underwent PPV with forceps removal [11]. If the IOFB has impacted the retina, the posterior hyaloid and vitreous base should be excised in order to limit the amount of traction and likelihood of post-operative retinal detachment. Gas or oil tamponade can be employed, depending on the number and location of retinal breaks and the ability of the patient to adequately position post-operatively. Post-operative retinal detachments have been reported to occur in up to 40% of cases, and can lead to a poor prognosis, although our patient did fantastically well [12].

Overall, IOFBs warrant expedited surgical repair. Visual potential remains guarded, especially if located in the posterior segment. The formation of an appropriate surgical approach relies on determining the location and if possible the composition of the IOFB. Regular and close follow-up is necessary, as complications such as post-operative retinal detachments and proliferative vitreoretinopathy can occur. Improved surgical techniques will hopefully limit these complications and lead to improved visual outcomes for these patients. Finally, secondary visual rehabilitation (IOL and pupil repair) is possible in such cases with significant improvement when staged appropriately.

29.9 Key Learning Points

- A significant proportion of open globe injuries include IOFBs.
- IOFBs pose a distinct challenge at every level including during the initial diagnosis, surgical approach, and management of late complications.
- Expedited surgical repair to close the globe and remove the IOFB is recommended.
- Through-and-through injuries must be considered when the IOFB cannot be visualized during vitrectomy.

References

1. Loporchio D, Mukkamala L, Gorukanti K, Zarbin M, Langer P, Bhagat N. Intraocular foreign bodies: a review. Surv Ophthalmol. 2016;61(5):582–96. https://doi.org/10.1016/j.survophthal.2016.03.005.
2. Jonas JB, Knorr HL, Budde WM. Prognostic factors in ocular injuries caused by intraocular or retrobulbar foreign bodies. Ophthalmology. 2000;107(5):823–8.
3. Zhang Y, Zhang M, Jiang C, Qiu HY. Intraocular foreign bodies in china: clinical characteristics, prognostic factors, and visual outcomes in 1,421 eyes. Am J Ophthalmol. 2011;152(1):66–73.e1. https://doi.org/10.1016/j.ajo.2011.01.014.
4. Fulcher TP, McNab AA, Sullivan TJ. Clinical features and management of intraorbital foreign bodies. Ophthalmology. 2002;109(3):494–500.
5. Potts AM, Distler JA. Shape factor in the penetration of intraocular foreign bodies. Am J Ophthalmol. 1985;100(1):183–7.
6. Lit ES, Young LHY. Anterior and posterior segment intraocular foreign bodies. Int Ophthalmol Clin. 2002;42(3):107–20.
7. O'Duffy D, Salmon JF. Siderosis bulbi resulting from an intralenticular foreign body. Am J Ophthalmol. 1999;127(2):218–9.
8. Modjtahedi BS, Rong A, Bobinski M, McGahan J, Morse LS. Imaging characteristics of intraocular foreign bodies: a comparative study of plain film X-ray, computed tomography, ultrasound, and magnetic resonance imaging. Retina. 2015;35(1):95–104. https://doi.org/10.1097/IAE.0000000000000271.
9. Laroche D, Ishikawa H, Greenfield D, Liebmann JM, Ritch R. Ultrasound biomicroscopic localization and evaluation of intraocular foreign bodies. Acta Ophthalmol Scand. 1998;76(4):491–5.
10. Peyman GA, Raichand M, Goldberg MF, Brown S. Vitrectomy in the management of intraocular foreign bodies and their complications. Br J Ophthalmol. 1980;64(7):476–82.
11. Mester V, Kuhn F. Ferrous intraocular foreign bodies retained in the posterior segment: management options and results. Int Ophthalmol. 1998;22(6):355–62.
12. Wickham L, Xing W, Bunce C, Sullivan P. Outcomes of surgery for posterior segment intraocular foreign bodies—a retrospective review of 17 years of clinical experience. Graefes Arch Clin Exp Ophthalmol. 2006;244(12):1620–6. https://doi.org/10.1007/s00417-006-0359-6.

Chapter 30
Case 25: Open Globe Injury with Posterior Foreign Body

Safa Rahmani and John B. Miller

30.1 History of Present Illness

A 53-year-old man with 3-week duration of eye irritation and loss of vision presents with concern for open globe of the right eye.

- 53-year-old mechanic presents with concern of possible foreign object getting into his eye while working in the shop. Immediately after the incident, the patient rinsed his eye with water, but did not seek immediate medical evaluation.
- The patient's vision and eye irritation did not improve over the next 3 weeks.
- He was seen by an outpatient ophthalmologist and noted to have a spontaneously closed Zone I open globe with concern for intraocular foreign body on dilated exam.
- The patient was transferred to Massachusetts Eye and Ear (MEE) for further evaluation and management.

30.2 Initial Trauma Evaluation

30.2.1 Visual Acuity (Without Correction)

OD: Hand motion
OS: 20/20

S. Rahmani, M.D., M.S. (✉) • J. B. Miller, M.D.
Vitreoretinal Surgery, Department of Ophthalmology, Harvard Medical School, Massachusetts Eye and Ear, Boston, MA, USA

S. Grob, C. Kloek (eds.), *Management of Open Globe Injuries*,
https://doi.org/10.1007/978-3-319-72410-2_30

30.2.2 Pupils

OD: Irregular, iris plugging temporal corneal wound, +afferent pupillary defect by reverse
OS: Reactive, no afferent pupillary defect

30.2.3 Intraocular Pressure

OD: 13
OS: 18

30.2.4 External Examination

Unremarkable

30.2.5 Slit Lamp Examination

	OD	OS
Lids and lashes	Mild upper eyelid edema	Normal
Sclera and conjunctiva	Diffuse 2+ conjunctival injection	Normal
Cornea	1 mm × 1 mm temporal peripheral corneal laceration with iris incarceration within the wound, Seidel negative	Normal
Anterior chamber	3+ cell, no hypopyon	Normal
Iris	Irregular with transillumination defect temporally, iris incarcerated and peaked temporally at 9 o'clock, posterior synechiae throughout (Fig. 30.1)	Normal
Lens	Traumatic 2+ nuclear sclerosis, cortical changes temporally	Normal
Vitreous	Poor view	Normal

30.2.6 Dilated Examination

Macula/Nerve OD: Poor view, a reflective foreign body by inferior arcade (Fig. 30.2)
Periphery OD: Poor view
Macula/Nerve: OS: Normal
Periphery OS: Normal

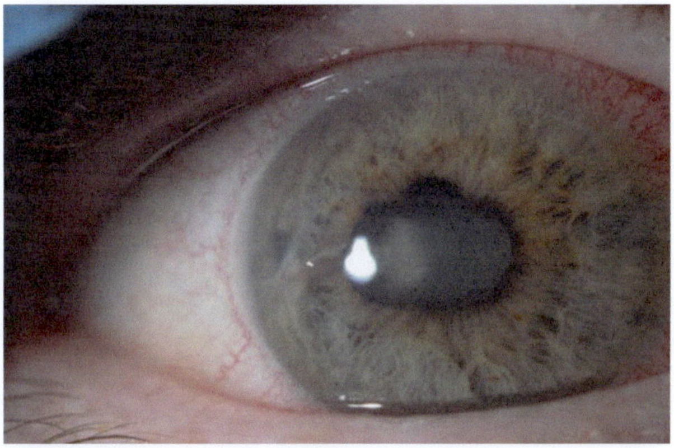

Fig. 30.1 Slit lamp photo of the right eye demonstrating closed corneal wound with iris incarceration, peaked pupil, and significant anterior chamber inflammation pre-operatively

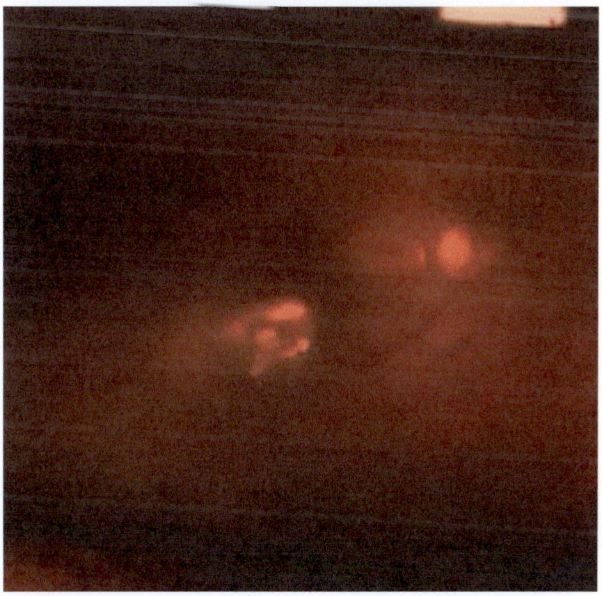

Fig. 30.2 Fundus photo of the right eye with the intraocular foreign body in the inferior macula. The posterior view is hazy secondary to cataract and vitritis

30.2.7 Radiographic Imaging

Computed tomography (CT) of the orbits showed a 2 mm metal foreign body in the vitreous cavity posteriorly in the right eye (Fig. 30.3).

30.3 Surgeon's Initial Assessment and Pre-Operative Plan

This case demonstrates a significant delayed presentation of retained metallic intraocular foreign body with associated severe uveitis. He was noted to have a spontaneously closed Zone I injury 3 weeks after the initial injury.

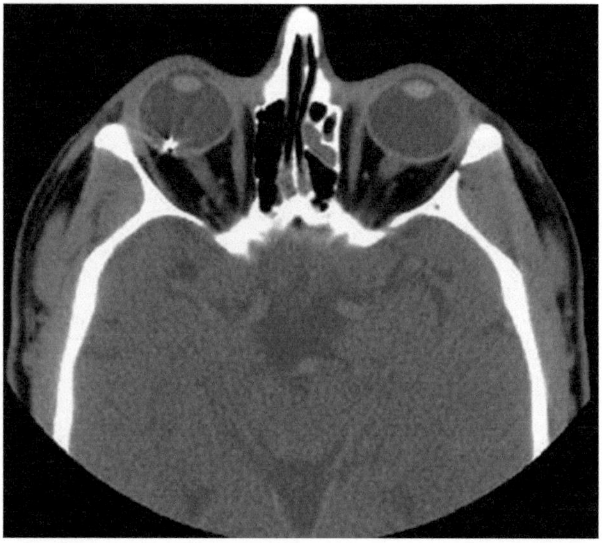

Fig. 30.3 Axial CT scan shows a metallic foreign body in the right eye

This case illustrates the delayed sequalae of intraocular foreign bodies. The most concerning potential complication is concurrent intraocular infection (endophthalmitis). Significant foreign body inflammation can also make surgical planning difficult and damage intraocular structures. Lastly, depending on the type of metal, there can be significant retinal toxicity and cellular damage prior to foreign body removal.

Initial pre-operative planning for this patient focused on treatment of the inflammation with extra coverage of possible early infection. Given poor historian and patient reliability, the decision was made to admit the patient for intravenous antibiotics with concurrent topical antibiotics and steroids prior to surgery.

The surgery was planned 48 hour after initial presentation to MEE to ensure complete coverage with antibiotics and time to control the inflammation with topical steroids. In addition, a tetanus shot was administered during initial evaluation.

The plan was to remove the traumatic cataract and perform pars plana vitrectomy with the removal of the intraocular foreign body.

30.4 Surgical Exploration and Repair: Operative Note

Informed consent was obtained and the operative eye was verified and marked. The uninjured left eye was taped and shielded for protection. The right eye was prepped and draped in the usual sterile ophthalmic fashion followed by placement of a lid speculum.

A superior 180° peritomy was made with Westcott scissors. A paracentesis was placed superonasally using supersharp blade. A superior temporal scleral tunnel was created with crescent blade and keratome. Provisc was used to break all the posterior synechiae. Iris hooks were placed. A central capsulorrhexis was created with a cystotome and Utrata forceps. The central nucleus was cleared with the phacoemulsification handpiece. The temporal corneal laceration was noted to be stable with iris adhesion. The track of the foreign body continued posteriorly through the anterior and posterior capsule. The irrigation and aspiration handpiece was used to remove most of the cortical cataract that remained.

Trocars were used to place cannulas in the inferotemporal, superotemporal, and superonasal quadrants through the pars plana. A 4 mm infusion cannula was placed through the inferonasal cannula and the infusion was confirmed in the vitreous cavity prior to turning it on. The remaining cortical material was removed by vitreous cutter taking care to keep anterior lens capsule intact. The posterior capsule was removed. At this time, a standard pars plana vitrectomy was performed. No retinal detachment was noted. There was dense vitreous hemorrhage inferiorly and an intraocular metallic-appearing foreign body embedded just inferior to the fovea within the arcades of the macula. There was underlying retinal whitening and small pockets of hemorrhage around the retinal strike site. The optic nerve was noted to be moderately pale and there was a blunted foveal reflex.

A core vitreous dissection was performed. Care was taken to clear all vitreous adhesions around the foreign body. A posterior vitreous detachment was created by gentle aspiration over the optic nerve. The vitreous was peeled past the equator in all quadrants. A thorough peripheral vitreous dissection was performed with scleral depression. No tears were noted.

Next, attention was directed to foreign body removal. A small pocket of perfluorocarbon liquid was injected to protect the fovea. Multiple attempts were made to remove the foreign body with max grip forceps and an intraocular magnet. Although the foreign body appeared metallic in appearance, the magnet was unable to create firm adhesion for removal (×2 separate magnets). An additional superior sclerotomy site was created with an MVR blade and the foreign body was successfully removed with intraocular foreign body forceps and max grip forceps. The foreign body was removed through the scleral tunnel and it measured approximately 3.5 mm in length.

The scleral tunnel was closed with 3 interrupted 10-0 nylon sutures. The superior sclerotomy site was closed with a butterfly suture using 9-0 nylon.

A repeat 360° scleral depression was performed and no tears or detachments were noted. The retinal strike site appeared closed with no breaks. A small shallow pocket of subretinal fluid was noted by the retinal strike site, tracking inferiorly (fluid pocket was approximately 4 disc diameters).

A complete fluid-air exchange was performed using a soft tip cannula. Residual fluid was removed from the posterior pole over the optic nerve using the soft tip cannula. A few drops of balanced salt solution was injected into the eye and residual perfluorocarbon liquid was removed. All iris hooks were removed.

The superonasal cannula was removed and sutured using 7-0 Vicryl in an interrupted fashion. Pure C_3F_8 gas was drawn up using a filter and then brought to a concentration of 14% using a second filter. This diluted gas was then exchanged into the vitreous cavity through the inferotemporal cannula, venting the air through the superotemporal cannula.

0.1 ml of ceftazidime and 0.1 ml of vancomycin were injected intravitreally through the supratemporal cannula using a 30 gauge needle.

The superotemporal cannula was removed followed by the infusion cannula. These sclerotomies were then sutured with 7-0 Vicryl in an interrupted fashion. The conjunctival peritomy was closed with separate 7-0 Vicryl sutures in an interrupted fashion. Incisions were noted to be water tight at the end of the case.

A subconjunctival injection of dexamethasone was administered. The lid speculum and drapes were removed. Drops of dexamethasone-neomycin-polymixin b ophthalmic ointment and atropine were applied. The eye was patched and shielded.

30.4.1 Surgical Exploration and Repair: Pearls

- Removal of a traumatic cataract is necessary for a clear view of the retina and to prevent intraocular inflammation associated with a violated lens capsule.
- Prophylactic intraocular injection of antibiotics is recommended given delayed presentation of an open globe and intraocular foreign body with significant intraocular inflammation.
- Multiple tools should be at a surgeon's disposal for intraocular foreign body removal. Magnets can be useful for metallic foreign bodies. A variety of intraocular forceps should also be available to assist with removal of an intraocular foreign body.
- The location of foreign body removal depends on the location of the original entry wound and where removal will cause the least amount of damage to the ocular structures. Pars plana is usually a safe zone with minimal damage to important intraocular structures.
- Perflourocarbon liquid can protect the central macula while attempting to remove a posterior intraocular foreign body [1].

30.5 Post-Operative Course

The patient was followed closely over the following 2 weeks by the retina service. The corneal wound remained stable without leaks. The importance of head positioning was extensively discussed with the patient. Since the retinal strike site was so posterior, good tamponade was needed to allow the surrounding retina to scar down. We were not as aggressive with laser given the close proximity to the fovea. Some retina specialists may argue that laser may have not been needed for repair of this posterior retinal defect, but in cases with foreign body removal, such approach is not recommended given the likely instability of the wound.

On follow up, the patient expressed difficulty with positioning, but the retina remained attached. Unfortunately, as the gas absorbed, he developed an inferior retinal detachment on post-operative month two (Fig. 30.4). There were no new

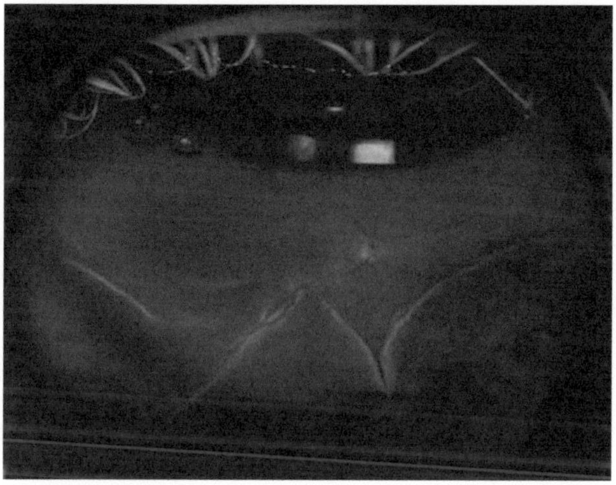

Fig. 30.4 Optos fundus photograph showing an inferior retinal detachment 2 months post-surgery. The detachment starts at original strike site by the inferior arcade. There is a superior gas bubble and the superior retina remains attached

tears or breaks. New scar tissue and proliferative vitreoretinopathy had developed around the posterior retinal strike site and detached the retina.

After extensive discussion with the patient, the decision was made to repair the retina by placement of a scleral buckle and repeat vitrectomy with insertion of silicone oil. Since the patient had difficulty with positioning after the first retinal repair, repeat placement of gas for tamponade was not recommended. We discussed that if the retina remained stable, the patient would need repeat surgery to remove the silicone oil.

30.6 Second Surgical Repair: Operative Note

In the operating room a time-out was performed to identify the correct patient, eye, procedure, and any allergies. The eye was prepped and draped in the usual sterile ophthalmic fashion followed by placement of a lid speculum.

A radial limbal incision was made nasally. A peritomy was then completed with blunt Wescott scissors 360° around the limbus. A radial incision was made temporally. Stevens scissors were used to bluntly dissect Tenon's capsule in each quadrant between the recti muscles. The quadrants were inspected carefully using a Schepens retractor. There were no signs of scleral thinning. The rectus muscles were isolated using a muscle hook and a 2-0 silk suture, passed after isolation with the Gass hook. Each recti muscle was inspected to ensure no muscle was split during passing. Tenon's capsule was dissected off the medial, inferior, and lateral rectus muscles using a cotton tip applicator. The 42 band scleral buckle was then brought on the field after being pre-soaked in polymyxin. The band was passed underneath the medial, inferior, lateral and superior rectus muscles using forceps. A 5-0 nylon suture was then passed in a horizontal mattress fashion in the bed of the buckle.

The 42 band was sutured in each of the 4 mid quadrants at the equator of the globe. A 70 sleeve was used to bring the band edges together in the superonasal quadrant.

Trocars were placed in the inferotemporal, superotemporal, and superonasal quadrants through the pars plana in a beveled fashion. A 4 mm infusion cannula was placed through the inferonasal cannula and the infusion was confirmed in the vitreous cavity prior to turning it on.

At this time, a standard three-port pars plana vitrectomy was performed. A core vitreous dissection had already been performed. A complete retinal detachment was noted. The previous inferior arcade retinal strike site was noted to have fibrosis and pre-retinal membranes. A thorough peripheral vitreous dissection was performed with scleral depression and no peripheral tears or breaks were noted. Mild proliferative vitreoretinopathy with pigment clumps were noted.

A small pocket of perfluorocarbon liquid was injected into the vitreous cavity and used to stabilize the detachment. Using max grip forceps, pre-retinal membranes were gently removed from the previous strike site. A posterior circular retinectomy was created around the strike site with intravitreal diathermy and a vitreous cutter. Dense subretinal fluid was aspirated. The perfluorocarbon liquid was aspirated out of the eye. An inferior peripheral iridectomy was created with a vitreous cutter.

Afterwards, a complete fluid-air exchange was performed using a soft tip cannula through the posterior retinectomy site. The retina was noted to flatten. Residual fluid was removed from the posterior pole over the optic nerve using the soft tip cannula. The endolaser probe was brought onto the field and was used to perform laser around the retinectomy.

Attention was directed back to the scleral buckle. The scleral buckle band was then tightened to the appropriate height. The buckle was trimmed to the appropriate length with the ends brought together in the superonasal quadrant.

The superonasal trocar was removed and the scleral defect was sutured using 7-0 Vicryl in an interrupted fashion. An exchange of silicone oil was then performed through the infusion cannula and vented through the superotemporal trocar. The superotemporal cannula was removed followed by the infusion cannula. These sclerotomies were then sutured with 7-0 Vicryl in an interrupted fashion.

The conjunctiva was closed over the scleral buckle with interrupted nasal and temporal 7-0 Vicryl sutures. Incisions were noted to be water tight at the end of the case.

Subconjunctival injections of Cefazolin and Dexamethasone were administered. The lid speculum and drapes were removed. The eye was patched and shielded.

30.6.1 Surgical Repair: Pearls

- Patients can develop significant scarring and proliferative vitreoretinopathy after trauma even if the original surgery was successful.
- Patient positioning can be very important in success of retinal surgical outcomes. It is important to inquire about the patients ability to comply with post-operative recommendations for surgical planning.

- Removing all scar tissue from the retina is key to eventual success.
- Silicone oil should be used in patients that need a longer tamponade agent or are unable to position post-operatively.

30.7 Post-Operative Course

The patient was followed closely over the following weeks. He was somewhat more compliant with positioning given his repeat surgery. He has remained attached 5 months after surgery with stable vision. There has been no evidence of repeat scar formation over the original strike site.

The plan will be silicone oil removal in the coming months and contact lens fitting for best visual potential given his current aphakia. If he does well with a contact lens, an intraocular lens placement can be discussed in the distant future.

30.8 Final Trauma Evaluation

30.8.1 Final Visual Acuity

OD: Count fingers (aphakic)
OS: 20/20

30.8.2 Pupils

OD: Irregular
OS: Normal

30.8.3 Slit Lamp Examination

	OD	OS
Lids and lashes	Normal	Normal
Sclera and conjunctiva	Mild conjunctival injection	Normal
Cornea	1 mm × 1 mm temporal peripheral old corneal wound with iridocorneal touch	Normal
Anterior chamber	Rare cell	Normal
Iris	Irregular with transillumination defect temporally, incarcerated and peaked temporally at 9 o'clock	Normal
Lens	Aphakia	Normal

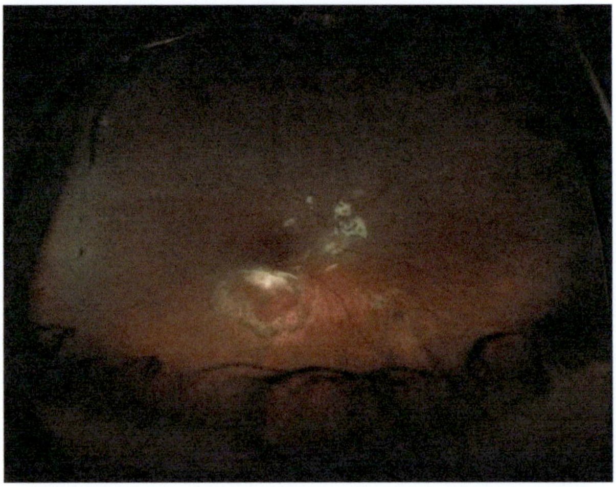

Fig. 30.5 Optos fundus photograph at 5 months post-operatively after the second retina surgery. The retina remains attached with scarring around the retinectomy site around the original retinal strike site

30.8.4 Dilated Examination

Macula/Nerve OD: Mild optic nerve pallor, fovea flat with mild epiretinal membrane, attached macula with inferior laser scars (Fig. 30.5)
Periphery OD: Scleral buckle elevation, retinectomy edges flat, retina attached (Fig. 30.5)
Macula/Nerve: OS: Normal
Periphery OS: Normal

30.9 Review and Lessons Learned

This 53-year-old man presented with a 3-week delayed, self-sealed Zone I open globe injury with a retained intraocular foreign body of the right eye. In open globe cases that present with intraocular foreign body, it is important to remove the foreign body timely in conjunction with globe repair. This case illustrates the delayed sequalae of retained intraocular foreign body. Most concerning is concurrent intraocular infection. Significant foreign body inflammation can also make surgical planning difficult and damage intraocular structures. Lastly, depending on the type of metal, there can be significant retinal toxicity and cellular damage prior to foreign body removal.

Our patient did have significant inflammation upon presentation. Fortunately, in this case there appeared to be no concurrent endophthalmitis at presentation. Due to high risk of infection, the patient was still treated with intravenous and intraocular antibiotics for complete coverage.

The original surgery focused on removing the traumatic cataract, removing the intraocular foreign body and repairing any retinal damage noted intraoperatively.

Although this foreign body appeared metallic on CT and clinical exam, it was unable to be removed with a magnet intraoperatively and was removed with foreign body forceps through a pars plana incision. Since it is very difficult to know prior to surgery what instruments will work best for removal, several options should be available and thought out prior to starting surgery.

Given the significant inflammation prior to surgery and subsequent patient difficulty with positioning, it was not entirely surprising that the patient detached 2 months following the original surgery. Scar formation occurs 6–8 weeks after surgery and this patient was at significant risk given his presentation. Removal of all retinal scar tissue and fibrosis is key to success with these traumatic open globe cases with vitreous or retinal findings [2, 3]. Close retinal follow up is needed in all these cases.

30.10 Key Learning Points

- Simultaneous removal of intraocular foreign body in conjunction with open globe repair is recommend.
- Delayed presentation of open globe and retained foreign body places an eye at significant risk for infection, inflammation, and possible retinal toxicity from components of intraocular foreign body.
- Eyes with a history of trauma are at significant risk for scar formation and retinal detachment.
- Multiple retinal surgeries may be needed in order to stabilize the eye and keep the retina attached. It is important to educate the patients about the risk of repeat detachment or need for more retinal surgery in the future.

References

1. Shah CM, Gentile RC, Mehta MC. Perflourocarbon liquids' ability to protect the macula from intraocular dropping of metallic foreign bodies: a model eye study. Retina. 2016;36(7):1285–91.
2. Nicoară SD, Irimescu I, Călinici T, Cristian C. Intraocular foreign bodies extracted by pars plana vitrectomy: clinical characteristics, management, outcomes and prognostic factors. BMC Ophthalmol. 2015;15:151.
3. Reed DC, Juhn AT, Rayess N, Hsu J, Chiang A. Outcomes of retinal detachment repair after posterior open globe injury. Retina. 2016;36(4):758–63.

Chapter 31
Case 26: Tissue Loss in Open Globe Injuries: A Case of an Open Globe Requiring Corneal Patch Graft

Jonathan C. Chou, Peter B. Veldman, and Seanna Grob

31.1 History of Present Illness

An 83-year-old man with a history of atrial fibrillation, rheumatoid arthritis, and prior open globe of his left eye secondary to a glass injury presented with concern for an open globe injury of the same eye.

- The patient reports he had a mechanical fall in the bathroom and hit his left eye and face on the metal railing of his shower.
- His baseline vision prior to this second eye trauma was hand motion.
- He was evaluated at an outside hospital and found to have significant left periorbital swelling and the computed tomography (CT) scan showed a ruptured globe of his left eye.
- He reports decreased vision and inability to see light in the left eye.

31.2 Initial Trauma Evaluation

31.2.1 Visual Acuity (With Correction)

OD: 20/30+2
OS: No light perception

J. C. Chou, M.D. (✉) • S. Grob, M.D., M.A.S.
Department of Ophthalmology, Harvard Medical School, Massachusetts Eye and Ear, Boston, MA, USA
e-mail: jonathan_chou@meei.harvard.edu

P. B. Veldman, M.D.
Cornea and Refractive Surgery, Department of Ophthalmology and Visual Science, University of Chicago, Chicago, IL, USA

S. Grob, C. Kloek (eds.), *Management of Open Globe Injuries*,
https://doi.org/10.1007/978-3-319-72410-2_31

31.2.2 Pupils

OD: Normal
OS: +Afferent pupillary defect by reverse

31.2.3 External Examination

Significant left-sided periorbital ecchymosis and edema

31.2.4 Slit Lamp Examination (Fig. 31.1)

	OD	OS
Lids and lashes	Normal	Significant periorbital ecchymosis, non-marginal laceration along the brow from the nasal edge to the center, left lower eyelid laceration laterally
Sclera and conjunctiva	Normal	Bullous subconjunctival hemorrhage
Cornea	Normal	Central corneal rupture with uveal prolapse
Anterior chamber	Normal	Complete hyphema
Iris	Normal	No view
Lens	Posterior chamber intraocular lens	No view
Vitreous	Normal	No view

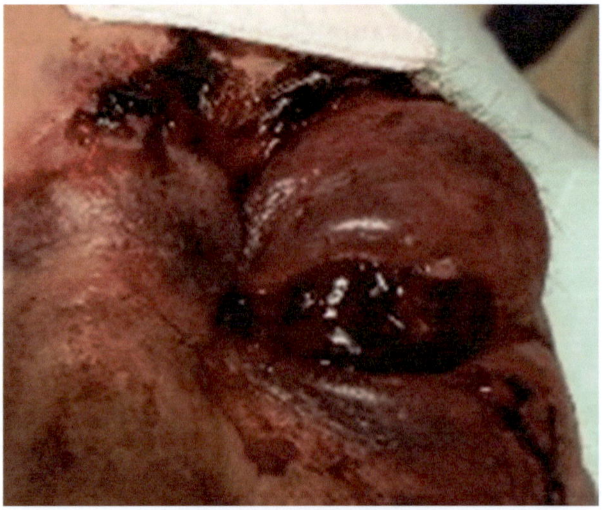

Fig. 31.1 External photograph showing significant periorbital edema and 360° of bullous subconjunctival hemorrhage of the left eye

31.2.5 Dilated Examination

Macula/Nerve OD: Normal
Periphery OD: Scattered pigmentary changes
Macula/Nerve: OS: No view
Periphery OS: No view

31.2.6 Radiographic Imaging

CT image showed a ruptured globe of the left eye with significant irregularity of the globe (Fig. 31.2), without evidence of an intraocular foreign body. There was associated hemorrhage and periorbital soft tissue swelling. No intracranial injury was identified.

31.3 Surgeon's Initial Assessment and Pre-Operative Plan

This patient had a Zone I open globe injury of the left eye with significant periorbital edema and ecchymosis. He had previously suffered an open globe injury to the same eye and as a result had a baseline visual acuity of hand motion. Although the patient understood the risks and the poor prognosis given his baseline low vision and presentation with no light perception vision, he was adamant about saving the eye.

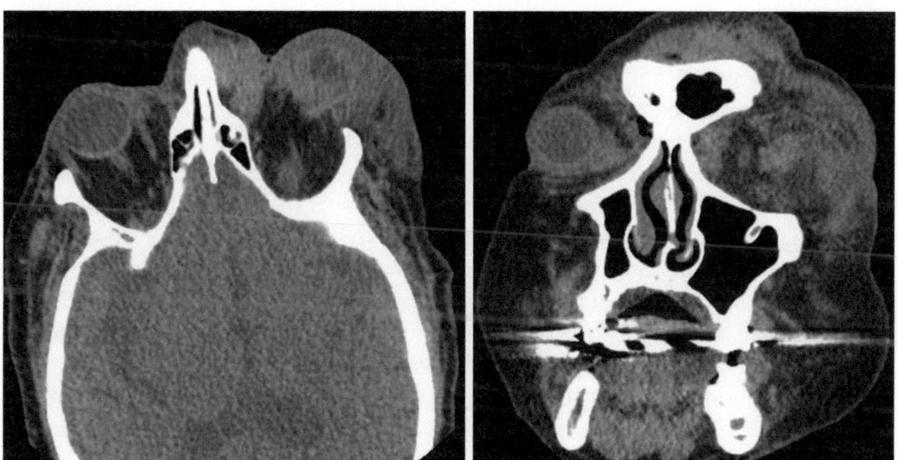

Fig. 31.2 CT of the orbits showing irregularity of the left globe with associated hemorrhage and periorbital soft tissue swelling

This case illustrates the importance of a detailed discussion regarding visual prognosis, as well as a discussion about the patient's goals. Some patients would like to do everything possible to save the eye, even if there is a very low chance of visual recovery. It is important to listen to the patient's wishes and concerns and inform them of the options and the risks and benefits of each. We did discuss the options of evisceration or enucleation versus repair of the globe, with the rare risk of sympathetic ophthalmia in addition to his poor visual prognosis given his no light perception vision pre-operatively and his baseline low vision due to a previous globe injury in that eye.

This case also demonstrates the importance of obtaining a past medical history prior to open globe repair. Since this patient had a prior ruptured globe, we were suspicious of a rupture of his previous corneal wound. Knowing this information can help the surgeon anticipate potential intraoperative challenges, including the possible need for supplemental tissue to facilitate wound closure.

31.4 Surgical Exploration and Repair: Operative Note

Surgical consent was obtained prior to surgery from the patient and health care proxy. After achieving satisfactory general anesthesia, the patient was prepped and draped in the usual sterile ophthalmic fashion. Jaffe lid speculums were placed on the left upper and lower lids. Examination of the eye under the operating microscope revealed significant prolapse of uveal tissue through a ruptured corneal flaplike defect likely in the area of his old corneal scar. The flap was all abnormal cornea which was very thin with lipid infiltrate. Uveal tissue was carefully replaced into the eye. Then, the flap was re-approximated with multiple 10-0 nylon sutures. It was noted throughout the process of placing the sutures that this flap of corneal tissue was very friable. The sutures were unable to be rotated because the flap of previously traumatized cornea was so friable. At this point, it was determined that this abnormal corneal tissue would not be sufficient to close the open globe and a corneal patch graft would be needed to appropriately close the open globe injury. The abnormal corneal tissue included most of the lateral half of the cornea, sparring only about a third of the nasal corneal tissue. The abnormal, friable corneal tissue was removed. An irradiated half-moon corneal graft was sutured over the large defect where there was no viable corneal tissue with multiple 10-0 nylon sutures. Suture passes were made with the intention of incorporating normal corneal tissue for stability of the graft. The wound was Seidel negative after placement of the graft. A 360° peritomy was performed with Wescott scissors with gentle exploration in all 4 quadrants to ensure the corneal wound did not extend past the limbus into sclera, and none was seen. The conjunctiva was closed with 8-0 Vicryl sutures. Subconjunctival injections of antibiotic and steroid were administered. The lid speculums were removed. The eye drape was then removed.

The patient was then re-prepped and draped for repair of his lacerations. After the blood clots were removed, two lacerations were noted, including one over the left brow on the forehead measuring approximately 2 inches and another smaller laceration on his nose that measured approximately 1 cm. The left forehead laceration was closed with three buried 5-0 Vicryl sutures and six 5-0 prolene interrupted sutures, and the nasal laceration was closed with three 5-0 plain gut sutures. Atropine and neomycin and polymyxin B sulfates and dexamethasone ophthalmic ointment were placed on the ocular surface. A sterile ophthalmic patch and shield were placed. The patient tolerated the procedure well.

31.4.1 Surgical Exploration and Repair: Pearls

- Corneal patch grafts may be necessary if the host's cornea is too abnormal (friable, infected, melting, missing) for primary closure. Tutoplast can be used as well if no other graft is available (see case below).
- It might not be obvious pre-operatively which patients will require replacement tissue, so it is important to be aware of the types of tissue you have access to and where they are located.

31.5 Post-Operative Course

Post-operatively, the patient's visual acuity remained no light perception. His periorbital ecchymosis and subconjunctival hemorrhage slowly improved over several weeks (Fig. 31.3). A B-scan ultrasound was performed the day after open globe repair that showed vitreoretinal scarring and choroidals with no obvious retinal detachments (Fig. 31.4). He underwent a retina evaluation and given the no light perception vision, no further surgery was recommended. Additionally, no further cornea surgery or intervention was recommended due to his no light perception vision. The post-operative course was directed by the goal of saving the eye and

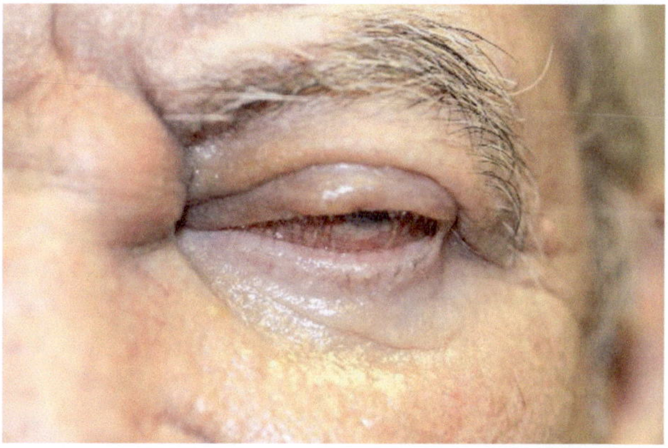

Fig. 31.3 External photograph showing improved periorbital ecchymosis and subconjunctival hemorrhage

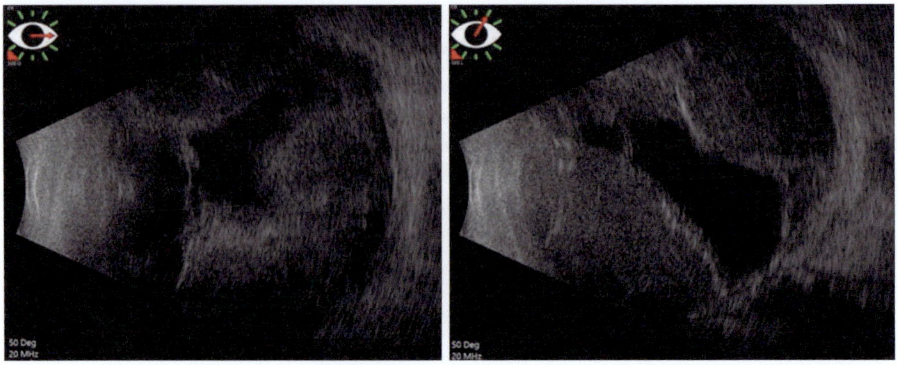

Fig. 31.4 B-scan ultrasound showing the vitreous containing scallop-shaped non-mobile membranous interfaces. No obvious mobile retinal detachment was identified

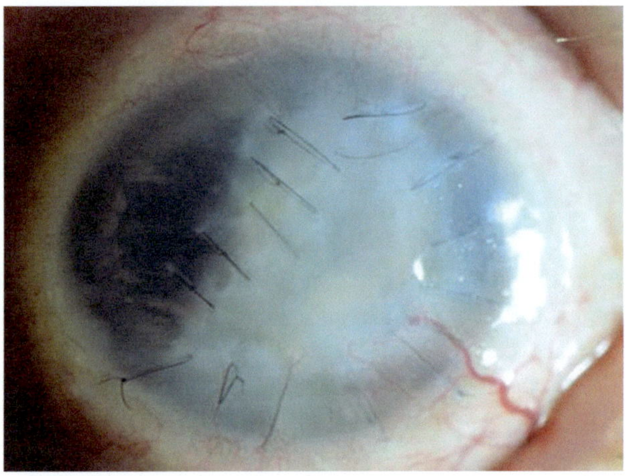

Fig. 31.5 Left eye with corneal patch graft well-positioned with nylon sutures at 6 months post-operatively. A number of these sutures have subsequently been removed, including the one with the suture knot visible at around 7 o'clock

patient comfort. Six months post-operatively, he had minimal pain and there was no change in visual acuity. The corneal patch graft remained in good position (Fig. 31.5) and the patient was happy that his eye was saved. The patient was given a prescription for polycarbonate glasses to protect both eyes.

31.6 Final Trauma Evaluation

31.6.1 Final Visual Acuity

OD: 20/25-1
OS: No light perception

31.6.2 Pupils

OD: none
OS: +Afferent pupillary defect by reverse

31.6.3 Slit Lamp Examination

	OD	OS
Lids and lashes	Ptosis, blepharitis, lower lid laxity	Ptosis, blepharitis, lower lid laxity
Sclera and conjunctiva	Normal	1+ injection
Cornea	Normal	Corneal patch graft well positioned, nylon sutures in place. No infiltrates or epithelial defects
Anterior chamber	Normal	Uvea behind patch graft, shallow
Iris	Normal	Poor view behind corneal graft, otherwise normal
Lens	Normal	No view
Vitreous	Normal	No view

31.6.4 Dilated Examination

Macula/Nerve OD: Normal
Periphery OD: Scattered pigmentary changes
Macula/Nerve: OS: No view
Periphery OS: No view

31.7 Review and Lessons Learned

There are special considerations in open globe injuries where there is inadequate viable tissue. In Zone I injuries, this can occur if there is underlying corneal pathology (e.g., corneal thinning from a non-healing ulcer), prior corneal surgeries or injuries (as in this case) or eye trauma that involves loss of corneal tissue or difficulty closing a round corneal wound (e.g., corneal hole from a penetrating nail or wire, delayed presentation open globe). In these situations, corneal patch grafts might be necessary for adequate closure of the globe.

Full-thickness corneal tissues can be used, similar to penetrating keratoplasty, for repair of dehisced corneal transplants, avulsed corneas, or in cases of significant corneal tissue loss [1, 2]. One disadvantage is that fresh corneal grafts must be obtained from an eye bank and are thus subject to availability and may not be available on an emergent basis if at all. Fortunately, a number of intermediate-term preserved corneal tissue options (e.g., Halo Sterile Tissues, Lions VisionGift, Portland, OR) exist and can be utilized when additional tissue may be required to close a corneal defect [3].

The process of irradiation sterilizes the tissue and enables room temperature storage of the tissue for over a year, making it an ideal option in the event of an unexpected need for patch tissue. It is important to note that irradiated tissue has no endothelial layer, which may result in significant cornea edema in larger full-thickness applications. Various irradiated corneal tissues are available in full corneas and half corneal tissues as well as full and split-thickness (having undergone trephination with a micro-keratome). We have used corneal patch grafts in cases where there are round corneal defects that cannot be closed without leaking, such as with large metal wires through the cornea, or in delayed or infected globes where part of the cornea has melted and cannot be sutured closed appropriately. Although we presented a case of an open globe with poor visual potential and the patch graft was placed because of the patient's strong desire to save the eye, we also have cases of open globe injuries requiring a corneal patch graft with great visual and aesthetic results (best-corrected visual acuity 20/20) (Fig. 31.6). Figure 31.7 illustrates a stepwise approach to creating a corneal patch graft.

In Zone II and III open globe injuries, significant damage or loss of the sclera may require additional tectonic support or tissue. Similar to the cornea, intermediate-term preserved scleral tissue can be used and is a cost-effective option. The scleral patch graft has been shown to be an effective option for preserving globe integrity in a variety of scenarios including patients with a history of necrotizing scleritis or traumatic injuries and is readily available as an off the shelf option [4]. Complications that can occur include post-operative endophthalmitis and graft dehiscence. The scleral graft is avascular and is thus, well tolerated with minimal inflammation. However, this characteristic is a double-edged sword as the area may be more prone

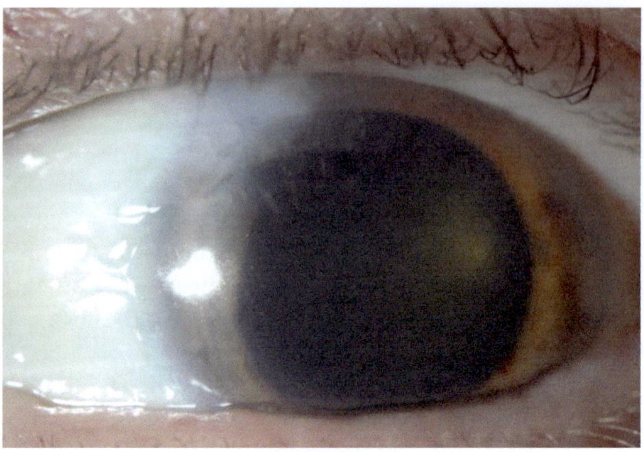

Fig. 31.6 Four year post-operative photo of a delayed presentation ruptured globe that required a split thickness corneal patch graft, made from an irradiated half moon cornea, in the superotemporal cornea

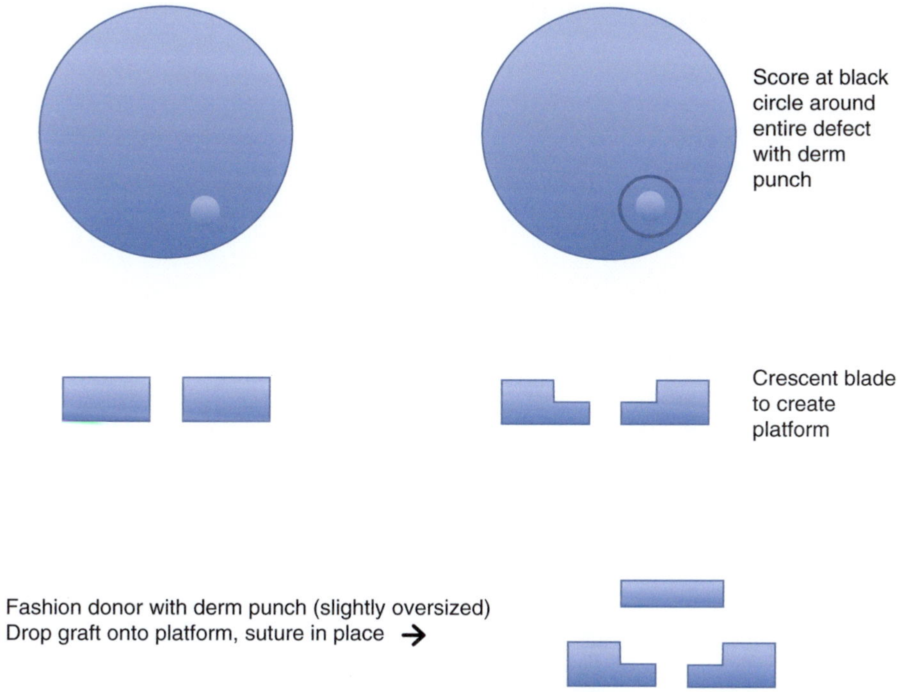

Fig. 31.7 Step-wise approach on inserting a split thickness corneal patch graft. (1) Mark the border of the cornea you will remove with a 3 mm derm punch (or a larger area if needed) and score a circle around the area of abnormal cornea or tissue loss; (2) Use a crescent blade to undermine and remove adjacent epithelium and superficial stromal layers up to the marked circular border to create a little platform out of the corneal stroma where the graft will sit; (3) Use a 3 mm derm punch to get an appropriate size graft (or larger graft if needed to fill the defect) from a split thickness corneal graft either using irradiated cornea or fresh tissue if available; (4) Drop the graft onto the platform and suture in place with 10-0 nylon. Sutures can either be placed radially around the graft like with a penetrating keratoplasty, or laid over the graft to hold it in position, or secured with tissue adhesives. *(Illustration courtesy of Dr. Yewlin Chee)*

to necrosis especially in eyes that are pro-inflammatory [5]. In some circumstances, the scleral patch graft may be too thick which may be a cosmetic issue [6].

Tutoplast® (IOP Ophthalmics, Denville, NJ) is an alternative to full-thickness scleral tissue. Similar to the corneal half-moon, Tutoplast is treated to be immunologically and biologically safe with a shelf life of 5 years. It is often used to cover glaucoma drainage implants, exposed scleral buckles or orbital implants. It has similar color and opacity to sclera, but is thinner, which may make patients more satisfied with the appearance for the eye [7]. However, some patients can notice the slight difference in color if it is used in a visible location more anteriorly. Tutoplast has been reported as an option in globe rupture cases at a previous trabeculectomy site [8]. Tutoplast can also be used for extensive corneal injuries if no other tissue is immediately available. Figure 31.8 shows an example of a patient that underwent a Tutoplast corneal patch graft after sustaining an ocular injury in

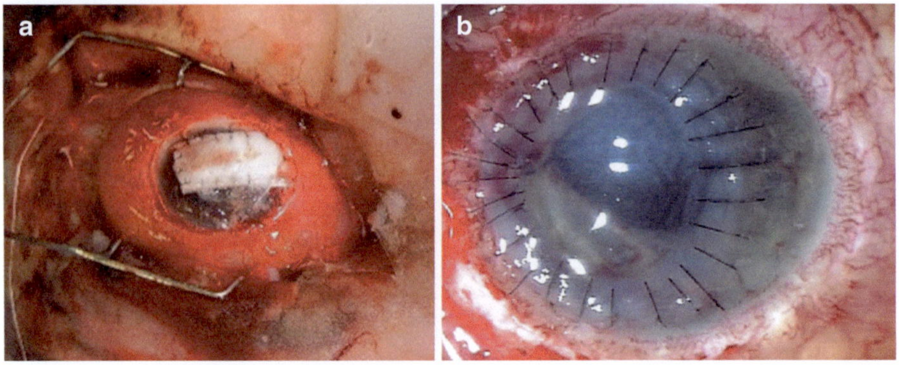

Fig. 31.8 (**a**) Tutoplast used as a corneal graft in a patient who sustained an injury while in combat at a combat field hospital. (**b**) The patient was eventually transferred and subsequently received a corneal transplant. *(Courtesy of Drs. Glenn Sanford, Marcus Colyer & Scot Bower)*

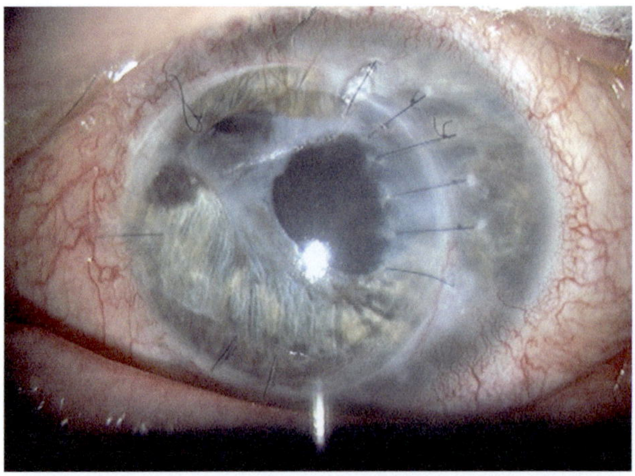

Fig. 31.9 Final clinical photo after visual rehabilitation surgeries and care with best-corrected visual acuity of 20/30. *(Courtesy of Drs. Glenn Sanford, Marcus Colyer & Scot Bower)*

the field while serving in the military. The patient was initially treated in a combat field hospital in Afghanistan. The corneal wound was unable to be closed due to tissue loss and significant corneal edema. The laceration was too large to glue and the only available tissue in the field was Tutoplast, so Tutoplast was used to cover and seal the corneal wound as a temporizing measure until the patient could be transferred and a corneal transplant could be completed. The patient ultimately received a penetrating keratoplasty and had a best corrected visual acuity of 20/30 on final follow up (Fig. 31.9). In our experience, we have also found Tutoplast to be a good option to help provide structural support in post-trauma patients with a prior trabeculectomy or glaucoma surgery. For example, we used Tutoplast in a case of an 85-year-old woman with dementia and severe bilateral glaucoma, status post bilateral trabeculectomy (baseline vision, count fingers at 1 ft. in each eye) who presented with trauma to the left eye. Upon exploration, she was found to have a damaged scleral trabeculectomy flap that was subsequently reinforced with Tutoplast. At 6 months post-operatively, the globe was well-formed and the patient reported no pain.

In summary, tissue loss or damage is an important issue to be prepared for in open globe injury repair. Depending on the site of tissue loss or damage (e.g., cornea, scleral), several tissue replacement options are available. Surgeons must balance each graft's pros and cons to determine which selection is optimal for each case.

31.8 Key Learning Points

- Consider patch grafts in trauma cases with tissue loss, damage that does not allow for direct closure or in which suture closure would cause undue tension and distortion/astigmatism. Figure 31.7 provides a step-wise approach on the use of a corneal-patch graft.
- Surgeons should be aware of the options available and their advantages and disadvantages.

References

1. Nobe JR, Moura BT, Robin JB, Smith RE. Results of penetrating keratoplasty for the treatment of corneal perforations. Arch Ophthalmol. 1990;108(7):939–41.
2. Krysik K, Dobrowolski D, Lyssek-Boron A, Jankowska-Szmul J, Wylegala EA. Differences in surgical management of corneal perforations, measured over six years. J Ophthalmol. 2017;2017:1582532.
3. Park JYSE. A case of tectonic lamellar corneal patch graft using acellular cornea in corneal ulcer perforation. J Korean Ophthalmol Soc. 2015;56(8):1278–83.
4. Sangwan VS, Jain V, Gupta P. Structural and functional outcome of scleral patch graft. Eye (Lond). 2007;21(7):930–5.
5. Nguyen QD, Foster CS. Scleral patch graft in the management of necrotizing scleritis. Int Ophthalmol Clin. 1999;39(1):109–31.
6. Smith MF, Doyle JW, Ticrney JW Jr. A comparison of glaucoma drainage implant tube coverage. J Glaucoma. 2002;11(2):143–7.
7. Novitskaya ES, Clifford L, Vivian AJ. Tutoplast pericardium patch graft for scleral thinning following strabismus surgery. Eye (Lond). 2013;27(5):682–3.
8. Shah BP, Clarke J. Donor pericardium graft repair of traumatic globe rupture at previous trabeculectomy site. Digit J Ophthalmol. 2014;20(3):48–50.

Chapter 32
Case 27: Zone I Open Globe Injury Requiring Corneal Glue

Catherine J. Choi and Alice C. Lorch

32.1 History of Present Illness

A 67-year-old man with history of hypertension and hyperlipidemia presents with concern for open globe of the right eye.

- The patient reports going deer hunting with a bow and arrow. While nocking an arrow, the arrow slipped and flipped up towards his right eye. He denied any significant pain or loss of vision and noted a mild foreign body sensation only.
- He presented to an outside hospital where he was examined and transferred to Massachusetts Eye and Ear (MEE) for further management.

32.2 Initial Trauma Evaluation

32.2.1 Visual Acuity (Without Correction)

OD: 20/25 + 2
OS: 20/25 + 2

C. J. Choi, M.D. (✉)
Bascom Palmer Eye Institute, University of Miami, Miami, FL, USA

A. C. Lorch, M.D., M.P.H.
Department of Ophthalmology, Harvard Medical School, Massachusetts Eye and Ear, Boston, MA, USA

S. Grob, C. Kloek (eds.), *Management of Open Globe Injuries*,
https://doi.org/10.1007/978-3-319-72410-2_32

32.2.2 Pupils

OD: Round, reactive to light, no afferent pupillary defect
OS: Round, reactive to light

32.2.3 External Examination

Within normal limits

32.2.4 Slit Lamp Examination

	OD	OS
Lids and lashes	Normal	Normal
Sclera and conjunctiva	Trace injection	Nasal pterygium
Cornea	0.5 mm stellate full-thickness limbal laceration at 12 o'clock, Seidel positive	Normal
Anterior chamber	1+ cell, early organizing fibrin centrally	Normal
Iris	Round	Normal
Lens	Normal	Normal
Vitreous	Normal	Normal

32.2.5 Dilated Examination

Macula/Nerve OD: Normal, myelinated nerve fiber layer at the inferior margin of the nerve
Periphery OD: Inferior and superior peripheral choroidal detachment, retina attached, no foreign body
Macula/Nerve: OS: Normal
Periphery OS: Normal

32.2.6 Radiographic Imaging

Computed tomography (CT) of the orbits showed preseptal swelling and relative shallowing of the anterior chamber of the right globe suggestive of an anterior globe rupture. No radiopaque bodies were identified (Fig. 32.1).

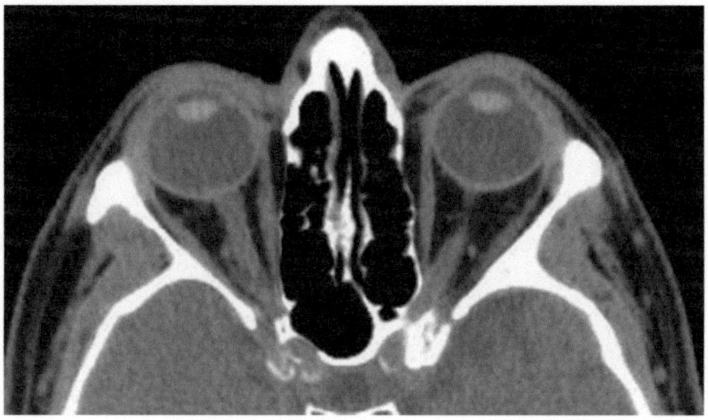

Fig. 32.1 Axial CT image showing a shallow anterior chamber on the right side and a normal globe on the left

32.3 Surgeon's Initial Assessment and Pre-Operative Plan

The patient presented with a Zone I limbal laceration of the right eye with mild shallowing of the anterior chamber and peripheral choroidal detachments.

The surgical approach was a standard Zone I repair with limited peritomy and a paracentesis (see earlier chapters for specifics on Zone I repair).

Important considerations for this case included anterior chamber depth and evaluation of the underlying iris, anterior chamber angle, and the peripheral lens. On slit lamp exam, the pupil was round and well dilated. There was no evidence of lens material, hyphema, or vitreous in the anterior chamber. The anterior chamber was shallow, without irido-corneal or lenticular touch.

Despite no overt signs of trauma to the deeper structures, complete evaluation was recommended at the time of surgery to ensure that the full extent of injury was addressed. Surgical planning should include appropriate placement of the paracentesis to allow for a cyclodialysis spatula, iris spatula, or an irrigating cannula to be used to sweep under the wound.

32.4 Surgical Exploration and Repair: Operative Note

Informed consent was obtained prior to the procedure. The operative eye was identified and marked. The patient was transported into the operating room where general anesthesia was induced. The non-operative eye was taped and shielded. The operative eye was prepped and draped in the usual sterile fashion. Jaffe lid speculum was placed and fixed with hemostats. Using a 27-gauge needle, the area of laceration was carefully inspected by lifting the laceration edges. A thorough exam and irrigation were performed to remove any debris and to confirm lack of iris prolapse. No foreign body or iris material was noted within the wound. A paracentesis was made with a 15° blade at the 10 o'clock position directed toward the wound.

A cyclodialysis spatula was used to sweep under the wound. No iris entrapment was noted. A limited peritomy was performed superiorly using blunt Westcott scissors. There was no extension of the laceration beyond the limbus under the conjunctiva. Three 10–0 nylon sutures were placed across the laceration to appropriately reappose the tissues. One 10–0 nylon suture was placed to close the paracentesis. The wound was then tested by palpating the globe to confirm a seal. Seidel negativity was confirmed again using a fluorescein strip. The anterior chamber was formed and deep. One 7–0 Vicryl suture was placed to re-appose the conjunctiva superiorly. The lid speculum and drapes were removed. Atropine and antibiotic-steroid ointment were applied to the surface of the eye. The eye was patched and shielded. The patient tolerated the procedure without any complications. General anesthesia was reversed and the patient was transported into the post-operative care unit in a stable condition.

32.4.1 Surgical Exploration and Repair: Pearls

- The entry wound should be carefully examined for any evidence of embedded foreign body or iris strands even in the absence of overt signs of iris trauma.
- A cyclodialysis spatula can be inserted from a paracentesis to allow access directly under the entry wound.

32.5 Post-Operative Course

The patient was admitted to MEE to complete a 48 hour course of intravenous antibiotics. On post-operative day 2, a new Seidel-positive leak from the center of the stellate wound with moderate flow was noted on exam. The three nylon sutures were in place with appropriate tension. A decision was made to apply cyanoacrylate corneal glue to seal the area of leak.

32.6 Procedure Note: Application of Corneal Glue to the Right Eye

Informed consent was obtained. The right eye was marked, prepped, and draped in the usual sterile fashion. Topical anesthetic and antibiotic drops were given. A 3 mm skin biopsy punch was used to cut a clear sterile plastic eye drape. A small dot of ophthalmic ointment was placed on the wooden end of a cotton tip applicator. The round 3 mm clear drape that was cut was placed on top of the dot of ophthalmic ointment. One drop of corneal cyanoacrylate glue was then applied to the 3 mm drape. The glue-coated circular drape was placed over the wound and allowed to dry. A small leak was noted temporally and additional glue was applied in the same fashion until the wound was Seidel negative. A bandage contact lens was placed over the glue-coated circular drape with additional topical ophthalmic antibiotic drops. Timolol was added to his medication regimen for aqueous suppression.

32.7 Post-Operative Course

At post-operative week 1, the patient returned with a dislodged glue patch and persistent Seidel positivity from the center of the stellate wound. No appropriate area for additional suture was present and additional corneal glue was applied, followed by a bandage contact lens. Prednisolone acetate was decreased and gentamicin drops were added to promote epithelial scar formation.

At post-operative week 10, the patient presented with 5 days of redness and pain and was noted to have elevated intraocular pressure at 37 mmHg, increased anterior chamber reaction, and engorged iris and limbal vessels (Fig. 32.2). Dilated fundus exam was within normal limits. Additional aqueous suppressive therapy was instituted and a new bandage contact lens was placed with improvement in intraocular pressure and inflammation.

By post-operative month 3.5, there was resolution of the iris vessels and at post-operative month 5, the bandage contact lens and corneal glue were removed without complications. The area under the glue was Seidel negative with diffuse neovascularization. Prednisolone acetate was restarted in an effort to promote regression of the corneal neovascularization. Corneal sutures were subsequently

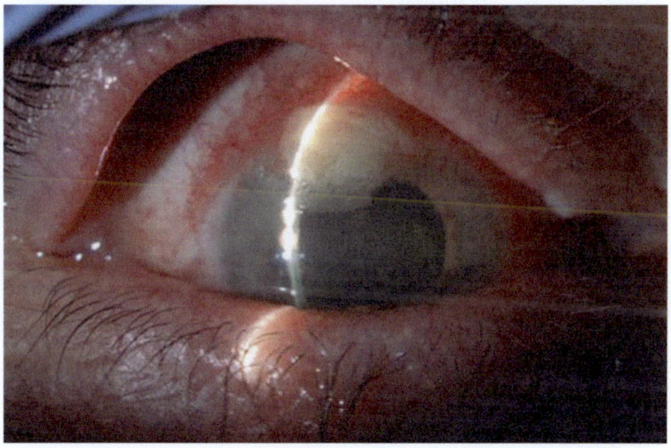

Fig. 32.2 Slit lamp photo of the right eye demonstrating the corneal glue at the superior limbus with adjacent area of conjunctival injection and early corneal neovascularization

removed at post-operative month 5.5 and there was complete regression of corneal neovascularization by post-operative month 7.

32.8 Final Trauma Evaluation

32.8.1 Final Visual Acuity

OD: 20/25 with correction
OS: 20/20 with correction

32.8.2 Pupils

OD: Round, reactive, no afferent pupillary defect
OS: Round, reactive

32.8.3 Slit Lamp Examination

	OD	OS
Lids and lashes	Normal	Normal
Sclera and conjunctiva	Normal	Nasal pterygium
Cornea	Regressed anterior stromal vessels, residual ghost vessels from deep stromal neovascularization, central cornea clear	Normal
Anterior chamber	Normal	Normal
Iris	Normal	Normal
Lens	1–2+ nuclear sclerosis, pigment on anterior lens capsule	1+ nuclear sclerosis
Vitreous	Normal	Normal

32.8.4 Dilated Examination

Macula/Nerve OD: Normal, myelinated nerve fiber layer at the inferior margin of the nerve
Periphery OD: Normal
Macula/Nerve: OS: Normal
Periphery OS: Normal

32.9 Review and Lessons Learned

Stellate corneal lacerations are typically more difficult to repair due to their configuration of having a central area of confluence of multiple radial lacerations with instability and limited room for placement of overlapping sutures. In this case, while a Seidel negative seal was achieved at the time of initial repair, a leak developed 2 days later from the center of the wound as the corneal edema began to resolve and the apices of the stellate wound retracted. A stellate corneal wound, a delayed presentation corneal wound, or a corneal wound with a retained foreign body can be difficult to close. In rare cases, it is necessary to place corneal glue in the operating room on initial repair for wounds that remain Seidel positive after several attempts to close the wound. It is helpful to place a small air bubble in the anterior chamber when placing glue so that the wound remains dry while the corneal glue dries and solidifies. More commonly, the wound is Seidel negative at the time of repair, but becomes Seidel positive as the corneal edema improves. These patients require further intervention in the form of bandage contact lens and aqueous suppression, corneal glue, or re-suturing.

Cyanoacrylate corneal glue can be applied either directly on the ocular surface, or by using a glue patch fashioned with a thin clear plastic drape. A glue patch allows for a more controlled and focal application of the glue, but does not conform to the curvature of the surface as readily. This is compared to directly applying glue to the cornea, which can result in a more diffuse spread on the surface of the eye [1].

While generally well tolerated, cyanoacrylate corneal glue can also incite acute and chronic inflammation secondary to local toxicity from its degradation products cyanoacetate and formaldehyde. This toxicity can lead to a range of intraocular and extraocular inflammation, including elevated intraocular pressure, anterior uveitis, and iris and corneal neovascularization [2]. In this patient, topical aqueous suppressants and steroids were instituted with a dramatic regression of corneal and iris vessels. Close monitoring is therefore essential in the setting of corneal glue, even in the setting of apparent stability with a good seal.

32.10 Key Learning Points

- Stellate-shaped corneal lacerations are more difficult to close than linear lacerations due to an area of central confluence of multiple segments of the laceration.
- Cyanoacrylate corneal glue is a useful adjunct method for treating small intraoperative or post-operative leaks and corneal wounds that are difficult to address with sutures alone.
- Longstanding cyanoacrylate glue application can induce an inflammatory reaction leading to the formation of corneal and iris neovascularization.
- Corneal neovascularization should be treated with aggressive topical steroid therapy to prevent extension into the central visual axis.

References

1. Rana M, Savant V. A brief review of techniques used to seal corneal perforation using cyanoacrylate tissue adhesive. Cont Lens Anterior Eye. 2013;36(4):156–8.
2. Tan J, Wechsler AW, Watson S. Long-term adhesion of cyanoacrylate on human cornea. Clin Exp Ophthalmol. 2014;42(8):791–3.

Chapter 33
Case 28: Zone I/II Open Globe Injury with Corneal Patch Graft and Corneal Glue

Michael Lin, Katherine E. Talcott, and Alice C. Lorch

33.1 History of Present Illness

A 53-year-old man with history of right eye corneal ulcer 6 years prior now presents with concern for open globe of the right eye.

- The patient reports that he was struck in the right eye by a barbed wire that he was cutting under tension while working on a fence at his tree farm. When he cut the barbed wire, a piece flew toward him and hit his right eye. He immediately noticed a "gush of fluid" from his eye after he was struck.
- He had immediate severe pain and reported whitening and blurring of his vision in the right eye.
- He was seen at an outside hospital, where he received a tetanus shot and was transferred to Massachusetts Eye and Ear (MEE) for further management of his eye trauma.

33.2 Initial Trauma Evaluation

33.2.1 Visual Acuity (Without Correction)

OD: 20/30 + 2
OS: 20/20

M. Lin, M.D. (✉) • A. C. Lorch, M.D., M.P.H.
Department of Ophthalmology, Harvard Medical School, Massachusetts Eye and Ear, Boston, MA, USA
e-mail: Michael_lin@meei.harvard.edu

K. E. Talcott, M.D.
Vitreoretinal Surgery, Wills Eye Hospital, Philadelphia, PA, USA

S. Grob, C. Kloek (eds.), *Management of Open Globe Injuries*,
https://doi.org/10.1007/978-3-319-72410-2_33

33.2.2 *Pupils*

OD: Irregular due to iris prolapse; no afferent pupillary defect by reverse
OS: Round and reactive

33.2.3 *External Examination*

No evidence of periorbital trauma. No lacerations, edema, or abrasions.

33.2.4 *Slit Lamp Examination*

	OD	OS
Lids and lashes	Normal	Normal
Sclera and conjunctiva	1-2+ diffuse injection without laceration or foreign body	Normal
Cornea	Peripheral stellate vertical full-thickness corneal laceration extending from 6 to 10 o'clock, approximately 5 mm vertically, iris prolapsed through inferior 3 mm of the wound, and the wound extends just slightly past the limbus	Normal
Anterior chamber	Shallow, inferior, layered hyphema approximately 3 mm in height, as well as scattered heme covering temporal iris, 3+ cell and flare	Normal
Iris	Iris prolapse through inferotemporal corneal laceration, no transillumination defects	Normal
Lens	Normal, no evidence of lens violation	Normal
Vitreous	Normal	Normal

33.2.5 *Dilated Examination*

Macula/Nerve OD: Hazy view, grossly normal
Periphery OD: Hazy view, gross normal
Macula/Nerve: OS: Normal
Periphery OS: Normal

33.2.6 *Radiographic Imaging*

Computed tomography (CT) of the orbits showed ruptured globe of the right eye, without evidence of an intraocular foreign body. There was a right temporal intraocular hyperdensity that was thought to represent a choroidal hemorrhage (Fig. 33.1).

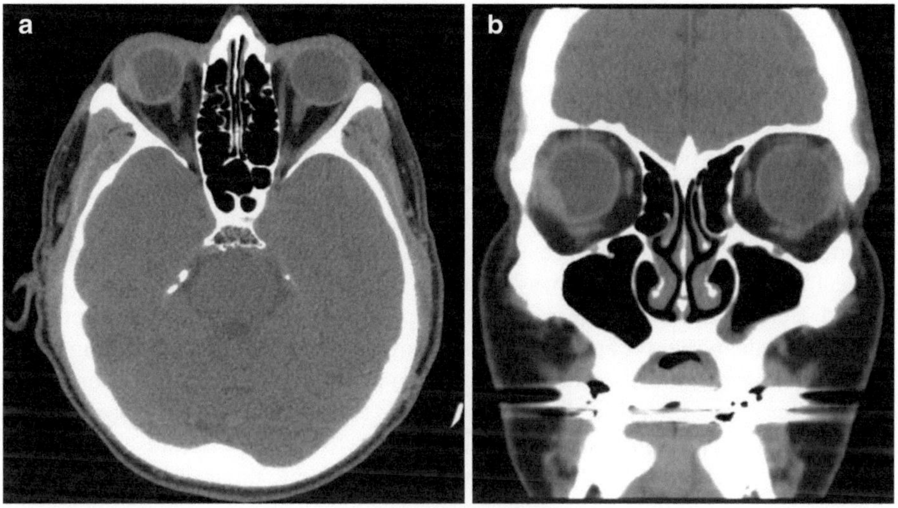

Fig. 33.1 Axial (**a**) and coronal (**b**) computed tomography images showing a choroidal hemorrhage of the right eye and a normal left eye. There is no evidence of intraocular foreign body

33.3 Surgeon's Initial Assessment and Pre-Operative Plan

The patient had a Zone I/II open globe injury of the right eye with a temporal full-thickness corneal laceration extending to the limbus and slightly extending past the limbus into the sclera of his right eye with uveal prolapse. The open globe was repaired approximately 17 hours after the initial injury, which still fit into the protocol at MEE for repair of open globes within 24 hours of the initial injury. During that time, the patient received intravenous vancomycin and ceftazidime per protocol for open globe injuries.

Though the patient had 20/30 vision at the time of his initial evaluation, he was counseled that he had suffered a very serious eye injury, and the surgery required to repair the wound would likely cause his vision to worsen in the immediate post-operative period due to corneal edema, astigmatism, and inflammation.

Even though this patient was repaired within 24 hours of initial injury, by the time he got to the operating room, it was clear that the corneal wound had become increasingly edematous and necrotic, concerning for possible infection. On further questioning with the patient, it was determined that the barbed wire that hit his eye was likely contaminated with manure. This increased the concern for corneal and intraocular infection. The plan would be to try and close the wound primarily with nylon sutures using long passes to incorporate normal, non-necrotic corneal tissue. Care would be taken to avoid full-thickness suture passes to prevent introduction of infected material intraocularly. The pre-operative plan also involved consideration for need of a possible corneal patch graft and/or corneal glue to close the necrotic wound, so these were available in the operating room at the start of the case. Additionally, intracameral antibiotics would be administered at the end of the case to help address the likely infected and contaminated wound.

33.4 Surgical Exploration and Repair: Operative Note

The risks, benefits, and alternatives were discussed with the patient pre-operatively, and he consented to proceed with the examination under anesthesia and globe repair. The right eye was prepped and draped in the usual sterile ophthalmic fashion with a Jaffe speculum to provide adequate exposure.

The wound was explored. The wound extended inferiorly to the limbus and was found to be newly opacified since examination the prior day, concerning for infected corneal tissue. Wound closure was therefore initiated at the superior aspect of the wound. Before any sutures were placed, the prolapsed iris was gently scraped with a Beaver blade to remove epithelial cells. A small piece of necrotic appearing iris at the inferior aspect of the wound was truncated and sent to pathology. Several 10-0 nylon sutures were then placed across the wound to help maintain the globe, and iris was reposited into the anterior chamber as sutures were placed. Sutures were placed over an iris spatula to avoid incorporation of iris tissue into the wound. After several sutures were placed, two paracenteses were made, one at 9 o'clock and one at 11 o'clock. The anterior chamber was inflated first with air, and a cyclodialysis spatula was used to try to sweep remaining iris out of the wound. As the chamber continued to collapse under air, Healon was injected into the anterior chamber. Again, the cyclodialysis spatula was used to sweep more iris out of the wound. More 10-0 sutures were placed along the superior aspect of the wound, until it was found to be well apposed and without prolapsed iris. At this time, a small gaping hole, less than 1 mm by 1 mm, was identified at the inferior extent of the wound. Sutured closure was attempted but was unsuccessful given the size of the hole, the astigmatism that was being induced, and the poor substrate of surrounding necrotic corneal tissue for suturing. Two pieces of this necrotic tissue were sent for culture. A limited conjunctival peritomy was made around the edge of the wound to improve visualization.

To repair this hole, a corneal patch graft was prepared from irradiated split thickness half moon cornea. A derm punch was used to prepare a 2 mm round corneal patch graft. The anterior corneal stroma surrounding the hole was undermined and excised to approximately 2 mm such that the patch graft could be placed on a corneal shelf and entirely cover the hole (please see earlier chapter for diagram, Fig. 31.7). 10-0 nylon sutures were used to secure the patch graft into position. Following successful placement of the patch graft, the patient was noted to have a persistent wound leak at the inferior aspect of the wound. Corneal glue attached to a clear piece of surgical drape was applied at first directly over the patch graft. This still did not stop the wound leak, and so a second piece of drape with corneal glue was placed. The glue was observed for 2 minutes to dry, and after this there was no further leakage. The conjunctiva was then closed using 8-0 Vicryl. A limited anterior chamber washout was performed, confirming that there was no remaining Healon in the eye. Intracameral antibiotics of vancomycin and ceftazidime were injected into the anterior chamber through the existing paracenteses. The paracenteses were found to be watertight. Topical moxifloxacin and atropine drops were applied. A patch was applied over the eye. The Jaffe speculum was then removed, followed by the surgical drape. The patient tolerated the procedure well.

33.4.1 Surgical Exploration and Repair: Pearls

- In cases with persistent corneal wound leak, a corneal patch graft for large defects, corneal glue for smaller defects or leakage, or a combination of both may be necessary to seal the wounds completely. This is more likely to occur in cases of necrotic or missing cornea.
- If there is suspicion of necrotic, infected tissue, sending samples for culture and pathology and addition of intracameral antibiotics may be considered. It is also advisable to delay initiation of steroid treatment.

33.5 Post-Operative Course

The patient was admitted to MEE to complete a 48 hour course of intravenous vancomycin and ceftazidime, as per standard practice at MEE. The frequency of his post-operative topical eyedrop antibiotic treatment was increased compared to standard practice because of the necrotic corneal appearance and concern for development of infection due to a contaminated wound caused by barbed wire from a fence on a farm. He was started on moxifloxacin one drop every hour and atropine one drop twice per day. Prednisolone acetate was deferred until there was less concern for infection. B-scan ultasound on post-operative day 1 showed right eye temporal choroidal hemorrhage and small non-hemorrhagic choroidals scattered elsewhere (Fig. 33.2). Vision on post-operative day 1 was counting fingers at 3 ft, significantly decreased from the patient's 20/30 pre-operative vision. This improved on post-operative day 8 to 20/200, at which point there was a nonappositional hemorrhagic choroidal detachment 360°. Culture of cornea and iris tissue showed no growth of infectious species. Gram stain showed rare epithelial cells, but no organisms or polymorphic neutrophils. Pathology was reported as loose edematous fibrocollagenous tissue with widely scattered lymphocytes. On post-operative day 8, the patient was started on prednisolone acetate 1% twice a day to the right eye, as cultures were negative, and there was no longer evidence of an infiltrate on slit lamp examination.

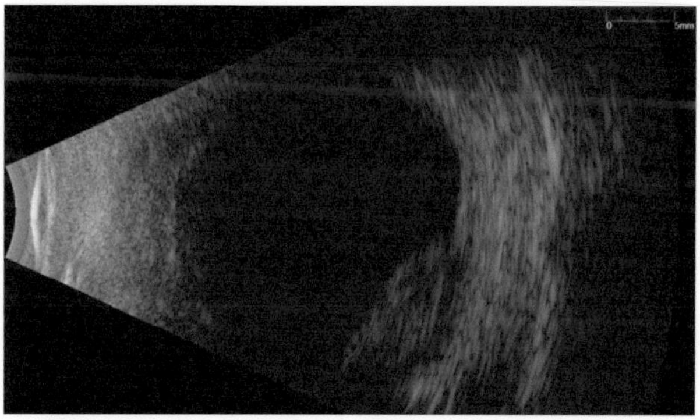

Fig. 33.2 B-scan on post-operative day 1 showed right eye temporal choroidal hemorrhage

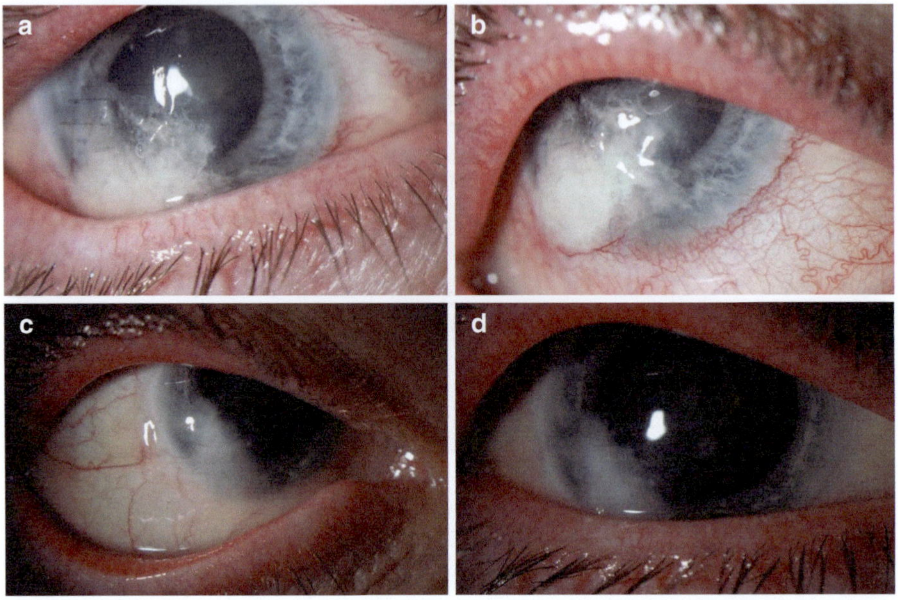

Fig. 33.3 External clinical images of the patient's right eye. (**a**) and (**b**) are taken at post-operative month 3 and show the area of inferotemporal corneal patch graft, glue, surgical drape, and sutures. (**c**) and (**d**) are taken at post-operative month 6 and show the eye with remaining inferotemporal scarring after removal of corneal glue and sutures. The central visual axis is clear of scarring

The patient was followed closely for several months after open globe repair. His intraocular pressure measured over his bandage contact lens (BCL) was 29 mmHg at 1.5 months after repair, and timolol was added. Two weeks later, pressure over his BCL was 38 mmHg, and brimonidine was added. At post-operative month 3, his BCL was removed, glue edges were trimmed, and a new BCL was placed (Fig. 33.3a, b). The next week, IOP was 26, latanoprost was added, and more glue was trimmed. In total, the patient had four visits for glue removal during post-operative months 3–4, and then sutures were removed over four visits from post-operative month 4–5. There was iridocorneal touch noted behind the corneal wound, but it always showed no leakage on Seidel testing. The patient was subsequently tapered off steroids and glaucoma medications.

33.6 Final Trauma Evaluation

33.6.1 Final Visual Acuity

OD: 20/30 without correction, 20/20 with +1.25−1.25 × 122 lens
OS: 20/20

33.6.2 Pupils

OD: Elongated in teardrop shape toward 7 o'clock, reactive, no afferent pupillary defect
OS: Round and reactive

33.6.3 Slit Lamp Examination

	OD	OS
Lids and lashes	Normal	Normal
Sclera and conjunctiva	Normal	Normal
Cornea	Diffuse inferotemporal stromal opacity with neovascular pannus, two inferotemporal suture remnants buried within stroma, no leakage on Seidel testing, and small, faint, round stromal scars centrally and close to neovascularization (Fig. 33.3c, d)	Normal
Anterior chamber	Inferotemporal iridocorneal touch, but otherwise deep and open to scleral spur, no cell	Normal
Iris	Corectopia with elongation of pupil toward 7 o'clock	Normal
Lens	Mild cortical cataract and pigment on anterior capsule	Normal
Vitreous	Normal	Normal

33.6.4 Dilated Examination

Macula/Nerve OD: Normal
Periphery OD: Normal
Macula/Nerve: OS: Normal
Periphery OS: Normal

33.7 Review and Lessons Learned

Any open globe repair follows specific surgical principles, but also must allow room for variation, requiring creativity and flexibility in the surgical approach. This case was unusual in the rapid progression of corneal opacification and the development of necrotic corneal tissue. Studies have suggested that repair of open globe injuries after delay of greater than 24 hours is associated with higher rates of endophthalmitis, and that is a contributing factor for consideration of intravitreal antibiotic injection at the time of primary repair, although this patient was taken to surgery within that window [1, 2]. A dirty wound is also a risk factor for endophthalmitis, and though this patient only developed corneal ulceration and necrosis without endophthalmitis, he may have been predisposed to these rapid changes due to the contaminated nature of his wound caused by a farm fence likely covered in manure. In cases of suspected infection, we often consider adding intracameral broad-spectrum antibiotics to our typical protocol of intravenous antibiotics with topical post-operative antibiotics, as was done in this case.

We always recommend trying to get the patient to the operating room for repair of a ruptured globe within 24 hours of injury. However, there are some times when it may be helpful to try and get the patient to the operating room as soon as possible: retained foreign body, contaminated or infected wound, uncontrolled pain, or a child who may not have the ability to understand the importance of not touching the injured eye. The cornea will become more edematous and hazy with time after an injury. This in itself can complicate repair. However, a contaminated corneal wound is at risk for corneal necrosis or melting and progression to endophthalmitis. These cases may benefit from surgical repair as soon as possible. If corneal necrosis or melting is more extensive than this case, a therapeutic corneal transplant may be necessary in order to remove unhealthy corneal tissue. For small defects or slow leaks, a corneal patch graft or glue can be a good tool for repair.

The subsequent necrosis of the cornea posed special challenges to the repair. Corneal glue has been utilized successfully in settings of wounds less than 1 mm in diameter [3]. Cyanoacrylate may be preferred over fibrin glue because fibrin may predispose to bacterial or fungal infections. Larger wounds may require grafts in order to seal the defect completely. After placement of a corneal patch graft with irradiated split-thickness half moon cornea, this patient still had a persistent wound leak, and therefore, a technique described by Vote and Elder was used to apply cyanoacrylate glue by cutting a piece of surgical drape, adhering it to the wooden end of a cotton tip applicator with lubricating jelly, applying glue to the other side of the drape, and then applying the glue surface to the wound [4]. In situations where emergent surgery is indicated, but there is no corneal tissue, amniotic membrane, or other appropriate biological graft available, temporary patch grafting with polyethylene film surgical drape and cyanoacrylate glue has been described as a temporizing measure before more definitive treatment [5]. Luckily, biologic material was available for this patient, and he healed well after surgery. Corneal sutures are usually removed starting at post-operative week 6, but this must be delayed in cases of compromised wound integrity.

33.8 Key Learning Points

- In cases of persistent corneal wound leak, corneal patch graft and/or corneal glue are necessary for surgical repair.
- If an infected wound and/or necrosis is suspected, send samples for gram stain, culture, and possibly also a tissue sample for pathology. In addition to intravenous

antibiotics, ophthalmologists should consider intracameral antibiotics at the time of open globe repair for these cases.

- Contaminated corneal wounds may need more immediate surgical repair to prevent tissue necrosis or melting.
- Corneal glue can be removed slowly over several visits if there is concern for a non-healing or leaking wound. The patient will need to continue wearing a bandage contact lens and using topical antibiotic drops until removal of the glue is complete.
- As discussed in an earlier case, patients with complicated corneal wounds should be counseled that even if their vision is not severely impaired at the time of injury, it will likely worsen immediately after surgery due to the surgical approaches required for repair. It is important to set realistic expectations and to provide appropriate warning regarding post-operative vision decrease, as patients may be alarmed that the surgical repair actually worsened their vision if they are not counseled to expect this.

References

1. Essex RW, Yi Q, Charles PG, et al. Post-traumatic endophthalmitis. Ophthalmology. 2004;111:2015–22.
2. Andreoli CM, Andreoli MT, Kloek CE, et al. Low rate of endophthalmitis in a large series of open globe injuries. Am J Ophthalmol. 2009;147:601–8.
3. Lekskul M, Fracht HU, Cohen EJ, et al. Nontraumatic corneal perforation. Cornea. 2000;19:313–9.
4. Vote BJ, Elder MJ. Cyanoacrylate glue for corneal perforations: a description of a surgical technique and a review of the literature. Clin Exp Ophthalmol. 2000;28:437–42.
5. Khalifa YM, Bailony MR, Bloomer MM, et al. Management of nontraumatic corneal perforation with tectonic drape patch and cyanoacrylate glue. Cornea. 2010;29:1173–5.

Chapter 34
Case 29: Traumatic Evisceration

Natalie Homer, Seanna Grob, Katherine E. Talcott, and Daniel R. Lefebvre

34.1 History of Present Illness

A 34-year old man with no past ophthalmologic history was sent for consultation regarding severe left-sided open facial fractures with severe eyelid soft-tissue trauma and concern for an open globe injury.

- On the evening of presentation, the patient was using a round metal wheel grinder at his workshop when the wheel shattered from the spool and flew up to strike the patient in the left face. Despite wearing safety glasses he sustained significant facial trauma.
- He was brought by ambulance to the Massachusetts General Hospital Emergency Department, where he was found to have a left orbital roof fracture resulting in pneumocephalus, multiple left-sided facial fractures of the orbit and midface that were open through numerous periorbital lacerations, and a severely deformed left globe with no normal structures visible.

34.2 Initial Trauma Evaluation

34.2.1 Visual Acuity (Without Correction)

OD: 23/30 pinhole 20/20
OS: No light perception

N. Homer, M.D. (✉) • S. Grob, M.D., M.A.S. • D. R. Lefebvre, M.D., F.A.C.S.
Department of Ophthalmology, Harvard Medical School, Massachusetts Eye and Ear, Boston, MA, USA
e-mail: natalie_homer@meei.harvard.edu

K. E. Talcott, M.D.
Vitreoretinal Surgery, Wills Eye Hospital, Philadelphia, PA, USA

S. Grob, C. Kloek (eds.), *Management of Open Globe Injuries*,
https://doi.org/10.1007/978-3-319-72410-2_34

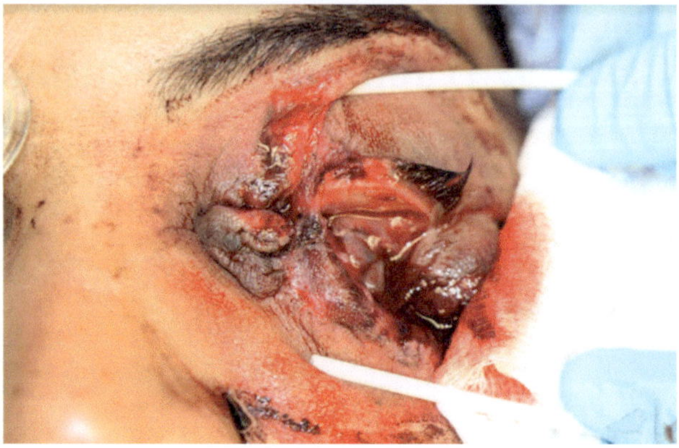

Fig. 34.1 Pre-operative photo displaying the numerous left periorbital and eyelid lacerations and grossly deformed and disorganized left globe

34.2.2 Pupils

OD: 2 mm → 1 mm, round and reactive
OS: Unable visualize, afferent pupillary defect by reverse

34.2.3 External Examination

Multiple periocular lacerations including a large inferior eyelid laceration involving the lower eyelid margin extending onto the cheek and a large superior eyelid laceration involving the upper eyelid margin (Fig. 34.1).

34.2.4 Slit Lamp Examination

	OD	OS
Lids and lashes	Normal	As above
Sclera and conjunctiva	Normal	Deformed, disorganized, with some scleral tissue seen
Cornea	Normal	Deformed, disorganized, with some corneal tissue seen
Anterior chamber	Normal	No anterior chamber visible
Iris	Normal	No iris tissue visible
Lens	Normal	No lens material visible
Vitreous	Normal	No view

34.2.5 Dilated Examination

Macula/Nerve OD: Macula flat. Disc with cup to disc ratio of 0.3, pink, and sharp margins
Periphery OD: Normal, no heme/tears/retinal detachment/commotio retinae
Macula/Nerve: OS: No view
Periphery OS: No view

34.2.6 Radiographic Imaging

Computed tomography (CT) of the orbits showed extensive left sided facial fractures involving the medial, superior and inferior walls of the orbit, all walls of the left maxillary sinus, the zyogmatic bone/inferior orbital rim, fracture through the left frontal sinus in association with the orbital roof fracture including fracture through the posterior sinus table into the intracranial space with associated pneumocephalus. The left globe appeared grossly deformed with no detectable intraocular structures (Figs. 34.2, 34.3 and 34.4).

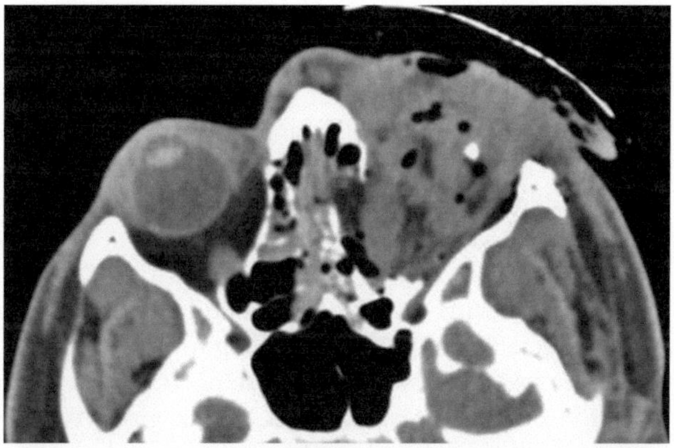

Fig. 34.2 Pre-operative axial CT scan with soft tissue image showing the extensive disorganization of the left globe anatomy, as well as left medial orbital wall disruption and left periorbital edema

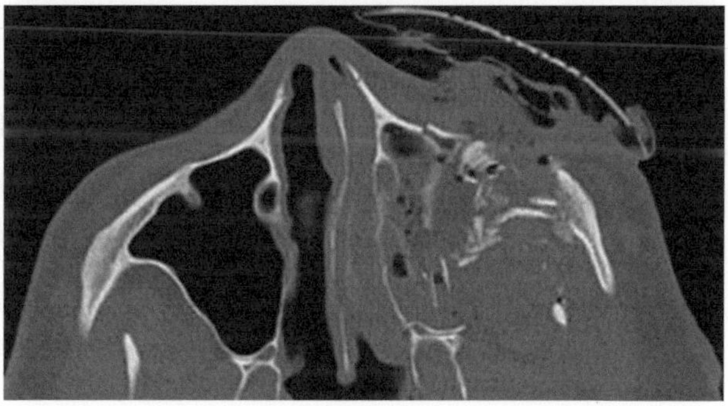

Fig. 34.3 Pre-operative CT scan, bone window, showing fractures of the walls of the left maxillary sinus, as well as disruption of the left zygomatic arch

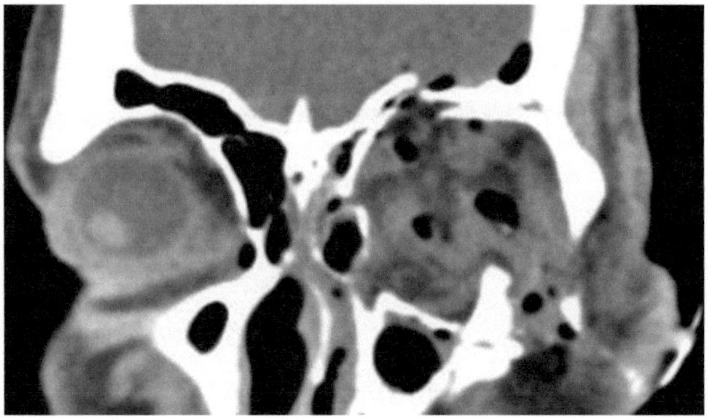

Fig. 34.4 Pre-operative CT scan, coronal view, soft tissue window showing a fracture of the left orbital roof with pneumocephalus, and fractures of the lateral wall, medial wall and orbital floor with comminuted fracture fragments extending from the inferior orbital rim into orbital soft tissues. Identifiable globe structure is not visualized

34.3 Surgeon's Initial Assessment and Pre-Operative Plan

The patient was started on pre-operative intravenous vancomycin and ceftazidime for open globe infection prophylaxis as per protocol. The patient was counseled regarding poor visual potential given the extent of the injury, complete deformity and disorganization of the globe, and pre-operative vision of no light perception, with the primary goal of surgery to close the eye and reduce the risk of infection. However, due to the extent of the injury, the patient was further counseled regarding the significant possibility of encountering an unsalvageable globe that would be best treated by primary evisceration or enucleation surgery with placement of an implant. The patient agreed to this plan and a consent for primary globe repair, with possible primary evisceration or enucleation with implant placement was reviewed and signed. Additionally, given that the facial fractures were open, consent was obtained for repair of facial fractures concurrently with repair of the periorbital soft-tissue lacerations.

In patients with severe open globe injuries, it is important to set expectations early, especially the poor visual prognosis. The globe should always be explored intraoperatively prior to any fracture or laceration repair to avoid manipulation and extrusion of intraocular contents. If the globe can be repaired, then ideally the fracture repair is delayed until visual potential can be evaluated and the globe has healed from the injury. If the globe cannot be primarily repaired or traumatic evisceration of the intraocular contents is identified, then orbital reconstruction and placement of an implant can occur during the first surgery or on follow up. Ideally this can be addressed all during one surgical intervention to decrease the patient's exposure to anesthesia.

The Oculoplastics team was contacted to aid in the repair of the complex eyelid lacerations, and the likely orbital reconstruction with placement of an orbital implant.

The remaining orbital roof fracture with pneumocephalus was evaluated by the Massachusetts General Hospital Neurosurgery Service, who recommended no acute neurosurgical intervention. It is important for patients with orbital roof fractures or other intracranial findings to be evaluated by the neurosurgery service prior to open globe repair as there may be more life-threatening issues that need to be addressed prior to globe repair. In some severe cases, an open globe repair may need to follow a neurosurgical intervention in the operating room as a combined case. Other times, no neurosurgical intervention is necessary, but recommendations may include starting Levetiracetam (Keppra) for seizure prophylaxis and/or taking care not to place any upward pressure on the orbital roof during globe repair.

34.4 Surgical Exploration and Repair: Operative Note

Informed consent was obtained and the operative eye was verified and marked. The uninjured right eye was taped and shielded for protection. The left eye was then prepped and draped in the usual sterile ophthalmic fashion. Given the significant lid lacerations, 4-0 silk sutures were used to retract the lids and explore the orbit. Further exploration of the injury under the microscope revealed extensive damage to the eye with multiple large lacerations involving the cornea and sclera, with partial shredding of the sclera, tracking back to the optic nerve. No intraocular or uveal contents were seen within or attached to the remaining sclera (Fig. 34.5). Given extrusion of all intraocular contents and extensive globe lacerations, attempts to surgically repair the globe were felt to be futile, and the decision was made to proceed with a modified primary evisceration in which the scleral remnants were sewn over a silicone sphere, attempting to preserve extraocular muscle attachments and position (Fig. 34.6a, b).

Further orbit exploration revealed significant bony abnormalities, including absent inferior orbital rim and orbital floor, entirely comminuted and shattered posterolateral maxillary wall and a skeletonized infraorbital neurovascular bundle. The inferior orbital rim was reconstructed with a Synthes single channel curved orbital rim titanium plate (Johnson & Johnson, New Brunswick, NJ) fixed with micro screws. The anterior maxillary fracture was repaired using a Synthes titanium

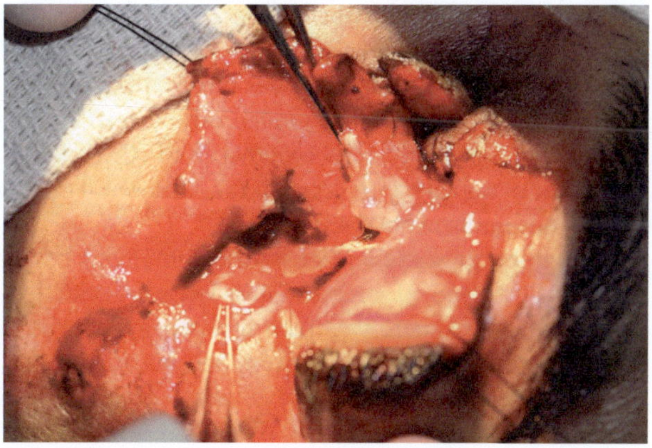

Fig. 34.5 Intraoperative photograph showing the scleral shell remnant being retracted using 0.2 mm forceps—uveal tissue is not visualized. Silk retraction sutures through the upper and lower eyelid margins are being used to retract the lacerated eyelid tissues for exposure of the globe without pressure on the globe

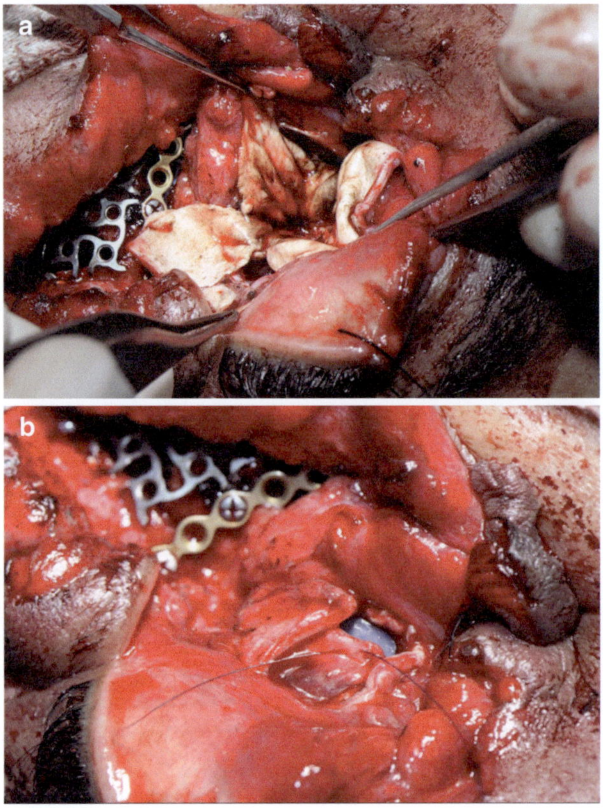

Fig. 34.6 Intraoperative photograph showing: (**a**) clean scleral shell prior to implant placement; (**b**) the silicone spherical implant within the scleral shell. Also can be seen is the reconstruction of the orbital floor with titanium mesh and the curved inferior orbital rim plate secured with micro screws

mesh fashioned into a "guitar pick"-shape to mimic the anatomical triangular configuration of the anterior maxilla, and secured into place with self-drilling micro screws—this was placed to provide a scaffold around which the severely comminuted bone fragments would consolidate. Finally, the orbital soft tissue contents were elevated out of the maxillary sinus and held within the orbital confines using a Stryker Medpor 3D preformed Titan Orbital Floor and Wall implant (Stryker, Billerica, MA). Care was taken in the placement of this implant to not be aggressive in addressing the medial orbital wall fracture superiorly out of concern for creating a possible cerebrospinal fluid (CSF) leak. The orbital roof was left to heal non-operatively with the plan for a future CT scan to ensure no development of latent sinus outflow obstruction.

The globe evisceration was then completed by carefully cleaning the inside surface of the residual scleral coat and treating with dehydrated ethanol solution. An 18 mm silicone sphere was then inserted into the scleral coat and secured with a combination of horizontal mattress and interrupted 6-0 Vicryl sutures. A posterior scleral release was performed to allow adequate laxity for full anterior scleral coverage of the sphere implant. Conjunctiva and Tenon's layers were subsequently

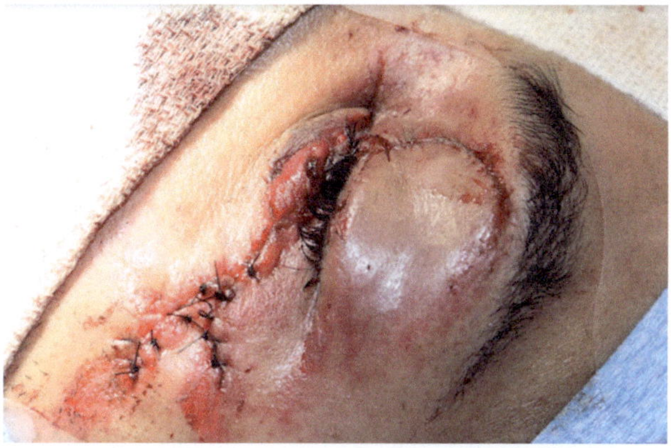

Fig. 34.7 Intraoperative photograph taken upon completion of repair of left periocular soft tissue lacerations with nonabsorbable sutures on the mid-face and absorbable sutures on the eyelid and eyelid margins

closed over the scleral coat using interrupted 6-0 Vicryl sutures. A medium rigid conformer was placed.

Finally, the complex eyelid and facial lacerations were explored and repaired in a layered fashion (Fig. 34.7). Upon completion of the case, the conjunctival surface and skin lacerations were covered in dexamethasone-neomycin-polymixin b (Maxitrol) ophthalmic ointment and dressed in sterile non-adherent pads, followed by eye pads.

34.4.1 Surgical Exploration and Repair: Pearls

- If facial and eyelid soft tissue lacerations are present, 4-0 silk traction sutures can be placed through the lid margin and retracted with a mosquito locking forceps to allow for adequate globe exposure.
- In cases with severely deformed globes where primary globe closure may not be possible, pre-operative discussions of possible need for primary evisceration or enucleation with implant placement should be undertaken with the patient.
- In the operating room, globe exploration should be completed first to determine if the globe can be repaired. If the globe can be repaired, then this would be our first option if the patient wishes.
- If the globe cannot be salvaged, then exploration will reveal the remaining ocular tissue. If the patient is found to have a traumatic evisceration, as in the present patient, the remaining scleral shell can be utilized for primary evisceration-type repair. If any small uveal contents remain, they should be removed and the shell cleaned. A spherical implant can then be placed in the shell and the shell closed with horizontal mattress Vicryl sutures.
- It is essential to restore orbital bony anatomy to allow for optimal globe or prosthetic globe support, as well as for facial function and cosmesis. If the globe is repaired primarily, then ideally fracture repair should be delayed until the globe has healed if there is potential for good vision. This does create a dilemma as

secondary (delayed) repair of facial fractures is more difficult and can often be associated with suboptimal outcomes. The timing of fracture repair in the setting of a repairable open globe thus needs to be discussed between the surgical services to arrive at a time-frame that maximizes the chance of good visual recovery and good facial skeleton reconstruction. If there is no hope for return of useful vision or if the globe is not salvageable, then fracture reconstruction should not be delayed.

34.5 Post-Operative Course

The patient recovered well from the surgery and was fitted 2 months post-operatively for a left ocular prosthesis. He was counseled on protection of his right eye, including daily use of polycarbonate eyeglasses and the need for a protective face shield and/or eye goggles while at work.

Several months after initial prosthetic fitting, the patient developed gradual left upper eyelid ptosis with medial eyelid peaking, as well as left lower eyelid retraction with forniceal shortening from cicatricial changes, causing problems with ocular prosthesis fit (Fig. 34.8).

Nine months following the patient's primary surgical repair, he underwent external levator repair of the left upper eyelid and an endoscopically-harvested nasal mucosal spacer graft of the left lower eyelid, as well as a left cheek scar revision, yielding an excellent cosmetic result (Fig. 34.9a, b).

The patient did experience significant chronic headaches following trauma, and these were not adequately alleviated by medical therapy. It was thought the headache pain could possibly be related to dura trapped within the left orbital roof fracture as there was no evidence of paranasal sinus obstruction on repeat imaging (Fig. 34.10). The patient subsequently underwent a frontal craniotomy for repair of the left orbital roof with release of entrapped dura and contouring of the orbital roof, performed 18 months following injury. Post-operatively there has been a good improvement of headaches.

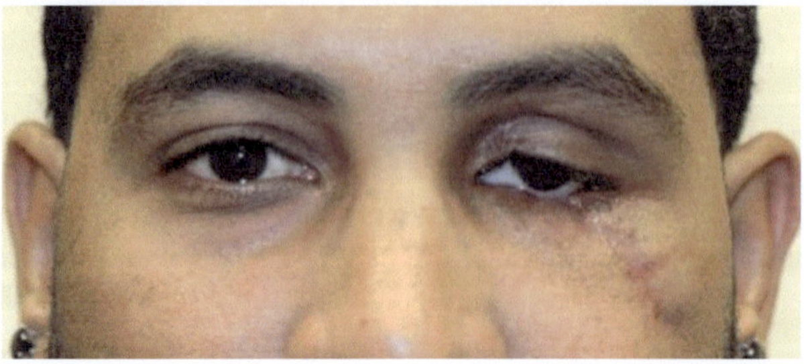

Fig. 34.8 Photograph of the patient 6 months after initial repair with left ocular prosthesis in place, showing left lateral upper eyelid ptosis with medial peak, and left lower eyelid retraction

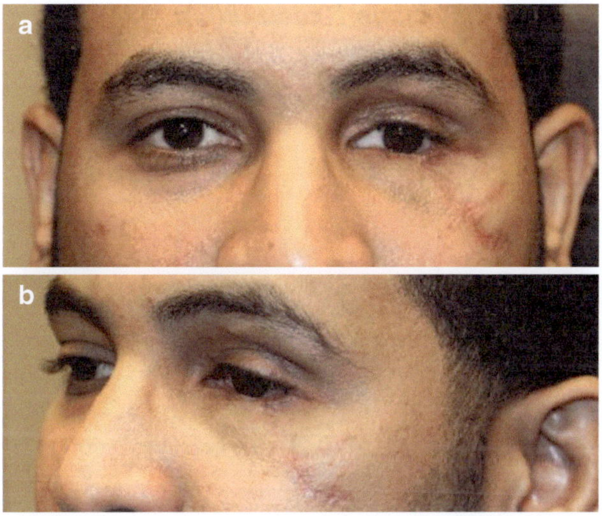

Fig. 34.9 (**a**, **b**) Patient photograph 10 months after primary injury and 4 months after subsequent oculoplastic external levator repair of left upper eyelid and nasal mucosal spacer graft to the left lower eyelid, as well as left cheek scar revision, with excellent cosmetic outcome achieved

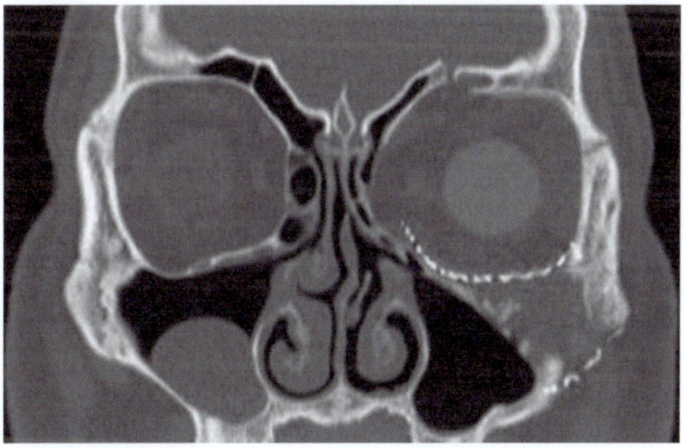

Fig. 34.10 Post-operative CT scan 10 months after the initial injury showing left inferior orbital rim and maxillary floor fracture repairs, with good orbital implant positioning. Left orbital roof non-union is seen with some bony projection towards subfrontal region

34.6 Final Trauma Evaluation

34.6.1 Final Visual Acuity

OD: 20/25
OS: Ocular prosthesis

34.6.2 Pupils

OD: Reactive
OS: Ocular prosthesis

34.6.3 Slit Lamp Examination

Hypesthesia over left cheek status post scar revision, with excellent cheek shape, contour and symmetry

	OD	OS
Lids and lashes	Normal	Good position and contour of left upper eyelid. Good position of left lower eyelid status post nasal mucosal posterior graft, holding prosthesis well
Sclera and conjunctiva	Normal	Inferior nasal graft in good position, slightly ectropic, prosthesis
Cornea	Normal	Prosthesis
Anterior chamber	Normal	Prosthesis
Iris	Normal	Prosthesis
Lens	Normal	Prosthesis
Vitreous	Normal	Prosthesis

34.6.4 Dilated Examination

Macula/Nerve OD: Normal
Periphery OD: Normal
Macula/Nerve: OS: Prosthesis
Periphery OS: Prosthesis

34.7 Review and Lessons Learned

In cases of extensive traumatic globe injury with severe globe deformity and/or absence of ocular tissue, primary globe closure for vision restoration may not be possible. Fortunately these cases are rare, with a recent retrospective study of 660 patients with open globe injuries finding that only 11 (1.7.%) required primary enucleation or evisceration [1]. However, a study of 99 open globe injuries with coexisting facial fractures reported a higher percentage at 19.6% of primary enucleation or evisceration for unsalvageable globes [2]. When such cases are encountered, it is essential to initiate pre-operative discussions with the patient regarding the possible need for primary enucleation or evisceration surgery with placement of an orbital implant to allow for optimal functional prosthesis potential and cosmesis, and to avoid complications of additional delayed surgery. These considerations should be discussed at length with the patient and family and documented in the procedure consent.

In the operating room, extensive exploration should be primarily undertaken to determine the extent of globe injury, which will determine whether primary globe closure should be attempted versus primary evisceration/enucleation. If extensive loss of ocular contents is noted and globe repair is not possible, evisceration or enucleation should be considered. If enough scleral tissue is present, as in this case, the remaining scleral shell tissue should be preserved and cleaned of any residual uveal tissue and utilized for support of the orbital implant.

Concomitant facial and orbital fractures are not uncommonly seen in patients presenting with open globe injuries. A single-center chart review of 300 consecutive patients presenting with open globe injuries found that 25.7% had coexisting orbital and/or adnexal injuries, 15.6% with orbital fractures specifically, most commonly following blunt injury. Those patients with concurrent orbital or adnexal injuries had worse vision outcomes, attributed to high incidence of posterior globe injuries in these patients [3, 4]. Zygomaticomaxillary complex fractures specifically have been found to be most frequently associated with blindness [2].

In cases in which significant orbital and facial bony anatomy is compromised, it is essential to restore the bony buttresses of the facial skeleton, for both general facial cosmesis and for globe or prosthetic support. This repair should be undertaken by a surgeon with proficient knowledge of normal facial and orbital bony anatomy and experience in use of orbital implants to perform the necessary reconstruction. In cases in which primary globe repair is undertaken, fracture repair should ideally be delayed until the globe has healed for a week or two if there is a chance for functional visual recovery, and care should be taken to minimize pressure to the globe during fracture repair surgery. Alternatively, in cases of an unsalvageable globe, fracture repair can be undertaken during the primary trauma surgery. Many cases such as this one present as open fractures which should be repaired expediently, again taking care to avoid any additional trauma or injury to a salvageable globe.

34.8 Key Learning Points

- In cases with extensive traumatic globe injury resulting in severe globe deformity and tissue loss, pre-operative consideration of primary enucleation or evisceration with implant placement should be considered and discussed with the patient and included in the surgical consent.
- A globe should be explored and repaired if possible, but if it is deemed unsalvageable after exploration, then primary enucleation or evisceration can be considered.
- Restoration of mid-face and orbital bony structure is essential to enable proper globe or prosthetic globe support and to maximize facial function and cosmesis. Reconstruction can be done primarily (or shortly after) if the globe is not salvageable; in cases of globe repair and expectation of return of useful vision,

timing of facial fracture repair needs to be such that the globe is not disrupted during the fracture repair, yet the facial skeleton is able to be fully reconstructed. This decision is made on an individual basis in a multidisciplinary fashion.
- Periorbital soft tissue injuries should be addressed after globe exploration and repair to avoid manipulation of an open globe.

References

1. Savar A, Andreoli MT, Kloek CE, Andreoli CM. Enucleation for open globe injury. Am J Ophthalmol. 2009;147(4):595–600.e1.
2. Vaca EE, Mundinger GS, Kelamis JA, Dorafshar AH, Christy MR, Manson PN, Rodriguez ED. Facial fractures with concomitant open globe injury. Plast Reconstr Surg. 2013;131(6):1317–28.
3. Rahman I, Maino A, Devadason D, Leatherbarrow B. Open globe injuries: factors predictive of poor outcome. Eye (Lond). 2006;20:1336–41.
4. Hatton MP, Thakker MM, Ray S. Orbital and adnexal trauma associated with open-globe injuries. Ophthal Plast Reconstr Surg. 2002;18:458–61.

Chapter 35
Case 30: Traumatic Enucleation

Liza M. Cohen, Alice C. Lorch, and Michael K. Yoon

35.1 History of Present Illness

A 24-week pregnant 41-year-old woman with a history of hypertension, anemia, varicose veins, scoliosis, substance abuse, anxiety, and depression presented with concern for severe open globe injuries of both eyes.

- The patient was a victim of physical domestic abuse, when she was attacked by her partner and strangled with loss of consciousness. She was unable to remember what happened to her eyes.
- She was seen at a local hospital and transferred to Massachusetts General Hospital for evaluation of her injuries. There were no injuries other than her ophthalmic issues. She was subsequently admitted to the Intensive Care Unit for close monitoring by the Obstetrics and Gynecology Service.
- She reported not being able to see any light in either eye.

35.2 Initial Trauma Evaluation

35.2.1 Visual Acuity (Without Correction)

OD: No light perception
OS: No light perception

L. M. Cohen, M.D. (✉) • A. C. Lorch, M.D., M.P.H.
Department of Ophthalmology, Harvard Medical School, Massachusetts Eye and Ear, Boston, MA, USA
e-mail: liza_cohen@meei.harvard.edu

M. K. Yoon, M.D.
Ophthalmic Plastic Surgery, Department of Ophthalmology, Massachusetts Eye and Ear Infirmary, Harvard Medical School, Boston, MA, USA

S. Grob, C. Kloek (eds.), *Management of Open Globe Injuries*,
https://doi.org/10.1007/978-3-319-72410-2_35

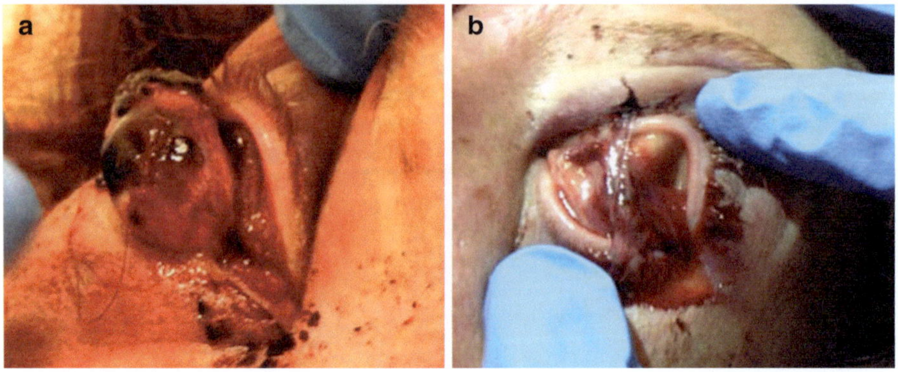

Fig. 35.1 (**a**) Clinical image of the patient's right eye on presentation showing a prolapsed, irregular globe. (**b**) The left eye had been traumatically enucleated without evidence of a globe with eyelid retraction

35.2.2 Pupils

OD: No view
OS: Not present

35.2.3 External Examination

The right globe was prolapsed outside of the right upper and lower eyelids and was irregular in shape and contour (Fig. 35.1a). The left eye had been traumatically enucleated, and there was no evidence of a globe (Fig. 35.1b). There was periorbital edema and ecchymosis bilaterally.

35.2.4 Slit Lamp Examination

	OD	OS
Lids and lashes	Globe grossly displaced anterior to the eyelid margins, eyelid edema and ecchymosis	Eyelid edema and ecchymosis
Sclera and conjunctiva	Globe grossly deformed with deflated appearance, 360 flat subconjunctival hemorrhage	Remnants of conjunctiva seen, no sclera noted
Cornea	Irregular, edematous, hazy	Not present
Anterior chamber	Shallow, layered hyphema several millimeters in height	Not present
Iris	Possible uveal tissue adjacent to globe	Not present
Lens	No view	Not present
Vitreous	No view	Not present

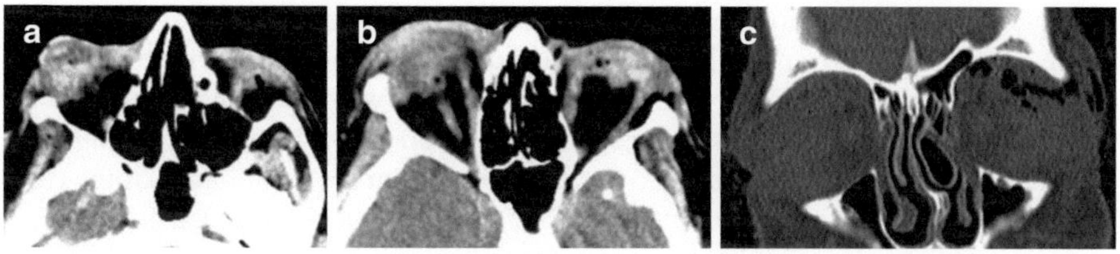

Fig. 35.2 Axial soft tissue window (**a**, **b**) and coronal bone window (**c**) CT images showing a proptotic, markedly deformed globe on the right and absence of a globe on the left

35.2.5 Dilated Examination

Macula/Nerve OD: No view
Periphery OD: No view
Macula/Nerve OS: Not present
Periphery OS: Not present

35.2.6 Radiographic Imaging

Computed tomography (CT) of the orbits showed a proptotic ruptured globe of the right eye (Fig. 35.2), with a 6.6 × 7.9 mm hyphema along the anterior inferior aspect directly adjacent to the lens, without evidence of an intraocular foreign body. There was no evidence of the left globe (Fig. 35.2). The optic nerve was not visualized on the left. There was a small hyperdensity along the lateral aspect of the left orbit, possibly representing an orbital hemorrhage. There was no intracranial injury.

35.3 Surgeon's Initial Assessment and Pre-Operative Plan

The patient had a proptotic, severely disfigured ruptured globe with hyphema in the right eye and a traumatic enucleation of the left eye due to assault.

This case illustrates several important areas of discussion beyond the standard repair of open globe injuries. These are the medical/surgical management of traumatic enucleation, management of bilateral severe open globe injuries, social aspects of assault, and psychological considerations in enucleating an eye.

Most cases of traumatic enucleation are caused by manual gouging injuries, either intentionally during an assault or self-induced. Some patients present with a proptotic globe from an assault or even a sports game where a teammate accidently sticks their finger into the orbit prolapsing the globe, but the globe and optic nerve are intact. In these cases, the eye can be gently placed back into the orbit. However, if there is concern for an open globe or the optic nerve is severed or severely damaged, it may be best to explore the globe and orbit in the operating room emergently prior to manipulating the globe. This patient had a traumatized prolapsed globe on the right and a complete traumatic enucleation on the left with bilateral no light perception vision. The extremely poor prognosis was discussed at length with the patient. Every attempt was going to be made to preserve the one remaining right eye. The decision was made to go to the operating room for exploration of the right globe with repair and repositioning. Since the left eye was not found, a globe repair was not possible, so orbital reconstruction with an orbital implant was discussed with the patient in detail.

Considerable force is required for removal of the globe from the orbit. Tension against the optic nerve can lead to tearing of the nerve at or near the chiasm, which can result in contralateral visual field defects and even hypothalamic dysfunction [1]. In this patient's case, it was not necessary to assess for contralateral visual field deficits given her complete loss of vision in the other eye as well. Tearing of the optic nerve can also lead to cerebrospinal fluid (CSF) leak, which carries a risk of developing meningitis [1–3]. Injury to the posterior ophthalmic artery can occur, which may result in subarachnoid hemorrhage [1–3]. Both of these potentially devastating complications necessitate a thorough neurological evaluation prior to surgical intervention. In this case, the patient was admitted to the Intensive Care Unit, where she underwent neurological examination that did not reveal evidence of injury.

Given the severity of injury in this patient's case with an open right globe with no light perception vision and traumatic enucleation of her left globe, the decision was made to pursue exploration in the operating room.

35.4 Surgical Exploration and Repair: Operative Note

Informed consent was obtained for bilateral exploration. General anesthesia was induced by a practitioner with experience in prenatal anesthesia. Both eyes were prepped and draped in the usual sterile manner for periocular and intraocular surgery.

Attention was first paid to the right globe, which was explored. It was found to have a formed anterior chamber with hyphema. However, the body of the globe appeared to be severely deflated. Upon further examination including a 360° peritomy, it was noted that only the inferior and lateral rectus muscle were intact. The likely bodies of the superior rectus and perhaps medial rectus muscles were also identified. A small laceration was discovered in the sclera under the lateral rectus muscle, and two interrupted 8-0 nylon sutures were used to close the rupture. The globe remained severely deflated, and sterile balanced salt solution was injected 4 mm from the limbus to re-inflate the globe. There were no other posterior lacerations identified and the globe remained formed. The conjunctiva was sutured to the limbus to maximize coverage of the globe. This was performed using 7-0 Vicryl (polyglactin) sutures. Two temporary tarsorrhaphies were placed to prevent globe proptosis and to protect the cornea. One was placed more laterally and the other more centrally, both using 4-0 Prolene (polypropylene) sutures.

For the left eye, exploration confirmed the absence of the globe. None of the extraocular muscles could be identified. A 20 mm silicone spherical implant was placed into the orbit. Tenon's capsule was closed over this to allow for watertight closure using 5-0 Vicryl (polyglactin) sutures in a buried, interrupted fashion in two layers. A 6-0 plain gut running suture was used to close the conjunctiva over the already closed Tenon's capsule. A conformer was placed in the socket, and a single 4-0 Prolene (polypropylene) suture was used for a temporary tarsorrhaphy.

35.4.1 Surgical Exploration and Repair: Pearls

- Temporary tarsorrhaphies can be used to mitigate corneal exposure in cases of traumatic proptosis.
- In cases of traumatic enucleation, careful orbital exploration should be carried out to evaluate for orbital foreign bodies and evidence of ocular structures. Any exposed extraocular uveal tissue should be removed.
- Even without identification of the extraocular muscles, an orbital implant can be placed to fill the volume of the orbit and allow for placement of a prosthesis in the future.

35.5 Post-Operative Course

Despite the patient's no light perception vision with poor potential for visual recovery in the right eye, the decision was made to avoid enucleation in an attempt to reduce psychological distress for the patient.

The patient returned to the floor, where she was admitted to the antepartum service. She continued to receive 48 hours of intravenous vancomycin and ceftazidime as per protocol for open globe injuries. On post-operative day 2, the more medial suture tarrsorhaphy was removed from the right eye, allowing limited view of the globe. On post-operative day 4, still with no light perception vision, the right eye became painful to touch, and the patient developed eyelid edema, conjunctival injection, diffuse corneal edema, and white haze in the anterior chamber, concerning for hypopyon. There was still no view to the fundus. B-scan ultrasound showed a disorganized globe with no optic nerve visualized. This presentation was concerning for endophthalmitis, so a retina specialist was consulted, and the patient was started on oral moxifloxacin in addition to continuing topical antibiotic eye drops. On post-operative day 5, the patient reported progressive right eye pain. After extensive discussion, the recommendation was made to enucleate the right eye given it was a blind painful eye with active infection. With the assistance of a social worker, counseling of the patient occurred, and she consented to enucleation knowing that she would not regain vision in the eye.

35.6 Second Surgical Repair: Operative Note

After informed consent was obtained, general anesthesia was induced, and the eyes were prepped and draped in the usual sterile manner for periocular and intraocular surgery.

For the right eye, a 360° limbal peritomy was performed. Dissection was carried out in the subconjunctival and Tenon's space in all four quadrants using Steven tenotomy scissors. Scar tissue was noted from her previous traumatic open globe repair. Only the inferior and lateral rectus muscles were identified. These were secured on double-armed 5-0 Vicryl (polyglactin) sutures before being disinserted from the globe. The superior and medial rectus muscles were not identified. An Allis clamp was used to clamp the medial rectus stump in order to rotate the globe laterally and apply traction to the optic nerve. The optic nerve was visualized attached to the globe. A hemostat was used to clamp the nerve as posterior in the orbit as possible. Enucleation scissors were then used to strum the nerve and cut it as posteriorly as possible. There was minimal bleeding. The globe was removed and any additional soft tissue attached to the globe was cut with scissors. A 20-mm silicone sphere was then inserted into the posterior orbit. Given that only the inferior and lateral rectus muscles were available, the sutures were cut, and these muscles were allowed to retract into the orbit. Tenon's capsule was then closed in two layers with interrupted 5-0 Vicryl (polyglactin) sutures in a buried, interrupted fashion. The conjunctiva was closed over Tenon's fascia using running 6-0 fast-absorbing plain gut suture. A conformer was placed, and a single temporary tarsorrhaphy was performed using 5-0 Prolene (polyprolylene).

The left suture tarsorrhaphy was released using scissors.

35.7 Post-Operative Course

The patient recovered well from surgery. On post-operative day 11 from enucleation of the left eye and post-operative day 4 from enucleation of the right eye, she was discharged to rehab with social services support and outpatient oculoplastics follow-up closer to home (out-of-state).

35.8 Final Trauma Evaluation

35.8.1 Final Visual Acuity

OD: No light perception
OS: No light perception

35.8.2 Pupils

OD: Anophthalmic
OS: Anophthalmic

35.8.3 Slit Lamp Examination

	OD	OS
Lids and lashes	Anophthalmic, conformer in place	Anophthalmic, conformer in place
Sclera and conjunctiva	Conjunctiva well-apposed over orbital implant without exposure	Conjunctiva well-apposed over orbital implant without exposure

35.8.4 Dilated Examination

Macula/Nerve OD: Anophthalmic
Periphery OD: Anophthalmic
Macula/Nerve OS: Anophthalmic
Periphery OS: Anophthalmic

35.9 Review and Lessons Learned

In cases of traumatic enucleation, there are important issues to consider beyond those required in managing a standard open globe.

The first is the risk for concurrent neurological injury, such as CSF leak due to tearing of the posterior optic nerve and subarachnoid hemorrhage due to injury to the posterior ophthalmic artery [1–3]. These potential complications necessitate neurologic consultation with a thorough neurologic examination on presentation and in the days following, as well as proper neuroimaging, in order to ensure that neurological disability does not occur.

Another important consideration is the risk of infection. Given that traumatic enucleations typically occur as a result of manual gouging injuries, the risk of infection from a dirty wound is high. It is therefore important to initiate treatment with broad-spectrum intravenous antibiotics and have a low threshold for suspecting infection. In our patient's case, the development of worsening pain, eyelid edema, conjunctival injection, corneal edema, and white haze in the anterior chamber was concerning for endophthalmitis, so a retina specialist was appropriately consulted, and treatment was augmented with oral moxifloxacin, which has been shown to have good vitreous penetration with a broad spectrum of coverage [4].

In surgical repair of traumatic enucleations, the choice of implant is a factor to consider. Due to the relative rarity of this scenario, there is currently no good evidence to suggest superiority of one type of implant over another in traumatic situations [5]. In routine enucleations, porous implants (e.g. hydroxyapatite, porous polyethylene) may be preferred to non-porous implants (e.g. silicone, acrylic, polymethylmethacrylate) due to fibrovascular ingrowth, which may reduce infection risk and improve extraocular motility [5]. However, in traumatic cases where the extraocular muscles cannot be identified and sutured to the implant, this potential benefit does not apply; therefore, either type of implant may be used. With the risk of ocular or orbital infection as in this case, a non-porous material is less likely to develop a deep-seated nosocomial infection. Finally, in situations with severe orbital inflammation or infection, the surgeon may elect not to place an implant at the time of enucleation and do so in a second operation.

In addition to the medical and surgical management of traumatic enucleations, the social and psychological aspects of these cases are just as important. Since cases of traumatic enucleation are most commonly a result of assault, it is important to screen for domestic violence and make sure the patient is safe at home. Social work should be involved early in the patient's care if deemed appropriate, as was done for our patient. Another common cause of traumatic enucleation is psychogenic auto-enucleation. With schizophrenia as the most common psychiatric condition associated with this form of self-mutilation, [6] psychiatric consultation should be acquired immediately in these cases. It is also important to consider the psychological distress of losing an eye, especially in a traumatic setting [3]. Patients should be counseled appropriately, and every effort should be made to save the eye, as long as it is deemed medically safe. This may provide the patient with hope and confidence that the surgeon has done all they can to save the eye. Psychiatry can assist in working with the patient to reduce psychological distress and provide treatment if necessary.

35.10 Key Learning Points

- Traumatic enucleation is most commonly due to manual gouging injury.
- In cases of traumatic enucleation, it is vital to do a thorough neurologic examination and obtain imaging to rule out life-threatening neurologic sequelae such as subarachnoid hemorrhage and CSF leak. One should also have a low threshold for suspecting and treating infections.
- There is no good evidence to support using one type of orbital implant over another; thus, this decision should depend on surgeon preference. If there is severe inflammation or infection, consider deferring placement of an implant until a later surgery.
- Cases of traumatic enucleation are usually due to assault; therefore, it is important to ask about domestic violence and obtain a social work consult to ensure the patient's safety.
- Enucleation, especially in a traumatic setting, can have potentially devastating psychologic consequences for the patient. It is important to counsel patients

appropriately and make sure they understand that every effort was made to save the eye. Even if the potential for recovering vision is poor bilaterally, if one eye can be safely left in place, consider deferring primary enucleation of both eyes at the same time due to the potential for psychological distress.

References

1. Shneck M, Oshry T, Marcus M, Lifshitz T. Attempted bilateral manual enucleation (gouging) during a physical assault. Ophthalmology. 2003;110:575–7.
2. Aboud ND, Shah P, Sullivan F. Assessment and management of manual traumatic enucleation. Aust N Z J Ophthalmol. 1995;23:55–7.
3. Tai AX, Mattern RM, Schaefer DP, Borke JA. Traumatic manual enucleation (gouging) from assault. Clin Exp Ophthalmol. 2016;44(7):628–30.
4. Hariprasad SM, Shah GK, Mieler WF, et al. Vitreous and aqueous penetration of orally administered moxifloxacin in humans. Arch Ophthalmol. 2006;124:178–82.
5. Schellini S, El Dib R, Silva LR, et al. Integrated versus non-integrated orbital implants for treating anophthalmic sockets. Cochrane Database Syst Rev. 2016;11:CD010293.
6. Large MM, Nielssen OB. Self-enucleation: forget Freud and Oedipus, it's all about untreated psychosis. Br J Ophthalmol. 2012;96(8):1056–7.

Chapter 36
Case 31: Delayed Presentation Zone I/II Open Globe Injury

J. Daniel Diaz, James A. Stefater, and Seanna Grob

36.1 History of Present Illness

A 28-year-old man with no prior ocular history presents with a potential open globe injury to the left eye.

- Patient reports that he was at work wearing safety glasses when he turned on a fan and felt something hit his left eye.
- He reports pain and blurred vision of the left eye.
- He initially presented to an outside urgent care center where he was diagnosed with a corneal abrasion.
- He continued to have worsening blurry vision and was seen at an outside hospital emergency room. Ophthalmology was consulted and the patient was ultimately transferred to Massachusetts Eye and Ear (MEE) with a concern for an open globe injury in the setting of a peaked pupil.

36.2 Initial Trauma Evaluation

36.2.1 Visual Acuity (Without Correction)

OD: 20/40 pinhole 20/25
OS: 20/60 pinhole 20/40

J. Daniel Diaz, M.D. (✉) • J. A. Stefater, M.D., Ph.D. • S. Grob, M.D., M.A.S.
Department of Ophthalmology, Harvard Medical School, Massachusetts Eye and Ear, Boston, MA, USA
e-mail: jose_diaz@meei.harvard.edu

S. Grob, C. Kloek (eds.), *Management of Open Globe Injuries*,
https://doi.org/10.1007/978-3-319-72410-2_36

36.2.2 Pupils

OD: Round and reactive
OS: Peaked pupil, no afferent pupillary defect

36.2.3 External Examination

Normal

36.2.4 Slit Lamp Examination

	OD	OS
Lids and lashes	Normal	Mild edema of the left upper eyelid
Sclera and conjunctiva	Normal	Bullous subconjunctival hemorrhage superiorly, flat subconjunctival hemorrhage from 3 to 5 o'clock
Cornea	Normal	Small focal full-thickness laceration at limbus 10:30 o'clock with iris prolapse plugging the wound
Anterior chamber	Normal	Formed, 1–2+ cell
Iris	Normal	Peaked pupil towards 10:30 o'clock, no transillumination defects
Lens	Normal	Normal, no lens capsule violation
Vitreous	Normal	Normal

36.2.5 Dilated Examination

Macula/Nerve OD: Normal
Periphery OD: Normal
Macula/Nerve: OS: Normal
Periphery OS: Normal, no intraocular foreign body seen

36.2.6 Radiographic Imaging

Computed Tomography (CT) imaging of the orbits showed no obvious evidence of globe rupture. No intraocular foreign body was identified.

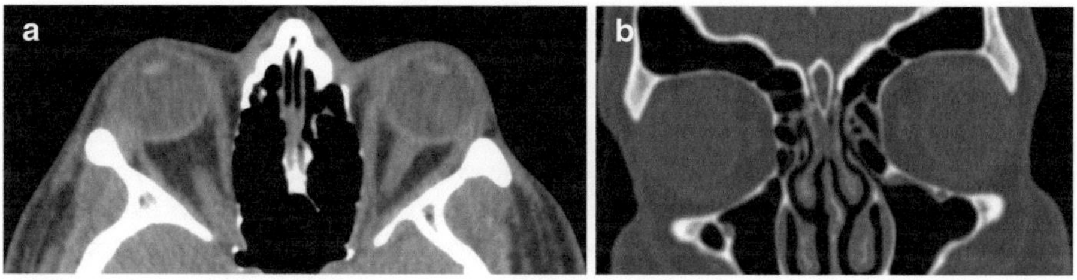

Fig. 36.1 Axial (**a**) and coronal (**b**) CT images showing normal and symmetric globe contours

36.3 Surgeon's Initial Assessment and Pre-Operative Plan

The patient appeared to have suffered a Zone I/II open globe injury of the left eye. Axial and coronal CT imaging showed no evidence of radio-opaque intraocular foreign bodies (IOFB) (Fig. 36.1a, b) Although no IOFBs were identified on CT imaging, it was important to keep in mind that nonmetallic foreign bodies may be missed, especially if small and not captured on thin CT cuts. Given the mechanism of injury in this patient with something flying out of a fan and hitting his eye, it was especially important to consider a foreign body.

The right eye appeared normal and the left eye had evidence of a full-thickness corneal laceration with uveal prolapse. The anterior chamber was formed and no violation of the lens capsule was evident. There was an adequate view of the posterior segment without evidence of vitreous hemorrhage or IOFBs.

The planned procedure entails a localized peritomy superiorly in the location of the laceration with careful blunt dissection in order to ensure no further ocular trauma was sustained. This is followed by gentle repositioning of iris tissue and subsequent suture repair of the corneal and scleral laceration.

In delayed presentation open globes, it is important to consider the possibility of infection either at the location of the laceration (e.g. corneal infiltrate) or endophthalmitis. Even if the wounds are not infected as in this case, corneal tissue around a laceration may be significantly edematous and friable depending on how delayed the patient presented.

36.4 Surgical Exploration and Repair: Operative Note

The patient was brought to the operating room where the anesthesia team proceeded with general anesthesia. A careful time-out was observed and the correct patient and eye were identified. The left eye was prepped and draped in the usual sterile ophthalmic fashion using a Jaffe speculum to provide adequate exposure. A temporal paracentesis was made with a supersharp blade. A 90° peritomy was initiated at 9 o'clock and extended to 12 o'clock with relaxing incisions at these clock hours.

Gentle exploration with blunt dissection using was performed with Westcott scissors to evaluate for posterior eye trauma.

The patient was found to have a 4 mm radial laceration at 11 o'clock extending 2 mm into the cornea and crossing the limbus and extending 2 mm posterior to the limbus with prolapse of iris through the wound. A cyclodialysis spatula was used to carefully remove the iris tissue from the wound and reposition into the eye. Filtered air was injected into the anterior chamber to maintain chamber depth. The limbus was then approximated with one 9-0 nylon suture. One additional 9-0 suture was placed adjacent to this to close the scleral portion of the laceration and then the corneal portion was approximated with one 10-0 nylon suture. A cyclodialysis spatula was used to sweep underneath the wound to ensure the iris was free from the wound. The suture knots were rotated. Fluorescein was used to check the integrity of the wound and it was found to be Seidel negative and the anterior chamber maintained good depth. A 10-0 nylon suture was also placed at the paracentesis site and was shown to be watertight.

The conjunctiva was then closed with multiple interrupted 8-0 Vicryl sutures. A subconjunctival steroid and antibiotic injection was performed inferiorly away from the laceration. The speculum was removed. The patient's drape was removed under the microscope. The patient tolerated the procedure well without any complications.

36.4.1 Surgical Exploration and Repair: Pearls

- Conjunctival peritomy and blunt dissection is crucial in ruling out evidence of posterior ocular trauma.
- A cyclodialysis spatula can be used to careful remove incarcerated iris tissue from wounds.
- Be aware of abnormal corneal tissue in delayed presentation cases. If the corneal tissue is friable, be sure to take longer suture passes to incorporate normal corneal tissue.

36.5 Post-Operative Course

The patient was admitted to complete a 48 hour course of intravenous antibiotics. On post-operative day one the patient had improved visual acuity to 20/40 with pinhole correction to 20/20. The patient was discharged uneventfully following his course of intravenous antibiotics. The patient was followed closely by the trauma service over the following weeks. At the 1 week follow-up the suture at the paracentesis wound was removed without complications. Six weeks after his injury, the one corneal suture was removed in the trauma clinic, per standard practice and the wound appeared well healed. The limbal and scleral suture were covered by conjunctiva and were not removed at this visit. The patient was very anxious during the suture removal and had to be carefully coached through the process. The limbal suture was removed 1 month later. The last remaining suture remained unexposed and covered by conjunctiva.

36.6 Final Trauma Evaluation

36.6.1 Final Visual Acuity (Without Correction)

OD: 20/40 pinhole 20/20
OS: 20/20-1

36.6.2 Pupils

OD: Round and reactive
OS: Round and reactive

36.6.3 Slit Lamp Examination

	OD	OS
Lids and lashes	Normal	Normal
Sclera and conjunctiva	Normal	1 nylon suture at 11 o'clock, covered by conjunctiva (Fig. 36.2)
Cornea	Normal	Seidel negative, mild endopigment
Anterior chamber	Normal	Formed, deep and quiet, slight iris elevation at 11 o'clock near wound site
Iris	Normal	Superonasal elevation
Lens	Normal	Pigment clumping on anterior lens capsule, no frank phacodonesis
Vitreous	Normal	Normal

36.6.4 Dilated Examination

Macula/Nerve OD: Normal
Periphery OD: Normal
Macula/Nerve: OS: Normal
Periphery OS: Normal

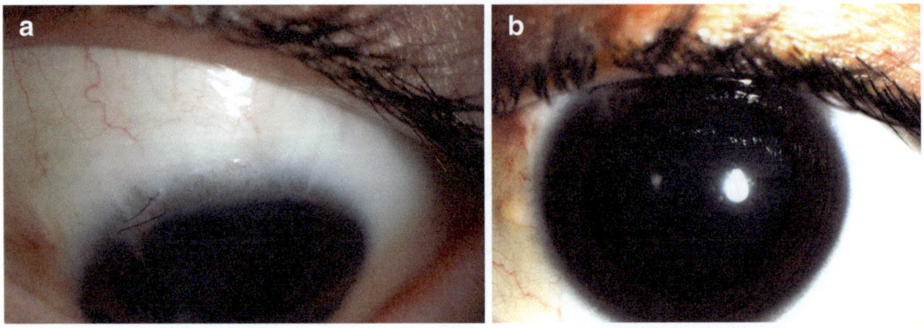

Fig. 36.2 (**a**) Anterior segment photograph showing a well-healed laceration prior to the removal of corneal sutures. (**b**) Anterior segment photograph showing a symmetrically round pupil

36.7 Review and Lessons Learned

This case highlights the importance of maintaining a high level of suspicion for an open globe injury in the setting of trauma. The pre-operative management of all open globe injuries includes collecting a detailed history. The history should emphasize several points, including: mechanism of injury, setting at which this injury occurred, date and time of injury, whether eye protection was used, when the patient last had something to eat or drink, allergies to medications, and whether any interventions were done since the injury. Delayed presentation of open globe injuries can occur for several reasons, and a detailed clinical history is crucial in identifying at risk patients. Patients sometimes do not experience debilitating pain or rapid changes in vision following trauma or open globe injuries. If the patient's history is suggestive of being in a high risk environment (i.e. using powered tools, projectile weapons, potential for high impact trauma, whether glasses are damaged, etc), physicians should be suspicious of a possible open globe injury [1–3].

After obtaining a detailed history, a complete external examination and ocular examination including visual acuity assessment, pupillary evaluation, slit lamp examination, and dilated fundus examination should be performed. Special care should be taken when attempting to obtain an intraocular pressure, as undue pressure on the globe may cause expulsion of ocular contents. If it is obvious an open globe injury has occurred, it is recommended to defer the measurement of intraocular pressure until the wound has been closed. Common clinical exam findings concerning for a ruptured globe include bullous subconjunctival hemorrhage, low intraocular pressure, shallow anterior chamber, and irregular pupillary contour (i.e. peaked). In cases where there may have been a full-thickness corneal laceration that is self-sealing, any of these clinical signs may be absent and an open globe injury may be missed.

In our case, the patient was initially seen at an outside urgent care center and misdiagnosed as a corneal abrasion. When he returned to a general emergency room, an ophthalmologist noticed the peaked pupil and immediately referred the patient to a tertiary care center. The iris plugging the corneal wound created a seal and limited the development of more significant and common ocular symptoms associated with open globe injuries. Careful evaluation of the pupil at his initial presentation would have prevented his delayed presentation.

Patients may present to a small local clinic for urgent evaluation after an eye trauma. Likely there are not slit lamps available for careful evaluation of the eye and ophthalmologists might not be on call at these centers. Usually fluorescein with a large blue light is used just with the naked eye to evaluate the cornea. A full-thickness corneal laceration and an abrasion will look the same with this mechanism. Therefore, as mentioned above, a detailed clinical history is key to determining high risk patients for full-thickness globe injuries. All patients with ocular trauma should be evaluated by an ophthalmologist to ensure more severe trauma is not missed [1, 2].

36.8 Key Learning Points

- A detailed clinical history is the first step in the pre-operative management of an open globe injury. Any ocular trauma associated with a projectile object raises concern for an open globe injury and potentially an intraocular foreign body as well.
- If a patient's clinical history is suggestive of a possible open globe injury, prompt assessment by an ophthalmologist is recommended.
- A peaked pupil is a concerning clinical finding for open globe injury.
- Careful external and slit lamp examination with attention to common clinical exam findings in patients with open globe injuries help prevent delayed presentations of open globe injuries.

References

1. Yeh S, Colyer MH, Weichel ED. Current trends in the management of intraocular foreign bodies. Curr Opin Ophthalmol. 2008;19(3):225–33. https://doi.org/10.1097/ICU.0b013e3282fa75f1.
2. Acuna OM, Yen KG. Outcome and prognosis of pediatric patients with delayed diagnosis of open-globe injuries. J Pediatr Ophthalmol Strabismus. 2009;46(4):202–9. https://doi.org/10.3928/01913913-20090706-04.
3. Cho W-K, Ko AC, Eatamadi H, et al. Orbital and orbitocranial trauma from pencil fragments: role of timely diagnosis and management. Am J Ophthalmol. 2017;180:46–54. https://doi.org/10.1016/j.ajo.2017.05.018.

Chapter 37
Case 32: Delayed-Presentation Zone I/II Open Globe Injury Requiring Corneal Glue

Seanna Grob, Shizuo Mukai, and Katherine E. Talcott

37.1 History of Present Illness

A 41-year-old man with a past medical history of bipolar disorder presents 5 days after hitting his right eye on the handle of a vacuum cleaner.

- The patient was bending over to pick something up off the floor and his right eye struck the handle of the vacuum cleaner.
- He noticed an immediate decrease in his vision with tearing, and pain.
- The patient was evaluated 5 days after the injury due to no improvement in vision and was transferred to Massachusetts Eye and Ear (MEE) from an outside hospital due to concern for an open globe injury.

37.2 Initial Trauma Evaluation

37.2.1 Visual Acuity (Without Correction)

OD: Count fingers at 3 feet
OS: 20/20

S. Grob, M.D., M.A.S. (✉) • S. Mukai, M.D.
Department of Ophthalmology, Harvard Medical School, Massachusetts Eye and Ear, Boston, MA, USA

K. E. Talcott, M.D.
Vitreoretinal Surgery, Wills Eye Hospital, Philadelphia, PA, USA

S. Grob, C. Kloek (eds.), *Management of Open Globe Injuries*,
https://doi.org/10.1007/978-3-319-72410-2_37

37.2.2 Pupils

OD: Peaked superiorly, no afferent pupillary defect
OS: Round and reactive

37.2.3 External Examination

Normal. No lacerations or other trauma noted.

37.2.4 Slit Lamp Examination

	OD	OS
Lids and lashes	Normal	Normal
Sclera and conjunctiva	2 × 4 mm area of uveal prolapse at the limbus	Normal
Cornea	2 × 4 mm area of uveal prolapse at the limbus	Normal
Anterior chamber	Vitreous to wound	Normal
Iris	Peaked superiorly	Normal
Lens	Not visualized	Normal
Vitreous	Vitreous to wound, vitreous hemorrhage	Normal

37.2.5 Dilated Examination

Macula/Nerve OD: Cup to disc ratio of 0.3, macula flat
Periphery OD: Grossly attached, very difficult view due to patient cooperation
Macula/Nerve: OS: Normal
Periphery OS: Normal

37.2.6 Radiographic Imaging

Computed tomography (CT) of the orbits showed the right eye without an intraocular lens, concerning for a ruptured globe. The scleral contour was fairly regular. There were no intraocular foreign bodies or fractures (Fig. 37.1).

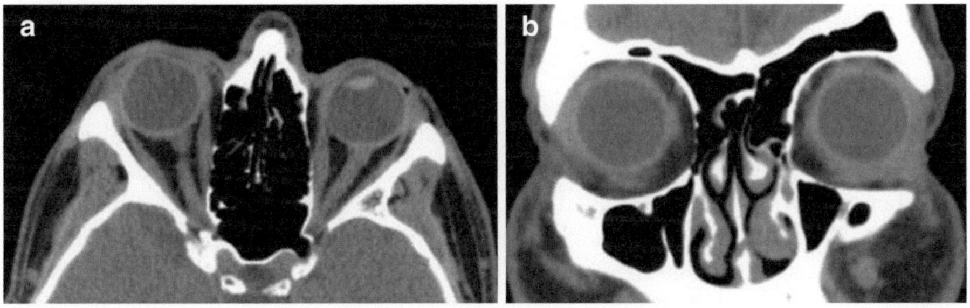

Fig. 37.1 Axial (**a**) CT image showing no sign of an intraocular lens in the right eye. Coronal (**b**) CT images showing no evidence of orbital fractures and generally normal scleral contour more posteriorly

37.3 Surgeon's Initial Assessment and Pre-Operative Plan

The patient had a delayed Zone I/II open globe injury of the right eye presenting 5 days after the initial injury.

Delayed-presentation open globes may offer greater challenges in surgical repair. In addition to the higher possibility of an infection on presentation, the tissue surrounding the laceration or rupture site is often very edematous and friable. Corneal melting may also be present. This can make primary closure with only nylon sutures difficult since the wound may leak or tissue may be lost. In these cases, it is important to have available supplemental tools for wound closure, including corneal glue or a patch graft. We keep a kit of supplies that are needed for corneal gluing and take this into the operating room in cases of delayed open globes or complex corneal lacerations. This includes a clear eye drape, dermal punches of different sizes, Q-tips, eye ointment, corneal glue, and a Kontur lens. It is also important to have available irradiated corneas or other tissues for a patch graft in case it is necessary. In our case, we discussed with the patient the possibility of needing corneal glue or a patch graft given the probable complexity of the wound closure based on the pre-operative appearance of the corneal tissue surrounding the rupture site.

Delayed-presentation open globes with uveal prolapse raise the concern for epithelial growth over the exposed uveal tissue and down the wound edges into the eye (epithelial downgrowth). It is helpful to rinse the exposed uveal tissue and even gently scrape the surface with a beaver or crescent blade prior to repositing it into the eye. This may help prevent the formation of intraocular epithelial membrane growth or downgrowth. In some cases, such as visible epithelialization or necrosis, one should consider resection of the prolapsed uvea.

This patient had no visible lens in the right eye on clinical examination or CT imaging. Likely it was expulsed from the eye from the blunt trauma. It is important to explore under the conjunctiva for lens material or an intraocular lens.

37.4 Surgical Exploration and Repair: Operative Note

Informed consent was obtained and the operative eye was verified and marked. The uninjured left eye was taped closed and shielded for protection. The patient was placed under general anesthesia. Examination revealed no lens in the anterior chamber, posteriorly, or underneath the conjunctiva. A dilated fundus examination was performed of the patient's right eye and this was normal. The patient was prepped and draped in the usual sterile ophthalmic fashion. Jaffe lid specula were inserted into the upper and lower eyelids for exposure. A superior limbal peritomy was initiated with blunt Westcott scissors. Gentle dissection was continued into the superior quadrants with blunt Westcott scissors. No lens material was found. A 4 mm Zone I/II full-thickness laceration was noted at the superonasal peripheral cornea that crossed the limbus but did not extend posteriorly. Uveal and vitreous prolapse was noted at the corneoscleral rupture site. The tissue surrounding the rupture site was friable and melting. Debris on the exposed iris was washed away with balanced-salt solution and removed with Weck-cels® (Beaver Visitec Inc., Waltham, MA). A Weck-cel vitrectomy was performed to remove prolapsed vitreous. A crescent blade was used to gently remove any epithelial cells that had coated the iris. A paracentesis was made temporally with a 15° super-sharp blade. A cyclodialysis spatula was used through the paracentesis to reposition the prolapsed uvea into the eye. Multiple 10-0 nylon sutures were placed to approximate the wound, and an iris spatula was used to prevent iris incarceration in the wound. The corneal and scleral tissue was noted to be very friable and soft during the suture placement. Despite multiple attempts to close the wound, it was found to be Seidel positive with a slow leak. The decision was made to apply corneal glue. Filtered air was injected into the anterior chamber. A dermal punch was used to cut out a round piece of a clear eye drape. Eye ointment was placed on the end of the back of a Q-tip and then the round piece of clear drape was placed on top of this. A small drop of corneal glue was placed onto the surface of the piece of clear drape on the opposite surface from that in contact with the ointment. Then the corneal glue and the piece of clear drape was applied to the wound and held for several seconds for it to dry and set into position. The filtered air was replaced with balanced salt solution. The paracentesis wound was hydrated and found to be watertight. The conjunctiva was sutured back into place with four 8-0 interrupted Vicryl sutures. A Kontur lens was placed. Subconjunctival injections of cefazolin and dexamethasone were placed inferotemporally away from the wound.

37.4.1 Surgical Exploration and Repair: Pearls

- Delayed presentation of open globe injuries can result in edematous and friable tissue along the edges of the laceration or rupture site. It is important to prepare for the possible need of corneal glue or a patch graft pre-operatively.

- Removal of vitreous prolapse from the corneal laceration or rupture site is important to relieve vitreous traction. This can be done with a gentle Weck-cel vitrectomy or if there is good visibility, with the vitrectomy handpiece.
- It is important to consider epithelial downgrowth in the delayed-presentation patients. Prolapsed uveal tissue and corneal wound edges can be gently scraped to remove epithelial cells.

37.5 Post-Operative Course

The patient was admitted to MEE to complete a 48 hour course of intravenous antibiotics. On post-operative day 1 he was hand motions vision without correction. A B-scan ultrasound showed no sign of an intraocular lens and an attached retina.

The contact lens fell out approximately two weeks post-operatively when he rubbed his eye and the corneal glue fell out soon afterwards. Without the glue, the wound was noted to be Seidel negative, so it was not replaced.

Six weeks after the open globe repair, his vision with a +12.00 diopter lens was 20/100 that improved with pinhole to 20/40. We decided to keep the sutures in place for a couple more weeks due to the complex wound repair. The patient returned 8 weeks after open globe repair for suture removal. This was attempted in the procedure room of the emergency department and despite pre-procedure lorazepam and coaching, he was not able to tolerate this. The patient was therefore taken to the operating room for removal of his corneal sutures under monitored anesthesia care (MAC) anesthesia that he tolerated well.

Six weeks after suture removal (14 weeks status post primary repair), the wound had healed well (Fig. 37.2). The patient was seen by optometry and was fitted for a scleral lens. He was found to be 20/30+2 with the contact lens. However, he was not able to tolerate putting in and removing the lens. The examination at that time also revealed residual vitreous to the wound, iris-to-cornea adhesions, and residual

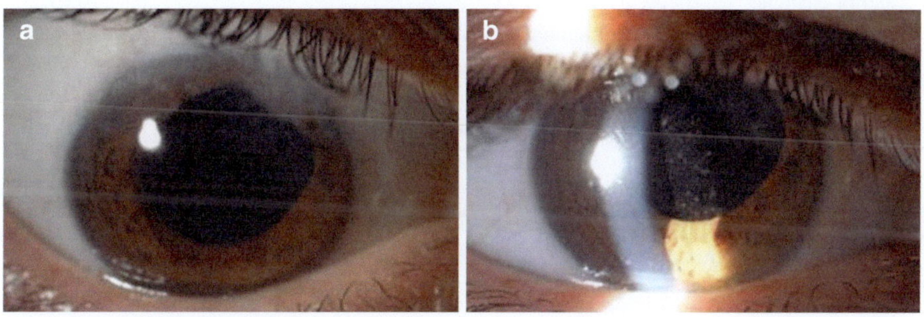

Fig. 37.2 (**a**) Slit lamp photograph showing a well-healed superonasal corneal scar with fine neovascularization with irregularity of the pupil superonasally. (**b**) Photo with a slit beam showing the anterior hyaloid face with pigment noted prior to his pars plana vitrectomy

vitreous hemorrhage. He was evaluated by a retinal specialist, and a vitrectomy was recommended to release the vitreous to the wound and the iris-to-cornea adhesions and clear the residual vitreous hemorrhage. The decision was made to insert a secondary anterior chamber intraocular lens (ACIOL) since he was not tolerating the aphakic contact lens. The footplates of the ACIOL were placed away from the area of the initial injury. At his follow up almost one year after the open globe injury, his vision was 20/50 that improved with pinhole to 20/20-2.

37.6 Final Trauma Evaluation

37.6.1 Final Visual Acuity

OD: 20/50 pinhole 20/20-2
OS: 20/20

37.6.2 Pupils

OD: More round, transillumination defect superonasally with slight irregularity
OS: Normal

37.6.3 Slit Lamp Examination

	OD	OS
Lids and lashes	Normal	Normal
Sclera and conjunctiva	Scleral tunnel wound well covered and healed	Normal
Cornea	Corneal scar superonasally with fine neovascularization	Normal
Anterior chamber	ACIOL	Normal
Iris	Transillumination defect nasally and irregularity superonasally	Normal
Lens	ACIOL	Normal
Vitreous	Status post pars plana vitrectomy	Normal

37.6.4 Dilated Examination

Macula/Nerve OD: Normal, cup to disc ratio of 0.3
Periphery OD: Vitreous opacity at vitreous base inferiorly, attached 360°
Macula/Nerve: OS: Normal
Periphery OS: Normal

37.7 Review and Lessons Learned

In delayed open globe injuries, it is important to rule out infection, either locally around the site of the laceration and/or endophthalmitis, since delayed treatment of the infection can lead to a poor visual prognosis [1]. These cases often have additional challenges for wound closure. Even after 24 hours, tissue around a corneal laceration can become very edematous, making it difficult to visualize the exact location of the laceration to close the wound. It can be helpful to draw the corneal laceration as soon as you examine the patient; if the cornea swells while you are waiting for the operating room, you will be able to remember its exact shape. With delayed open globes, you will not have this chance, and the cornea can have significant edema and melting at the wound. In these cases, it is important to know about adjunctive options for closing the wound if it will not close with sutures alone. Open globes with delayed presentation are prone to wound leaks [2]. Preparing for the possible need for corneal glue or patch graft is helpful in these cases. Educating the patient pre-operatively about these possibilities is also important.

Patients may present after the recommended 24 hour time for a number of reasons. They can be scared and want to avoid evaluation for fear of need for intervention and a poor prognosis. Some patients are worried about burdening family and friends to take them to an ophthalmologist for evaluation. Some patients are seen at outside facilities that do not have an eye care specialist, and they can be diagnosed inappropriately with a corneal abrasion for example instead of an open globe. They are then sent home with antibiotic drops or ointment perhaps even without a follow-up appointment and may not present to an eye specialist until several days later when they don't think their eye is getting any better. Kids are often at risk for delayed presentation as they are difficult to examine at an outside emergency department or clinic or may not be able to verbalize the extent of their vision loss or eye symptoms [3].

Pediatric patients are often taken back to the operating room for corneal suture removal. However, older children and most adults are able to tolerate suture removal at the slit lamp in the exam room. Some might need some additional coaching while other patients like to turn on music. We have found that music of the patient's choice can often help distract or calm patients enough to get them through the procedure if they are anxious. However, there are some adult patients that have difficulty cooperating with the procedure despite best attempts. It is safer and wiser to take the patient back to the operating room and remove the sutures under MAC or even general anesthesia if necessary.

37.8 Key Learning Points

- Delayed globes can pose challenges for wound closure. Being prepared pre-operatively for the possibility of needing to use corneal glue or even a patch graft is important.

- If corneal sutures cannot be removed safely in the examination room or in a procedure room due to patient anxiety or cooperation, consider taking the patient back to the operating room for suture removal. It will be safer and more comfortable for the patient and minimizes the chance of broken retained sutures or injury.

References

1. Nicoara SD, Irimescu I, Calinici T, Cristian C. Outcome and prognostic factors for traumatic endophthalmitis over a 5-year period. J Ophthalmol. 2014;2014:747015.
2. Kong GY, Henderson RH, Sandhu SS, Essex RW, Allen PJ, Campbell WG. Wound-related complications and clinical outcomes following open globe injury repair. Clin Exp Ophthalmol. 2015;43(6):508–13.
3. Acuna OM, Yen KG. Outcome and prognosis of pediatric patients with delayed diagnosis of open globe injuries. J Pediatr Ophthalmol Strabismus. 2009;46(4):202–7.

Chapter 38
Case 33: Delayed Zone I Open Globe Injury with Corneal Ulcer and Hypopyon

Yewlin E. Chee and Alice C. Lorch

38.1 History of Present Illness

A 63-year-old man with history of Hepatitis C presents with one and a half days of right eye pain.

- The patient reports he was using a crowbar to help a friend dismantle an old wood shed when a large piece of wood broke off and hit him in the right eye. He had immediate pain. He tried to rinse the eye with artificial tears then went to sleep. He awoke the following morning with more eye pain, then presented to an outside hospital, where he was subsequently referred to Massachusetts Eye and Ear (MEE).
- He presents to MEE approximately 34 hours after his injury.
- He reports persistent pain with decreased vision in his right eye.

38.2 Initial Trauma Evaluation

38.2.1 Visual Acuity (Without Correction)

OD: Count fingers
OS: 20/70 pinhole 20/50

Y. E. Chee, M.D. (✉)
Vitreoretinal Surgery, Department of Ophthalmology, University of Washington, Seattle, WA, USA

A. C. Lorch, M.D., M.P.H.
Department of Ophthalmology, Harvard Medical School, Massachusetts Eye and Ear, Boston, MA, USA

S. Grob, C. Kloek (eds.), *Management of Open Globe Injuries*,
https://doi.org/10.1007/978-3-319-72410-2_38

38.2.2 Pupils

OD: Irregular, no afferent pupillary defect
OS: Round, no afferent pupillary defect

38.2.3 External Examination

Normal

38.2.4 Slit Lamp Examination

	OD	OS
Lids and lashes	Normal	Normal
Sclera and conjunctiva	Diffuse, flat subconjunctival hemorrhage	Normal
Cornea	6 mm, horizontally oriented, shelved, full-thickness laceration in the inferior paracentral cornea. 1 mm × 1 mm infiltrate at nasal aspect of wound. Slowly seidel positive. No foreign bodies in wound	Normal
Anterior chamber	3+ WBC, fibrin, 0.3 mm layered hypopyon. Shallow nasally	Normal
Iris	Inferior and temporal iridocorneal touch, transillumination defects at 3:30 and 9	Normal
Lens	Posterior chamber intraocular lens (PCIOL)	PCIOL
Vitreous	Difficult view secondary to cornea, no obvious cell	Clear

38.2.5 Dilated Examination

Macula/Nerve OD: Grossly normal
Periphery OD: Grossly attached, no foreign body
Macula/Nerve: OS: Normal
Periphery OS: Attached

38.2.6 Radiographic Imaging

Computed tomography (CT) of the orbits showed a formed globe with no evidence of a radiopaque intraocular foreign body (Fig. 38.1).

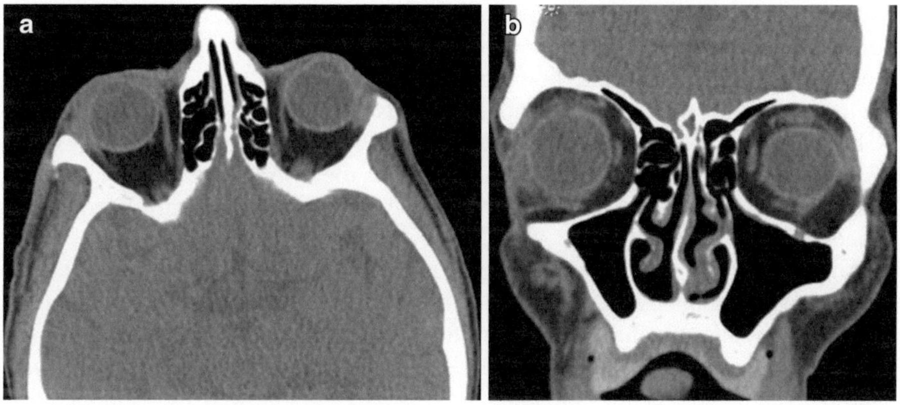

Fig. 38.1 Axial (**a**) and coronal (**b**) CT images showing a normal globe contour in both eyes with no evidence of radiopaque foreign body

38.3 Surgeon's Initial Assessment and Pre-Operative Plan

The patient had a delayed presentation Zone I open globe injury of the right eye with corneal infiltrate and intraocular inflammation with a layered hypopyon.

This case illustrates two important areas of discussion beyond the standard repair of a Zone I laceration (see earlier cases in this book for examples). These are the management of corneal laceration with an associated corneal ulcer, and management of a delayed presentation open globe injury with concern for possible endophthalmitis.

The integrity of corneal tissue is compromised in the setting of infection, and special considerations need to be made when repairing a corneal wound with an associated corneal ulcer. Suture passes should be placed such that the infected tissue is avoided; depending on the configuration of the corneal wound, this can be achieved by offsetting the sutures such that they cross the laceration but are away from the corneal infiltrate, or in certain cases, longer suture passes can be used to cross both the laceration and a small infiltrate at the edge of the wound with the needle entering and exiting through healthy cornea. If a suture is placed with the needle passing through infected corneal tissue, there is concern that the infectious material could be dragged into the anterior chamber and/or the suture will tear through the compromised tissue and the wound could remain open. If necessary, cyanoacrylate glue has intrinsic bactericidal properties and can be used to help repair focal defects in infected corneal tissue [1].

Delay in wound closure of greater than 24 hours is a known risk factor for traumatic endophthalmitis after open globe injury [2, 3]. A high index of suspicion for endophthalmitis must be maintained in any eye after penetrating or perforating injury, particularly if there is delay in presentation. It can be difficult to differentiate the signs of early endophthalmitis and expected inflammation in the setting of trauma, but the presence of a hypopyon and/or vitritis is concerning for endophthalmitis and warrants treatment. In this particular case, there was a corneal laceration, a corneal ulcer, and a small, layered hypopyon. No obvious vitritis was seen on exam, however the view to the anterior vitreous was compromised by the corneal wound. As this patient presented to MEE over 30 hours after his injury, he was at higher risk for endophthalmitis and the presence of a hypopyon prompted consultation with the vitreoretinal service, who recommended treatment for presumed endophthalmitis with intravitreal vancomycin and ceftazidime.

Another known risk factor for post traumatic endophthalmitis is a retained intraocular foreign body [2, 3]. Although this patient underwent a pre-operative CT scan of the orbits, his injury was from a broken piece of wood, and nonmetallic foreign bodies are sometimes undetectable on CT imaging [4]. In these cases, careful examination at the slit lamp pre-operatively followed by intraoperative inspection of the wound with copious irrigation of the cornea and possible anterior chamber washout should be performed.

The surgical plan was to proceed with corneal scraping for microbiology, globe exploration and careful inspection of the wound and anterior segment for possible foreign bodies, followed by closure of the corneal laceration, acquisition of aqueous and vitreous samples to send for gram stain and culture, and injection of subconjunctival and intravitreal antibiotics.

38.4 Surgical Exploration and Repair: Operative Note

The risks, benefits, and alternatives were discussed pre-operatively and informed consent was obtained. The patient was brought to the operating room and placed under general anesthesia. The operative eye was identified. Corneal scrapings for gram stain and cultures were obtained using a #15 blade and sterile cotton swabs at the site of the corneal ulcer. Then, the eye was prepped and draped in the usual sterile ophthalmic fashion. A Lieberman speculum was placed.

The shelved corneal laceration was inspected under the operating microscope. The laceration was explored with a cannula and irrigated to remove any debris from the wound. Two 10-0 nylon sutures were placed away from the nasal stromal infiltration. Fluorescein was applied to confirm that the wound was watertight.

A paracentesis was created superotemporally. A cannula was inserted into the anterior chamber to aspirate the hypopyon mostly located inferotemporally and the sample was labeled. The anterior chamber was reinflated with balanced salt solution (BSS) and the anterior chamber was irrigated thoroughly with BSS to washout the fibrin, inflammation, and debris. No foreign bodies were found. A caliper set at 3.5 mm was used to identify the pars plana inferotemporally where a 27 gauge needle was used to retrieve a 0.1 mL vitreous sample. Intravitreal vancomycin (1 mg/0.1 mL) and intravitreal ceftazidime (2 mg/0.1 mL) were injected intravitreally 3.5 mm posterior to the limbus. The anterior chamber and vitreous samples were sent to microbiology for gram stain and culture. The corneal wound was checked again and remained Seidel negative.

Subconjunctival injections of vancomycin 25 mg/0.5 mL and ceftazidime 100 mg/0.5 mL were performed. Gatifloxacin drops and erythromycin ointment were applied topically. The speculum was removed. The eye was patched and shielded. The patient was transferred to the post-operative area in stable condition. The patient tolerated the procedure well without any complications.

38.4.1 Surgical Exploration and Repair: Pearls

- Obtain corneal scrapings prior to prepping the eye with povidone iodine in order to maximize the yield of the sample.
- Consider wound exploration and anterior chamber washout if there is concern for radiolucent foreign material.
- Pass corneal sutures through healthy corneal tissue. Avoid suturing through an area with a corneal infiltrate.
- If the intraocular volume of the eye is manipulated after a laceration is sutured, recheck the wound to ensure that it remains watertight.

38.5 Post-Operative Course

The patient was admitted to MEE to complete a 48 hour course of intravenous antibiotics. On post-operative day one his vision was 20/320 and his corneal wound was Seidel negative (Fig. 38.2). The corneal infiltrate measured 0.8 mm × 1 mm with an overlying epithelial defect and there was 1+ anterior chamber cell and flare but no layered hypopyon. Corneal scraping cultures grew abundant *Staphylococcus aureus*, resistant to penicillin and ampicillin, and sensitive to vancomycin and levofloxacin. Anterior chamber and vitreous samples demonstrated polymorphonuclear lymphocytes but no growth on culture.

He was started on hourly topical fortified vancomycin to treat his corneal ulcer in addition to atropine 1% twice daily and prednisolone acetate 1% twice daily. A B scan ultrasound was performed on post-operative day 1, which demonstrated scant vitreous debris and an attached retina. The vitreoretinal service at MEE reevaluated him and as his inflammation was improving, and there was no evidence of endophthalmitis clinically or on his ultrasound, advised continued monitoring without additional intravitreal antibiotics.

Initially he was examined daily until his corneal ulcer demonstrated signs of improvement with consolidation of the infiltrate and decrease in size of the overlying epithelial defect. During this time, he remained an inpatient in order to ensure compliance with his eye drop regimen. He was discharged on post-operative day 5 and continued to be followed closely as an outpatient. At his post-operative month 1 visit, his vision in his right eye was 20/40 pinholing to 20/30, the corneal epithelial defect had resolved, and his fortified vancomycin eyedrops were discontinued (Fig. 38.3).

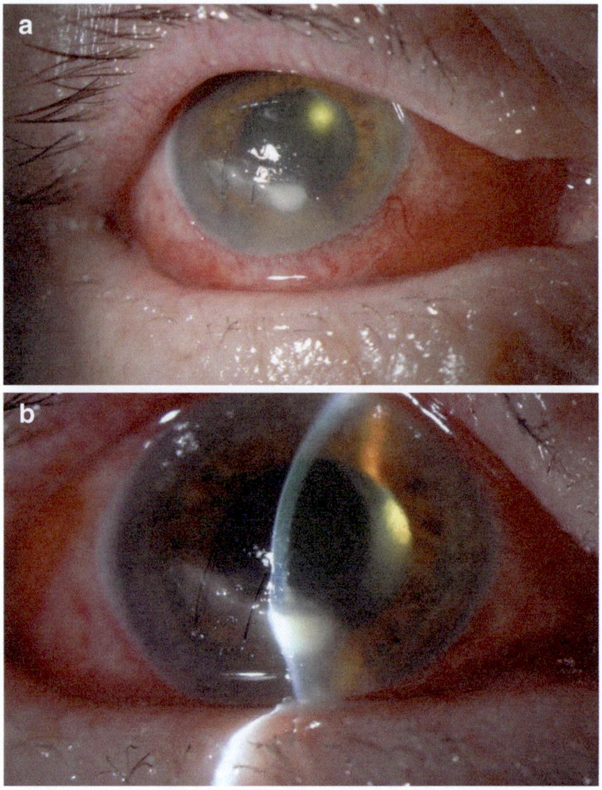

Fig. 38.2 Post-operative day 1 anterior segment photos with diffuse (**a**) and slit beam (**b**) illumination. The full-thickness, shelved corneal laceration was closed with two interrupted nylon sutures positioned away from the nasal corneal ulcer

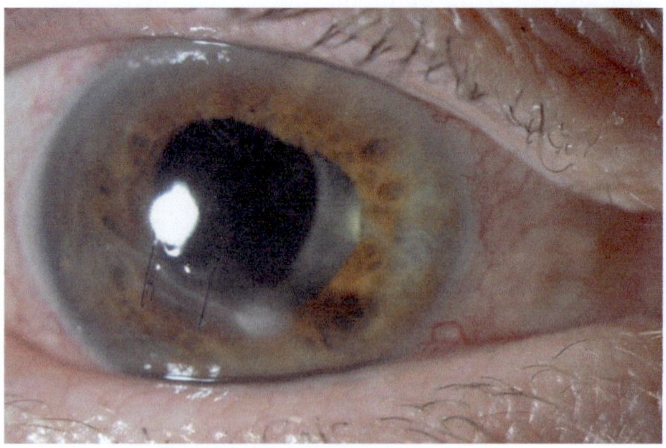

Fig. 38.3 Post-operative month 1 anterior segment photo taken prior to the development of a central suture abscess

He returned at his post-operative month 2 visit complaining of 1 week of increased eye pain and blurred vision. Although he was instructed to seek care when his pain started, he was unable to obtain transportation to the emergency ward. His vision had declined to 20/200 pinholing to 20/100 and he was found to have a suture abscess at his central suture with associated corneal thinning of 20%. Corneal scrapings were sent for gram stain and culture and the patient was empirically started on fortified topical vancomycin and ceftazidime eye drops. Due to concern for treatment noncompliance, he was admitted to the inpatient unit until his corneal infiltrate and epithelial defect demonstrated clear improvement.

Suture removal was deferred while his suture abscess was being treated. Once the infiltrate and epithelial defect improved, his two corneal sutures were removed. His topical antibiotics were gradually tapered and stopped. He ultimately was refracted to 20/20 with a contact lens 8 months after his initial injury.

38.6 Final Trauma Evaluation

38.6.1 Final Visual Acuity

OD: 20/25– without correction, 20/20 with +1.50–1.25 × 095 correction
OS: 20/20+ without correction

38.6.2 Pupils

OD: Round, no afferent pupillary defect
OS: Round

38.6.3 Slit Lamp Examination

	OD	OS
Lids and lashes	Normal	Normal
Sclera and conjunctiva	Normal	Normal
Cornea	1.8 mm V × 2.8 H mm scar (40% thinned); band of fibrotic and neovascular tissue at 9 o'clock mid periphery	Normal
Anterior chamber	Normal	Normal
Iris	Posterior synechiae at 9 o'clock	Normal
Lens	PCIOL	PCIOL
Vitreous	Mild vitreous debris	Normal

38.6.4 Dilated Examination

Macula/Nerve OD: Normal
Periphery OD: Normal
Macula/Nerve: OS: Normal
Periphery OS: Normal

38.7 Review and Lessons Learned

Any eye with history of an open globe injury is at increased risk of traumatic endophthalmitis. Risk factors for traumatic endophthalmitis include delay in wound closure of greater than 24 hours, retained intraocular foreign body, rural setting of injury, and disruption of the crystalline lens capsule [2]. A high index of suspicion must be maintained, and if there are clinical signs of possible endophthalmitis such as the presence of a hypopyon and/or vitritis, treatment with broad-spectrum intravitreal antibiotics should be initiated.

The presence of a concomitant corneal ulcer with a Zone I laceration can complicate wound closure. Prior to sterilization of the operative eye, obtain corneal scrapings to send for gram stain and culture. Care should be taken to avoid passing sutures through a corneal infiltrate in order to decrease the likelihood of introducing infectious material into the anterior chamber and to increase the integrity of the wound closure. If necessary, cyanoacrylate glue has intrinsic bactericidal properties and can be used if appropriately placed sutures are inadequate [1]. Post-operatively, frequent topical broad-spectrum antibiotic eye drops should be administered, and then the antibiotic choice can be narrowed with guidance based on the corneal culture results. Patients must be counseled regarding signs of infection and recurrence of infection and instructed to return immediately if there is any increase in eye pain, redness, photophobia, and/or decrease in vision. Suture removal generally should be delayed beyond the standard 6 weeks after wound repair if there is concern for an active infection at or adjacent to the wound. In the case of this patient, suture removal was delayed until post-operative month 4 when the patient's secondary suture abscess was improving and the suture associated with the infiltrate had loosened. Despite his complex presentation and prolonged recovery, this patient regained excellent visual acuity.

38.8 Key Learning Points

- Delayed wound closure of greater than 24 hours and retained intraocular foreign body are risk factors for traumatic endophthalmitis.

- The signs of early traumatic endophthalmitis can be difficult to differentiate from inflammation after open globe injury; treatment with intravitreal antibiotics should be administered if endophthalmitis is suspected.
- Corneal sutures need to be carefully placed in the setting of a concomitant corneal ulcer such that suture passes are through healthy cornea.
- Counsel patients regarding the potential for infection in the post-operative recovery period and the need for urgent evaluation if they experience new symptoms such as increased pain and/or decreased vision after their open globe repair.
- Consider inpatient admission for patients who require frequent medication administration when there is concern for treatment noncompliance.

References

1. de Almeida Manzano RP, Naufal SC, Hida RY, Guarnieri LOB, Nishiwaki-Dantas MC. Antibacterial analysis in vitro of ethyl-cyanoacrylate against ocular pathogens. Cornea. 2006;25(3):350–1. https://doi.org/10.1097/01.ico.0000183490.16131.e3.
2. Ahmed Y, Schimel AM, Pathengay A, Colyer MH, Flynn HWJ. Endophthalmitis following open-globe injuries. Eye (Lond). 2012;26(2):212–7. https://doi.org/10.1038/eye.2011.313.
3. Reynolds DS, Flynn HWJ. Endophthalmitis after penetrating ocular trauma. Curr Opin Ophthalmol. 1997;8(3):32–8.
4. Moisseiev E, Last D, Goez D, Barak A, Mardor Y. Magnetic resonance imaging and computed tomography for the detection and characterization of nonmetallic intraocular foreign bodies. Retina. 2015;35(1):82–94. https://doi.org/10.1097/IAE.0000000000000266.

Chapter 39
Case 34: Globe Injury with Concurrent Intracranial Injury

Seanna Grob, Yoshihiro Yonekawa, Alison Callahan, Yewlin E. Chee, Carolyn Kloek, David Wu, Dean Eliott, and John B. Miller

39.1 History of Present Illness

A 40-year-old man with no significant past medical history who presents with concern for a penetrating open globe of the right eye.

- One week prior to presentation, the patient was using a nail gun and he felt like the gun flew back and hit him in the right cheek.
- He developed significant periorbital edema and lost vision in his right eye after the incident, but thought it would improve over time. He did not lift his eyelid during this time to check his vision.
- Over the subsequent days, he started to have increasing pain without improvement of his periorbital edema, so he went to an outside eye doctor for evaluation who transferred the patient to Massachusetts General Hospital for emergent evaluation.

S. Grob, M.D., M.A.S. (✉) • A. Callahan, M.D. • C. Kloek, M.D. • D. Wu, M.D., Ph.D.
Department of Ophthalmology, Harvard Medical School, Massachusetts Eye and Ear, Boston, MA, USA

Y. Yonekawa, M.D.
Vitreoretinal Surgery, Harvard Medical School, Massachusetts Eye and Ear and Boston Children's Hospital, Boston, MA, USA

Y. E. Chee, M.D.
Vitreoretinal Surgery, Department of Ophthalmology, University of Washington, Seattle, WA, USA

D. Eliott, M.D. • J. B. Miller, M.D.
Vitreoretinal Surgery, Department of Ophthalmology, Harvard Medical School, Massachusetts Eye and Ear, Boston, MA, USA

S. Grob, C. Kloek (eds.), *Management of Open Globe Injuries*,
https://doi.org/10.1007/978-3-319-72410-2_39

39.2 Initial Trauma Evaluation

39.2.1 Visual Acuity (Without Correction)

OD: Light perception
OS: 20/20

39.2.2 Pupils

OD: Fixed, non-reactive pupil at approximately 4 mm, afferent pupillary defect by reverse
OS: Round and reactive

39.2.3 Intraocular Pressure

OD: 25
OS: 10

39.2.4 Color Testing

OD: 0/8
OS: 8/8

39.2.5 Extraocular Movements

OD: Restricted movements in all directions of gaze
OS: Normal

39.2.6 External Examination

Two healing 3–4 mm lacerations on the right lower eyelid-cheek junction

39.2.7 Slit Lamp Examination

	OD	OS
Lids and lashes	Ptosis with poor upper eyelid elevation	Normal
Sclera and conjunctiva	360° bullous chemosis	Normal
Cornea	Hazy with significant corneal edema, no apparent corneal abrasions or lacerations	Normal
Anterior chamber	Hazy view, formed	Normal
Iris	Normal	Normal
Lens	Normal	Normal
Vitreous	Hazy view from vitreous hemorrhage	Normal

39.2.8 Dilated Examination

Macula/Nerve OD: No view
Periphery OD: No view
Macula/Nerve: OS: Normal
Periphery OS: Normal

39.2.9 Radiographic Imaging

Computed tomography (CT) of the orbits showed an 8.2 cm nail originating within the inferior right lateral orbit, directed cephalad and medially, extending into the right frontal lobe of the brain (Fig. 39.1).

Gentle B-scan ultrasonography of the right eye: irregular globe contour due to a linear foreign body that sonographically appeared to penetrate or perforate the globe along the eye wall, entering at 7 o'clock about 12 mm posterior to iris, and exiting at 10 o'clock about 20 mm posterior to iris. There was dense vitreous hemorrhage and shallow choroidal effusions (Fig. 39.2). Note: A B-scan was done in this case to better assess the integrity of the globe as there was question whether the nail penetrated the globe or passed through the orbit adjacent to the globe based on the CT scan. Although a B-scan was done in this case, it is generally contraindicated to do ocular ultrasound when a open globe may be present given the risk for expulsion of intraocular contents.

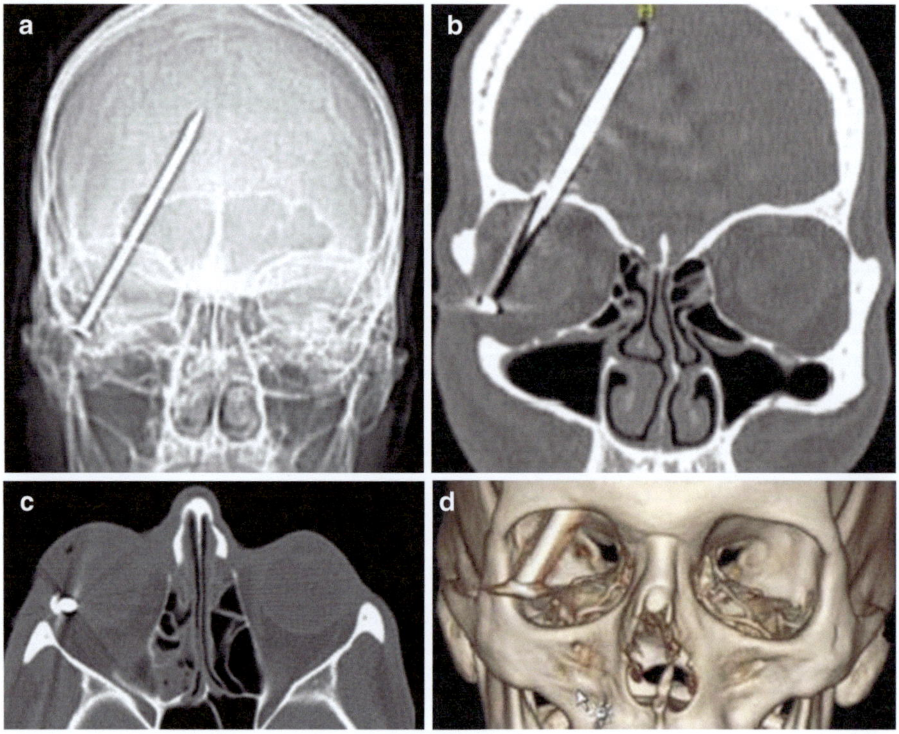

Fig. 39.1 Coronal (**a**) X-ray and (**b**) CT images showing the metallic nail both within the right orbit and right frontal lobe. Axial (**c**) CT image showing the nail coursing through the lateral orbit. Coronal view of a 3D reconstruction (**d**) showing the trajectory of the nail through the lateral orbit

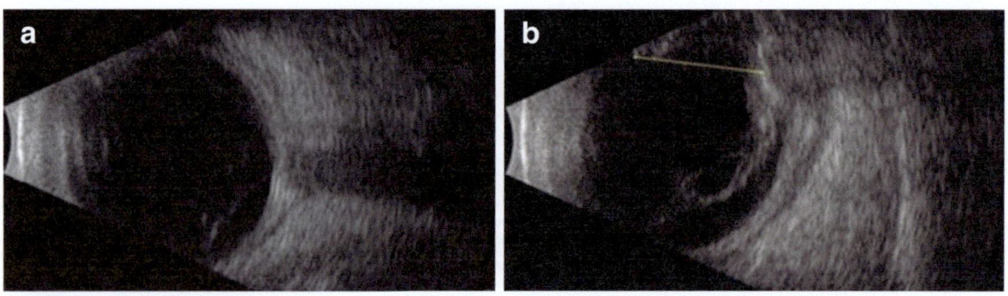

Fig. 39.2 B scan ultrasound showing vertical disc view (**a**) with attached retina and temporal view (**b**) showing irregularity to the globe contour in the area of trajectory of the nail

39.3 Surgeon's Initial Assessment and Pre-operative Plan

This patient had an intraorbital and intracranial foreign body with concern for an open globe injury on CT and ultrasound imaging.

This case illustrates an important area of discussion beyond the standard open globe exploration and repair—the management of globe injuries with concurrent intracranial injuries. These patients need to be urgently evaluated by neurosurgery and subsequent management needs to be done with careful communication with the neurosurgical service. Do not dilate the patient until neurosurgery has evaluated the patient and given permission for dilation. The pupillary light reflexes are an important exam tool that neurosurgery uses to assess the patient for progressive intracranial edema or hemorrhage. Fortunately if you only dilate one eye and the contralateral eye is without pathology, you can assess for a relative afferent pupillary defect by reverse after dilation. These patients often have to be carefully monitored with serial CT imaging so open globe exploration and repair might need to be delayed until the imaging shows no signs of progressive edema or hemorrhage. Sometimes these patients require neurosurgical intervention in the operating room prior to open globe repair. It is important if there is concern for a life-threatening injury, that it be addressed first. A rigid eye shield can be placed over the eye to protect it until it is safe to address the globe.

We usually do not recommend checking intraocular pressure when there is concern for an open globe injury, as there is a risk of extrusion of intraocular contents with pressure on the globe. However, in rare cases it may provide additional information. In this case, there was uncertainty about whether the foreign body actually penetrated or perforated the globe versus transversed the orbit without injuring the globe. The intraocular pressure was mildly elevated in this case likely due to the intraorbital foreign body and periorbital and orbital edema. The high pressure a week after injury may have supported that the globe was intact, however, this does not rule out an open globe. There are cases of normal or high intraocular pressure with an open globe injury on exploration. If there is concern for a possible open globe injury, only exploration of the globe can rule out an open globe injury.

This particular case required a team-based approach to surgical repair, including neurosurgery, oculoplastics, and ocular trauma. The most urgent concern was to ensure that there was no sign of progressive intracranial bleeding or hemorrhage. The patient had notably had this foreign body in place for a week prior to presentation and was neurologically intact on presentation. Given the location of the foreign body through the orbit and into the frontal lobe, it was decided that the nail would be removed by both the oculoplastics and neurosurgical team through an orbital approach. A craniotomy would be done initially and the brain would be carefully monitored intraoperatively by the neurosurgeons while the nail was extracted. Subsequently, the ocular trauma team would explore the globe for injury and repair. Neurosurgery would remain in the room to monitor the patient.

On both CT and ultrasound imaging there was concern for possible globe penetration or perforation, but it was very difficult to know for sure since there was no intraocular view on dilated examination due to dense vitreous hemorrhage. Therefore, the patient was consented for exploration of the globe after removal of the foreign body and globe repair if any injury was found. We made sure to have a

Gass muscle hook and 2-0 silk suture available to hook the rectus muscles and allow for more posterior exploration temporally in the location of the foreign body trajectory. A Schepens retractor and/or thin malleables can be helpful for improved visualization of posterior injuries as well.

39.4 Surgical Exploration and Repair: Operative Note

After informed consent was obtained the patient was brought to the operating room where general anesthesia was induced. Neurosurgery first performed a craniotomy in preparation for removal of the intracranial and orbital foreign body.

The area was palpated and CT imaging scrutinized to determine the best approach to the foreign body. The decision was made to make an inferotemporal orbital entry through a lower eyelid crease incision. An incision was made with a #15 blade. Hemostasis was achieved using the unipolar electrocautery. Toothed forceps and double-pronged retractors were used for exposure. Curved scissors were used to explore with blunt and sharp dissection. The orbital septum was opened. The orbital soft tissue was retracted using orbital and malleable retractors. Cotton-tipped applicators were used to dissect delicately. After entering into the inferotemporal orbit, the orbit floor was encountered. Proceeding along the orbital floor superolaterally, along the lateral wall, the foreign body was encountered. Additional fibrotic tissue was dissected away using toothed forceps and curved scissors. Ultimately, the head of the nail was identified and was secured with heavy toothed forceps.

Before retrieving the foreign body, neurosurgery exposed the brain through the craniotomy site and watched the brain tissue and the foreign body as it was removed. It was delicately pulled out uneventfully and sent for cultures. There was no significant additional bleeding. There was no bleeding identified intracranially. The wound was left open to allow for drainage in the event of bleeding or infection.

Attention was then turned to the globe. The uninjured left eye was taped and shielded for protection. The right eye was then prepped and draped in the usual sterile ophthalmic fashion. Jaffe lid speculums were placed for eyelid retraction. A 360° conjunctival peritomy was completed using blunt Westcott scissors. All four quadrants were explored with gentle blunt dissection using blunt Westcott scissors followed by curved Stevens tenotomy scissors. There was significant temporal and inferotemporal scarring corresponding to the area of orbital violation by the foreign body. This scar limited safe blunt dissection of the temporal sclera from the overlying soft tissues. Further inspection of the temporal globe was then achieved by securing the inferior and superior rectus muscles. A Gass muscle hook was passed under the superior and inferior rectus muscles and secured with a 2-0 silk suture. The silk sutures were used to retract the globe nasally to better visualize the temporal globe and the location of the trajectory of the foreign body.

A Gass muscle hook was used to hook the lateral rectus muscle but no muscle remained at the expected insertion site as measured from the temporal limbus with calipers. The dissection was then carefully extended posteriorly to try to identify a possible laceration site. A partial-thickness scleral laceration was found temporally. This was the same area where the lateral rectus muscle should have inserted onto the globe so we suspected that it was disinserted during the nail's course through the orbit. Upon careful dissection of the surrounding scarred conjunctiva and Tenon's, part of the lateral rectus muscle was found. These lateral rectus muscle fibers were isolated and secured using a double-armed 6-0 Vicryl suture on an S-29 needle in an imbricating fashion. The globe was then further explored and no other lacerations were noted. The remaining lateral rectus muscle was then reinserted at its approximate insertion site. The 2-0 silk sutures were removed from the superior and inferior rectus muscles and the conjunctiva was closed using 8-0 Vicryl sutures in an interrupted fashion with an episcleral pass at the temporal limbus. Subconjunctival antibiotic and steroid were injected.

Neurosurgery then continued with closure of the craniotomy site.

The eyelids were cleaned and atropine and antibiotic eye ointment was placed into the operative eye. We then placed a sterile eye patch and shield in the usual ophthalmic fashion.

39.4.1 Surgical Exploration and Repair: Pearls

- For patients with intracranial injuries or hemorrhage, it is important to work closely with the neurosurgeons in assessment and management of the patient. Life threatening injuries should be addressed prior to open globe exploration and repair. Sometimes it is necessary to do combined cases with neurosurgery, as in this case, or the patient might require a craniotomy or other neurosurgical procedures prior to open globe repair.
- If there is concern on imaging that a foreign body is close to the globe with possible globe penetration or perforation and there is no intraocular view on dilated examination, it is necessary to explore the globe for possible full-thickness injuries.
- If you are having trouble hooking a muscle, it could be because the rupture site is just posterior to the muscle insertion or because the muscle has been injured. If the muscle is found to be injured or severed, try to locate the muscle and suture it to the best approximate location of the insertion site.

39.5 Post-operative Course

The patient was admitted for close neurological monitoring and to complete a 48 hour course of intravenous antibiotics. On post-operative day one he still had count fingers vision, with no view to the posterior pole. Infectious disease was consulted due to the high risk of infection from 1 week of an intraorbital and intracranial foreign body who recommended broad spectrum antibiotics including vancomycin, cefepime, and metronidazole (for anaerobic coverage given likely contact with the sinuses). The nail came back positive for coagulase negative staphylococcus. The patient remained stable without signs of infection or other issues and was discharged with a 10-day course of amoxicillin-clavulanate 4 days after his surgery.

The patient followed up with the retina service 4 days after his surgery. A B-scan ultrasound showed shallow choroidals temporally. Dilated examination showed whitening temporally concerning for sclopeteria with subretinal scarring and

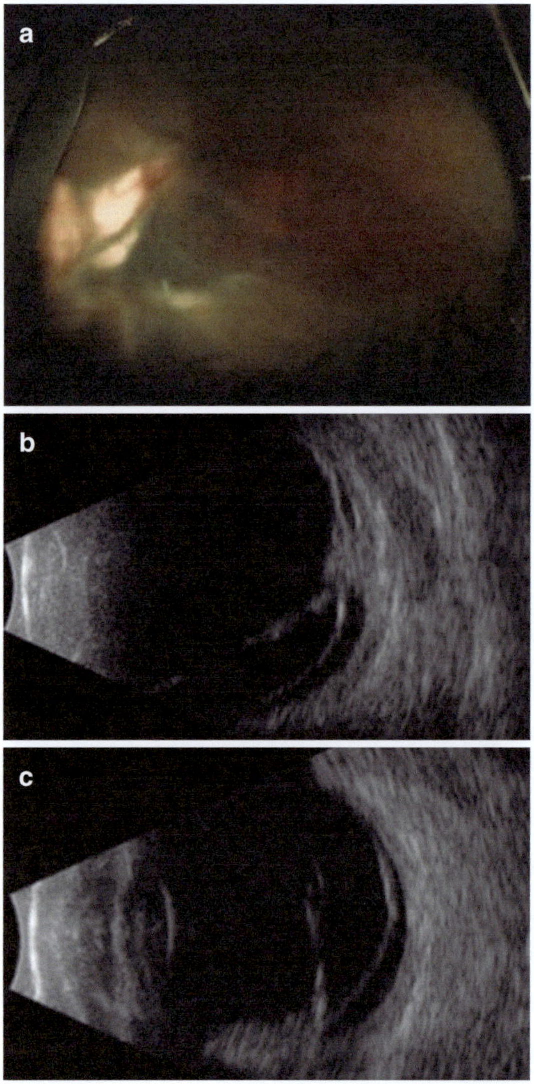

Fig. 39.3 (**a**) Optos widefield image showing whitening temporally and an inferior and temporal retinal detachment. B scan ultrasound showing a retinal detachment both temporally (**b**) and inferiorly (**c**)

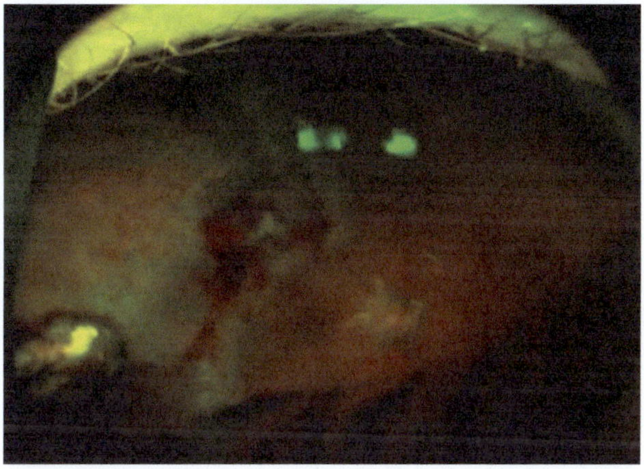

Fig. 39.4 Optos widefield image 1 week post-operatively after the initial retinal detachment repair showing an attached retina with the temporal and inferotemporal retinectomy with temporal hemorrhage

hemorrhage in this area as well. The patient was asked to return a week later for repeat evaluation. At this follow up visit the patient was found to have hand motions vision with concern for a retinal detachment temporally (Fig. 39.3) and the patient was consented for repair of the retinal detachment.

Nineteen days after initial surgical repair, the patient underwent a pars plana vitrectomy and lensectomy, membrane peel, relaxing retinectomy, perfluorocarbon, endolaser, air/fluid exchange, and silicone oil injection. (Fig. 39.4) Post-operatively, the patient had to return to the operating room twice for recurrent retinal detachment repair, once approximately 1 month after the initial retinal surgery in which an inferior 180° retinectomy was completed and again 4 months later when a larger retinectomy was completed to flatten and reattach the retina. Four months following the final repair the patient remained attached with count fingers vision (improved compared to his vision on presentation).

39.6 Final Trauma Evaluation

39.6.1 Final Visual Acuity

OD: Count fingers at 1 foot
OS: 20/15

39.6.2 Pupils

OD: Irregular, afferent pupillary defect by reverse
OS: Normal

39.6.3 Slit Lamp Examination

	OD	OS
Lids and lashes	Normal	Normal
Sclera and conjunctiva	Normal	Normal
Cornea	Normal	Normal
Anterior chamber	+0.5 cells	Normal
Iris	Peripheral iridotomy	Normal
Lens	Aphakic	Normal
Vitreous	Status post pars plana vitrectomy	Normal

39.6.4 Dilated Examination

Macula/Nerve OD: Mild optic nerve pallor, epiretinal membrane
Periphery OD: Large retinectomy, attached remaining retina
Macula/Nerve: OS: Normal
Periphery OS: Normal

39.7 Review and Lessons Learned

In cases that present with concurrent intracranial injury, it is important to facilitate urgent imaging and evaluation by the neurosurgical service. These injuries could include an intracranial foreign body (as in this case), intracranial hemorrhage, orbital roof facture with hemorrhage and/or pneumocephalus, or other associated cranial or intracranial injuries. These patients need to be closely co-managed with neurosurgery. It is important to wait to dilate the patient until obtaining permission from neurosurgery and to coordinate the safest time for open globe exploration and repair.

Patients will need urgent CT imaging of the head +/− neck with thin cuts to evaluate for intracranial injury, head, face and neck injuries and for an open globe injury. If there is concern for a metallic foreign body, magnetic resonance imaging (MRI) is contraindicated. If there is no concern for a metallic foreign body, the neurosurgeons might request a MRI and/or magnetic resonance angiography (MRA) to evaluate for vascular injury as well. MR imaging can also be helpful in cases of wooden foreign bodies or other non-metallic material. The patient also might require serial CT images to monitor for progression of intracranial edema and hemorrhage. Active communication with the neurosurgery service is necessary to ensure that adequate imaging is obtained pre- and post-operatively.

Intracranial penetration by foreign bodies that traverse the orbit represent an unusual form of traumatic brain injury. Much is as stake with these high-risk injuries including cranial nerve injury, neurovascular injury, and globe injury. Obtaining a careful history and establishing a high level of suspicion based on the history and physical examination is vital in diagnosis of these cases [1]. Be aware that the external wounds may appear trivial compared to the severity of these injuries. Transorbital intracranial injuries often result from a projectile injury or a stab injury from assault or fall onto the object [2]. These injuries have been reported with chopsticks [3], bamboo shoots [4], a toothbrush [5], pens and pencils [1, 6], glasses [7], and a nail [8]. Some of these injuries are self-inflicted and may represent an attempted suicide or a state of psychosis and urgent psychological evaluation may be necessary [7, 9]. These traumas may also represent domestic violence and patients should be screened accordingly [5].

Open globes with intracranial foreign bodies or injuries can present delayed as in this case. Our patient had this foreign body in place for a week prior to evaluation and was alert and orientated on presentation. There are even cases of long-standing intracranial foreign bodies presenting with infection or altered mental status years later [10]. Therefore, it is important to consider intracranial foreign bodies or intracranial injuries in the setting of open globe injuries, especially in cases with high velocity projectiles such as with nail guns or BB guns.

Although we routinely give patients intravenous ceftriaxone and vancomycin for 48 hours after their injury, patients with transorbital intracranial foreign bodies might need additional coverage. Our patient was also given metronidazole for anaerobic coverage since the foreign body might have had contact with the sinuses. An infectious disease specialist should be consulted for recommendations regarding appropriate antibiotic coverage. The foreign bodies, once retrieved, should be sent to the microbiology lab for cultures.

Removal of transorbital intracranial foreign bodies should be removed in coordination with neurosurgery. Some cases may best be managed with direct visualization via a craniotomy [8], as was done in our case, and others may be managed with removal and close neurological monitoring and post-operative imaging. Sometimes neurosurgery does not recommend retrieval of the foreign body, like a BB, if the risks outweigh the benefits of removal. Like was completed in our case, often transorbital intracranial foreign bodies are removed via an orbital approach [1, 3]. Therefore, we recommend consultation of oculoplastic surgery for assistance with the orbital dissection. After removal of the foreign body, the globe should be closely explored for any evidence of open globe injury and repaired if an injury is found. This case was not found to have an open globe, however, the potential risk of concurrent open globe was high given the initial examination.

Another case with an intracranial foreign body that did have open globe injury includes a 14 year-old-boy who was hit with a BB from a BB gun who presented with no light perception vision in the left eye with the BB lodged in the left frontal lobe (Fig. 39.5). Neurosurgical intervention was deferred due to the risk of retrieving the BB. The patient then underwent open globe repair and was found to have an entry site at the temporal limbus and also a very posterior exit wound superiorly. The patient remained no light perception post-operatively and subsequently underwent enucleation for a blind painful eye.

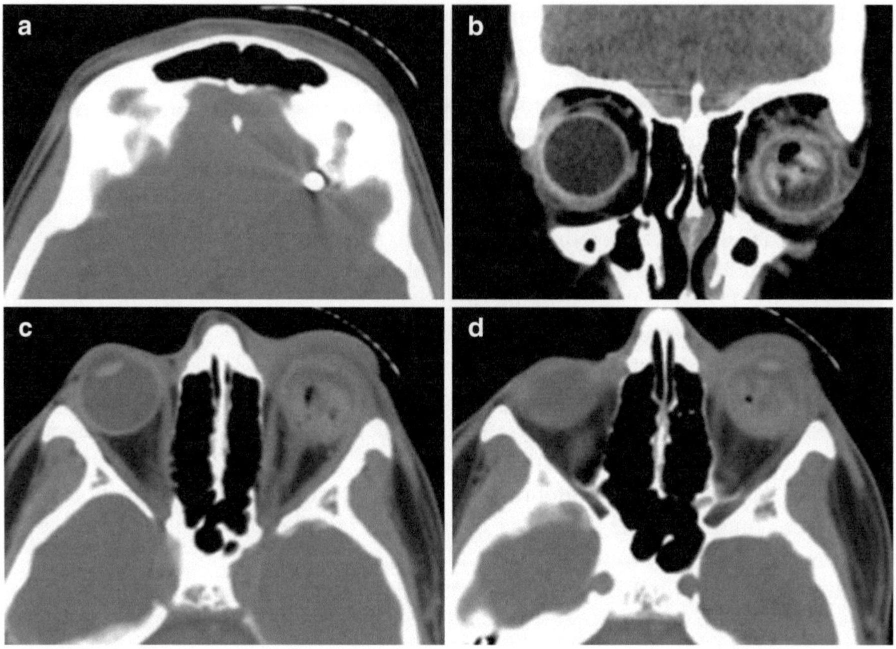

Fig. 39.5 Axial CT image (**a**) of a 14 year-old-boy who was hit with a BB that traversed the left globe and was found in the left inferior frontal lobe. Coronal (**b**) and axial (**c**, **d**) CT images showing irregular contour to the left globe with intraocular air and hemorrhage concerning for an open globe injury

Sclopetaria, or a large area of choroidal and retinal rupture and necrosis with significant subretinal, retinal and vitreous hemorrhage, can result from a high-speed missile injury to the orbit. As the blood resorbs overtime, extensive scar formation and pigmentary changes are seen. The ocular damage is thought to be caused by the shock waves that are generated by the deceleration of the high-speed projectile passing close to the globe. Most groups have found that retinal detachment rarely occurs with sclopetaria [11, 12]. However, our group recently reported on three consecutive cases of retinal detachment from sclopeteria [13]. These patients need to be given careful retinal detachment precautions and should be monitored closely by a retina specialist after the injury.

39.8 Key Learning Points

- A high level of suspicion should be established for transorbital intracranial foreign bodies based on the history and mechanism of injury, as a patient's external injuries may be trivial compared to the severity of their injury.

- Pupillary light reflexes are critical to a multi-system traumatic evaluation and should be carefully reviewed by both neurosurgery/neurology and ophthalmology before dilation. It is important to discuss dilation with neurosurgery prior to dilation and inform all members of the medical team when dilation drops are placed.
- In cases with concurrent intracranial injury, it is important to facilitate urgent imaging and neurosurgical evaluation. These patients will need to be closely co-managed with the neurosurgical team to coordinate the safest time for surgical intervention, combined surgical procedures, and post-operative neurological monitoring. Combined surgeries may require that the ophthalmic surgeon adapt to an unusual microscope, instruments, and patient position due to patient safety requirements.
- Patients with sclopetaria should be observed carefully over the months following eye trauma due to the risk of retinal detachment.

References

1. Ahmad SS, et al. 5-year-old girl with left upper eyelid swelling. Digit J Ophthalmol. 2012;18(4):15–7.
2. Turbin RE, et al. Patterns of transorbital intracranial injury: a review and comparison of occult and non-occult cases. Surv Ophthalmol. 2006;51(5):449–60.
3. Shin TH, et al. Transorbital penetrating intracranial injury by a chopstick. J Korean Neurosurg Soc. 2012;52(4):414–6.
4. Parajuli A, et al. A case of transorbital intracranial injury presenting with subtle neurological deficit. Nepal J Ophthalmol. 2015;7(14):186–90.
5. Skoch J, Ansay TL, Lemole GM. Injury to the temporal lobe via medial transorbital entry of a toothbrush. J Neurol Surg Rep. 2013;74(1):23–8.
6. Schreckinger M, et al. Transorbital penetrating injury: case series, review of the literature, and proposed management algorithm. J Neurosurg. 2011;114(1):53–61.
7. Strub WM, Weiss KL. Self-inflicted transorbital and intracranial injury from eyeglasses. Emerg Radiol. 2003;10(2):109–11.
8. Riley JP, et al. The role of intraoperative cerebral angiography in transorbital intracranial penetrating trauma: a case report and literature review. World Neurosurg. 2017;**97**:761 e5–761 e10.
9. Lunetta P, Ohberg A, Sajantila A. Suicide by intracerebellar ballpoint pen. Am J Forens Med Pathol. 2002;23(4):334–7.
10. Wieland AM, et al. Management of a long-standing organic intracranial foreign body. Skull Base. 2010;20(6):487–90.
11. Ahmadabadi MN, et al. Clinical presentation and outcome of chorioretinitis sclopetaria: a case series study. Injury. 2010;41(1):82–5.
12. Martin DF, et al. Treatment and pathogenesis of traumatic chorioretinal rupture (sclopetaria). Am J Ophthalmol. 1994;117(2):190–200.
13. Papakostas TD, et al. Retinal detachment associated with traumatic chorioretinal rupture. Ophthalmic Surg Lasers Imaging Retina. 2014;45(5):451–5.

Chapter 40
Case 35: Orbital Foreign Body with Concern for Open Globe Requiring Exploration

Isaiah Giese, Thanos D. Papakostas, Seanna Grob, and John B. Miller

40.1 History of Present Illness

A 17-year-old healthy man presents with concern for open globe of the right eye.

- That morning he was hammering a nail into a plaster wall without eye protection when he felt pain and decreased vision in the right eye.
- He immediately went to an outside hospital where a computed tomography (CT) scan demonstrated concern for an intraocular foreign body, and the patient was transferred to Massachusetts Eye and Ear for further management.

40.2 Initial Trauma Evaluation

40.2.1 Visual Acuity (Without Correction)

OD: Counting fingers at 2 feet
OS: 20/20

I. Giese, M.D. (✉) • T. D. Papakostas, M.D. • S. Grob, M.D., M.A.S.
Department of Ophthalmology, Harvard Medical School, Massachusetts Eye and Ear, Boston, MA, USA
e-mail: Isaiah_giese@meei.harvard.edu

J. B. Miller, M.D.
Vitreoretinal Surgery, Department of Ophthalmology, Harvard Medical School, Massachusetts Eye and Ear, Boston, MA, USA

S. Grob, C. Kloek (eds.), *Management of Open Globe Injuries*,
https://doi.org/10.1007/978-3-319-72410-2_40

40.2.2 Pupils

OD: Mid-dilated, sluggish, minimally reactive, no afferent pupillary defect by reverse
OS: Reacts briskly to light

40.2.3 Intraocular Pressure

OD: 14 mmHg
OS: 17 mmHg

40.2.4 External Examination

Unremarkable

40.2.5 Slit Lamp Examination

	OD	OS
Lids and lashes	Normal	Normal
Sclera and conjunctiva	Nasal conjunctival laceration with seemingly intact sclera	Normal
Cornea	Clear	Normal
Anterior chamber	4+ red blood cells, no hyphema	Normal
Iris	Mid-dilated, no peaking	Normal
Lens	Normal	Normal
Vitreous	1+ vitreous hemorrhage	Normal

40.2.6 Dilated Examination

Macula/Nerve OD: Disc drusen, macular hole (Figs. 40.1a and 40.2)
Periphery OD: Extensive commotio retinae, diffuse inferonasal pre-retinal hemorrhage (Fig. 40.1a)
Macula/Nerve: OS: Disc drusen
Periphery OS: Normal (Fig. 40.1b)

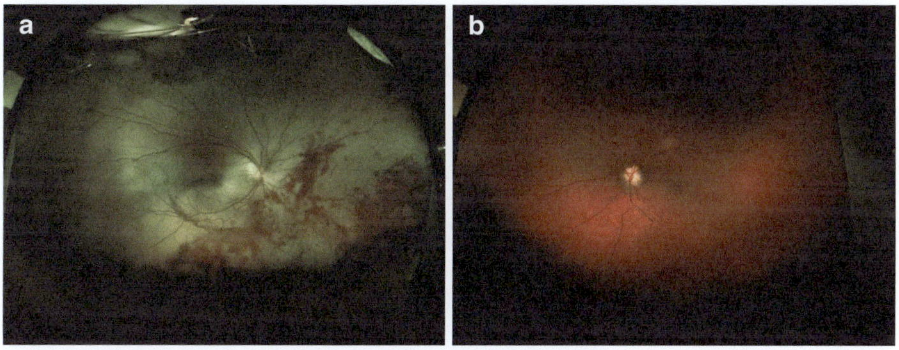

Fig. 40.1 Optos fundus photographs of the right (**a**) and left (**b**) eyes. The fundus photograph of the right eye (**a**) shows diffuse retinal whitening suggesting significant commotio retinae and scattered vitreous and retinal hemorrhage inferiorly and inferonasally. The fundus photograph of the left eye shows a normal fundus

Fig. 40.2 OCT macula of the right eye showing a traumatic macular hole

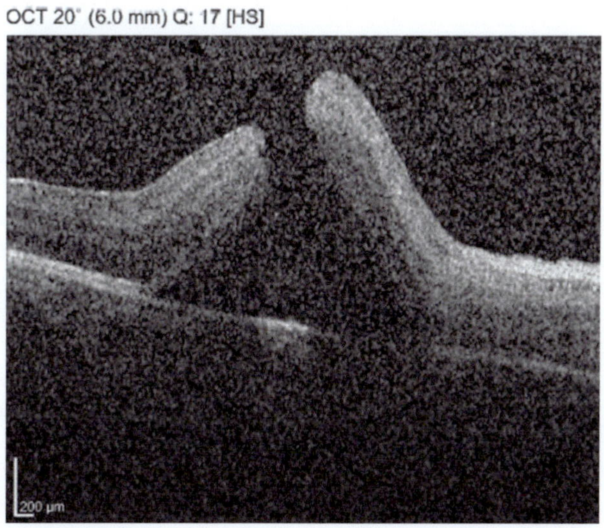

40.2.7 Radiographic Imaging

CT of the orbits demonstrated an inferonasal intraorbital foreign body directly adjacent to the globe with scatter artifact (Fig. 40.3). There was no fracture. Optic nerve head drusen was also noted bilaterally.

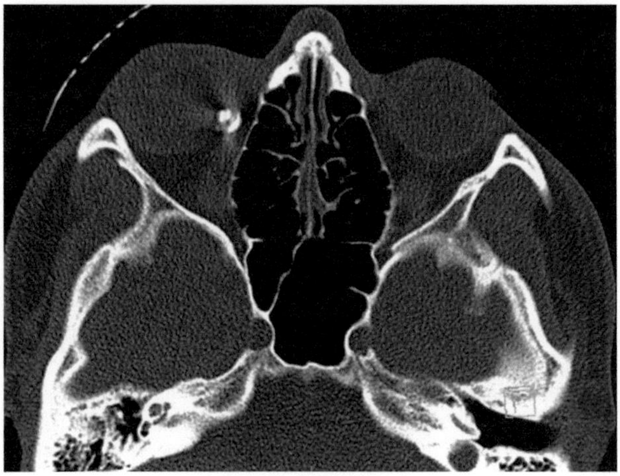

Fig. 40.3 Maxillofacial CT scan, bone window and axial cut, showing a medial metallic intraorbital foreign body immediately adjacent to the right globe with scatter artifact

40.3 Surgeon's Initial Assessment and Pre-Operative Plan

This patient presented with a high-velocity projectile injury to the right orbit and a medial conjunctival laceration. There was no visible evidence of scleral laceration on slit lamp examination and exploration of the conjunctival laceration. The intraocular pressure was normal. The inferonasal view of the retina was obscured by vitreous and pre-retinal hemorrhage. A CT scan of the orbit demonstrated a retrobulbar foreign body, though the metallic foreign body produced scatter artifact that again made it difficult to evaluate the contour of the globe. Given that the metallic foreign body appeared to be abutting the globe on imaging and there was not a clear view to this area intraocularly due to hemorrhage, surgical exploration was performed for definitive evaluation of the globe.

This case illustrates two important points: (1) the necessity of surgical exploration in orbital trauma where there is uncertainty regarding the integrity of the globe, and (2) the intraocular injuries and complications that result from periocular trauma.

The first goal in the management of ocular trauma is establishing the magnitude of injury. A critical first step is the expedited assessment of whether one is dealing with an open globe injury or closed globe injury. Many cases of open globe injuries are unequivocal, such as clear penetrating or perforating injuries with expulsion of intraocular contents, or a grossly deflated globe on CT imaging. Alternatively, some cases are more nuanced, such as conjunctival lacerations that tunnel posteriorly, injuries such as hyphema or vitreous hemorrhage that limit the view of the fundus, and injuries in children where poor cooperation makes evaluation in an examination room nearly impossible. The case presented here included a nasal conjunctival laceration with an inferonasal foreign body in the posterior orbit on CT imaging. Fundoscopic assessment of the region of interest (the inferonasal retina) was obscured by hemorrhage. In cases such as this, the only way to definitively rule out an open globe is to perform a peritomy whereby the conjunctiva is reflected away from the globe and an intact sclera is confirmed with direct visualization. There was a clear intraocular view to the superior retina which did not show any full-thickness lacerations, so the area that required exploration intraoperatively was the inferior and nasal quadrants, specifically inferonasally where the track of the foreign body was noted.

40.4 Surgical Exploration and Repair: Operative Note

The risks, benefits, and alternatives were discussed with the patient pre-operatively and the patient consented to proceed with exploration and repair of a potential open globe injury. The patient was brought to the operating room where the anesthesia team proceeded with general anesthesia. A careful time-out was observed and the correct patient and the eye were identified. The right eye was prepped and draped in the usual sterile ophthalmic fashion using a Jaffe speculum to provide adequate exposure.

A 270° peritomy was initiated from 12 o'clock until 9 o'clock. Gentle exploration with blunt dissection into 3 quadrants (superonasal, inferonasal, inferotemporal) was performed initially with Westcott scissors followed by curved Stevens scissors to evaluate for posterior eye trauma. The medial and inferior rectus were hooked with a Gass muscle hook followed by a 2-0 silk suture and the sclera beneath the muscle insertions was examined carefully. The patient was found to have an intact globe. There was no evidence of scleral injury on examination. The eye maintained its pressure throughout the surgical exploration. The orbital foreign body was not identified during the globe exploration.

The conjunctiva was then closed with interrupted 8-0 Vicryl sutures. A subconjunctival steroid and antibiotic injection was performed temporally. The speculum was removed. The patient's drape was removed under the microscope. The patient tolerated the procedure well without any complications.

40.4.1 Surgical Exploration and Repair: Pearls

- In cases of unclear globe injury (i.e. 360° bullous subconjunctival hemorrhage, tunneled conjunctival lacerations, foreign bodies abutting the globe, obscured intraocular view due to hemorrhage), especially in the setting of a projectile injury, the patient should be taken to the operating room and a peritomy performed with scleral exploration to directly visualize the status of the globe.

40.5 Post-Operative Course

Once an open globe injury was ruled out, the patient was subsequently managed primarily by the retina service. Spontaneous closure of the traumatic macular hole occurred by the second week visit, and the extensive area of commotio retinae and sclopeteria was observed by the retina service. Unfortunately, the patient developed proliferative vitreoretinopathy and tractional membranes that created a tractional retinal detachment (Fig. 40.4).

The tractional detachment was repaired surgically by careful dissection, elevation and removal of the pre-retinal membranes. Heavy barricade laser was applied nasally in order to wall off the nasal area of sclopeteria, hemorrhage, and shallow subretinal fluid. Given the patient's young age and unclear compliance with the strict positioning required of gas, the retinal detachment was tamponaded with silicone oil. The retina flattened and the nasal area and associated laser scarred down nicely. Five months later the patient underwent silicone oil removal. At 12 months after his initial injury, the patient's visual acuity had improved to 20/200 and his retina remained attached (Fig. 40.5).

The patient was also evaluated by the oculofacial surgery service who elected to observe the orbital foreign body as it was not causing the patient significant complications. Furthermore, the high pressure required to explore the deep orbit should be avoided, if possible, in the setting of multiple intraocular surgeries.

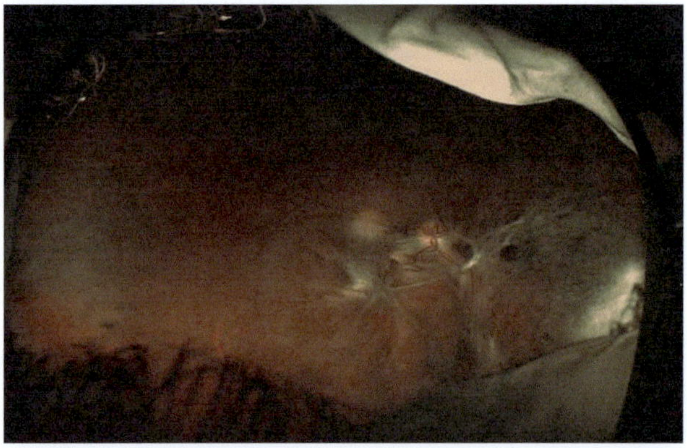

Fig. 40.4 Optos fundus photos at 3 months after trauma showing an inferonasal tractional retinal detachment

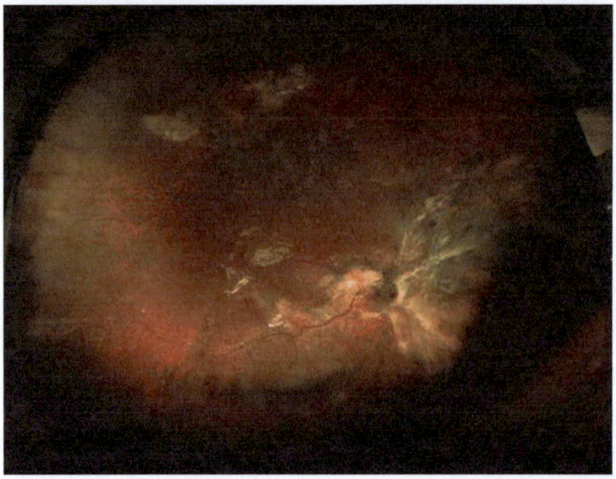

Fig. 40.5 Optos fundus photos at 12 months after trauma showing inferonasal evidence of sclopetaria with scarring

40.6 Final Trauma Evaluation

40.6.1 Final Visual Acuity (Without Correction)

OD: 20/200
OS: 20/20

40.6.2 Pupils

OD: Dilated (pharmacologic, on atropine)
OS: Reacts briskly to light

40.6.3 Slit Lamp Examination

	OD	OS
Lids and lashes	Normal	Normal
Sclera and conjunctiva	Vicryl conjunctival sutures intact	Normal
Cornea	Normal	Normal
Anterior chamber	3+ cell, 1+ flare	Normal
Iris	Pharmacologically dilated	Normal
Lens	Clear silicone oil emulsification on posterior capsule, 1+ posterior subcapsular cataract	Normal
Vitreous	Status post pars plana vitrectomy, silicone oil	Normal

40.6.4 Dilated Examination

Macula/Nerve OD: Disc drusen, epiretinal membrane with pigment changes
Periphery OD: Sclopeteria nasally. Traction nasally and subretinal fluid with some hemorrhage. Good laser reaction inferiorly and nasally, and otherwise attached retina (Fig. 40.5)
Macula/Nerve: OS: Disc drusen
Periphery OS: Normal

40.7 Review and Lessons Learned

Suspected open globe injuries require a thorough history, comprehensive ophthalmology exam, and ancillary testing when indicated, such as an orbital CT scan. If there is uncertainty of an open globe injury, then patients should undergo exploratory surgery for confirmation, including takedown of the conjunctiva and/or hooking of the extraocular muscles and examination of the sclera posterior to the muscle insertion sites to directly visualize the entire globe for injury.

Intraorbital foreign bodies can be challenging to recover intraoperatively. When foreign bodies pose a risk to the patient, such as with organic matter at high risk for infection, persistent inflammation, or strabismus, then they should be removed. Alternatively, inorganic intraorbital foreign bodies can often be observed without consequence to the patient [1].

Even in the absence of an open globe injury, orbital trauma and intraorbital projectiles can result in severe vision loss. Once an open globe injury is ruled out, attention was subsequently turned to investigating concurrent sight threatening injuries, such as macular holes and commotio retinae as seen in this case. Traumatic macular holes are one of the complications of closed globe injuries and can cause severe vision loss. While some traumatic macular holes do require surgical intervention, an initial period of observation is typically recommended. A recent large case series showed that approximately 40% of traumatic macular holes will close spontaneously, with even higher closure rates seen in the pediatric population [2]. Commotio retinae is an injury to the outer retinal layers following orbital trauma that results in retinal whitening on exam. Macular involvement frequently causes vision loss. Fortunately, many patients experience some improvement in visual acuity following injury, however, many do not experience a full recovery to their pre-injury baseline acuity [3].

40.8 Key Learning Points

- If the clinical ophthalmological exam cannot rule out an open globe injury (i.e. 360° bullous subconjunctival hemorrhage with no view posteriorly, tunneled conjunctival laceration and/or foreign bodies abutting the globe on imaging with no clear view intraocularly to rule out full-thickness lacerations, obscured intraocular view due to hemorrhage), then a patient should undergo surgical exploration for definitive evaluation.
- Projectile injuries that do not violate the globe can nonetheless result in significant intraocular injury, such as commotio retinae, sclopetaria, traumatic macular holes, and vitreous hemorrhage. Visual outcomes from these injuries is variable, and management can often span multiple ophthalmological subspecialties.

References

1. Callahan AB, Yoon MK. Intraorbital foreign bodies: retrospective chart review and review of literature. Int Ophthalmol Clin. 2013;53(4):157–65.
2. Miller JB, Yonekawa Y, Eliott D, Kim IK, Kim LA, Loewenstein JI, Sobrin L, Young LH, Mukai S, Vavvas DG. Long-term follow-up and outcomes in traumatic macular holes. Am J Ophthalmol. 2015;160(6):1255–8.
3. Blanch RJ, Good PA, Shah P, Bishop JR, Logan A, Scott RA. Visual outcomes after blunt ocular trauma. Ophthalmology. 2013;120(8):1588–91.

Chapter 41
Case 36: Bilateral Open Globe Injury Stemming from an Assault

Tomasz P. Stryjewski, Tavé van Zyl, John B. Miller, and Seanna Grob

41.1 History of Present Illness

A 53-year-old male prisoner with a past medical history of atrial fibrillation on warfarin, hepatitis C, and hypertension was transferred to the Massachusetts General Hospital after suffering extensive facial trauma, including bilateral open globe injuries, following a prison assault.

- The assault occurred using a makeshift prison weapon (a padlock within a sock, swung like a flail, striking the victim's face).
- He was transferred to an outside hospital where he underwent a computed tomography (CT) scan (Figs. 41.1 and 41.2) and was transferred to Massachusetts General Hospital (MGH) for further care. On arrival to MGH, bilateral canthotomy and cantholysis procedures were performed by a different subspecialty service.
- Ophthalmology was then consulted and the patient was found to have a Zone I/II open globe injury (rupture) with uveal prolapse of the right eye (Fig. 41.3), a Zone I/II/III open globe injury (rupture) with uveal prolapse of the left eye (Fig. 41.4), and a left orbital floor, zygomaticomaxillary complex (ZMC), and nasal bone fracture.

T. P. Stryjewski, M.D. (✉) • T. van Zyl, M.D. • S. Grob, M.D., M.A.S.
Department of Ophthalmology, Harvard Medical School, Massachusetts Eye and Ear, Boston, MA, USA
e-mail: Tomasz_stryjewski@meei.harvard.edu

J. B. Miller, M.D.
Vitreoretinal Surgery, Department of Ophthalmology, Harvard Medical School, Massachusetts Eye and Ear, Boston, MA, USA

S. Grob, C. Kloek (eds.), *Management of Open Globe Injuries*,
https://doi.org/10.1007/978-3-319-72410-2_41

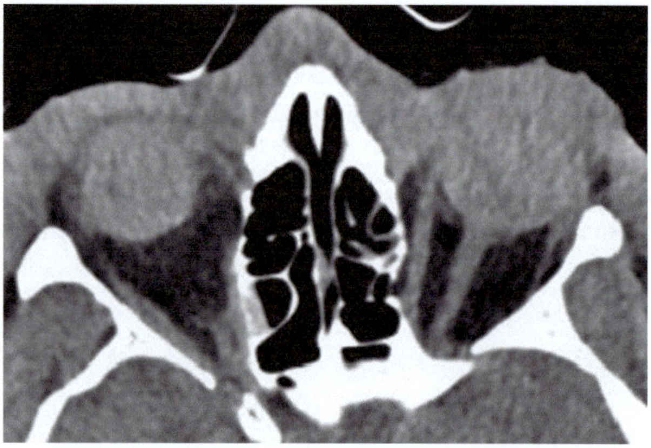

Fig. 41.1 Axial CT imaging showing irregular globe contours bilaterallay with diffuse intraocular hyperdensity

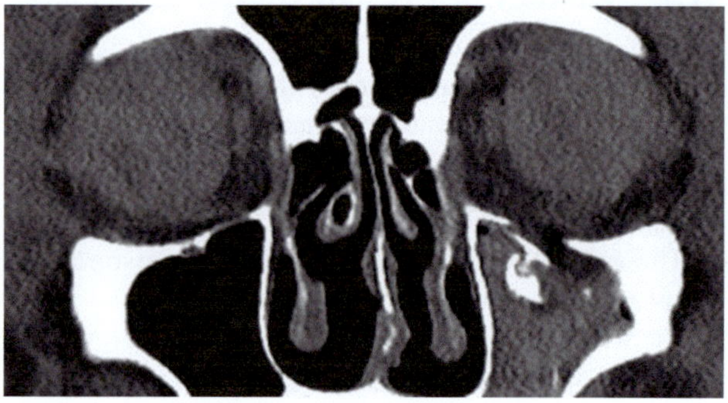

Fig. 41.2 Coronal CT image demonstrating similar findings with deformed globe contour, as well as a left orbital floor fracture

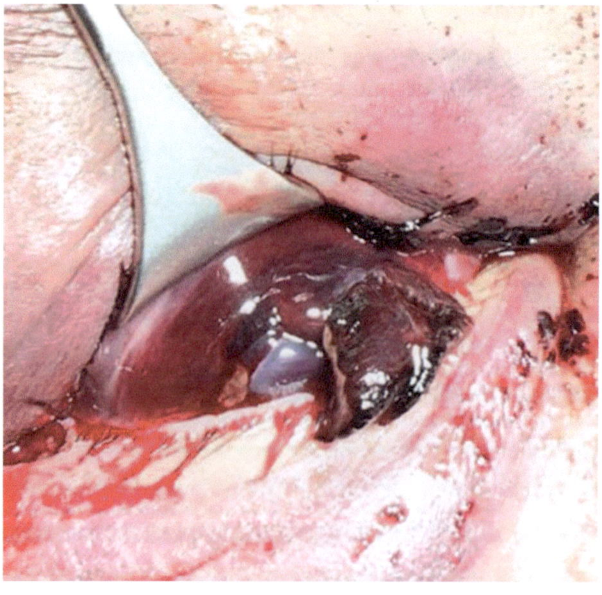

Fig. 41.3 Pre-operative photo of the right eye showing periobital edema and ecchymosis requiring gentle Desmarres retraction for clinical exam with 360° subconjunctival hemorrhage and extensive uveal prolapse superiorly

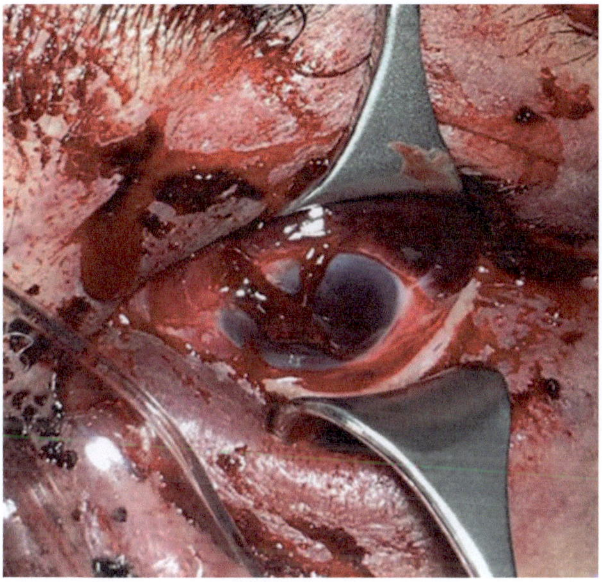

Fig. 41.4 Pre-operative photo of the left eye showing periobital edema and ecchymosis requiring gentle Desmarres retraction for clinical exam with 360° subconjunctival hemorrhage with a limbus to limbus oblique full-thickness corneal laceration extending through the limbus superonasally

41.2 Initial Trauma Evaluation

41.2.1 Visual Acuity (Without Correction)

OD: No light perception
OS: Light perception

41.2.2 Pupils

OD: Not visible due to hemorrhage
OS: Not visible due to hemorrhage

41.2.3 External Examination

OD: Periorbital edema, ecchymosis, status post lateral canthotomy
OS: Periorbital edema, ecchymosis, 4 cm brow laceration laterally, 1 cm brow laceration medially, status post lateral canthotomy

41.2.4 Slit Lamp Examination

	OD	OS
Lids and lashes	Right lower lid non-marginal laceration; status post lateral canthotomy	Status post lateral canthotomy
Sclera and conjunctiva	Bullous subconjunctival hemorrhage	Bullous subconjunctival hemorrhage
Cornea	Edematous, covered by prolapsed uveal tissue	Limbus to limbus laceration from 10:00 to 5:00 o'clock
Anterior chamber	Total hyphema	Total hyphema
Iris	No view	No view
Lens	No view	No view
Vitreous	No view	No view

41.2.5 Dilated Examination

No view bilaterally

41.2.6 Radiographic Imaging

CT of the orbits (Figs. 41.1 and 41.2) showed a left orbital floor blowout fracture and ZMC and nasal bone fractures and diffuse hyperdensities within both globes, suggestive of intraocular hemorrhage, and moderate soft tissue swelling overlying the bilateral aspects of the frontal bones extending into the periorbital regions bilaterally.

41.3 Surgeon's Initial Assessment and Pre-Operative Plan

Bilateral open globe injuries are rare, catastrophic events and are associated with a high risk of irreversible blindness [1, 2]. This case was particularly severe with no light perception in one eye and light perception only in the other eye. Setting appropriate expectations is prudent in all cases of open globe trauma but is especially pertinent in bilateral cases where the probability of blindness is high. The visual acuity should be checked and repeated to confirm the pre-operative visual acuity. This patient was consistently seeing light in the left eye pre-operatively with no light perception on the right. Due to this finding and the pre-operative examination showing severe open globe injuries bilaterally, an extensive discussion regarding the poor visual prognosis was completed prior to proceeding to the operating room.

All attempts to salvage the eyes should be undertaken in cases of severe bilateral globe injuries, as these patients especially need any possible level of visual acuity preserved. Even light perception vision is important so these patients can determine the time of day (day or night).

Patients who have been assaulted need a full trauma survey prior to proceeding to the operating room. More severe, life-threatening injuries, such as an intracranial hemorrhage, need to be ruled out prior to open globe repair. Depending on the trauma burden, other surgical specialties may need to intervene surgically prior to open globe repair. If this is the case, then fox shields should be placed over both eyes and all other services involved should be contacted and notified of the open globe injuries and the importance of not manipulating the eyes or periocular area. If the patient is stable for open globe repair, then these patients should proceed to the operating room as soon as possible for bilateral open globe repair.

The significant periocular hemorrhage on presentation in this patient concerned the evaluating team for potential retrobulbar hemorrhage, leading to bilateral canthotomies. However, in cases concerning for open globe injury, the least amount of periocular manipulation is important in preventing extrusion of intraocular contents.

41.4 Surgical Exploration and Repair: Operative Note

The patient was brought to the operating room where the anesthesia team proceeded with general anesthesia. A careful time-out was observed and the correct patient and both eyes were identified.

The left eye was repaired first since the patient was able to see light out of this eye prior to surgery (compared to no light perception in the right eye). The left eye was prepped and draped in the usual sterile ophthalmic fashion using a Jaffe speculum to provide adequate exposure. The patient was found to have a limbus to limbus corneal laceration with uveal prolapse extending from 5:30 to 11 o'clock. Then it crossed the limbus and extended into the superotemporal quadrant approximately 8 mm posterior to the limbus. First the limbus was approximated at 11 o'clock using a 9-0 nylon suture. The uveal tissues was gently reposited into the eye. Then the corneal laceration was repaired using multiple interrupted 10-0 nylon sutures. The iris spatula was used while suturing to prevent uveal incarceration in the wound. Once all the sutures were placed, they were adjusted to similar tension and then tied down and the knots were rotated. A peritomy was initiated superiorly around 12 o'clock and extended to about 8 o'clock. Gentle exploration with blunt dissection was performed with Westcott scissors followed by Stevens scissors to evaluate the posterior extent of the lesion. The end of the rupture site was found approximately 8 mm posterior to the limbus in the superonasal quadrant. Multiple 8-0 nylon sutures were placed to close the scleral rupture. Further exploration was completed to ensure complete closure of the rupture site. A fluorescein strip was then used to check for any corneal wound leaks and none were noted. The conjunctiva was then closed with interrupted 8-0 Vicryl sutures. A subconjunctival steroid and antibiotic injection was performed temporally away from the rupture site. The speculum was removed. Atropine and maxitrol ointment were placed in the eye.

Then attention was turned to the periocular lacerations on the left. The left upper eyelid lesion was repaired using 5-0 plain gut interrupted sutures. The left brow laceration was repaired using multiple deep interrupted 5-0 Vicryl sutures to approximate the wound edges. Then multiple interrupted 5-0 plain gut sutures were placed to repair the laceration. The patient's drape was removed under the microscope. The periocular area was cleaned. A sterile eye pad and shield were placed over the left eye.

Then attention was turned to the right eye. The staff and surgeons re-scrubbed and a new set of ophthalmic instruments was used for the right eye. The right eye was prepped and draped in the usual sterile ophthalmic fashion using a Jaffe speculum to provide adequate exposure. Extensive uveal prolapse was noted from the superior rupture site. A large portion of ciliary body was visible in this uveal tissue. The eye was noted to be significantly deflated. A peritomy was initiated at 3 o'clock and extended until 7 o'clock. A large corneoscleral laceration was noted extending from 8 o'clock to 1 o'clock following the limbus and then extended further into the sclera towards the superonasal quadrant for approximately 4 mm. The uveal tissue was gently reposited into the intraocular space. The limbus was reapproximated with a 9-0 nylon suture at 1 o'clock. The scleral rupture was repaired with several interrupted 8-0 nylon sutures. Then multiple sutures radial to the limbus were placed to approximate the corneoscleral laceration that followed the limbal contour. The iris spatula was used to prevent uveal incarceration in the wound. The suture knots were rotated away from the visual axis. Further exploration into the quadrants was then completed to ensure complete closure of the rupture. The sclera was noted to be significantly irregular since the eye was deflated, but no other scleral ruptures were noted. The conjunctiva was then closed with interrupted 8-0 Vicryl sutures. A subconjunctival steroid and antibiotic injection was performed inferiorly away from the rupture site. The speculum was removed. Atropine and maxitrol ointment were placed in the eye.

Then attention was turned to the periocular laceration on the right. The right lower eyelid lesion was repaired using 6-0 plain gut interrupted sutures. The patient's drape was removed under the microscope. The periocular area was cleaned. A sterile eye pad and shield were placed over the right eye.

41.4.1 Surgical Exploration and Repair: Pearls

- When performing bilateral same day eye surgery, it is important to use entirely separate instruments and re-prep when switching to the other eye.
- Consider repairing the better seeing eye first.

- Make sure a fox shield is placed over the eye not being operated on in every case, but this is especially important in bilateral open globe cases so that pressure is not accidently placed on the eye under the surgical drape.

41.5 Post-Operative Course

Interestingly, the vision post-operatively was consistently light perception in the right eye and no light perception in the left eye (opposite of pre-operative vision) (Figs. 41.5 and 41.6). The left eye was deemed non-operative due to the consistent no light perception vision.

An ultrasound performed of the right eye showed choroidal hemorrhages and a funnel retinal detachment that was referred to retina for repair (Fig. 41.7).

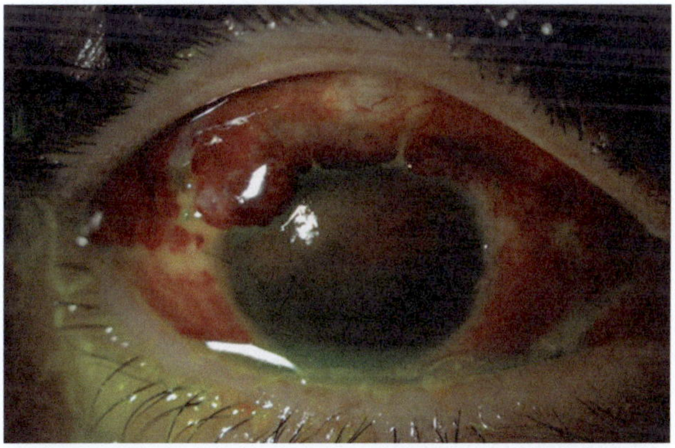

Fig. 41.5 Right eye, post-operative week 1 showing 360° improving subconjunctival hemorrhage with the limbal repaired rupture site well-covered by conjunctiva superiorly, corneal edema, and a poor intraocular view due to intraocular hemorrhage

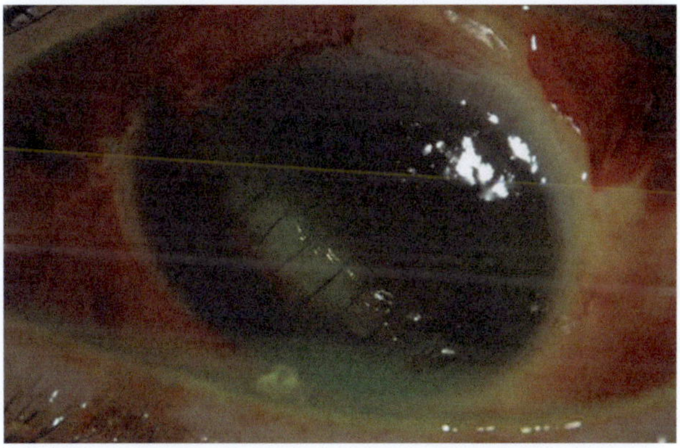

Fig. 41.6 Left eye, post-operative week 1 showing 360° improving subconjunctival hemorrhage with a repaired limbus to limbus oblique corneal laceration with nylon sutures in place and the scleral laceration well-covered by conjunctiva superonasally

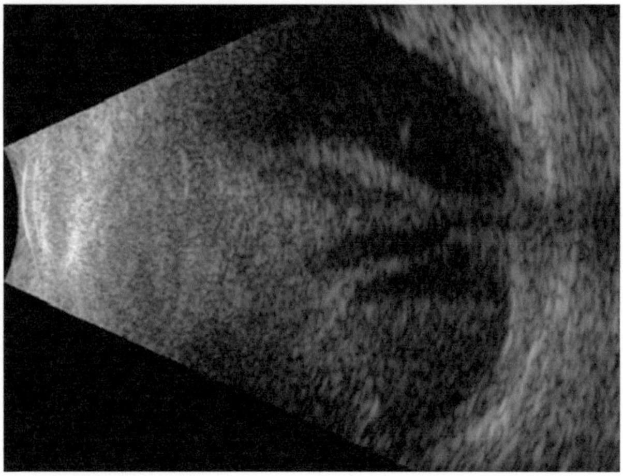

Fig. 41.7 B scan ultrasound of the right eye showing a retinal detachment overlying the optic nerve

For the right eye, 5 weeks after initial globe repair, the patient underwent choroidal drainage and 23 gauge pars plana vitrectomy for a funnel retinal detachment, but ultimately the retina could not be reattached. The patient expired due to unrelated causes 3 months later.

41.6 Final Trauma Evaluation

41.6.1 Final Visual Acuity

OD: Light perception
OS: No light perception

41.6.2 Pupils

Irregular and poorly reactive bilaterally

41.6.3 Slit Lamp Examination

	OD	OS
Lids and lashes	Healing laceration	Normal
Sclera and conjunctiva	Subconjunctival hemorrhage; good conjunctival apposition at limbus	White and quiet

	OD	OS
Cornea	2+ Descemet membrane folds	Well apposed limbus to limbus laceration
Anterior chamber	Total hyphema	Total hyphema
Iris	No view	No view
Lens	No view	No view
Vitreous	No view	No view

41.6.4 Dilated Examination

Poor view bilaterally

41.7 Review and Lessons Learned

If there is a high suspicion for an open globe injury on clinical exam, it is extremely important that ophthalmology be contacted immediately. A protective shield should be placed over the eye and the least amount of manipulation of the eye should be encouraged. Further manipulation of the globe or the periorbital tissues can cause extrusion of intraocular contents. Procedures of the eyelids or face should be avoided if possible if an open globe is suspected.

All efforts should be made to obtain a pre-operative visual acuity. If the vision is found to be no light perception (NLP), then the vision should be rechecked to confirm this finding, as this will often change the pre-operative discussion with the patient. However, pre-operative vision in the setting of severe eye trauma may be somewhat unreliable at times. Patients are often very scared about the prognosis of their eye. It may be difficult for them to cooperate with a vision test. However, even if a patient refuses to open their eye, you can still check light perception vision through the eyelid. There are times, as with this case, where a patient is noted to be NLP prior to surgery and light perception (LP) after. The cause of this is uncertain, but may be due in part to the state of mind of the patient. This is mentioned because we recommend making every attempt to close an open globe even if it is NLP, as sometimes, light perception or other vision is noted post-operatively. When LP vision is noted post-operatively, then patients are referred to the retina service for evaluation of secondary surgeries for vision rehabilitation. If NLP vision persists post-operatively, then options can be discussed with the patient. It is more common though to see the opposite, where a patient comes in with LP or bare LP vision and over the early post-operative days this is lost. This should be communicated to the patient prior to open globe repair.

Bilateral simultaneous open globe injuries are much less common than unilateral open globe injuries and can be devastating. As discussed previously, every attempt should be made to close the globes and save the remaining vision. Extra precautions should be taken in the operating room as well. As is often done with bilateral cataract surgery cases, we recommend treating each eye separately and re-scrubbing and prepping after completion of globe repair on one side. We also open a separate sterile table and instrument set for the second eye. We also address the better seeing eye first during globe repair. A protective shield should always be placed over the eye that is not being operated on (which we do even in cases that are not bilateral open globes). If visual prognosis is poor bilaterally, then patients should be referred to social work or other hospital services to help them get connected to the Commission for the Blind or other organization early.

41.8 Key Learning Points

- Bilateral open globe injuries are rare and often catastrophic occurrences.
- Canthotomies should be avoided in cases of suspected open globe injury due to the risk of iatrogenic damage to the globe and further expulsion of intraocular contents.
- When operating on both eyes the same day, the surgeon should re-prep before operating on the second eye and utilize new gowns and instrument trays.

References

1. Knyazer B, Bilenko N, Levy J, Lifshitz T, Belfair N, Klemperer I, Yagev R. Open globe eye injury characteristics and prognostic factors in Southern Israel: a retrospective epidemiologic review of 10 years experience. Isr Med Assoc J. 2013;15(3):158–62.
2. Nguyen HV, Talcott KE, Lorch A, Chee Y, Kloek C, Eliott D, Grob SR. 2017. Bilateral open globe injuries at a Tertiary Care Center. ARVO Annual Conference, Poster Number 5950, Poster Board Number: B0713, Baltimore, MD.

Chapter 42
Case 37: Zone I/II/III Open Globe Injury with Orbital Fractures

Ashley A. Campbell, Eric D. Gaier, Alice C. Lorch, and Yewlin E. Chee

42.1 History of Present Illness

A 29-year-old man with no past ocular history presents with concern for an open globe injury of the left eye.

- He was playing softball on the evening of presentation when a line drive hit him in the left eye.
- He noted that his vision went dark and he had immediate pain.

42.2 Initial Trauma Evaluation

42.2.1 Visual Acuity (Without Correction)

OD: 20/20
OS: Light perception

A. A. Campbell, M.D. (✉)
Department of Ophthalmology, Johns Hopkins University School of Medicine, Baltimore, MD, USA

A. C. Lorch, M.D., M.P.H. • E. D. Gaier, M.D., Ph.D.
Department of Ophthalmology, Harvard Medical School, Massachusetts Eye and Ear, Boston, MA, USA

Y. E. Chee, M.D.
Vitreoretinal Surgery, Department of Ophthalmology, University of Washington, Seattle, WA, USA

S. Grob, C. Kloek (eds.), *Management of Open Globe Injuries*,
https://doi.org/10.1007/978-3-319-72410-2_42

42.2.2 Pupils

OD: Reactive
OS: +Afferent pupillary defect by reverse

42.2.3 External Examination

Laceration measuring 3 cm over left maxilla and diffuse periorbital ecchymosis.

42.2.4 Slit Lamp Examination

	OD	OS
Lids and lashes	Normal	1 cm non-marginal left upper eyelid laceration
Sclera and conjunctiva	Normal	Diffuse chemosis and subconjunctival hemorrhage, most prominent temporally
Cornea	Normal	Limbus to limbus full-thickness corneal laceration from approximately 5 o'clock to 11:30 o'clock
Anterior chamber	Normal	Flat
Iris	Normal	Prolapsed uveal tissue nasally
Lens	Normal	No view, but possible prolapse of lens material inferiorly out of corneal wound
Vitreous	Normal	Not visualized

42.2.5 Dilated Examination

Macula/Nerve OD: Normal
Periphery OD: Normal
Macula/Nerve: OS: No view
Periphery OS: No view

42.2.6 Radiographic Imaging

Non-contrast computed tomography (CT) of the orbits showed a comminuted fracture involving the inferior wall and lateral wall of the left orbit. There were fractures of the anterior and lateral walls of the left maxillary sinus with an air-fluid level within the left maxillary sinus. There was a transverse fracture involving the superior confluence of the left pterygoid plates. There were several fractures involving the left zygomatic arch without substantial displacement. There was a

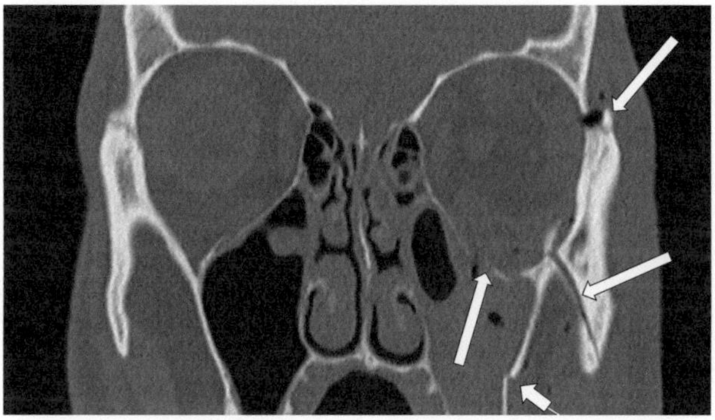

Fig. 42.1 CT Maxillofacial coronal view with arrows marking the left orbital floor fracture and the left zygomaticomaxillary complex fracture (see arrows)

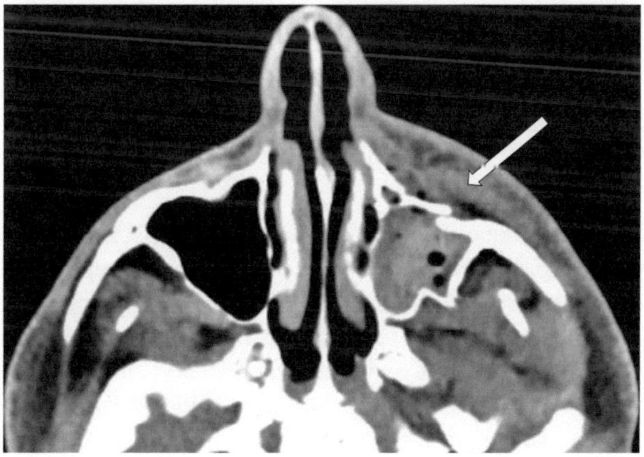

Fig. 42.2 CT Maxillofacial Axial view demonstrates inward displacement of the left anterior maxillary face (see arrow)

left-sided nasal bone fracture. There was soft tissue swelling overlying the left globe with deformation of ocular contour. The left lens was not visualized (Figs. 42.1 and 42.2).

42.3 Surgeon's Initial Assessment and Pre-operative Plan

A 29 year-old male presented status-post high velocity blunt trauma to the left eye from a softball sustaining an open globe injury and multiple left-sided facial fractures including the zygomaticomaxillary complex (ZMC) and orbital floor. He was admitted for intravenous antibiotics per protocol. The plan was for repair of the open globe injury and facial lacerations within 24 hours of his injury. The patient was counseled regarding the poor visual prognosis of the left eye given the severe nature of the injury with poor initial visual acuity and presence of an afferent pupillary defect and the possibility of future surgeries for the eye and facial fractures. The plan for the exploration and repair of the Zone I/II/II is similar to previous similar cases (see earlier chapters).

Once the open globe is suspected, it is important to place a shield over the eye and inform other services to refrain from manipulating the eye. Often in multi-trauma cases, there are several services examining the patient and minimizing manipulation of the eye is very important. Ideally, fracture repair should be postponed until the open globe has been explored and repaired and has had time to heal. Fracture repair can place pressure on the globe that could further extrude intraocular contents or uveal components. Unless the face or airway is unstable requiring urgent repair or any other emergent situation, it is recommended that the fracture repair is delayed until the globe has been repaired and has had time to heal. If the patient undergoes enucleation primarily or early after repair due to a severe open globe injury with no light perception vision, then it can be an option to repair the fractures at that time. In patients with visual potential, we would often wait at least 6 weeks before fracture repair if possible (and if repair was necessary) and potentially longer if the patient required additional eye surgeries for visual rehabilitation.

42.4 Surgical Exploration and Repair: Operative Note

The risks, benefits, and alternatives were discussed with the patient pre-operatively and the patient wished to proceed with globe repair. The patient was brought to the operating room where the anesthesia team placed the patient under general anesthesia. A careful timeout was observed and the correct patient and the eye were identified. The left eye was prepped and draped in the usual sterile ophthalmic fashion using a Jaffe speculum to provide adequate exposure.

On inspection of the globe, it was noted that there was an approximately 10 mm corneal full-thickness laceration from 11:30 to 5:00 o'clock across the central axis. A 9-0 nylon suture was placed at the limbus at 11:30 followed by adjustable interrupted sutures along the corneal laceration with 10-0 nylon sutures. After the corneal laceration was closed, filtered air was injected into the eye through a paracentesis created at the 2:00 o'clock position to reform the anterior chamber of the eye. At that time, it appeared that the cornea was closed. Attention was then turned to the scleral laceration. A 360° peritomy was created with a pair of blunt Westcott scissors. Exploration of the globe was continued posteriorly with blunt Wescott scissors followed by curved Stevens scissors. Inspection of the laceration was then made and it was noted to go far posteriorly along the superior globe. An 8-0 nylon suture was then used to place interrupted sutures along the scleral wound until the end was found, which was approximately 12 mm posterior to the limbus. The rest of the quadrants of the globe were inspected carefully with Stevens tenotomy scissors for exposure to ensure that the extent of the injury had been repaired. No other wounds were noted. An 8-0 Vicryl suture was then used to repair the conjunctiva. A fluorescein strip was then applied to all of the lacerations to ensure that the wound was sealed. The wound was noted to be Seidel negative. A subconjunctival steroid and antibiotic injection was provided.

Attention was then turned to the left upper eyelid and left upper cheek laceration. A 6-0 interrupted fast gut suture was placed at the laceration site. Steri-strips were then applied over the wounds.

The speculum was removed and the patient's drape removed under the microscope. The patient tolerated the procedure well without any complications.

42.4.1 Surgical Exploration and Repair: Pearls

- In this case, adjustable sutures were placed in the cornea so that the tension could be adjusted as the corneal laceration was closed. As mentioned previously, this is a helpful technique for long corneal lacerations.
- The Zone I portion of the laceration should be repaired prior to the Zone II/III portions in order to minimize tissue prolapse during the globe manipulation required to repair more posterior lacerations.
- Make sure to align the limbus first!
- Delay repair of facial lacerations until after the open globe has been repaired.
- Ideally, fracture repair should be postponed until after the open globe has been repaired and has had a chance to heal.

42.5 Post-operative Course

Following surgery, the patient was noted to have light perception vision and corneal sutures were intact (Fig. 42.3). He stayed admitted to the hospital to continue his course of intravenous antibiotics. He underwent a B-scan ultrasound that demonstrated a total retinal detachment with no anterior attachment points, likely representing a giant retinal tear. Hemorrhagic choroidals with clots were also present (Fig. 42.4). Five days after the initial injury, the Retina Service evaluated the patient. While counseling him that visual prognosis was poor, the patient was offered retinal detachment repair via pars plana vitrectomy with concomitant penetrating keratoplasty. After also undergoing consultation with the Cornea Service, the patient decided to not pursue further surgery.

A week after the initial injury, the patient was evaluated by facial plastics for his left ZMC fracture and orbital floor fracture. He was noted to have left midface

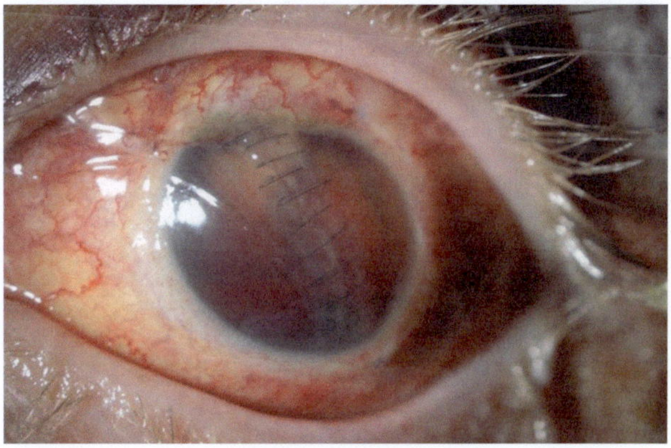

Fig. 42.3 Anterior segment photo taken on post-operative day 5 of the left eye demonstrating limbal to limbal corneal laceration after repair with 10-0 nylon sutures in place

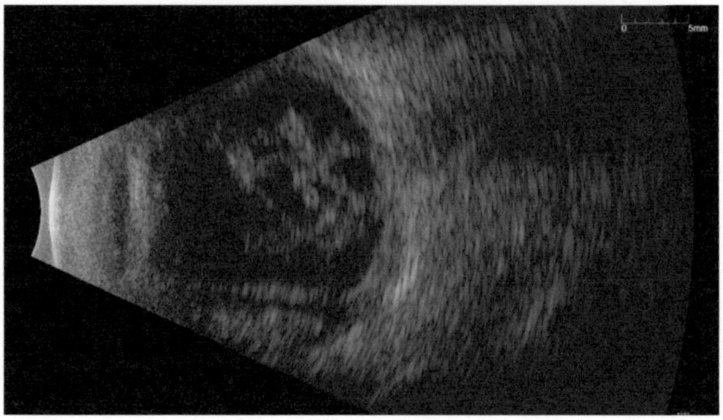

Fig. 42.4 B-scan ultrasound of the left eye 1 week after initial globe repair demonstrating a total retinal detachment with no anterior attachment points, likely representing a giant retinal tear. Hemorrhagic choroidals with clots also present

numbness. There was no malocclusion and he was able to breathe well out of his nose. Given that the ZMC fracture was minimally displaced, he was felt to not be at risk for loss of malar projection or arch depression. In addition, the orbital floor fracture was thought to be small and thereby unlikely to lead to enophthalmos. Given these findings, surgery to repair the facial fractures was not recommended.

His corneal sutures were removed over a few visits between post-operative week 6 and 12. Over time, the patient developed an exodeviation of the left eye. He was evaluated by the Contact Lens Service for a cosmetic lens but deferred given the expense. He developed neovascularization of the iris and angle and presented with a hyphema 16 months after the initial injury. The intraocular pressure remained under good control, however, and the patient was not in any pain. Given the pre-phthisical state of the eye, the patient was offered an enucleation or evisceration for cosmetic rehabilitation. At this time, the patient preferred to keep his eye.

42.6 Final Trauma Evaluation

22 months after initial injury

42.6.1 Final Visual Acuity

OD: 20/15
OS: Light perception with projection

42.6.2 Pupils

OD: Reactive
OS: +Afferent pupillary defect by reverse

42.6.3 Extraocular Muscle Exam

Small degree of exotropia.

42.6.4 External Exam

Enophthalmos of the left eye.

42.6.5 Slit Lamp Examination

	OD	OS
Lids and lashes	Normal	Left upper eyelid ptosis
Sclera and conjunctiva	Normal	Superonasal scleral sutures intact and covered under conjunctiva
Cornea	Normal	Limbal to limbal corneal scar from 5 to 11 o'clock status-post suture removal, pigment/heme on endothelium inferiorly, +deep neovascularization into the wound
Anterior chamber	Normal	Quiet, no hyphema or cell present
Iris	Normal	Irregular pupil, extensive neovascularization of the iris, dilates poorly, also with neovascularization of the angle on gonioscopy
Lens	Normal	Aphakic
Vitreous	Normal	Poor view

42.6.6 Dilated Examination

Macula/Nerve OD: Normal, cup to disc ratio 0.2
Periphery OD: Normal
Macula/Nerve: OS: Poor view
Peripheral OS: Poor view, appears detached

42.7 Review and Lessons Learned

In this case, high velocity blunt trauma from a softball line drive resulted in both a severe open globe injury and multiple facial fractures. The visual prognosis for patients with open globe injuries and concomitant orbital fractures is worse compared to patients with an open globe injury alone. In one study, it was reported that only 4.8% of patients with both an open globe and facial fractures recovered a vision of 20/400 or better after injury [1]. In a more recent study, the authors found that 29% of patients with concomitant facial fractures and open globe injuries had final visual acuities of counting fingers or better, arguing that the open globe injury should be priority in the early stages of these patients' care to optimize their visual outcomes.

The poor visual prognosis in cases of concomitant facial fractures with open globe injuries likely relates to the mechanism of injury, which is more often from blunt trauma in these cases [2]. As a result, the rupture more frequently affects multiple open globe zones compared to isolated open globe injuries [2]. Based on the (albeit limited) evidence available, it is our recommendation to make repair of the eye the primary focus in this setting, with repair of the fractures as the secondary consideration, as was followed in this case.

Before considering repair of the associated fracture, one should first answer whether repair is warranted. In the case of ZMC fractures, pertinent exam findings include the presence of malocclusion and whether the patient is at risk for developing loss of malar projection or arch depression. In the case of orbital floor fractures, the size of the fracture, whether any extraocular muscles are incarcerated within in the fracture, and whether there is any risk of developing enophthalmos must be considered. If it is deemed necessary to proceed with fracture repair to prevent cosmetic and/or functional deficit, the next question is when to proceed with repair. If possible, the repair should be delayed as long as possible, although this risks difficulty in repair and suboptimal healing of the fracture. If a fracture repair is undertaken, considerable effort should be made to minimize pressure on the globe as much as possible.

42.8 Key Learning Points

- Defer repair of facial/orbital fractures, if possible, in the setting of an open globe injury until after the open globe injury is addressed.
- If fracture repair is undertaken, it should be ensured that there is minimal pressure placed on the globe intraoperatively.
- Visual prognosis is poor in these settings given the nature of the injury, which is often a blunt, causing a large or posterior rupture.

References

1. Vaca EE, Mundinger GS, Kelamis JA, Dorafshar AH, Christy MR, Manson PN, Rodriguez ED. Facial fractures with concomitant open globe injury: mechanisms and fracture patterns associated with blindness. Plast Reconstr Surg. 2013;131(6):1317–28.
2. Gaier ED, Tarabishy S, Wolkow N, Gardiner M, Lefebvre DR, Grob S. Open globe injury associated with orbital fracture carries a poor prognosis. ARVO poster 2016.

Chapter 43
Case 38: Self-sealing Open Globe Injury

Kristine Lo, Danielle Trief, and Yewlin E. Chee

43.1 History of Present Illness

A 51-year-old man presents with blurred vision after a metallic foreign body in the right eye.

- The patient reports he was hammering metal when a piece of metal flew into his right eye. He went to a local hospital where a metallic foreign body was removed from his cornea. He was sent home on antibiotic ointment.
- Two days later, he presents to Massachusetts Eye and Ear (MEE) with persistent blurry vision. He is found to have a self-sealed corneal laceration, an iris transillumination defect, and a traumatic cataract.
- A computed tomography (CT) scan confirms the presence of an intralenticular foreign body.

43.2 Initial Trauma Evaluation

43.2.1 Visual Acuity (Without Correction)

OD: 20/40−2
OS: 20/20

K. Lo, M.D. (✉)
Department of Ophthalmology, Harvard Medical School, Massachusetts Eye and Ear, Boston, MA, USA
e-mail: Kristine_lo@meei.harvard.edu

D. Trief, M.D., M.Sc.
Department of Ophthalmology, Columbia University Medical Center, New York City, NY, USA

Y. E. Chee, M.D.
Vitreoretinal Surgery, Department of Ophthalmology, University of Washington, Seattle, WA, USA

S. Grob, C. Kloek (eds.), *Management of Open Globe Injuries*,
https://doi.org/10.1007/978-3-319-72410-2_43

43.2.2 *Pupils*

OD: Round, no afferent pupillary defect
OS: Round, no afferent pupillary defect

43.2.3 *External Examination*

Normal external exam

43.2.4 *Slit Lamp Examination*

	OD	OS
Lids and lashes	Normal	Normal
Sclera and conjunctiva	1+ diffuse conjunctival injection	Normal
Cornea	1.3 mm shelved full-thickness corneal laceration with focal Descemet folds at 10 o'clock, wound is Seidel negative	Normal
Anterior chamber	2+ cell, formed	Normal
Iris	Transillumination defect at 10 o'clock	Normal
Lens	Focal lens opacity at 10 o'clock, wedge-shaped anterior and posterior subcapsular opacification	Normal
Vitreous	Normal	Normal

43.2.5 *Dilated Examination*

Macula/Nerve OD: Normal
Periphery OD: Normal
Macula/Nerve: OS: Normal
Peripheral OS: Normal

43.2.6 *Radiographic Imaging*

CT of the orbits showed a bright metallic intraocular foreign body in the temporal aspect of the crystalline lens (Fig. 43.1).

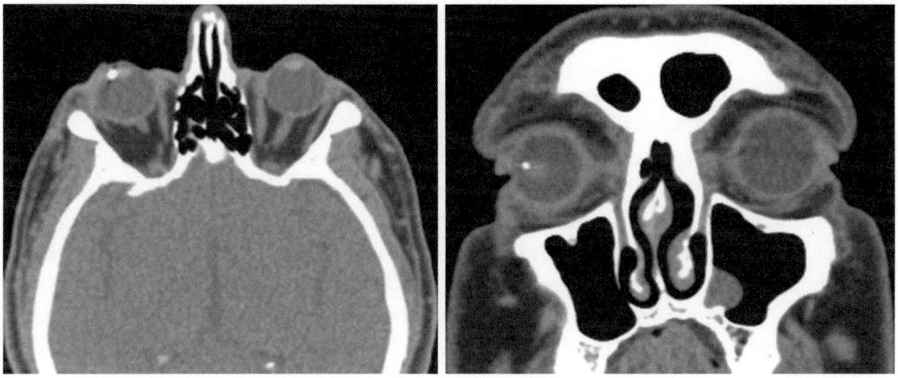

Fig. 43.1 Axial and coronal CT images showing a metallic foreign body imbedded in the right crystalline lens

43.3 Surgeon's Initial Assessment and Pre-operative Plan

The patient had a Zone I self-sealing corneal laceration, an intralenticular foreign body, and a traumatic cataract. The corneal laceration alone would not have required surgical repair. The presence of a likely metallic intraocular foreign body, however, necessitated urgent removal.

This case illustrates three areas of discussion: the management of self-sealing corneal lacerations, the management of an intralenticular foreign body and traumatic cataract, and timing of intraocular lens implantation.

Patients who present with metallic foreign body injury should be examined carefully for the presence of an intraocular foreign body. An iris transillumination defect is an important clue to the presence of an intraocular foreign body, therefore examination of the iris must be performed prior to pupillary dilation at the slit lamp. When in doubt, a CT scan of the orbits should always be ordered.

Corneal lacerations should be checked for wound leakage. If no wound leakage is found, the laceration may not need to be repaired. Although a self-sealing corneal laceration might not require surgical intervention, an open globe injury still occurred and the patient is at increased risk of endophthalmitis as a result. As such, appropriate antibiotic coverage should be considered. Other factors that influence the decision to operate on the patient include the presence of an intraocular foreign body or a traumatic cataract with capsular violation. In this patient, the presence of an intralenticular foreign body and traumatic cataract prompted surgical intervention.

43.4 Surgical Exploration and Repair: Operative Note

Informed consent was obtained and the operative eye was verified and marked. The uninjured left eye was taped and shielded for protection. Two iris hooks were placed temporally in the area of the full-thickness corneal laceration. The iris was retracted and an intralenticular foreign body was seen at the temporal aspect of the lens close to the zonules. There were posterior synechiae in this area. A paracentesis was made in the inferior cornea and Healon was used to lyse the posterior synechiae. Additional viscoelastic was used to fill the anterior chamber and surround the foreign body. The paracentesis wound was enlarged. Max grip forceps were used to free the foreign body and deliver it through the enlarged wound. The lens was inspected and was found to have residual rust and debris within as well as a traumatic cataract. Thus, the decision was made to remove the lens with plans for secondary intraocular lens implantation at a later date. Additional iris hooks were then placed to retract the iris. A separate paracentesis was made temporally. Trypan blue was used to stain the capsule. A continuous curvilinear capsulorrhexis was performed central to the area of capsule violation. Gentle hydrodissection and hydrodelineation were performed. The nucleus was then prolapsed anteriorly and removed with phacoemulsification. The cortex was removed with the irrigation and aspiration handpiece. The posterior capsule was polished. The residual viscoelastic was removed. The eye was brought to physiologic pressure. A 10-0 nylon suture was placed to close the wound. Wounds were checked and were watertight. A subconjunctival injection of antibiotic and steroid was injected away from the wounds. The corneal laceration site remained watertight throughout the procedure and did not need to be sutured.

43.4.1 Surgical Exploration and Repair: Pearls

- Viscoelastic is helpful for gentle synechiolysis.
- Iris hooks are helpful in cases where pupillary dilation is limited or when you need to retract the iris to explore for an intraocular foreign body or an area of capsule violation.
- A traumatic cataract should be removed if there is residual rust or debris that could not be manually removed with forceps. Violation of the anterior lens capsule with prolapse of lenticular material into the anterior chamber is also a reason to consider primary lensectomy at time of open globe repair. The patient may be left aphakic temporarily and intraocular lens implantation done secondarily.

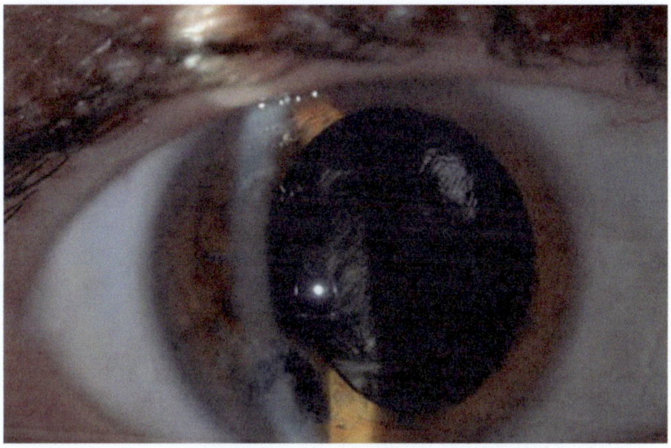

Fig. 43.2 Slit lamp photograph showing a small corneal scar at 10 o'clock and focal synechiae to the anterior capsule temporally

43.5 Post-operative Course

The patient was admitted to MEE to complete a 48 hour course of intravenous antibiotics. On post-operative day 1 he had counting fingers vision. He was discharged on a topical steroid, antibiotic, cycloplegic agent, and nonsteroidal anti-inflammatory drop (NSAID).

He then followed up a week later and his visual acuity was 20/25+2 with a +10 diopter lens. The cycloplegic agent and antibiotic drops were discontinued. The steroid drop was tapered and the NSAID was continued for a month.

A month later, his best corrected visual acuity was 20/20−. The cornea had healed nicely. There were posterior synechiae to the lens capsule at 7 o'clock (Fig. 43.2). The posterior capsule was intact. The options for aphakic correction were discussed with the patient. These included aphakic contact lens and secondary intraocular lens placement. The patient opted for intraocular lens placement as he did not have the dexterity for contact lens placement.

43.6 Secondary Intraocular Lens Implantation: Operative Note

Informed consent was obtained. A peribulbar block was performed. The operative eye was prepped and draped in the usual sterile ophthalmic fashion. A paracentesis incision was created at 2 o'clock. Viscoelastic was injected in the anterior chamber and into the ciliary sulcus. The iris was noted to be adherent to the capsule from 8 to 10 o'clock. Synechiolysis was performed using a cyclodialysis spatula and microsurgical technology (MST) forceps. After successful synechiolysis, a clear corneal incision was created at 10 o'clock and slightly enlarged to fit the cartridge for a 3-piece lens. A three-piece intraocular lens was injected into the sulcus and dialed into position. The viscoelastic was removed. The wounds were hydrated. A 10-0 nylon suture was used to secure the incision.

43.6.1 Secondary Intraocular Lens Implantation: Pearls

- In cases where the iris is adherent to the underlying lens capsule, a viscoelastic can be used to try and lyse the synechiae, or if more adherent, MST forceps or scissors may facilitate synechiolysis.
- If it is difficult to re-inflate the capsular bag, implanting the intraocular lens in the sulcus is a reasonable option provided a three piece intraocular lens is used.

43.7 Final Trauma Evaluation

43.7.1 Final Visual Acuity

OD: 20/20–
OS: 20/20

43.7.2 Pupils

OD: Irregular, no afferent pupillary defect
OS: Round, no afferent pupillary defect

43.7.3 Slit Lamp Examination

	OD	OS
Lids and lashes	Foamy lid margins	Normal
Sclera and conjunctiva	Normal	Normal
Cornea	Small full-thickness corneal scar at 10 o'clock	Normal
Anterior chamber	Rare cell	Normal
Iris	Iris atrophy inferotemporally, transillumination defects revealing the presence of the sulcus intraocular lens	Normal
Lens	Sulcus 3-piece intraocular lens, mild posterior capsule fibrosis	Normal
Vitreous	Normal	Normal

43.7.4 Dilated Examination

Macula/Nerve OD: Normal
Periphery OD: Normal
Macula/Nerve: OS: Normal
Periphery OS: Normal

43.8 Review and Lessons Learned

In cases that present with high velocity corneal foreign body, it is important to perform a thorough examination to look for corneal perforation and intraocular foreign body. If there is any doubt, a CT scan should be ordered. Ultrasound biomicroscopy (UBM) may be a useful adjunct in cases where the intraocular foreign body is found in the posterior chamber.

Small self-sealing wounds may be treated medically with topical antibiotics [1]. We recommend considering a course of intravenous antibiotics for all suspected open globe injuries. A bandage contact lens may be used in larger wounds or even to decrease leakage of aqueous prior to going to the operating room. Patching and aqueous suppressants can also be used to manage very small lacerations [2]. If there is any concern that the wound has not self-sealed or will not close, then the patient should be taken to the operating room for repair of the full-thickness laceration, as a leaking corneal wound puts the patient at higher risk for endophthalmitis.

Intraocular foreign bodies should always be removed. A CT scan and/or UBM are helpful in determining the location of the foreign body.

The timing of traumatic cataract removal and intraocular lens implantation should be considered carefully. Focal lens injuries without capsular violation can remain stable for an extended period of time, and delayed removal can be considered in these cases. In contrast, injuries with capsular violation have less post-operative inflammation and morbidity when the lens is removed during the primary repair. However, if the view through the cornea is insufficient after trauma to safely perform a primary lensectomy, or if there is known violation of the posterior capsule with vitreous prolapse, it is often safer to wait until the view improves for the lensectomy or for the lens to be removed by a vitreoretinal surgeon by pars plana lensectomy.

As discussed in earlier cases, the timing for intraocular lens implantation should be considered carefully. Primary intraocular lens implantation at the time of open globe repair and lensectomy may benefit the patient by shortening rehabilitation time, reducing the number of surgical procedures and promoting early binocular function [3]. However, it may expose the patient to: increased risk for infection as the intraocular lens may act as a nidus for infection, increased post-operative inflammation, and increased risk for retinal detachments [4]. Primary intraocular lens placement is a risk factor for endophthalmitis as shown in a case series by Andreoli et al. [5]. Axial length and keratometry measurements are challenging in the setting of acute eye trauma and can change after corneal laceration repair and suture removal. Secondary intraocular lens implantation can allow for more careful surgical planning and selection of the most appropriate lens implant.

43.9 Key Learning Points

- Not all corneal perforating injuries need to be repaired. Self-sealing wounds oftentimes can be treated with topical antibiotics, however, the patient is still at risk of endophthalmitis given their history of open globe injury and a high index of suspicion needs to be maintained during their recovery period. A course of intravenous or oral antibiotics should be considered as well.
- Intraocular lens implantation can be performed as a secondary procedure, allowing for appropriate corneal healing, lens measurements, and surgical planning.

References

1. Hamill MG. Corneal and scleral trauma. Ophthalmol Clin North Am. 2002;15:185–94.
2. Vora GK, Haddadin R, Chodosh J. Management of corneal lacerations and perforations. Int Ophthalmol Clin. 2013;53(4):1–10.
3. Baykara M, Dogru M, Ozcetin H, et al. Primary repair and intraocular lens implantation after perforating eye injury. J Cataract Refract Surg. 2002;28:1832–5.
4. Shah AS, Turalba AV. Intraocular lens implantation in penetrating ocular trauma. Int Ophthalmol Clin. 2010;50(1):43–59.
5. Andreoli DM, Andreoli MT, Kloek CE, et al. Low rate of endophthalmitis in a large series of open globe injuries. Am J Ophthalmol. 2009;147(4):601–8.

Chapter 44
Case 39: Delayed Presentation Zone I Open Globe Injury at Site of Previous Trauma

Tavé van Zyl and Seanna Grob

44.1 History of Present Illness

A 31-year-old otherwise healthy man presents with concern for open globe of the right eye.

- While at work as an HVAC (Heating, Ventilation and Air Conditioning) technician the morning prior, the patient stood up from a crouching position and struck his eye on the corner of a hard, plastic drawer.
- He presented to a primary care office after work due to "mildly blurry vision" and irritation and was referred to ophthalmology the following day, after which he was referred to Massachusetts Eye and Ear (MEE) due to concern for open globe injury (>24 hours after injury).
- The patient recalls history of recurrent unilateral "conjunctivitis" of the right eye since age 12, occurring approximately 3–4 episodes per year, treated to the extent of symptom resolution each time by primary care provider with topical antibiotics.
- He does not recall any specific prior trauma to the eye, but has had history of issues with that eye for many years.

44.2 Initial Trauma Evaluation

44.2.1 Visual Acuity (Without Correction)

OD: 20/30
OS: 20/20

T. van Zyl, M.D. (✉) • S. Grob, M.D., M.A.S.
Department of Ophthalmology, Harvard Medical School, Massachusetts Eye and Ear, Boston, MA, USA
e-mail: tave_vanzyl@meei.harvard.edu

S. Grob, C. Kloek (eds.), *Management of Open Globe Injuries*,
https://doi.org/10.1007/978-3-319-72410-2_44

44.2.2 Pupils

OD: 4 mm minimally reactive, no afferent pupillary defect by reverse
OS: 3 mm briskly reactive, no afferent pupillary defect

44.2.3 External Examination

Normal without lacerations, edema or ecchymosis

44.2.4 Slit Lamp Examination

	OD	OS
Lids and lashes	Normal	Normal
Sclera and conjunctiva	Mild injection, prominent conjunctival/episcleral vessels nasally leading to limbus	Normal
Cornea	Horizontal full-thickness corneal defect 6.5 mm in length, running from 4 o'clock at the limbus temporally across the cornea, neovascularization and pigment noted within the wound, Seidel positive without provocation.	Normal
Anterior chamber	1+ cell	Normal
Iris	Posterior synechiae at 6 o'clock, large sectoral transillumination defect from 5 to 8 o'clock, associated prominent iris vessels, round but mid-dilated pupil, no iris to wound.	Normal
Lens	Normal without cataract or capsule violation	Normal
Vitreous	No pigment or red blood cells	Normal

44.2.5 Dilated Examination

Macula/Nerve OD: Normal
Periphery OD: Normal
Macula/Nerve: OS: Normal
Periphery OS: Normal

44.2.6 Radiographic Imaging

Computed tomography (CT) of the orbits showed no orbital fractures and no intraocular foreign body. The globes appeared symmetric and well-formed.

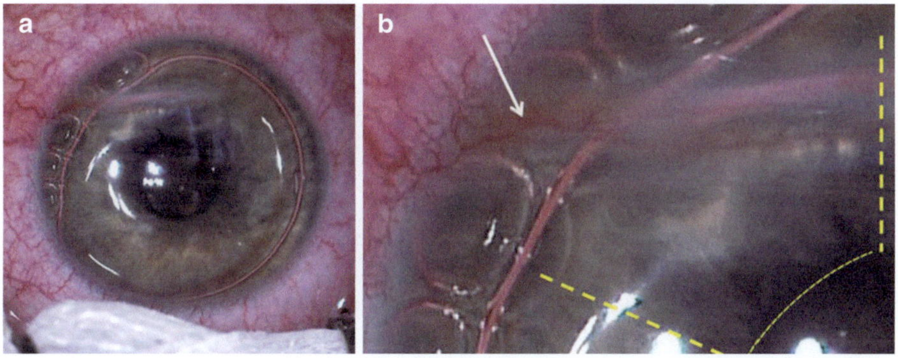

Fig. 44.1 Intraoperative photo (surgeon's view) taken prior to open globe repair (following instillation of filtered air to maintain anterior chamber). Prominent episcleral/conjunctival vessels are noted feeding into the corneal wound suggestive of chronicity and there is corneal whitening around the wound (**a**). Higher magnification view of peripheral aspect of wound demonstrating blood vessel (arrow) within the cleft of the full-thickness corneal defect. A sectoral transillumination defect of the iris was also noted (yellow dashed outline) (**b**)

44.3 Surgeon's Initial Assessment and Pre-operative Plan

The patient has a Zone I open globe injury after a presumed blunt rupture upon standing up from crouching position. The history of "recurrent conjunctivitis" in the injured eye and the findings of a linear corneal abnormality with corneal neovascularization within the wound is suggestive of a chronic corneal wound—possibly even a full-thickness, self-sealing defect from a previous injury—which was ruptured acutely during the patient's most recent blunt eye trauma (Fig. 44.1a, b). He also has an area of sectoral iris atrophy just posterior to the corneal abnormality also suggesting a possible previous trauma (Fig. 44.1b). Since he had an already abnormal area of corneal tissue, the blunt trauma from the corner of the drawer caused a full-thickness wound in this area of "weakened" cornea.

Complexities related to repairing a delayed presentation Zone I injury include wound epithelialization and friable corneal tissue. We planned to debride the wound edges with a #67 blade to remove aberrant epithelium, promote healing and prevent epithelial downgrowth, which could have devastating visual consequences beyond persistent wound leakage [1]. We also made sure to have a bandage contact lens on hand for the end of the case to provide additional protection in the early post-operative period.

44.4 Surgical Exploration and Repair: Operative Note

The risks, benefits, and alternatives were discussed with the patient pre-operatively and the patient consented to proceed with exploration and repair of the open globe injury. The patient was brought to the operating room where the anesthesia team

proceeded with general anesthesia. A careful time-out was observed and the correct patient and the eye were identified. The right eye was prepped and draped in the usual sterile ophthalmic fashion using a Jaffe speculum to provide adequate exposure.

The anterior segment was inspected. The patient was found to have a 6.5 mm shelved, full-thickness corneal laceration inferonasally at the limbus at approximately 4:30 o'clock extending horizontally towards the visual axis. There was prominent neovascularization growing from the limbus into the cornea along approximately 1/3 of the length of the wound. There was whitening of the cornea around the area of the wound. The wound was actively Seidel positive. There was no iris incarceration in the wound although a faint line of pigmentation was noted within the wound. There were posterior synechiae at 6 o'clock.

Wound repair was initiated (Fig. 44.2a–i). A paracentesis was fashioned temporally at 9 o'clock with a 15° blade. Filtered air was injected into the anterior

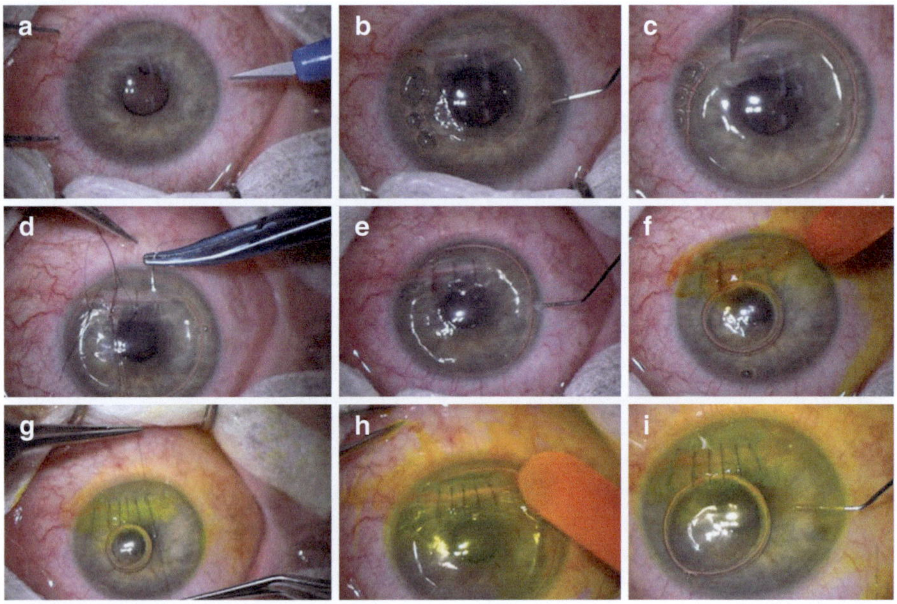

Fig. 44.2 Montage of critical steps during repair of acute rupture of a chronic corneal wound. A paracentesis was made away from the wound (**a**) and filtered air was injected on a 27 G blunt-tipped cannula to maintain anterior chamber stability (**b**). The wound was debrided with a #67 blade to remove aberrant epithelium and debris (**c**). Initial 10-0 nylon sutures were placed and tied using adjustable tension slipknots, which were secured and trimmed after all sutures were tied at the desired tension (**d**). There was bleeding during the corneal suture passes due to intrastromal neovessels (**e**). The wound was Seidel positive due to friable corneal stroma in the setting of a chronic wound; leakage was noted from the suture tracts as well as from the main wound (**f**). Additional sutures were placed (**g**). The wound was Seidel negative (**h**). Balanced salt solution was injected once again as another means of confirming the closure was intact (**i**)

chamber. Using a #67 blade, the wound edges were debrided. Then, the wound was closed with six interrupted 10-0 nylon sutures. The cornea was noted to be friable, consistent with a delayed presentation wound, and there was bleeding during the corneal suturing due to corneal neovascularization. After adequate approximation of the wound edges, a Seidel test was performed with a fluorescein strip to confirm the wound was watertight. A Kontur bandage contact lens, diameter 16.0 mm, was placed as a safety measure given the observed friability of the corneal tissue and delayed nature of presentation.

A subconjunctival steroid and antibiotic injection was performed temporally and inferiorly away from the laceration. The speculum was removed. The patient's drape was removed under the microscope. The patient was extubated and transported to the recovery area, having tolerated the procedure well without any complications.

44.4.1 Surgical Exploration and Repair: Pearls

- Filtered air is an excellent tool for maintaining anterior chamber stability while suturing corneal wounds.
- A small residual air bubble can be left in the eye and may help with wound integrity; one must, however, ensure the bubble does not obstruct the entire pupil and cause an intraocular pressure spike secondary to pupillary block.
- Delayed presentation wounds may benefit from debridement prior to closure to ensure proper healing and to prevent epithelial downgrowth.
- Delayed presentation wounds may require more sutures than anticipated to achieve watertight closure.
- It is important to inspect the wound prior to repair for abnormalities suggestive of a more chronic issue, such as neovascularization.

44.5 Post-operative Course

The patient was admitted to complete a 48 hour course of intravenous antibiotics. His post-operative day 1 visual acuity was 20/200 pinhole 20/60−1. The wound was secure, Seidel negative and the bandage contact lens was in place. There was mild corneal edema with striae at the wound.

On post-operative week 6, half (3/6) corneal sutures were removed. On post-operative week 8, the remaining three sutures were removed without issue (Fig. 44.3). At the most recent follow-up visit, 3 months following repair, the patient described his vision as "essentially back to normal." He reported wearing safety glasses 100% of the time at work, and polycarbonate eyewear "about two-thirds" of the time while not at work.

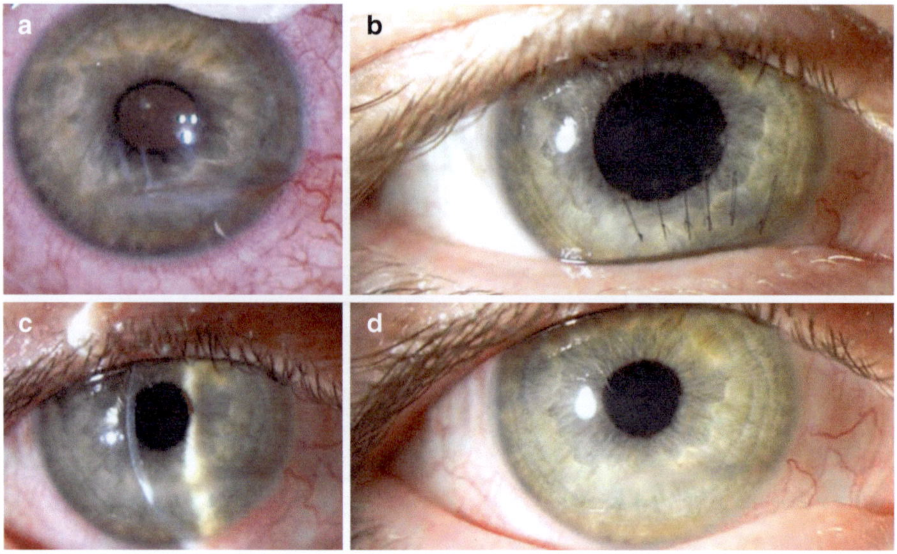

Fig. 44.3 External photos of delayed presentation Zone I open globe injury at a site of suspected prior trauma over 10 years prior. Pre-operative photo shows the wound extending horizontally below the visual axis from the limbus at 4 o'clock. There are associated prominent vessels extending from the perilimbal conjunctiva into the corneal wound and also corneal whitening around the wound (**a**). Post-operative month 1 photo showing secure wound with 10-0 nylon sutures intact; pupil contour is irregular from 4 to 7 o'clock secondary to atrophy from suspected longstanding, chronic low grade inflammation/infection (**b**). Post-operative month 3 photos demonstrating corneal scar and pupil irregularity; the prominent vessels are partially regressed (**c, d**)

44.6 Final Trauma Evaluation

44.6.1 Final Visual Acuity

OD: 20/20
OS: 20/15

44.6.2 Pupils

OD: 4 mm reactive, no afferent pupillary defect
OS: 4 mm reactive

44.6.3 Slit Lamp Examination

	OD	OS
Lids and lashes	Normal	Normal
Sclera and conjunctiva	Prominent but somewhat regressed perilimbal vessels at 4:30 o'clock	Normal
Cornea	6 mm horizontal wound from 4 o'clock at the limbus extending centrally status post repair, now with corneal scar, less prominent deep blood vessels in the wound (compared to prior to globe repair) and growing in from the limbus approx. 5.5 mm, Seidel negative.	Normal
Anterior chamber	Normal	Normal
Iris	Posterior synechiae at 6 o'clock. Large sectoral transillumination defect from 5 to 8 o'clock.	Normal
Lens	Normal	Normal
Vitreous	Normal	Normal

44.6.4 Dilated Examination

Macula/Nerve OD: Normal
Periphery OD: Normal
Macula/Nerve: OS: Normal
Periphery OS: Normal

44.7 Review and Lessons Learned

By history, the patient's injury occurred more than 24 hours prior to presentation at MEE, qualifying him as a delayed presentation. His relatively preserved visual acuity and anterior site of injury are consistent with a large proportion of late presenters encountered at MEE. In a retrospective chart review of 823 open globe injuries at MEE over 9 years, patients presenting >24 hours after injury (n = 58) were more likely to have better presenting visual acuity and less likely to have a hyphema or posterior (Zone III) injury ($p = 0.0028$, 0.0308 and <0.0001, respectively) [2]. This is likely attributable in large part due to patients' underestimation of the severity of their ocular injury. In this study, there were no cases of endophthalmitis among this group of late presenters. These patients also tended to have better post-operative visual acuities.

Our patient offers an even more extreme example of a late presentation open globe, potentially having had a prior ocular injury that was not previously treated.

Due to the self-perceived minimal extent of his eye problem he had never before sought evaluation by an eye care provider. It is unknown whether the patient had a history of a full-thickness self-sealing laceration or a partial-thickness laceration; however, the transillumination defect behind the corneal wound would suggest a possible full-thickness laceration. Regardless of the prior insult, this patient had an area of "weakened" corneal tissue susceptible to rupture with blunt trauma. The chronic intermittent low-grade infection and/or inflammation he experienced in this area over an extended time period likely promoted the corneal neovascularization that was noted on presentation and bled during repair. It likely also contributed to the notably friable corneal tissue encountered intraoperatively, i.e. when the main wound continued to be Seidel positive after multiple sutures that otherwise would have been sufficient for a fresh corneal wound, and also the persistent slow leak through the corneal suture tracks. Intraoperative debridement of the wound ensured fresh wound edges, encouraged healing and also prevented epithelial downgrowth that could lead to post-operative leakage.

This case highlights two important opportunities for effective patient counseling. As mentioned previously, patients who present with an open globe injury and relatively good visual acuity will inevitably emerge from the repair with worse visual acuity due to a variety of short-term post-operative sequelae of the surgery including corneal edema, suture-induced astigmatism, residual intraocular air bubble, or hyphema. They are likely to be disappointed, concerned, alarmed or even angry if they are not adequately prepared for this in advance. Taking special care and additional time during the consent process to counsel the patient and their families to expect this short-term outcome prior to repair will go a long way towards an optimal recovery. Finally, patients with open globe injuries are at high risk of recurrent injury years later due to inherent weakness at the original site of injury even if appropriately repaired and fully healed. These patients should be routinely and repetitively counseled about the importance of using full-time polycarbonate eye protection to serve the dual purpose of preserving the uninjured eye and also preventing re-injury to the injured eye.

44.8 Key Learning Points

- Avoid patient disappointment: open globe injury patients presenting with relatively preserved visual acuity require dedicated pre-operative counseling that their vision will initially be worse post-operatively.
- Be wary of delayed presentation corneal wounds: they may require additional sutures during repair and/or a bandage contact lens after repair and an extended post-operative healing time with staged suture removal.
- Repeat open globe injuries occur every year: ensure consistent and repetitive counseling of patients regarding the importance of full-time polycarbonate eye protection.

References

1. Chen SH, Pineda R II. Epithelial and fibrous downgrowth: mechanisms of disease. Ophthalmol Clin North Am. 2002;15(1):41–8.
2. Trief D, Andreoli M, Shah A, Yonekawa Y, Andreoli C. Outcomes and characteristics of open-globe injuries with delayed presentation. Invest Ophthalmol Vis Sci. 2013;54(15):4435.

Chapter 45
Case 40: Iridodialysis Repair Following a Zone I Open Globe Injury

Natalie Wolkow, Seanna Grob, and Roberto Pineda

45.1 History of Present Illness

A 64-year-old female construction worker with a history of hypertension and posterior vitreous detachment presented with concern for open globe of the left eye.

- The patient was removing shingles from a house. She pulled very hard on a shingle thinking it would require a lot of force to remove, but it was loosely attached, and she hit herself in the left eye with her knuckles.
- She went to an outside hospital because of decreased vision, and was transferred to Massachusetts Eye and Ear (MEE) due to a high probability of an open globe injury.

45.2 Initial Trauma Evaluation

45.2.1 Visual Acuity (Without Correction)

OD: 20/100 pinhole 20/25−1
OS: Hand motion at 2 feet

N. Wolkow, M.D., Ph.D. (✉) • S. Grob, M.D., M.A.S.
Department of Ophthalmology, Harvard Medical School, Massachusetts Eye and Ear, Boston, MA, USA
e-mail: natalie_wolkow@meei.harvard.edu

R. Pineda, M.D.
Cornea and Refractive Surgery, Department of Ophthalmology, Harvard Medical School, Massachusetts Eye and Ear, Boston, MA, USA

S. Grob, C. Kloek (eds.), *Management of Open Globe Injuries*,
https://doi.org/10.1007/978-3-319-72410-2_45

45.2.2 Pupils

OD: Round, brisk, no afferent pupillary defect
OS: No afferent pupillary defect by reverse

45.2.3 External Examination

Normal

45.2.4 Slit Lamp Examination

	OD	OS
Lids and lashes	Normal	Normal
Sclera and conjunctiva	Normal	Superonasal subconjunctival hemorrhage and conjunctival laceration
Cornea	Normal	Central corneal laceration, thick white wavy film overlying the cornea (likely extruded iris tissue or ciliary body)
Anterior chamber	Normal	Total hyphema
Iris	Normal	Unable to evaluate
Lens	1+ NS	Unable to evaluate
Vitreous	Normal	Unable to evaluate

45.2.5 Dilated Examination

Macula/Nerve OD: Cup to disc ratio 0.3, peripapillary atrophy, posterior vitreous detachment, flat macula
Periphery OD: Normal
Macula/Nerve: OS: Unable to evaluate
Periphery OS: Unable to evaluate

45.2.6 Radiographic Imaging

Computed tomography (CT) of the orbits showed a slightly shallow left anterior chamber and a slightly flattened left globe concerning for globe rupture. There was mild left periorbital soft tissue swelling. No facial fractures or radiopaque foreign bodies were seen.

45.3 Surgeon's Initial Assessment and Pre-operative Plan

The patient had a blunt injury to her left eye from a significant amount of force, resulting in a corneal laceration with uveal extrusion (Fig. 45.1). Additionally, there was a hyphema and vitreous hemorrhage limiting the view of the posterior pole.

In our experience, blunt injuries commonly result in larger and more extensive open globe injuries with uveal prolapse than injuries with sharp objects [1]. Often, large blunt injuries carry a poorer long term visual outcome than limited injuries from sharp objects. The patient should be counseled pre-operatively about the high likelihood of poor visual outcome.

In larger injuries, the limbus is often involved. When such is the case, during wound repair, the limbus should be approximated first in order to aid with alignment of the wound.

The patient has a large amount of uveal extrusion, either iris or ciliary body. With uveal extrusion, a decision needs to be made as to whether the uveal tissue should be reposited, partially truncated, or completely excised. If the tissue appears to be viable, clean and healthy, it should be reposited. If it appears to be necrotic, dirty, or overgrown with epithelium, it usually needs to be to be partially or completely excised. Attempts should be made to preserve iris and ciliary body, as this will provide a better opportunity to preserve production of aqueous humor and prevent hypotony. On the other hand, non-viable or contaminated uvea can predispose to infection, and uvea with epithelial overgrowth can introduce epithelium into the anterior chamber, leading to epithelial downgrowth (See Chap. 51 for a more extensive discussion on this topic).

There is vitreous hemorrhage present without adequate visualization of the posterior pole. Post-operatively, the patient will need a B-scan to assess the status of the retina. Pre-operative B-scan is contraindicated as it would apply unnecessary pressure onto the globe.

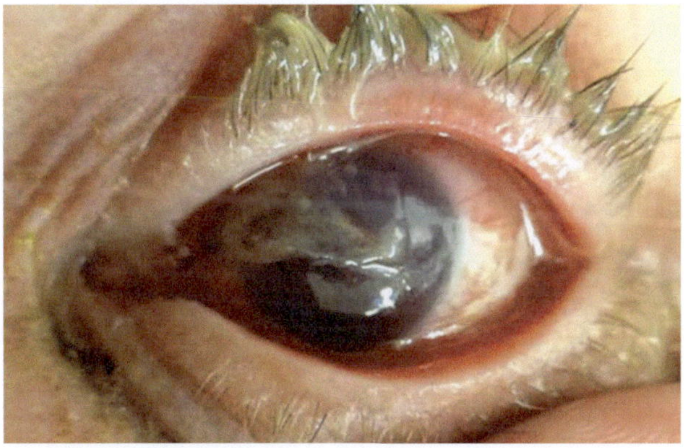

Fig. 45.1 External photograph of the patient's left eye, obtained in the operating room prior to surgery. Extruded uveal tissue is seen on the surface of the cornea

45.4 Surgical Exploration and Repair: Operative Note

The risks, benefits, and alternatives were discussed with the patient pre-operatively and the patient consented to proceed with exploration and repair of the open globe injury. In the pre-operative area, the patient was identified and the left eye was marked. The patient was brought to the operating room where the anesthesia team proceeded with general anesthesia. A careful time-out was observed and the correct patient and the eye were identified. The patient was prepped and draped in the standard ophthalmic surgical fashion and Jaffe lid specula were used to retract the eyelids.

The globe was inspected and a single shelved curvilinear corneal wound was noted to extend from the 10 o'clock limbus to almost the 2 o'clock limbus. The wound curved down into the visual axis. There was a significant amount of pale iris tissue protruding onto the corneal surface. The inferior portion of the anterior chamber was filled with blood, and the lens could not be visualized due to heme. Superonasally, the conjunctiva was lacerated and there were 6 eyelashes within the laceration. The eyelashes were removed and the conjunctiva was irrigated to remove any additional debris in the area.

A paracentesis was made at the 1 o'clock limbus with a 15° supersharp blade. The extruded iris was gently repositioned through the corneal wound into the anterior chamber using an iris spatula and a cyclodialysis spatula, using the paracentesis wound to assist with the repositioning. Next, a conjunctival peritomy was made from 7 o'clock to 2 o'clock with Westcott scissors, and blunt dissection was used to inspect the globe. No additional areas of globe rupture were noted, and the corneal laceration at the 10 o'clock limbus did not extend beyond the limbus. The 10 o'clock limbus was then re-approximated with a 9-0 nylon suture. Then, nine additional interrupted 10-0 nylon corneal sutures were placed to close the corneal laceration. Care was taken not to incarcerate any iris tissue within the suture passes. The wound was tested with a fluorescein strip and found to be Seidel negative.

Next, the globe was once again re-explored using blunt dissection with Westcott and Stevens scissors to aid in visualization. No additional lacerations were found. The conjunctiva was re-approximated with four 8-0 Vicryl sutures, using episcleral bites near the limbus to secure the conjunctiva. A subconjunctival injection of cefazolin-dexamethasone was administered. The Jaffe lid specula were removed under microscopic visualization. The eye was gently cleaned, and an atropine drop and maxitrol ointment were applied, followed by a sterile patch and shield. The patient tolerated the procedure well, without any complications, and was transferred to the post-operative area for recovery.

45.4.1 Surgical Exploration and Repair: Pearls

- If a wound involves the limbus, align the limbus first, as you would a vermilion border in a lip laceration. This improves wound alignment and facilitates with closure of the rest of the wound.

- If extruded uveal tissue appears viable and free of epithelial overgrowth, it may be reposited into the globe during repair. Dirty or necrotic uveal tissue, on the other hand, should be excised.

45.5 Post-operative Course

On the first post-operative day the patient's vision in the surgical eye was hand motions at 1 ft. B-scan ultrasound revealed that the retina was attached.

In subsequent post-operative visits, her wounds were healing well, but her vision remained poor at count fingers at 1–2 ft, as the repositioned iris tissue was bunched together centrally over the visual axis, and a superotemporal iridodialysis was present from 11 to 4 o'clock (Fig. 45.2).

At post-operative week 7, five of the ten corneal sutures were removed (Fig. 45.3). Two weeks later, the remaining five corneal sutures were removed. A repeat B-scan demonstrated that the retina was still attached, which together with the continued absence of a relative afferent pupillary defect by reverse, suggested that there was potential for visual improvement. The patient was referred to a corneal specialist for visual rehabilitation.

Examination by a corneal specialist at three and a half months post open globe injury revealed that the corneal incision was well healed (Fig. 45.4). An iridodialysis was present from 11 to 4 o'clock, with iris and ciliary body tissue resting on the lens paracentrally. There were adhesions present from the iris to the superonasal and central corneal wound, and posterior synechiae were present from the iris to the 5 o'clock lens anterior capsule. The lens had both a nuclear and posterior subcapsular cataract component, the zonules appeared mostly intact, and there was no phacodonesis. Review of corneal topography revealed irregular astigmatism. Cataract extraction with intraocular lens implant, iridoplasty and a limbal relaxing incision from 120 to 130° were planned. A-scan was performed to determine axial length, and average keratometry readings of 47.00 were used to determine the lens power. The refractive

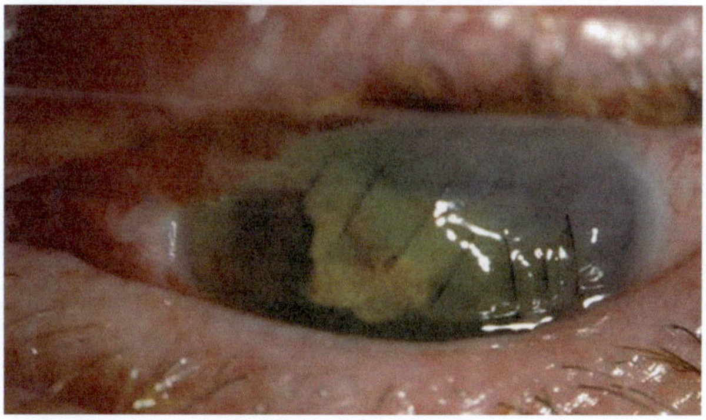

Fig. 45.2 External photograph of the left eye, 1 week after open globe injury repair, demonstrating corneal wound repair with an underlying central iris tissue

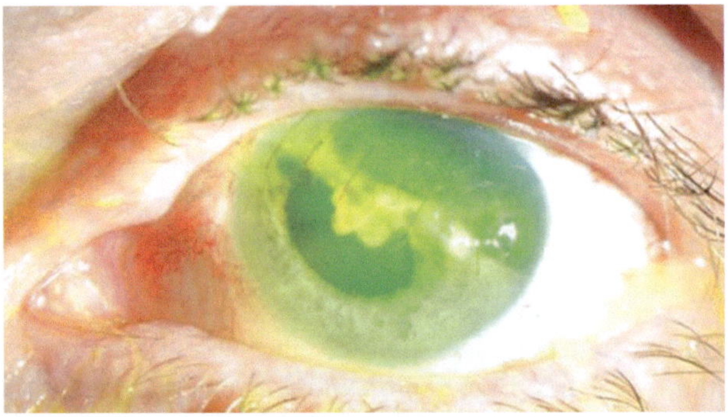

Fig. 45.3 External photograph of the left eye, 2 months after repair of open globe injury, after five of the ten corneal sutures had been removed. The superotemporal iridodialysis is clearly visible, with iris blocking the visual axis

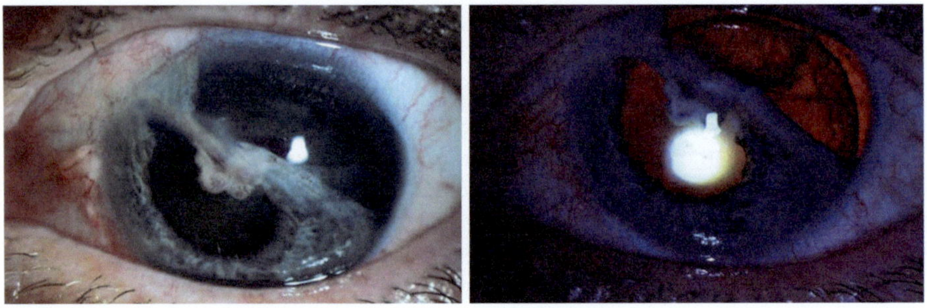

Fig. 45.4 External photographs of the left eye, 4 months after repair of open globe injury, demonstrating the (**a**) well-healed corneal laceration with uveal tissue blocking the central visual axis, and (**b**) the intraocular lens well-centered, but with cataractuous changes on transillumination

target was aimed myopic at −0.9. Five months after the initial open globe injury, the patient underwent surgery for the purpose of rehabilitating her vision.

45.6 Second Surgical Repair: Operative Note

After proper identification, the left eye was marked. The patient was given a peribulbar injection of anesthesia by the anesthesia staff in the holding area. The patient was then taken into the operating room, where she was positioned and monitored anesthesia with sedation was begun. The patient was prepped and draped in typical sterile ophthalmic fashion.

The surgeon sat in the superior position. An eyelid speculum was placed and the eye was examined. Several features were noted including a white traumatic cataract, an iridodialysis from 12 to 5 o'clock, and a corneal scar with uveal tissue attached to the corneal scar.

A toric marker was used to ink the 120° location, and a 4-mm limbal relaxing incision was made centered at 120° with a preset 600 μm guarded blade. Two peritomies were made, one superotemporally and one inferotemporally. Then, in the locations of the peritomies, two 3-mm scleral grooves were created 2-mm behind the limbus with a crescent blade. A paracentesis was made at 9 o'clock with a 15° super blade. Trypan blue was injected into the anterior chamber to stain the anterior capsule, and the residual dye was washed out with balanced saline solution. Viscoat was injected into the anterior chamber to break the uveal attachments from the corneal scar and the posterior synechiae.

A temporal clear corneal incision was made. It was noted that there was vitreous prolapsing from the clear corneal incision, and this vitreous was cut with Wescott scissors. Two double-armed 10-0 polypropylene sutures were used to repair the iridodialysis between the 12 and 2 o'clock and 3–5 o'clock hours. The sutures were trimmed, tied, and buried into the previously made scleral grooves.

A cystotome needle and Utrata forceps were used to create an anterior continuous curvilinear capsulorrhexis. Balanced saline solution on a blunt tipped cannula was used for hydrodissection and hydrodelineation. Using the phacoemulsification unit, the lens nucleus was removed from the eye. Using irrigation and aspiration, the remaining cortical material was removed from the eye. A small capsular bag dehiscence was seen superiorly during this time.

The capsular bag was then inflated with viscoelastic material. A Bausch and Lomb LI60AO +18.5 diopter lens was placed into the capsular bag and dialed into position with a Sinskey hook. The remaining viscoelastic material was removed from the eye with irrigation and aspiration. Balanced saline solution on a blunt tipped cannula was used to hydrate all the wounds. The wounds were checked with Weck-cels and were found to be watertight and free of vitreous.

The peritomies were closed with 8-0 Vicryl sutures. At the end of the case, the lens appeared to be in good position, and the intraocular pressure was palpated to be physiologic. A subconjunctival injection of cefazolin and dexamethasone was administered at the end of the case. The eyelid speculum was then removed. Tobramycin-dexamethasone ointment was applied to the eye. An eye patch and shield were placed over the eye. The patient was brought into the recovery room in stable condition.

45.6.1 Surgical Repair: Pearls

- When performing cataract surgery in a patient with a prior open globe injury with irregular astigmatism, a three piece design and neutral aspheric lens may provide a better visual outcome, if it is available.
- Iridodialysis repair may allow better visualization for subsequent cataract surgery.

45.7 Post-operative Course

On post-operative day 1 the patient's vision had improved to 20/200, pinhole 20/125. The iridodialysis repair was intact, the lens well centered, and there was dense posterior capsular opacification. By post-operative week 1, the patient's vision was pinhole 20/50. Three and a half months after cataract surgery, the patient underwent YAG capsulotomy, with further improvement of best-corrected visual acuity to 20/40 (Fig. 45.5). A Pentacam at 4 months post operatively revealed approximately 3 diopters of astigmatism, with 2.5 diopters of astigmatism on manifest refraction.

45.8 Final Trauma Evaluation

45.8.1 Final Visual Acuity

OD: 20/20−2
OS: 20/60−1 pinhole 20/40−2

45.8.2 Pupils

OD: Round
OS: Surgical, no afferent pupillary defect by reverse

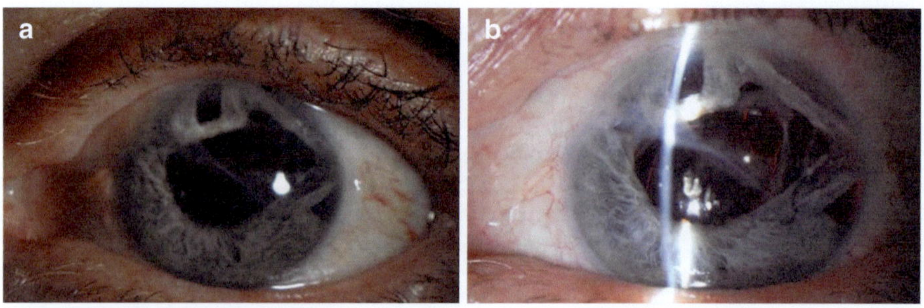

Fig. 45.5 External photographs after cataract extraction, iridodialysis repair, limbal relaxing incision and YAG capsulotomy. The visual axis is no longer obstructed by iris tissue, allowing for significant improvement in visual acuity

45.8.3 Slit Lamp Examination

	OD	OS
Lids and lashes	Blepharitis	Blepharitis
Sclera and conjunctiva	Normal	2 superotemporal sutures immediately outside the limbus, well covered
Cornea	Normal	Superotemporal phaco wound; limbal relaxing incision at 120–130°; Healed limbus to limbus corneal laceration from 10 to 4. Sutures all out.
Anterior chamber	Normal	Deep, quiet, tiny vitreous strand to wound at 1 o'clock
Iris	Normal	Status post pupilloplasty, iridodialysis repair from 12-2 and 3-5 o'clock
Lens	1+ NS	3 piece posterior chamber intraocular lens, well centered, open posterior capsule
Vitreous	Posterior vitreous detachment, old cells	Posterior vitreous detachment

45.8.4 Dilated Examination

Macula/Nerve OD: Normal, cup to disc ratio 0.5, macula flat
Periphery OD: Normal
Macula/Nerve: OS: Normal, cup to disc ratio 0.6, peripapillary atrophy, macula flat
Periphery OS: Normal

45.9 Review and Lessons Learned

In corneal injuries that involve the limbus, the limbus should first be approximated prior to closing the rest of the corneal wound for better alignment.

Uveal extrusion is more common in blunt mechanism injuries than in sharp injuries [2]. When iris or ciliary body is extruding through a wound, every effort should be made to return it to its normal place to prevent complications such as hypotony [2]. If iris or ciliary body is visibly necrotic or contaminated, or has epithelial overgrowth, those portions should be excised, and as much viable tissue as possible returned into the anterior chamber [2]. Excision of uveal tissue can lead to bleeding, inflammation and hypotony, as the ciliary body is necessary for aqueous production. Although it is best to preserve as much normal tissue as possible, the primate eye is, surprisingly, able to compensate for the loss of a significant portion of the iris and ciliary body. Studies in monkeys, where 6, 7, or 8 clock hours of normal iris and ciliary body were surgically excised, demonstrated that the eye is able to regain and maintain normal ocular tension when up to 6 clock hours are excised [3]. If more than 6 clock hours are excised, the intraocular pressure never returns to the pre-operative level and remains low [3].

It is not necessary to repair iridodialyses as part of the primary open globe repair, as it is safer to perform these types of repairs at a later time in a more controlled environment. Multiple techniques have been described for repair of iridodialysis [2, 4–10], and it is up to the surgeon to determine which type of repair is most appropriate for the patient. Scleral fixation techniques vary and one has not proven superior to the others. Usually, scleral fixation is necessary every 3 clock hours for an iridodialysis repair.

Untreated iridodialysis may cause unwanted symptoms of glare, may interfere with vision and may produce a poor cosmetic effect. Treatment options for iridodialysis included surgical repair of the dialysis, surgical insertion of an iris prosthesis, colored contact lenses or corneal tattooing over the affected area.

After open globe injury repair, patients often may have visually significant astigmatism. Hard contact lenses are often used to treat the astigmatism; however, in certain cases a limbal relaxing incision or arcuate keratotomy may be beneficial. Corneal topography is usually helpful in directing the best option if indicated.

45.10 Key Learning Points

- Blunt-mechanism injuries are often accompanied by uveal extrusion.
- Extruded uvea should be reposited whenever possible. Only excise tissue that is dirty, necrotic, or epithelialized.
- Iridodialysis repair should be performed after the primary open globe injury repair if the patient is symptomatic.

References

1. Wolkow N, Gaier ED, Tarabishy S, Grob S, Lefebvre DR, Gardiner M. Open globe injury associated with orbital fracture carries a poor prognosis. Poster, program # 5949-B0712. ARVO conference. Baltimore, MD. May 2017.
2. Dalma-Weiszhausz J. Chapter 16. Extrabulbar tissue prolapse from ocular trauma: principles and practice. Thieme 2011:123–30.
3. Barrada A, Peyman GA, Palacio MN. Limitation of iris and ciliary body resection in primates. Retina. 1984;4(2):119–22.
4. Pandav SS, Gupta PC, Singh RR, Das K, Kaushik S, Raj S, Ram J. Cobbler's technique for iridodialysis repair. Middle East Afr J Ophthalmol. 2016;23(1):142–4.
5. Zeiter JH, Shin DH, Shi DX. A closed chamber technique for repair of iridodialysis. Ophthalmic Surg. 1993;24:476–80.

6. Bardak Y, Ozerturk Y, Durmus M, Mensiz E, Aytuluner E. Closed chamber iridodialysis repair using a needle with a distal hole. J Cataract Refract Surg. 2000;26:173–6.
7. Kaufman SC, Insler MS. Surgical repair of a traumatic iridodialysis. Ophthalmic Surg Lasers. 1996;27:963–6.
8. Wachler BB, Krueger RR. Double-armed McCannell suture for repair of traumatic iridodialysis. Am J Ophthalmol. 1996;122:109–10.
9. Kervick GN, Johnston SS. Repair of inferior iridodialysis using a partial-thickness scleral flap. Ophthalmic Surg Lasers. 1991;22:354–5.
10. Nunziata BR. Repair of iridodialysis using a 17-millimeter straight needle. Ophthalmic Surg Lasers. 1993;24:627–9.

Chapter 46
Case 41: Zone I Open Globe Injury with Retained Corneal Foreign Body and Lens Capsule Violation

Lisa A. Cowan, Catherine J. Choi, Katherine E. Talcott, and Seanna Grob

46.1 History of Present Illness

A healthy 31-year-old man was referred by an outside hospital with a retained piece of wood lodged into his right cornea.

- Earlier that day, he had been using a power drill at work when a splinter of wood hit his right eye.
- He was not wearing eye protection at the time of the accident.

46.2 Initial Trauma Evaluation

46.2.1 Visual Acuity (Without Correction)

OD: 20/200
OS: 20/20

L. A. Cowan, M.D., Ph.D. (✉)
Department of Ophthalmology, Southern California Permanente Medical Group, Bakersfield, CA, USA

C. J. Choi, M.D.
Bascom Palmer Eye Institute, University of Miami, Miami, FL, USA

K. E. Talcott, M.D.
Vitreoretinal Surgery, Wills Eye Hospital, Philadelphia, PA, USA

S. Grob, M.D., M.A.S.
Department of Ophthalmology, Harvard Medical School, Massachusetts Eye and Ear, Boston, MA, USA

S. Grob, C. Kloek (eds.), *Management of Open Globe Injuries*,
https://doi.org/10.1007/978-3-319-72410-2_46

46.2.2 Pupils

OD: No afferent pupillary defect, round reactive
OS: No afferent pupillary defect, round reactive

46.2.3 Intraocular Pressures

OD: Deferred
OS: 14

46.2.4 External Examination

Normal, no external lacerations

46.2.5 Slit Lamp Examination

	OD	OS
Lids and lashes	Normal	Normal
Sclera and conjunctiva	Trace injection	Normal
Cornea	Full-thickness corneal laceration with retained wooden foreign body spanning exterior and interior surfaces of cornea through visual axis extending 1–2 mm into anterior chamber	Normal
Anterior chamber	1–2 + pigmented/nonpigmented cells, extension of lodged foreign body into anterior chamber	Normal
Iris	Normal	Normal
Lens	Anterior lens capsular violation nasally, faint opacification of underlying lens material, no posterior capsular violation	Normal
Vitreous	Normal	Normal

46.2.6 Dilated Examination

Macula/Nerve OD: Normal
Periphery OD: Normal, attached
Macula/Nerve: OS: Normal
Periphery OS: Normal, attached

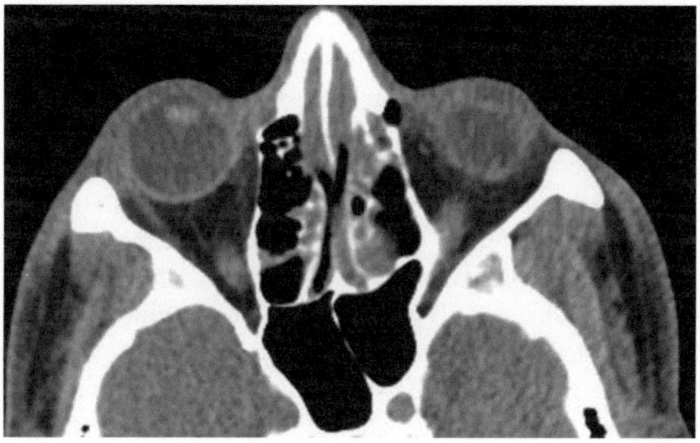

Fig. 46.1 Axial CT image from the day of presentation showing preservation of globe contour on the right despite clinically apparent corneal laceration and retained wooden foreign body

46.2.7 Radiographic Imaging

Computed Tomography (CT) of the orbits showed preservation of the globe contour on the right and absence of an intraocular foreign body in posterior segment (Fig. 46.1).

46.3 Surgeon's Initial Assessment and Pre-operative Plan

This patient is a 31-year-old man with a Zone I open globe injury from a wooden splinter with capsular violation and early cataract formation. The clinical findings included an obvious wooden foreign body extending through the cornea and into the anterior chamber. He also had an anterior lens capsular violation with faint opacification of the underlying lens material. No posterior capsular violation was noted and no posterior segment pathology was detected. The CT scan was normal without any indication of an open globe injury as the globe contour was intact (Fig. 46.1).

Discussion of this case highlights the risks of delayed presentation and retained intraocular foreign material, special concerns in open globe repair with capsular violation, and consideration of secondary intraocular lens implantation.

The goal of his initial surgery was to remove the wooden splinter, explore the wound and debride any retained foreign material, close the corneal laceration, and prophylactically treat with intracameral and intravenous antibiotics to minimize infection risk.

46.4 Surgical Exploration and Repair: Operative Note

Informed consent was obtained for open globe repair and the operative eye was verified and marked. General anesthesia was induced. The surgical field was prepped and draped in the usual sterile fashion for ophthalmic surgery. Jaffe specula were placed to retract the lids. The wooden foreign body was noted to be impaling the cornea superonasally with the deeper aspect in the anterior chamber. Mucus strands around the foreign body were removed. The foreign body was then firmly grasped with forceps, removed, and sent to gross pathology. There was immediate egress of aqueous. The edges of the corneal wound were carefully examined to ensure that no residual foreign material remained. The corneal wound was noted to be approximately triangular in shape with an apex directed superiorly. Filtered air was injected to help reform and maintain the anterior chamber. Three 10-0 nylon sutures were placed in a simple interrupted fashion to appose the wound, which was approximately 1.5 × 1.5 mm in greatest dimensions. Intracameral vancomycin 1 mg/0.1 mL and ceftazidime 2 mg/0.1 mL were injected on a 30-gauge needle into the anterior chamber. A fluorescein strip was used to check for water tightness of the wound closure. The wound was found to have a very slow leak, at the time of elevated intraocular pressure after antibiotic injections. At physiologic pressure, on provocation, the anterior chamber was maintained, and the leak did not increase in briskness. A subconjunctival injection of dexamethasone was administered in the superotemporal quadrant. The specula were removed and a 18 mm bandage contact lens was placed onto the ocular surface. Atropine and gatifloxacin were instilled over the ocular surface, followed by a sterile eye patch and a shield. Anesthesia was reversed. The patient tolerated the procedure well without any complications.

46.4.1 Surgical Exploration and Repair: Pearls

- Removal of a full-thickness corneal or scleral foreign body should be attempted in the operating room under controlled conditions.
- Intracameral antibiotics were used as this patient was at high risk of infection given a retained intraocular wooden foreign body and lens capsule violation.
- The anterior capsular lens violation and early cataract formation were not addressed at this initial surgery since the corneal laceration and edema after repair undermined the visibility of underlying structures.

46.5 Initial Post-operative Course

Our patient was admitted post-operatively for intravenous antibiotics for 48 hours, as is our standard of care. On post-operative day 1 his vision in the right eye was 20/800 without correction and 20/70 with pinhole (pre-operative vision 20/200). Intraocular pressure by palpation was approximately 15 mmHg. Slit lamp examination of his right cornea showed a paracentral, stellate, shelved corneal laceration status post repair with 3, 10-0 nylon sutures and a bandage contact lens in

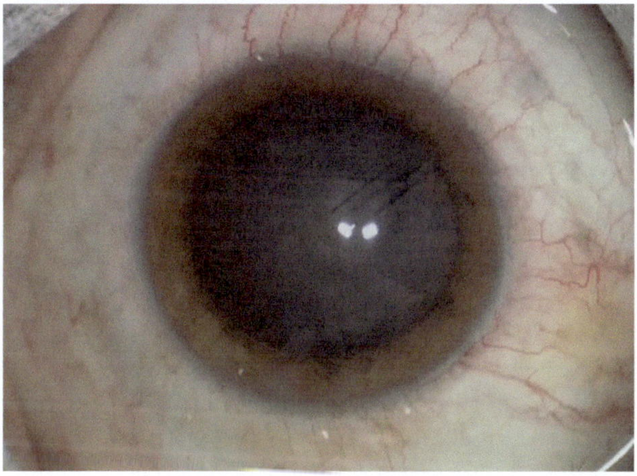

Fig. 46.2 Intraoperative photo before cataract extraction showing the corneal laceration with three 10-0 nylon sutures and a traumatic cataract

place (Fig. 46.2). His anterior chamber was formed with ½+ cell and no frank lens material. The lens violation noted pre-operatively was again appreciated now with anterior subcapsular opacification paracentrally. His bandage contact lens was left in place given the slow leak noted intraoperatively. He was started on prednisolone acetate one drop eight times daily, gatifloxacin four times daily and atropine twice daily all in the right eye.

Post-operative day 5 he noted mild discomfort in the right eye and sensitivity to light. At that point the vision in his right eye was 20/200 with pinhole acuity of 20/70 without correction. His intraocular pressure by applanation was 21 mmHg. His anterior chamber was found to have rare cell with no lens material; however, his early subcapsular cataract had rapidly progressed to mild nuclear opacification throughout the entire lens. Given the scarcity of inflammation, his prednisolone acetate was tapered down to six times daily.

On his post-operative week 2 visit, his vision on pinhole had decreased to 20/400 without correction and his eye pressure increased to 24 mmHg. His bandage contact lens was removed and his shelved stellate corneal wound was found to be briskly Seidel positive. Lens material clumped inferiorly and was found to be expressing out of anterior capsular lens violation. The anterior capsular violation had elongated compared to initial presentation. His cataract had progressed compared to his examination 1 week prior. He was started on dorzolamide/timolol ophthalmic solution twice daily for aqueous suppression, prednisolone acetate was increased to eight times daily, and gatifloxacin and atropine were continued. His bandage contact lens was replaced. Cataract extraction for increasing intraocular pressure and lens material in the anterior chamber was discussed with the patient with the goal to leave the eye aphakic given his history of retained wooden foreign body and risk of infection. Discussed options of an aphakic contact lens versus possible placement of an intraocular lens in the future.

46.6 Cataract Extraction: Operative Note

Informed consent was verified and the operative eye was verified and marked. General anesthesia was induced (per patient's request) after a careful time-out. He was prepped and draped in the usual sterile ophthalmic fashion for ophthalmic surgery. A lid speculum was placed to retract the lids and fluorescein strip was used to check for leaks over the corneal wound that had been repaired 2 weeks prior. No leak was found on fluorescein Seidel testing in the operating room.

Attention was turned to the cataract extraction. A paracentesis was created at the 2 o'clock position and the 8 o'clock position. Chopstick irrigation/aspiration instruments were introduced into the paracenteses and the loose lens material was removed. Trypan blue was introduced through the paracentesis, followed by balanced salt solution. Ophthalmic viscosurgical device was used to inflate the anterior chamber. Next, a corneal keratome 2.85 mm blade was used to create a triplanar incision at 10 o'clock. A cystotome was used to initiate a tear in the capsule inferior to the margin of the lens capsule violation. Next, a flap was raised and propagated with Utrata forceps to create a capsulorhexis with incorporation of the capsular wound inferotemporally to superotemporally. Next, microsurgical technology (MST) scissors were introduced into the eye to create a flap to continue the capsulorhexis inferonasally to superonasally. Both edges of the capsulorrhexis were able to incorporate the wound from the original trauma. Next, the lens nucleus was hydrodelineated with balance salt solution on a cannula. The phacoemulsification hand piece was introduced into the eye on epinuclear settings and the soft lens material was removed. Next, ophthalmic viscosurgical device was introduced to visco-dissect the cortical material off of the lens capsule. The irrigation/aspiration hand pieces was introduced for cortical removal. The cortical material was removed and the ophthalmic viscosurgical device was then aspirated from the anterior chamber. Next, the balanced salt solution cannula was used to hydrate all wounds (main incision and two paracentesis wounds). A 10-0 nylon suture was placed in the main wound. The corneal laceration from the original open globe trauma was checked with fluorescein and was again found to be Seidel negative. Cefazolin and decadron were injected in the subconjunctival space. A bandage contact lens was placed over the surface of the eye and found to fit well. The speculum and the drapes were removed. Gatafloxacin and atropine were instilled over the ocular surface and the patient was patched and shielded. The patient tolerated the procedure well. General anesthesia was reversed.

46.6.1 Cataract Extraction: Pearls

- Trypan blue is helpful for staining a torn anterior lens capsule and finding the exact location of the tear. Once the tear is identified, then a plan can be made to construct the best possible capsulorrhexis.

- It is best to try to incorporate the anterior capsular violation into the capsulorrhexis. If this cannot be done to achieve a continuous capsulorrhexis, MST scissors, a cystotome, and Utrata forceps can be used to create the best possible capsulorrhexis.
- Consider leaving the patient aphakic in the early trauma setting given the risk of endophthalmitis.

46.7 Post-operative Cataract Extraction Follow Up

On post-operative day 1, his vision was count fingers at three feet without correction with an eye pressure of 19 mmHg. Vision improved to 20/50 with a +18.0 diopter lens. His bandage contact lens and corneal sutures were all in good position. He had ½+ cell in the anterior chamber with small strands of retained cortex nasally and an intact posterior capsule. He was aphakic (as planned given risk of endophthalmitis from prior wooden foreign body). He was continued on gatifloxacin four times a day, prednisolone acetate six times daily, and atropine twice daily as well as dorzolamide/timolol for aqueous suppression and intraocular pressure control. His bandage contact lens was left in place.

At his post-operative week 1 visit, his vision was 20/100 with a +12.0 D lens and 20/40−1 with pinhole. His bandage contact lens was removed and his wounds were found to be Seidel negative. His prednisolone acetate regimen was tapered off starting at four times daily for 1 week then reducing frequency of administration by one drop at each subsequent week. Gatifloxacin and dorzolamide/timolol were stopped at post-operative week 1. His vision at his post-operative week 6 exam was 20/70 with +12.0 D lens. His decrease in vision was attributed to posterior capsular wrinkling. At his post-operative month 2 exam, slit lamp and intraocular pressure findings were stable. At this point, all four corneal sutures were removed. He was referred to optometry for evaluation of an aphakic contact lens.

He was fit with a rigid gas permeable contact lens with 20/30− vision, but due to discomfort, concern for infection given his dusty work environment, and binocular diplopia, he only used the lens for 3 days. At his 4-month follow up visit from his cataract extraction (5 months after globe repair), he was noted to have hypertropia and exotropia of his left eye with full ductions and versions bilaterally. It was felt his tropias were likely present prior to eye trauma and were brought out due to dissociation from decreased vision in the right eye. On further questioning, he had previous head traumas when racing, but no recent trauma. His vision was 20/125+1 with +11.5 D lens, 20/60−2 with pinhole. Stromal scarring was noted in the superonasal aspect of the cornea and extending into visual axis. He was aphakic and the posterior capsule was intact but now had extensive wrinkling and opacification. Given that he had failed a contact lens trial, intraocular lens implantation was discussed. It was discussed that his vision would most likely be better with a contact lens compared to an intraocular lens given his irregular corneal surface. There was also concern for the possibility of post-operative diplopia since this was present with the contact lens.

Table 46.1 Lenstar measurements after cataract extraction, prior to secondary lens implantation

	OD	OS
Axial length (mm)	23.28	23.38
Anterior chamber depth (mm)	4.46	3.28
Corneal power, K1 (D)	43.95	43.53
Corneal power, K2 (D)	45.22 at 129°	44.59 at 015°

Biometry measurements were obtained in preparation of a secondary sulcus intraocular lens aiming for a refractive goal of −0.5 D (Table 46.1).

46.7.1 Auto Refraction Measurements

OD: +11.25 − 0.75 × 089
K1: 44.25 D
K2: 45.00 D at 154
Cyl +0.75 D at 154

46.8 Secondary IOL Implantation: Operative Note: (6 Months After Initial Trauma)

In the pre-operative area the patient was correctly identified and the right eye was marked. The anesthesia team performed a peribulbar block and the patient was brought into the operating room. A time-out was performed and the lens implant was verified. Under the microscope the pupil was well dilated, without synechiae between the iris and lens capsule. A paracentesis was created with a supersharp blade at 2 o'clock. The anterior chamber was filled with ophthalmic viscosurgical device, which was also deposited in the sulcus to ensure that there was adequate space in the sulcus for lens insertion. Next, a clear corneal incision was created at 11:30 o'clock with a 2.4 mm keratome. This was enlarged to accommodate the lens inserter. An MA60AC +21.0 D was inserted into the sulcus, using a Y-hook and a Sinsky hook to rotate it into position. Careful irrigation/aspiration was performed to remove the viscoelastic material. Miochol was then instilled to constrict the pupil. The wounds were hydrated with balanced salt solution and were found to be secure. Subconjunctival cefazolin and decadron was administered and the speculum was removed. Maxitrol ointment was placed in the right eye and a sterile eye patch and shield were applied.

46.9 Secondary IOL Follow Up Evaluation

Post-operative visit month 1 status post secondary intraocular lens, post-operative month 7 after open globe repair (Figs. 46.3, 46.4, and 46.5):

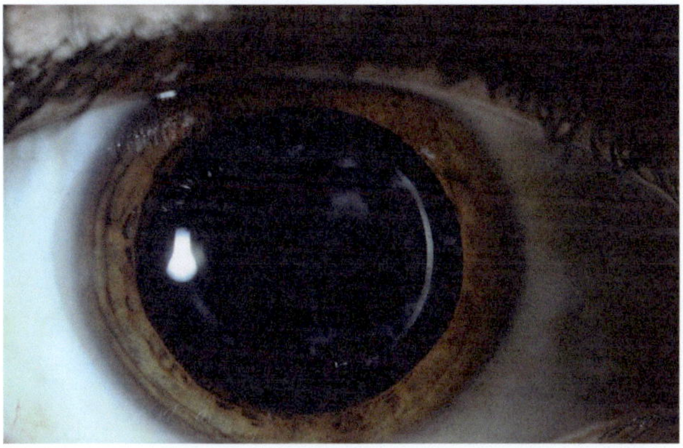

Fig. 46.3 Three piece lens in the sulcus in the right eye 1 month after secondary lens implantation

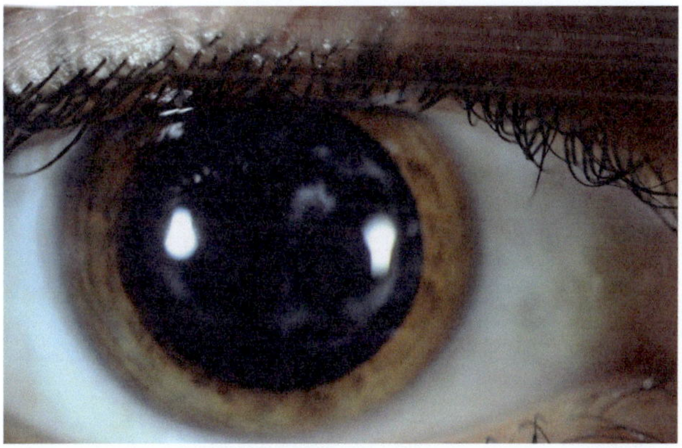

Fig. 46.4 Corneal scar superonasal to visual axis from open globe injury of the right eye 1 month after secondary lens implantation and 7 months after open globe repair

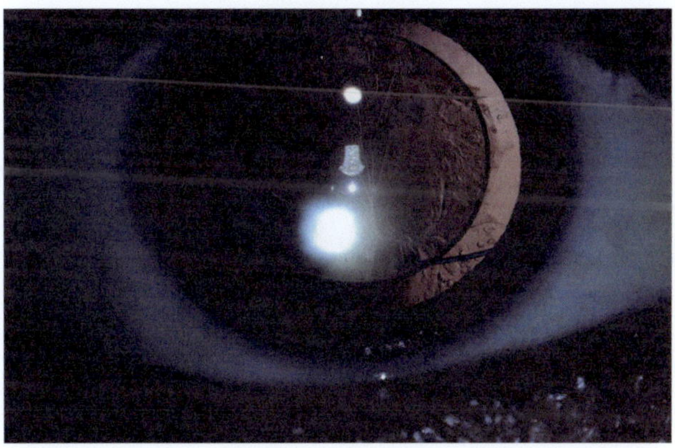

Fig. 46.5 Posterior capsular opacification and wrinkling 1 month after secondary lens implantation in the right eye

46.9.1 Refraction

OD: Plano −1.50 × 95 (20/30−)
OS: −0.75 − 1.75 × 5 (20/20−)

46.9.2 Visual Acuity (with correction)

OD: 20/30−1 ph 20/20−2
OS: 20/30−2

46.9.3 Pupils

OD: Round, reactive
OS: Round, reactive

46.9.4 Slit Lamp Examination

	OD	OS
Lids and lashes	Normal	Normal
Sclera and Conjunctiva	Normal	Normal
Cornea	Wounds Seidel negative, superonasal corneal scarring	Normal
Anterior chamber	Normal	Normal
Iris	Normal	Normal
Lens	Sulcus 3-piece lens in position, posterior capsule intact with slight wrinkling	Normal
Vitreous	Normal	Normal

46.9.5 Dilated Examination

Macula/Nerve OD: Normal
Periphery OD: Small area of chorioretinal scarring
Macula/Nerve: OS: Normal
Peripheral OS: Normal

46.10 Follow Up

At post-operative month 8 (after secondary IOL), he underwent a YAG capsulotomy and his vision improved to 20/20 with spectacle correction. His prior symptoms of diplopia had resolved.

46.11 Review and Lessons Learned

Our patient had a very high risk of developing endophthalmitis given his relatively delayed presentation with an intraocular wooden foreign body and lens capsular violation. Luckily, he did not develop an infection, but prophylactic intracameral antibiotics (vancomycin and ceftazidime) at the time of open globe repair and 48 hours of intravenous antibiotics (vancomycin and ceftazidime) were utilized.

Post-traumatic acute infectious endophthalmitis usually occurs within a week of open globe trauma [1]. Risk factors for post-traumatic endophthalmitis include presence of an intraocular foreign body, lens violation, delay to repair (>24 hours), laceration-type injury, and trauma with contaminated objects [1–5]. Some studies have found early primary repair and prolapse of intraocular tissue and self-sealing of wounds protective against development of post-traumatic endophthalmitis [3, 6].

The rate of post-traumatic endophthalmitis ranges in the literature with and without prophylactic antibiotics (0.9–17%) and evidence loosely supports that prophylactic oral and/or intravenous antibiotic administration reduces the risk of endophthalmitis [1–3, 5–7], but the recommended standardized prophylactic antibiotic protocol administration modality is not well established [5, 8].

Du Toit et al. published a randomized controlled non-inferiority trial of prophylactic antibiotic treatment (established intravenous[IV]/oral prophylaxis [IV cefazolin and oral ciprofloxacin] versus only oral ciprofloxacin and cefuroxime each for 3 days from admission) in open globe injuries and found that the incidence of endophthalmitis was 2–3% across both treatment arms [1]. Furthermore, the difference in post-traumatic endophthalmitis between IV/oral antibiotics [2%, 3 patients out of 150] and oral only antibiotics [2.7%, 4 patients out of 150] was not significant [$p = 0.703$] [1]. In their study, patients which were high risk for infection were excluded (those with an intraocular foreign body, dirty injuries caused by contaminated or organic objects). Tabatabaei et al. also found no significant difference between oral (ciprofloxacin) and intravenous (ceftazidime and vancomycin) antibiotic prophylaxis for open globe injuries in their prospective study on 1255 consecutive patients. The overall rate of endophthalmitis in their study was 2.2% [9]. However, our protocol with intravenous antibiotics has shown a very low rate of endophthalmitis at 0.9% [7].

Although our patient did not develop an infection, he did develop an increase in eye pressure, related to anterior lens capsular violation, which was treated successfully with cataract extraction. Again, out of concern for his high risk of developing infection, he was left aphakic. The incidence of ocular hypertension after open globe injury ranges in the literature (from 2% to 43%) [10].

One retrospective, case-control study reviewed records of consecutive open globe injuries and found that out of 382 patients with 2 months of follow-up, 65 (17%) developed ocular hypertension (>22 mmHg) [11]. Risk factors for developing ocular hypertension identified from that same study were increased age, hyphema, lens injury, and Zone II injury [11]. Another large prospective cohort study obtained data from the United States Eye Injury Registry regarding 3627 patients with penetrating ocular injury [12]. This study, by Girkin et al, showed a 2.67% incidence of post-traumatic glaucoma, as identified by the treating physician on the 6-month report form based on increased intarocular pressure, optic disk, or visual field abnormality consistent with glaucoma, with risk factors including advancing age, lens injury, poor baseline visual acuity, and inflammation [12]. A retrospective chart review of patients admitted for open globe injury over the course of 15 years showed a 5.3% incidence of developing post-traumatic glaucoma (41 patients out of 775) [13]. Osman et al. found Zone II injury, penetrating ocular trauma, lens injury, vitreous hemorrhage, and the presence of an intraocular foreign body were associated with post-traumatic glaucoma. Another retrospective observational case series, which reviewed over 13 years of data, noted traumatic ocular hypertension in 23.3% (120/515 eyes) and glaucoma in 6.2% (32/515 eyes) [10]. Bojikian et al. found associations between traumatic intraocular pressure elevation and glaucoma with older age, prior penetrating keratoplasty, vitreous hemorrhage, Zone II injury, and penetrating keratoplasty after open globe repair [10].

46.12 Key Learning Points

- Delayed presentation and lens violation especially in the setting of retained organic foreign body is very high risk for endophthalmitis and must be considered an emergency for urgent surgical repair.
- For any open globe injury, ongoing routine examinations are essential including gonioscopy as increases in eye pressure can occur.
- Increases in intraocular pressure may occur after lens capsule violation and patients should be watched closely for pressure spikes.
- Intracameral/intravitreal antibiotics should be considered in open globe injuries presenting with infection or with high risk for infection.
- Sulcus intraocular lenses are a viable alternative for patients unable to tolerate an aphakic contact lenses.

References

1. Du Toit N, Mustak S, Cook C. Randomised controlled trial of prophylactic antibiotic treatment for the prevention of endophthalmitis after open globe injury at Groote Schuur Hospital. Br J Ophthalmol. 2017;101(7):862.
2. Bhagat N, Nagori S, Zarbin M. Post-traumatic infectious endophthalmitis. Surv Ophthalmol. 2011;56:214–51.
3. Zhang Y, Zhang MN, Jiang CH, Yao Y, Zhang K. Endophthalmitis following open globe injury. Br J Ophthalmol. 2010;94(1):111–4.
4. Duch-Samper AM, Chaques-Alepuz V, Menezo JL, Hurtado-Sarrio M. Endophthalmitis following open-globe injuries. Curr Opin Ophthalmol. 1998;9:59–65.
5. Huang J, Pansick AD, Blomquist PH. Use of intravenous vancomycin and cefepime in preventing endophthalmitis after open globe injury. J Ocul Pharmacol Therap. 2016;32(7):437–41.
6. Faghihi H, Hajizadeh F, Esfahani MR, Rasoulinejad SA, Lashay A. Posttraumatic endophthalmitis: report no. 2. Retina. 2012;32(1):146–51.
7. Andreoli CM, Andreoli MT, Kloek CE, Ahuero AE, Vavvas D, et al. Low rate of endophthalmitis in a large series of open globe injuries. Am J Ophthalmol. 2009;147(4):601–8.
8. Lorch A, Sobrin L. Prophylactic antibiotics in posttraumatic infectious endophthalmitis. Int Ophthalmol Clin. 2013;53:167–76.
9. Tabatabaei SA, Soleimani M, Behrooz MJ, Sheibani K. Systemic oral antibiotics as a prophylactic measure to prevent endophthalmitis in patients with open globe injuries in comparison with intravenous antibiotics. Retina. 2016;36(2):360–5.
10. Bojikian KD, Stein AL, Slabaugh MA, Chen PP. Incidence and risk factors for traumatic intraocular pressure elevation and traumatic glaucoma after open-globe injury. Eye. 2015;29:1579–84.
11. Turalba AV, Shah AS, Andreoli MT, Andreoli CM, Rhee DJ. Predictors and outcomes of ocular hypertension after open-globe injury. J Glaucoma. 2014;23(1):5–10. https://doi.org/10.1097/IJG.0b013e318265bb4a.
12. Girkin CA, McGwin G Jr, Morris R, Kuhn F. Glaucoma following penetrating ocular trauma: a cohort study of the united states eye injury registry. Am J Ophthalmol. 2005;139:100–5.
13. Osman EA, Al-Fawaz N, Al-Otaibi AG, Al-Mansouri SM, Mousa A, et al. Glaucoma after open globe injury at a tertiary care university hospital in Central Saudi Arabia. Cumulative incidence and risk factors. Saudi Med J. 2013;34(4):374–8.

Chapter 47
Case 42: Open Globe Rupture and Retinal Detachment with Retinal Incarceration from Baseball Injury

Avni P. Finn, Catherine J. Choi, and Dean Eliott

47.1 History of Present Illness

A 56-year-old man presented with concern for globe rupture after being struck in the right eye by a baseball.

- He was coaching his son's baseball team and was hit with a high-speed ball immediately after it was struck by the bat.
- He reported immediate loss of vision on impact.
- Computed Tomography (CT) was consistent with an open globe injury.

47.2 Initial Trauma Evaluation

47.2.1 Visual Acuity (Without Correction)

OD: Hand motion
OS: 20/20

A. P. Finn, M.D., M.B.A. (✉)
Vitreoretinal Surgery, Duke Eye Center, Durham, NC, USA

C. J. Choi, M.D.
Bascom Palmer Eye Institute, Miami, FL, USA

D. Eliott, M.D.
Vitreoretinal Surgery, Department of Ophthalmology, Harvard Medical School, Massachusetts Eye and Ear, Boston, MA, USA

S. Grob, C. Kloek (eds.), *Management of Open Globe Injuries*,
https://doi.org/10.1007/978-3-319-72410-2_47

47.2.2 Pupils

OD: Poor view with afferent pupillary defect by reverse
OS: Round and reactive

47.2.3 Slit Lamp Examination

	OD	OS
Lids and lashes	5 mm sub-brow upper eyelid laceration	Normal
Sclera and conjunctiva	360° subconjunctival hemorrhage	White and quiet
Cornea	Clear	Clear
Anterior chamber	Shallow with diffuse total hyphema	Deep and quiet
Iris	Poor view, appears round	Round and reactive
Len	Poor view, appears intact	1+ nuclear sclerosis
Vitreous	Poor view, vitreous hemorrhage	Clear

47.2.4 Dilated Examination

Macula/nerve OD: No view
Periphery OD: No view
Macula/nerve OS: Normal, cup to disc ratio 0.3, sharp
Periphery OS: Normal

47.2.5 Radiographic Imaging

CT scan on presentation showed findings consistent with a posterior rupture with flattened contour of the posterior globe, nondisplaced fractures of the medial wall and orbital floor, and no intraocular foreign body (Fig. 47.1).

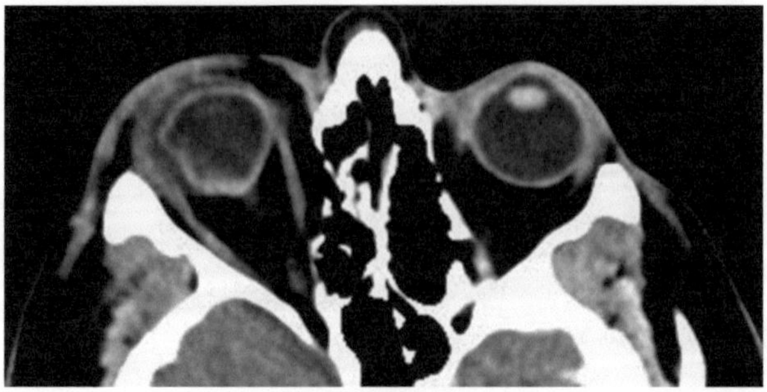

Fig. 47.1 An axial CT image showing a deformed and flattened globe contour temporally consistent with a posterior scleral rupture

47.3 Surgeon's Initial Assessment and Discussion on Pre-operative Planning

This patient sustained a blunt trauma with concern for a Zone III rupture. The clinical findings including 360° subconjunctival hemorrhage and total hyphema, combined with CT scan findings were concerning for a blunt rupture. As discussed earlier in the book, a rupture is a full-thickness eyewall wound caused by a blunt object such as a baseball. The impact results in a momentary increase in intraocular pressure and an inside-out mechanism of injury. A scleral rupture may be occult and hidden under conjunctiva, Tenon's capsule, or the rectus muscles as in this case. CT may be useful in these cases, showing flattening of the posterior contour of the sclera or a "flat tire" sign [1].

This case illustrates three important areas of discussion, including identifying and closing a posterior rupture, planning for retina surgery after initial globe closure, and addressing retinal detachment and retinal incarceration with vitreoretinal surgery.

The primary goal of the initial surgery was to explore the eye to find the posterior rupture and to close the globe to the greatest extent possible. This entails a 360° peritomy, exploration of all four quadrants of the eye and under the rectus muscles, and closure of the rupture to prevent infection and decrease the risk of sympathetic ophthalmia. As discussed in an earlier case with blunt trauma and associated fractures, these cases often are associated with a worse visual prognosis and patients need to be appropriately educated before globe repair.

47.4 Surgical Exploration and Repair: Operative Note

Informed consent was obtained for open globe exploration, repair of the open globe injury, and repair of upper eyelid laceration for the right eye. The uninjured left eye was protected with a taped shield and the right eye was prepped and draped in the usual sterile ophthalmic fashion using a Jaffe speculum to provide adequate exposure.

A 360° limbal peritomy was then initiated with a relaxing incision at 9 o'clock and was extended along the entire circumference of the cornea. Each quadrant of the globe was then explored using first Westcott scissors and then curved Stevens scissors. Each rectus muscle was hooked with a Gass muscle hook followed by a 2-0 silk suture and the area behind the muscle explored. The patient was found to have a posterior full-thickness scleral rupture temporally beginning posterior to the lateral rectus muscle. The rupture was noted to begin 12 mm from the limbus under the lateral rectus at 9 o'clock and noted to extend circumferentially in the inferotemporal direction, diving inferiorly and posteriorly under the inferior oblique muscle. The lateral rectus muscle was hooked and isolated using 2-0 silk suture. The inferior oblique was also hooked.

However, this did not provide adequate exposure to close the rupture. The lateral rectus was then imbricated using double armed 6-0 Vicryl suture on an S-29 spatulated needle and disinserted using Westcott scissors to allow for improved exposure of the rupture site. Care was taken to evaluate the orientation of the muscle so it could be replaced to its originally position after repair of the scleral rupture.

Approximately 9 mm of the rupture was re-approximated using interrupted 8-0 nylon sutures on a spatulated needle. Care was taken to carefully reposit uveal tissue with an iris spatula during this process and any vitreous at the wound was carefully cut using a Weck-cel sponge and Westcott scissors. However, the rupture was noted to continue posteriorly and the full extent of the wound could not be safely visualized or re-approximated despite maximal exposure. No continuation was found from the nasal side.

The lateral rectus muscle was reinserted at its original insertion using the double armed 6-0 Vicryl suture. The conjunctiva was then closed with 8-0 Vicryl sutures. A subconjunctival injection of steroid and antibiotics was then performed superonasally away from the wound. The speculum was carefully removed. The drape was removed under the microscope.

Attention was then turned to the right upper eyelid laceration. This was closed using deep interrupted 6-0 Vicryl sutures followed by 6-0 plain gut interrupted sutures.

Topical atropine and dexamethasone-neomyxin-polymixin b ophthalmic ointment were applied and the eye was patched and a shield was placed. Topical erythromycin was applied to the eyelid laceration.

47.4.1 Surgical Exploration and Initial Globe Repair: Pearls

- In cases of a posterior rupture, the scleral wound may be located under the rectus muscles or extend under the muscles. In these cases, a muscle hook may be used to lift the muscle out of the way. If this does not provide adequate exposure, the muscle may be isolated and cut from the globe. After the repair the muscle is re-sutured to its original location.
- Uveal tissue must be reposited by the assistant while the surgeon closes the overlying sclera. If vitreous has extruded it should be cut with sharp scissors flush to the sclera.
- We make every attempt to close every open globe wound in its entirety; however, in very posterior ruptures the full extent of the wound may be extremely difficult to close despite achieving optimal exposure. In such cases, it is safer to allow the very posterior extent of the wound to heal by secondary intent once most of the wound has been closed, rather than subject the globe to excess pressure, rotation, and manipulation.

47.5 Initial Post-operative Course

The patient was admitted and completed a 48 hour course of intravenous antibiotics. On post-operative day (POD) 1, vision was light perception (LP), intraocular pressure was 14 mm Hg, there was diffuse corneal edema with Descemet's membrane folds, 4 mm layered hyphema, and nuclear sclerosis (Fig. 47.2). There was no view of the posterior segment and B-scan showed lens capsule violation, dense vitreous hemorrhage, and total retinal detachment with evidence of retinal incarceration with membranes tracking towards the inferotemporal incarceration site (Fig. 47.3).

He was evaluated by the retina service for consideration of repair of the retinal detachment. Options were discussed with the patient including complex retinal detachment repair involving possible pars plana lensectomy and vitrectomy, retinectomy, and silicone oil. The need for an extensive surgery and extremely guarded prognosis were discussed in detail with the patient and his family. This included a discussion of the possible progression to blindness or loss of the eye, even with surgery, and the possible need for additional operations. The patient elected to undergo surgery and 10 days later was brought to the operating room.

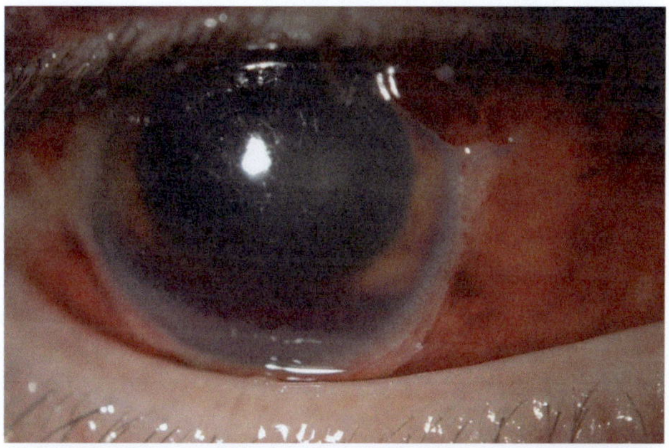

Fig. 47.2 POD #2 external slit lamp photos of the right eye showed peritomy sutured closed, formed anterior chamber with resolving hyphema and nuclear sclerotic cataract

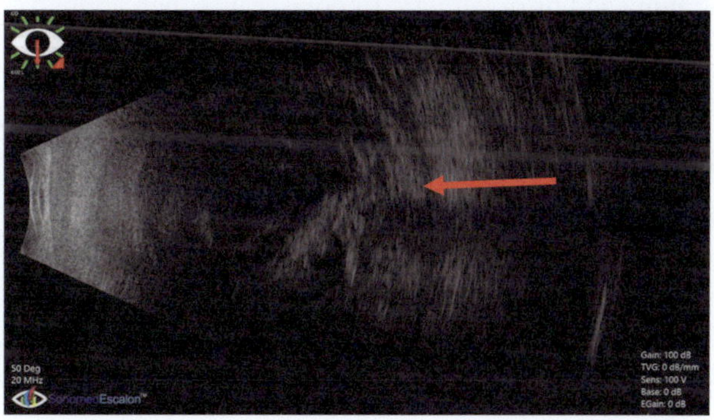

Fig. 47.3 B-scan on POD #2 demonstrates thickened choroid, retinal detachment, and membranes tracking towards the site of retinal incarceration (red arrow)

47.6 Retina Surgery: Operative Note

After informed consent was obtained, the patient was brought to the operating room and general anesthesia was induced. The right eye was prepped and draped in routine sterile fashion. A wire lid speculum was placed. A 23-gauge surgery was performed. Points were marked 3.0 mm posterior to the limbus in the usual locations. Cannulas and trocars were placed.

There was blood in the anterior chamber and this was washed out to improve visualization. A pars plana lensectomy was carried out. After complete removal of lens nucleus and cortex, the lens capsule was removed with forceps. The entire capsule was removed.

Pars plana vitrectomy was carried out with the vitreous cutter and the fiberoptic light source. There was very dense hemorrhage that was carefully cleared with the vitreous cutter before the posterior hyaloid could be visualized. The retina was completely detached on initial inspection. The posterior hyaloid was elevated except for temporally where it was attached to retina which was incarcerated in the scleral wound. The posterior hyaloid membrane was elevated and stripped to the extreme periphery. Meticulous membrane peeling was performed along the edge of the retinal incarceration. Then it was obvious that the retina needed to be cut to remove it from the wound and a relaxing retinectomy was performed along the incarceration site with intraocular scissors. There were subretinal membranes and subretinal hemorrhage present in the macular region which were removed and washed out.

Eventually after completing these tedious maneuvers, it could be seen that the retina was completely free of traction and nicely relaxed. Scleral depression was then performed for 360° and no additional retinal breaks were noted. An inferior peripheral iridectomy was performed with the vitreous cutter. A fluid-air exchange was performed with the soft-tipped cannula and the fiberoptic light source.

Drainage was performed through the posterior extent of the retinectomy, just temporal to the fovea, without the use of perfluorocarbon. The retina flattened without traction remaining anywhere. Prior to performing the fluid air exchange, an attempt at scleral buckle was performed; however, we were unable to isolate the lateral rectus muscle due to the significant scarring that was present from the initial trauma and prior surgery. Endolaser was then applied confluently along the edge of the retinectomy, achieving a good endolaser pattern.

Each of the three sclerotomies were sutured with 7-0 Vicryl interrupted sutures. Prior to placing the final sutures, silicone oil was placed up to the pupil plane. A good oil fill was achieved. The conjunctiva was closed with multiple interrupted Vicryl sutures. Subconjunctival injections of cefazolin and dexamethasone were given. The pressure was checked at the conclusion of the procedure and was normal. The eye was flushed with betadine and then dressed with dexamethasone-neomyxin-polymixin b ophthalmic ointment and a patch and shield were placed and the patient was extubated and transferred to the recovery room in good condition, having tolerated this procedure well.

47.6.1 Retina Surgery: Pearls

When vitrectomy is performed in the case of ocular trauma the following are the goals of surgery:

1) Clearing the ocular media by removing the cataractous lens and/or vitreous hemorrhage to allow adequate visualization.
2) Removing the posterior hyaloid to release vitreoretinal traction and minimize future scaffold for proliferative vitreoretinopathy.
3) Identifying and treating all the retinal breaks with endolaser.
4) Relaxing retinectomy may be necessary to fully allow the retina to relax in cases of severe proliferative vitreoretinopathy (PVR) or retinal incarceration.

47.7 Post-operative Course and Final Evaluation

The silicone oil was removed 9 months later in the setting of emulsified silicone oil and elevated intraocular pressure. Best corrected vision 1 year after initial ruptured globe injury had improved to 20/320 from hand motion pre-operatively and the retina remained attached (Figs. 47.4 and 47.5).

47.7.1 Final Visual Acuity (With Refraction)

OD: 20/320
OS: 20/20

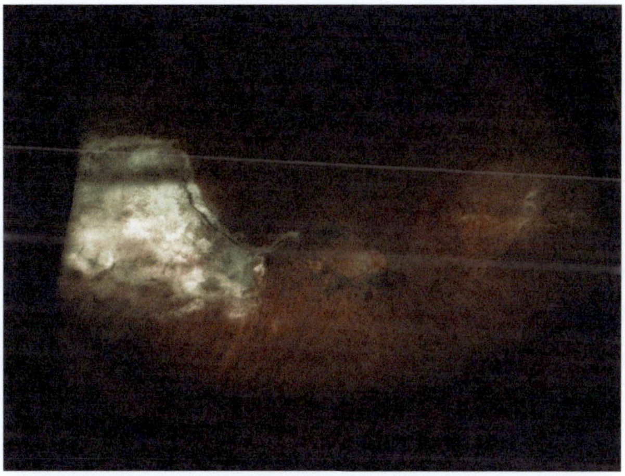

Fig. 47.4 Optos fundus photo of the right eye demonstrates attached retina 1 year post-operatively with a triangular area where the relaxing retinotomy was performed at the site of prior retinal incarceration. There are pigmentary changes in the macula and nasal atrophy

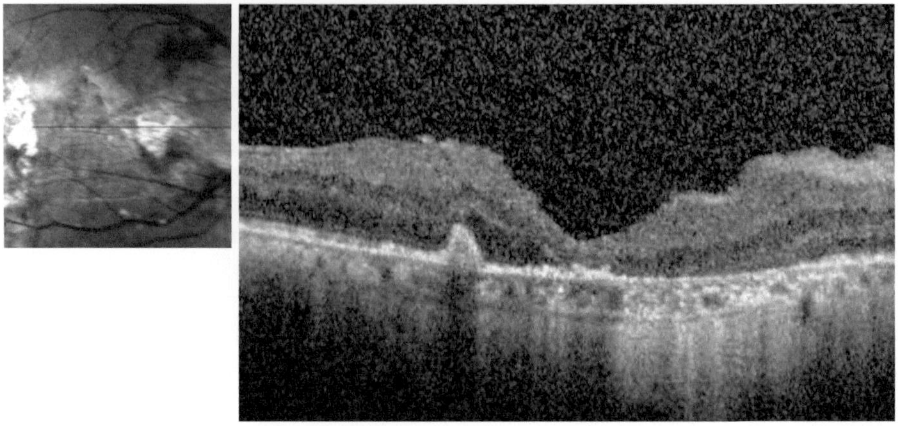

Fig. 47.5 Optical coherence tomography (OCT) shows attached macula, no cystoid macular edema, loss of the foveal outer retinal layers, and trace epiretinal membrane with irregular inner retinal contour

47.7.2 Pupils

OD: Surgical, inferior peripheral iridectomy, afferent pupillary defect by reverse
OS: Round and regular

47.7.3 Slit Lamp Examination

	OD	OS
Lids and lashes	Small right upper eyelid scar	Normal
Sclera and conjunctiva	White and quiet	White and quiet
Cornea	Clear	Clear
Anterior chamber	Deep and quiet	Deep ad quiet
Iris	Inferior peripheral iridectomy	Round and reactive
Lens	Aphakic	1+ Nuclear sclerosis
Vitreous	Status post pars plana vitrectomy	Clear

47.7.4 Dilated Examination

Macula/nerve OD: Trace epiretinal membrane (ERM), flat macula, cup to disc ratio 0.4
Periphery OD: Temporal retinectomy with lasered edges, attached, pigmentary changes nasally (Fig. 47.4).
Macula/nerve OS: Normal, cup to disc ratio 0.3, sharp
Periphery OS: Normal

47.8 Review and Lessons Learned

If anterior segment abnormality or vitreous hemorrhage obscures examination of the retina as in this case, ultrasonography plays a critical role in pre-operative decision making for vitreoretinal surgery. B-scan is useful for determining the presence of a retinal detachment, posterior vitreous detachment, occult scleral rupture, choroidal detachment, retinal tears, or retinal incarceration. When ultrasound demonstrates membranes emanating or tracking to an equatorial location, vitreous or retinal incarceration may be inferred as in this case.

Most vitreoretinal surgeons advocate for vitrectomy in cases of severe ocular trauma necessitating retinal detachment repair within 2 weeks [2–4]. Repair within 2 weeks allows the eye to heal from the initial open globe injury so that an intraocular pressure may be maintained during vitrectomy and the posterior hyaloid can be removed. It also allows for intervention prior to extensive intraocular membrane formation [5].

If anterior chamber opacity or lens opacity does not allow the surgeon to start the surgery through the pars plana, an anterior chamber infusion may be placed at the limbus to allow the surgeon to clear the media and allow a view to place a pars plana infusion. A decision must be made on whether to perform lensectomy. Often the lens is violated or cataractous from the time of injury and must be removed and other times it may be subluxated or dislocated. The surgeon should be careful to remove all of the lens capsule as it may serve as a nidus for future PVR leading to a higher rate of recurrent retinal detachment or hypotony.

Once the anterior segment is cleared and the posterior pathology can be visualized, it is critical to remove as much of the posterior cortical vitreous as possible. When a posterior vitreous detachment is not present, one is created with aspiration using the vitreous cutter to lift the hyaloid. A pic or forceps may useful to help completely peel and remove the cortical vitreous if it is very adherent.

Additionally, tangential and anterior-posterior traction must be relieved by either extensive membrane peeling and if needed a relaxing retinectomy. Retinal incarceration is one of the most challenging situations in ocular trauma, producing complex and difficult to repair retinal detachment. Vitrectomy, combined with scleral buckling and/or relaxing retinectomy is necessary in these cases to repair the retinal detachment. If the retinal incarceration is located posteriorly as in this case, scleral buckling cannot support the area, and retinectomy is recommended. In an anterior incarceration, scleral buckling may be more advantageous. Han et al. report their experience with retinal incarceration and recommend retinectomy when the scleral buckle is not sufficient to relieve traction or when the incarceration is too posterior to be treated adequately with scleral buckling. In the situation of posterior incarceration, relaxing retinectomy circumscribing the area of incarceration was performed much the same in the case described above. Seventy-three percent of the eyes (11 of 15 eyes) achieved anatomic success but only 6 eyes regained visual acuity of 5/200 or better [6].

In most cases of ocular trauma, particularly those with inferior pathology, long acting tamponade such as silicone oil is preferred [7]. Patients with severe ocular trauma including those with vitreous hemorrhage, large retinal tears, retinal incarceration, large retinal detachments, choroidal detachments and choroidal ruptures are at increased risk for severe proliferative vitreoretinopathy. A scleral buckle, usually a 3.5 mm or 4 mm encircling band, is a useful adjunct in cases of ocular trauma to decrease the risk of subsequent re-detachment in the setting of PVR. However, in this case a buckle could not be placed due to extensive scarring of the lateral rectus muscle, which was disinserted and reinserted at the time of initial repair. Some other adjunctive treatments, such as high dose steroids, low molecule weight heparin, 5-fluorouracil and methotrexate, have been used with variable success to prevent PVR, though there is further research to be done [8, 9].

Even when aggressive and prompt management is carried out with multiple specialists, eyes with retinal detachment in the setting of open globe injury have a guarded prognosis and an extensive discussion with the patient is of utmost importance.

47.9 Key Learning Points

In this case, our patient had an extensive, very posterior blunt rupture in Zone III. Despite best efforts to expose the area of rupture the entire site could not be closed. Additionally, there was a total retinal detachment with retinal incarceration. The incarceration may have resulted from uvea in the area that was not closed during the initial repair or occurred in the area of repair despite the surgeon's best attempt to reposit uveal tissue at the time of globe closure.

- Retinal incarceration is most likely to occur in posterior scleral wounds such as the case in this patient and careful repositing of uveal tissue must always be employed to attempt to avoid this potential complication.
- While disinsertion of a muscle may be necessary for maximal exposure to repair an open globe injury, the surgeon should be aware that the scarring that ensues may preclude isolation of the muscles in the case that a scleral buckle is needed.
- Retinal incarceration is best managed by scleral buckling +/– relaxing retinotomy for anterior incarceration and relaxing retinotomy for posterior incarceration.
- Proliferative vitreoretinopathy is the most common cause for recurrent detachment in cases of ocular trauma and may be minimized with meticulous removal of the posterior hyaloid, extensive membrane peeling, and the use of adjuvant encircling buckle.

References

1. Sevel D, Krausz H, Ponder T, Centeno R. Value of computed tomography for the diagnosis of a ruptured eye. J Comput Assist Tomogr. 1983;7(5):870–5.
2. Ryan SJ, Allen AW. Pars plana vitrectomy in ocular trauma. Am J Ophthalmol. 1979;88(3 Pt 1): 483–91.

3. Coles WH, Haik GM. Vitrectomy in intraocular trauma. Its rationale and its indications and limitations. Arch Ophthalmol (Chicago, Ill 1960). 1972;87(6):621–8.
4. Coleman DJ. Early vitrectomy in the management of the severely traumatized eye. Am J Ophthalmol. 1982;93(5):543–51.
5. Winthrop SR, Cleary PE, Minckler DS, Ryan SJ. Penetrating eye injuries: a histopathological review. Br J Ophthalmol. 1980;64(11):809–17.
6. Han DP, Mieler WF, Abrams GW, Williams GA. Vitrectomy for traumatic retinal incarceration. Arch Ophthalmol (Chicago, Ill 1960). 1988;106(5):640–5.
7. Spiegel D, Nasemann J, Nawrocki J, Gabel VP. Severe ocular trauma managed with primary pars plana vitrectomy and silicone oil. Retina. 1997;17(4):275–85.
8. Pennock S, Haddock LJ, Eliott D, Mukai S, Kazlauskas A. Is neutralizing vitreal growth factors a viable strategy to prevent proliferative vitreoretinopathy? Prog Retin Eye Res. 2014;40:16–34.
9. Krader CG. Effective drug management of PVR remains unfulfilled goal. 2017. http://modernretina.modernmedicine.com/modern-retina/news/effective-drug-management-pvr-remains-unfulfilled-goal?page=0,2. Accessed 29 May 2017.

Chapter 48
Case 43: Large Zone III Open Globe from a Finger Injury While Playing Basketball

Elizabeth J. Rossin, Yewlin E. Chee, Peter B. Veldman, and Dean Eliott

48.1 History of Present Illness

A 57-year-old man with history of cardiac disease presents with concern for open globe of the left eye.

- The patient reports he was playing basketball and was struck by a fellow player's finger in the left eye.
- He was brought to an outside hospital where computed tomography (CT) revealed a dislocated lens and collapsed globe.
- He complains of left eye pain, especially on eye movement, and decreased vision on the left.

E. J. Rossin, M.D., Ph.D. (✉)
Department of Ophthalmology, Harvard Medical School, Massachusetts Eye and Ear, Boston, MA, USA
e-mail: Elizabeth_rossin@meei.harvard.edu

Y. E. Chee, M.D.
Vitreoretinal Surgery, Department of Ophthalmology, University of Washington, Seattle, WA, USA

P. B. Veldman, M.D.
Cornea and Refractive Surgery, Department of Ophthalmology and Visual Science, University of Chicago, Chicago, IL, USA

D. Eliott, M.D.
Vitreoretinal Surgery, Department of Ophthalmology, Harvard Medical School, Massachusetts Eye and Ear, Boston, MA, USA

S. Grob, C. Kloek (eds.), *Management of Open Globe Injuries*,
https://doi.org/10.1007/978-3-319-72410-2_48

48.2 Initial Trauma Evaluation

48.2.1 *Visual Acuity (Without Correction)*

OD: 20/15
OS: Light perception

48.2.2 *Pupils*

OD: Round, reactive
OS: No view, no afferent pupillary defect by reverse

48.2.3 *External Examination*

3-mm left cheek laceration

48.2.4 *Slit Lamp Examination*

	OD	OS
Lids and lashes	Normal	Diffusely ecchymotic and tender to palpation
Sclera and conjunctiva	Normal	360 bullous subconjunctival hemorrhage
Cornea	Normal	Normal
Anterior chamber	Normal	Total hyphema
Iris	Normal	No view
Lens	Normal	No view
Vitreous	Normal	No view

48.2.5 *Dilated Examination*

Macula/Nerve OD: Normal
Periphery OD: Normal
Macula/Nerve: OS: No view
Periphery OS: No view

48.2.6 Radiographic Imaging

Outside CT of the orbits revealed a collapsed globe of the left eye with poorly visualized and dislocated lens, very distorted globe contour, and high density material in both the anterior and posterior segments suggestive of hemorrhage. There was no orbital fracture or skull base fracture. There were no intraocular foreign bodies.

48.3 Surgeon's Initial Assessment and Pre-operative Plan

The patient presented with a large Zone III rupture from blunt trauma due to a finger.

In eyes with significant trauma, as is the case here, a view to the posterior pole is often obscured by a complete "eight-ball" hyphema in the anterior chamber or by vitreous hemorrhage. As discussed in earlier chapters, if there is bullous subconjunctival hemorrhage and no view to the posterior pole due to a hyphema and/or vitreous hemorrhage, globe exploration must be performed in the operating room in order to rule out an open globe injury. Ultrasound B-scan should not be done at initial assessment due to risk of extruding intraocular contents with pressure from the ultrasound probe. The primary focus should be on globe repair and this approach should not differ from standard repair previously described (see previous chapters in this book).

Once the initial repair is completed, B scan ultrasound should be done without delay to assess for vitreous hemorrhage, vitreous traction, retinal detachment and/or choroidal hemorrhage. All eyes with history of Zone III injury with vitreous hemorrhage with or without retinal detachment should be referred promptly to a vitreoretinal surgeon for serial examinations with B scan ultrasound, as secondary vitrectomy surgery can potentially yield a more favorable visual outcome. Generally, secondary vitrectomy surgery should be performed within 7–14 days of the initial trauma.

The secondary vitrectomy surgery is often difficult due to post-traumatic complications, including media opacity and proliferative vitreoretinopathy. These cases often involve incarcerated vitreous and retina at the site of the original scleral wound. Indications for secondary vitrectomy after open globe repair include persistent media opacity, progressive vitreoretinal traction, retinal detachment, and/or retinal incarceration. Secondary vitrectomy can aid in the removal of hemorrhage and inflammatory mediators that can hamper healing and induce proliferative membranes.

48.4 Surgical Exploration and Repair: Operative Description from Open Globe Repair

Informed consent was obtained and the operative eye was verified and marked. The left eye was prepped and draped in the usual sterile ophthalmic fashion using a Jaffe speculum to provide adequate exposure.

Examination revealed a 360° bullous subconjunctival hemorrhage and a soft eye with a total hyphema. A 360° peritomy was performed using 0.12 forceps and Westcott scissors. The preliminary examination of the sclera suggested that the globe injury was most likely temporal. The superior rectus, medial rectus and inferior rectus were hooked and secured using 2-0 silk suture. The lateral rectus was then hooked and isolated using 6-0 Vicryl double-armed suture in an imbricating fashion. The muscle insertion was marked. The lateral rectus insertion was then dissected from the globe. It was noted that the superior portion of the lateral rectus had been split. This portion of the lateral rectus was also imbricated and removed from the globe. Examination of the sclera at this time revealed an extensive Zone III rupture site extending from 12:00 o'clock to 6:00 o'clock and beginning 8 mm posterior to the limbus at the 12:00 o'clock position and spiraling outwards to 11 mm posterior to the limbus at the most inferior 6:00 o'clock position. There was extrusion of uveal tissue. The lens was found underneath the conjunctiva inferotemporally and removed and sent to pathology. The scleral defect was closed using interrupted 8-0 nylon sutures with repositing of uveal contents, taking care not to incorporate the uveal tissue into the wound. The inferior portion of the lateral rectus was reattached to the globe at its original insertion site initially by passing partial thickness scleral bites at the insertion site. Then, the additional 6-0 double-armed Vicryl suture in the superior section of the lateral rectus was also secured at its appropriate insertion site. The conjunctiva was re-approximated using 8-0 Vicryl suture. Balanced saline solution on a 30-gauge needle was used to refill the eye through a corneal paracentesis. A subconjunctival injection of Cefazolin and Dexamethasone were administered superiorly. The patient tolerated the procedure well and was awakened from anesthesia. He was taken to the post-operative holding area in stable condition.

48.5 Post-operative Course

On post-operative day 1, the globe was formed and the patient maintained light-perception vision. B scan ultrasound that day revealed a membrane extending from the optic nerve in all four quadrants concerning for a total retinal detachment with retinal incarceration in the scleral wound (Fig. 48.1). One week post-operatively, the patient was evaluated by the retina service who confirmed via repeat B scan ultrasound a total retinal detachment as well as evidence of an inferotemporal choroidal detachment with choroidal effusion. The decision was made to proceed with vitrectomy and retinal detachment repair. The retinal surgery occurred 10 days after the initial globe repair.

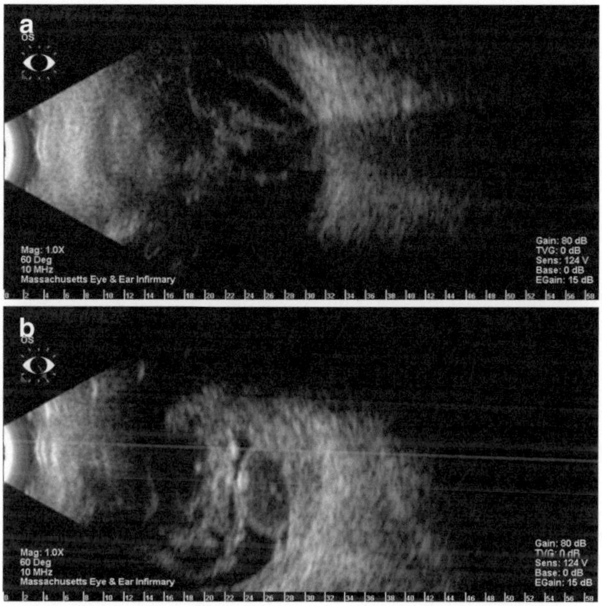

Fig. 48.1 Contact B scan ultrasound showing normal globe contour post-primary repair surgery, (**a**) a corrugated membrane extending off the optic nerve in all quadrants suggestive of a total retinal detachment with retinal incarceration, and (**b**) an inferotemporal dome-shaped elevation with a shallow annular extension suggestive of a choroidal detachment and effusion

48.6 Second Surgery: Operative Note from Retinal Detachment Repair 1 Week Later

After informed consent was obtained, the patient was brought to the operating room and induced under general anesthesia. The left eye was prepped and draped in routine sterile fashion. A wire lid speculum was placed. Points were marked 3.0 mm posterior to the limbus in the usual locations. Cannulas and trocars were placed. Using the vitreous cutter and fiberoptic light source, hemorrhagic, axial and peripheral vitreous were removed. This was extremely difficult as there were multiple layers of hemorrhage and the view was limited. The patient was aphakic. Eventually it could be seen that there was a total retinal detachment with multiple folds. The retina was pulled taut and incarcerated in the temporal scleral wound for 180°. There were tears inferotemporally and below the tears there was a localized choroidal hemorrhage. Eventually after meticulous dissection, a 360° relaxing retinectomy was performed. Scleral depression was performed for 360° to facilitate vitreous base dissection. Eventually all traction was relieved and the membranes were peeled from the surface of the peripheral retina. The retina was flipped over and one subretinal band membrane was removed. Perfluorocarbon liquid was then placed over the posterior pole and the retina flattened nicely with no traction remaining anywhere. After perfluorocarbon liquid flattened the retina, endolaser was applied for 360° around the edge of the retinectomy. This was difficult in the area of the choroidal hemorrhage as the view was limited on the down slope of the hemorrhage.

An inferior peripheral iridectomy was performed with the vitreous cutter. Then, a fluid/air exchange was performed using the soft tipped cannula and the fiberoptic light source. The retina remained attached with no traction remaining anywhere. Perfluorocarbon liquid was washed free from the posterior pole with balanced salt solution. Each of the three sclerotomies were sutured with 7-0 Vicryl after small incisions were made in the overlying conjunctiva. Prior to placing the final sutures, oil was placed up to the pupil plane. Conjunctiva was closed with multiple interrupted sutures. Subconjunctival injections of cefazolin and dexamethasone were given. During this procedure, it was necessary to remove the central corneal epithelium with a Beaver blade. The pressure was checked at the conclusion of the procedure and it was normal. The eye was flushed with betadine and then dressed with dexamethasone-neomycin-polymyxin b ointment and a sterile patch and shield. The patient was extubated and transferred to the recovery room in good condition having tolerated this procedure well.

48.7 Post-operative Course After Second Surgery

In summary, the patient underwent pars plana vitrectomy, removal of retinal incarceration, 360° retinectomy with endolaser and silicone oil placement (Fig. 48.2). The attending surgeon noted how technically difficult this surgery was due to extensive pre- and sub-retinal proliferative membranes. On post-operative day 1, his vision was hand-motion in the left eye and the retina was attached. By 3 months post-op his vision had improved to 20/480 with pinhole to 20/100. His retina was attached. He underwent silicone oil removal 10 months later. Two years later his retina remained attached (Fig. 48.3) and his best corrected visual acuity with a contact lens was 20/80 in the left eye.

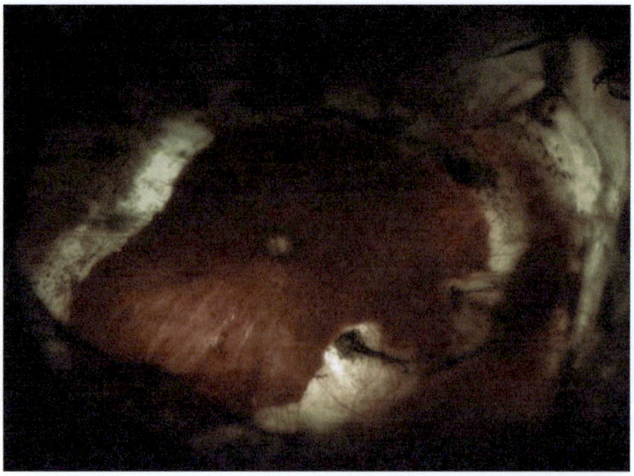

Fig. 48.2 Optos fundus photo of the left eye after retinal detachment repair. The patient is 1 month status post vitrectomy, 360° relaxing retinectomy and placement of silicone oil. He remains attached. Visual acuity is 20/200−2

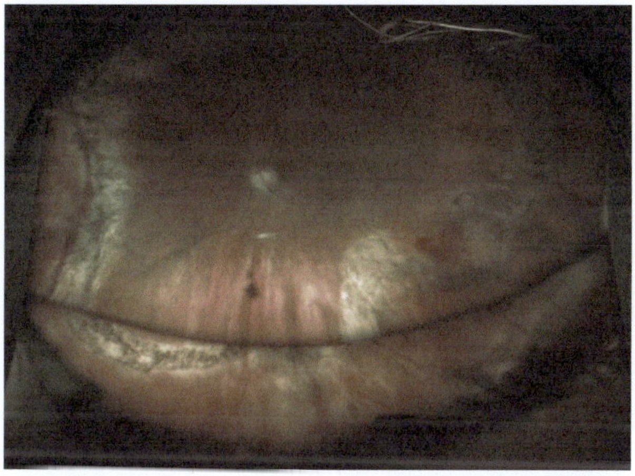

Fig. 48.3 Optos photo of left fundus after silicone oil removal. Visual acuity 20/80 with a contact lens

48.7.1 Surgical Exploration and Repair Parts I and II: Pearls

- For Zone III ruptures without a posterior view, it is critical to obtain a B scan ultrasound after repair of the ruptured globe to assess the status of the vitreous and retina. Early referral to a retina specialist for secondary vitrectomy within 7–14 days can potentially improve the visual prognosis after trauma.
- Indications for secondary vitrectomy after open globe repair include persistent media opacity, progressive vitreoretinal traction, retinal detachment, and/or retinal incarceration.
- For many Zone III repairs with vitreous and uveal prolapse, the retina becomes incarcerated at the time of injury or during the repair despite meticulous effort to reposition the uveal contents.
- Relaxing retinectomy at the site of incarceration followed by silicone oil tamponade should be used for complicated detachments such as this one with a total retinal detachment, suprachoroidal hemorrhage and retinal incarceration.
- The surgery is often difficult, requiring meticulous dissection of pre-retinal and sub-retinal membranes.

48.8 Final Trauma Evaluation

48.8.1 Final Visual Acuity

OD: 20/20+2
OS: 20/300−2 pinhole 200−3, with contact lens 20/80

48.8.2 Pupils

OD: Round, reactive
OS: Irregular

48.8.3 Slit Lamp Examination

	OD	OS
Lids and lashes	Normal	Normal
Sclera and conjunctiva	Normal	Normal
Cornea	Normal	Normal
Anterior chamber	Normal	1+ pigment, emulsified oil
Iris	Normal	Post-surgical with irregular contour, absent iris temporally, peripheral iridectomy inferiorly
Lens	Normal	Aphakic
Vitreous	Normal	Tiny emulsified oil droplets

48.8.4 Dilated Examination

Macula/Nerve OD: Normal
Periphery OD: Normal
Macula/Nerve: OS: Attached, mild epiretinal membrane with striae temporally
Periphery OS: Attached, 360° retinectomy

48.9 Review and Lessons Learned

Retinal detachment (RD) occurs in up to 30% of all open globe trauma [1–3]. The detachment occurs at the time of trauma (as is likely in this case) or later when vitreous membranes form and exert traction on the retina. 70% of retinal detachments occur within 1 month of the original trauma [1, 3]. These detachments are often complicated as they frequently involve retinal incarceration as well as preretinal and even sub-retinal membranes that must be carefully dissected and make vitrectomy technically very challenging. Previously, these eyes were deemed inoperable and were enucleated. However, it has become clear that surgery to reattach the retina and remove some of the inflammatory mediators that are present helps to promote healing with fewer tractional membranes and help to prevent phthisis [4, 5].

Though surgical techniques in repairing the detachment will vary, prompt referral to a vitreoretinal surgeon is critical. The surgical approach should be focused on clearing membranes that often form, removing vitreous and retinal traction, and reattaching the retina. Techniques that are frequently used in the setting of RD repair after trauma can include scleral buckle, membrane peeling, retinectomy, and silicone oil tamponade, and as every trauma case is unique, the techniques used will vary by case. Some have reported that with ruptures one can use a vitrectomy with scleral buckle [4]; however, the additional use of retinectomy with silicone oil tamponade is preferable if there is proliferative vitreoretinopathy (PVR), giant retinal tear, total RD, suprachoroidal hemorrhage, or multiple breaks [2, 6]. Silicone oil has been shown to result in better visual outcomes than sulfur hexafluoride (SF6) gas in eyes with complicated detachments from trauma [2].

The timing of retinal detachment surgery is still under debate. The main distinction is between primary surgery (at the time of open globe repair or shortly thereafter) and delayed retinal surgery. The argument for waiting is that it allows time for the globe to heal, a complete posterior vitreous detachment to develop, and there is a decreased risk of severe intraoperative hemorrhage [7]. However, postponing the surgery for too long increases the risk of severe vitreous membranes and PVR formation which can lead to more extensive detachment, complicated retinal surgery and post-operative re-detachment. Orban et al. reported no difference in the reattachment rate or the improvement in visual acuity when comparing early (<7 days) to late (≥7 days) RD repair in traumatic RD patients with open globes [5]; however, others have found benefit in early reattachment [8]. In our experience, secondary vitrectomy after open globe repair should occur within approximately 7–14 days.

48.10 Key Learning Points

- Retinal detachment following an open globe, either immediate or delayed, is common and requires prompt referral to a vitreoretinal specialist.
- The retinal detachment surgery should be performed within approximately 7–14 days.
- All patients should undergo vitrectomy, and we suggest subsequent retinectomy to relieve incarcerated retina followed by oil tamponade for complicated cases such as this one.

References

1. Xia T, Bauza A, Soni NG, Zarbin MA, Langer PD, Bhagat N. Surgical management and outcome of open globe injuries with posterior segment complications: a 10-year review. Semin Ophthalmol. 2016:1–6.

2. Nowomiejska K, Choragiewicz T, Borowicz D, Brzozowska A, Moneta-Wielgos J, Maciejewski R, et al. Surgical management of traumatic retinal detachment with primary vitrectomy in adult patients. J Ophthalmol. 2017;2017:5084319.
3. Stryjewski TP, Andreoli CM, Eliott D. Retinal detachment after open globe injury. Ophthalmology. 2014;121(1):327–33.
4. Wei Y, Zhou R, Xu K, Wang J, Zu Z. Retinectomy vs vitrectomy combined with scleral buckling in repair of posterior segment open-globe injuries with retinal incarceration. Eye. 2016;30(5):726–30.
5. Orban M, Islam YFK, Haddock LJ. Timing and outcomes of vitreoretinal surgery after traumatic retinal detachment. J Ophthalmol. 2016;2016:4978973.
6. Lucke K. Silicone oil in surgery of complicated retinal detachment. Ophthalmol Z Dtsch Ophthalmol Ges. 1993;90(3):215–38.
7. Orban M, Islam YFK, Haddock LJ. Timing and outcomes of vitreoretinal surgery after traumatic retinal detachment. J Ophthalmol [Internet]. 2016 [cited 29 May 2017];2016. Available from: https://www-ncbi-nlm-nih-gov.ezp-prod1.hul.harvard.edu/pmc/articles/PMC5141321/.
8. Kuhn F. The timing of reconstruction in severe mechanical trauma. Ophthalmic Res. 2014;51(2):67–72.

Chapter 49
Case 44: Severe Zone I/II Open Globe Injury with Stellate Wound Repair Followed by Enucleation

Grayson W. Armstrong, Tavé van Zyl, and Seanna Grob

49.1 History of Present Illness

A 22-year-old man without any past medical or ocular history presented after facial trauma with concern for a left-sided open globe injury.

- The patient had been walking his pitbull when he tripped and fell and hit his left eye on broken glass on the ground, causing multiple facial lacerations.
- The patient denied any loss of consciousness from the head strike, but did note significant vision loss in the left eye.
- The patient had difficulty opening the left eye and had significant left eye pain.

49.2 Initial Trauma Evaluation

49.2.1 Visual Acuity (Without Correction)

OD: Count fingers (patient too distressed to perform a reliable visual acuity test)
OS: Light perception through the eyelid (unable to assess reliably due to poor patient cooperation, as the patient refused to open the eye)

G. W. Armstrong, M.D., M.P.H. (✉) • T. van Zyl, M.D. • S. Grob, M.D., M.A.S.
Department of Ophthalmology, Harvard Medical School, Massachusetts Eye and Ear, Boston, MA, USA
e-mail: grayson_armstrong@meei.harvard.edu

S. Grob, C. Kloek (eds.), *Management of Open Globe Injuries*,
https://doi.org/10.1007/978-3-319-72410-2_49

49.2.2 Pupils

OD: Round and reactive
OS: Unable to assess due to poor patient cooperation (refused to open eye)

49.2.3 External Examination

Right nose laceration, as well as a full-thickness upper lip laceration involving the vermilion border.

49.2.4 Slit Lamp Examination

	OD	OS
Lids and lashes	Lower eyelid laceration with sutures in place	Normal
Sclera and conjunctiva	Normal	Conjunctival injection, subconjunctival hemorrhage
Cornea	Normal	Complex corneal laceration, difficult examination due to poor patient cooperation
Anterior chamber	Normal	Unable to assess
Iris	Normal	Unable to assess
Lens	Normal	Unable to assess
Vitreous	Normal	Unable to assess

49.2.5 Dilated Examination

Macula/Nerve OD: Normal
Periphery OD: Normal
Macula/Nerve OS: Unable to assess
Periphery OS: Unable to assess

49.2.6 Radiographic Imaging

Computed tomography (CT) of the orbits showing marked contour irregularity along the posterior and superior aspects of the left globe with loss of volume consistent with open globe rupture (Fig. 49.1a–c). Hyperdense material was present within the left globe consistent with vitreous hemorrhage (Fig. 49.1a, c). The left

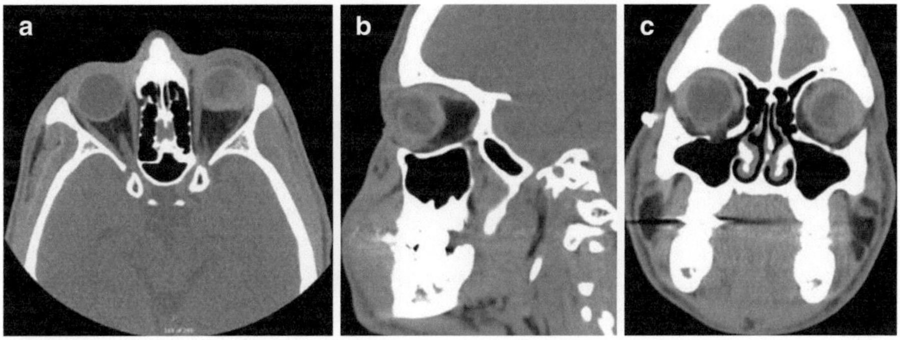

Fig. 49.1 Pre-operative CT orbit images after suspected open globe injury. Axial view showing irregular left globe contour with intraocular hyperdensities consistent with hemorrhage (**a**); Sagittal view showing discontinuity of anterior eye wall and lack of intraocular lens (**b**); Coronal view showing lentiform hyperdensity suggestive of hemorrhage in the left eye (**c**)

lens was not visualized, likely secondary to lens extrusion. No significant retrobulbar hematoma was identified. The extraocular muscles were grossly normal. The right globe was unremarkable.

There was a defect in the right orbital floor with mild herniation of intraorbital fat, but no evidence of inferior rectus muscle entrapment, likely either congenital or sequela of prior trauma.

49.3 Surgeon's Initial Assessment and Pre-operative Plan

This patient has a complex Zone I/II open globe injury of the left eye with multiple facial lacerations caused by trauma resulting from a fall on glass.

This case provides an example of three important concepts: (1) repair of an open globe where the initial pre-operative clinical exam is severely limited, (2) coordination with other surgical subspecialties, such as Otolaryngology (ENT), and (3) the importance of counseling and support in a patient's decision to undergo enucleation in an eye with a poor prognosis, despite the possibility for preservation of some level of low vision.

Pre-operative examination of the extent of globe injury was severely limited in this patient. He presented to the emergency department in significant pain and distress and even with appropriate pain medications, the patient would not cooperate with an examination. Fleeting views of the left eye and CT imaging were enough to confirm an open globe injury requiring exploration and repair. Similar to a pediatric case, in which patients may not be cooperative for a clinical exam, pre-operative surgical planning is limited. If a patient is in significant pain and distress, trying to force an eye exam could make matters worse, as prying open the eyelids or pressing on the eye could extrude intraocular contents. If suspicion is high for ruptured globe and CT imaging rules out an intraocular foreign body, then it is best to proceed to the operating

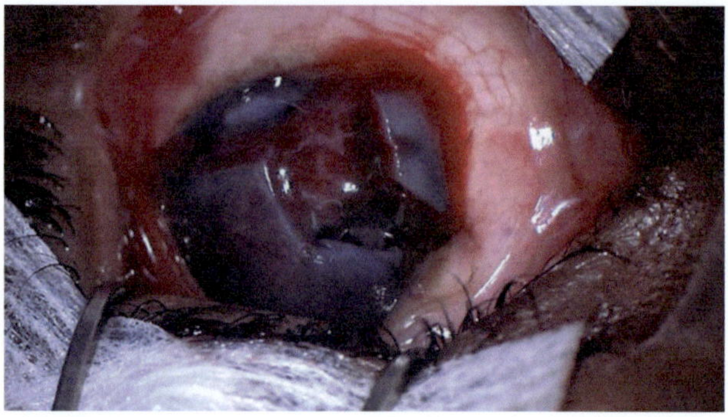

Fig. 49.2 Pre-operative external photo of the left eye showing a complex stellate corneal laceration and subconjunctival hemorrhage. Notably, no obvious scleral lacerations are visible at this time

room for exploration and repair. If the open globe injury is severe and the vision is no light perception, then it may also be important to discuss the possibility of primary enucleation to the patient if the globe trauma is too severe for repair. This could then be written in the consent as "exploration and possible repair of ruptured globe, possible evisceration or enucleation". This all needs to be discussed in detail with the patient and any family members they wish to have involved. However, we recommend that every effort is made to close the eye primarily, as this can be psychologically important for the patient. If the vision remains no light perception post-operatively, then enucleation or evisceration can be considered in the subsequent weeks.

This patient had a Zone I/II open globe injury and, in general, repair of the globe would proceed similar to cases discussed in prior chapters of this book. However, on initial evaluation in the operating room, it was clear this patient had a very complex stellate corneal laceration (Fig. 49.2). As discussed in early Zone I cases, it is important to align the limbus and all of the apices of the laceration first, which was key in this case. Also, there was significant prolapse of uveal tissue and likely retinal tissue anteriorly, which needs to be carefully repositioned into the eye and kept out of the corneal wound repair. Sometimes it is necessary to place some sutures that will ultimately be removed, just to hold tissues closer together to prevent significant uveal prolapse.

On initial exam, multiple facial lacerations were noted. The ENT Service was consulted for repair of the upper lip laceration involving the vermilion border to ensure appropriate repair and alignment for a good cosmetic result. It can be helpful to consult other subspecialty services prior to going to the operating room to coordinate any necessary intraoperative care. Periocular lacerations are often easily addressed by an ophthalmologist, but complex lacerations involving the nose, lip, ear, or face may need to be addressed by oculoplastics, ENT, or facial plastics.

49.4 Surgical Exploration and Repair: Operative Note

The risks, benefits, and alternatives were discussed with the patient pre-operatively and the patient consented to proceed with exploration and repair of the open globe injury. The patient was brought to the operating room where the anesthesia team

proceeded with general anesthesia. A careful time-out was observed and the correct patient and the eye were identified. The left eye was prepped and draped in the usual sterile ophthalmic fashion using a Jaffe speculum to provide adequate exposure.

During surgical prep, the face was cleaned and inspected. The patient was found to have a moderately deep upper lip laceration approximately 2 cm perpendicular to and involving the vermillion border. Repair of this wound was performed by the ENT service at the conclusion of the globe repair. The patient was also found to have a non-marginal, non-canalicular left lower eyelid laceration medially and a nearby laceration along the left side of the nose. There was also a very superficial laceration near the left lateral canthus. These lacerations were repaired by the eye trauma service at the conclusion of the globe repair.

The globe was then inspected. The patient was found to have an extensive stellate corneal wound extending across the inferior portion of the cornea from approximately 4 o'clock to 10 o'clock. There was extensive prolapse of intraocular contents including retina, vitreous, and uveal tissue through the corneal laceration (Fig. 49.2). A lens was not identified. The intraocular contents were gently reposited into the eye and a few initial 10-0 nylon sutures were placed in the cornea to stabilize the intraocular contents. It was noted at this time that the corneal laceration was an intricate laceration with multiple stellate components with several triangular sections coming together at 6 o'clock at the limbus, at 5 o'clock just anterior to the limbus, paracentrally and also at around 10 o'clock adjacent to the limbus.

A 270° peritomy was initiated exposing the nasal, inferior and lateral aspect of the limbus. Gentle exploration with blunt dissection was performed with Westcott scissors and Vannas scissors to identify the posterior-most aspect of the corneoscleral lacerations. The laceration extended across the limbus approximately 2 mm at around 10 o'clock, 2 mm at around 6 o'clock and 3 mm around 4 o'clock. A 9-0 nylon suture was used at each of these three locations to re-approximate the limbus. In an interrupted fashion, twenty-eight 10-0 nylon sutures were placed to close the corneal wound (Fig. 49.3a–c). Some of these were placed and then replaced in order to carefully align all the triangular lacerations. An iris spatula was used throughout the suturing to prevent uveal incarceration in the wound (Fig. 49.3a, b). Multiple 8-0 nylon sutures were used to close the scleral aspect of the laceration both temporally, inferiorly, and nasally. Upon completion of the wound closure, a Seidel test was performed to ensure that the wounds were water tight and the globe was found to be Seidel negative (Fig. 49.3d).

The conjunctiva was then closed with interrupted 8-0 Vicryl sutures. A Kontour lens (18 mm diameter) was placed for patient comfort, given the extensive corneal trauma and patient's pre-operative pain. A subconjunctival steroid and antibiotic injection was performed inferiorly away from the laceration and with care not to disrupt the contact lens. The specula were removed. The patient's drape was removed under the microscope.

At this point, the face was re-prepped and draped in the usual sterile fashion for repair of the facial lacerations. The lower eyelid laceration was inspected and it was confirmed to be both non-canalicular and non-marginal. A lacrimal probe was used to confirm no canalicular involvement. This eyelid laceration along with the lateral canthal laceration were repaired with 6-0 plain gut sutures in an interrupted fashion.

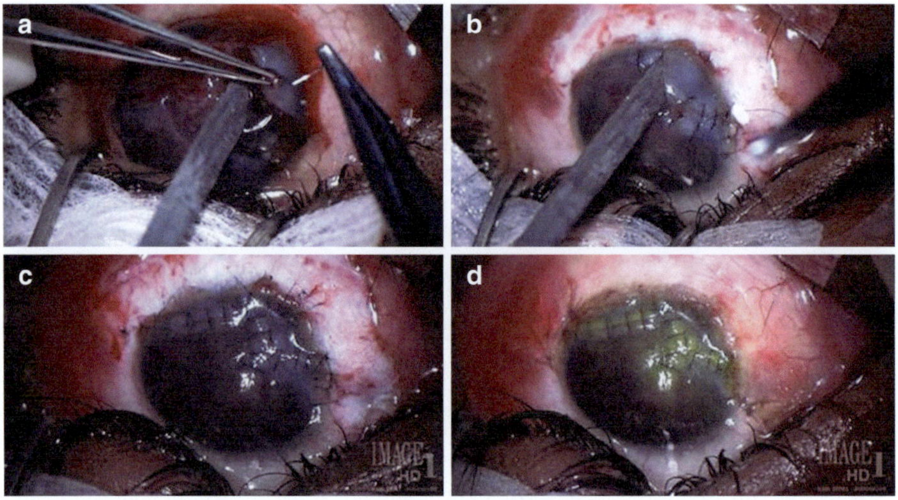

Fig. 49.3 Intraoperative photos showing the use of iris spatula to protect uveal contents of the globe during corneal suturing with 10-0 nylon (**a**, **b**). The globe was successfully repaired with both scleral and corneal sutures (**c**) and was Seidel negative at the completion of the case (**d**)

The nasal laceration was repaired with interrupted 5-0 Vicryl (deep) and 5-0 nylon for the skin.

The upper lip laceration was repaired by the ENT service. After hemostasis was achieved, multiple 5-0 Vicryl deep sutures, followed by 5-0 nylon for the skin. Care was taken to re-align the vermillion border, lip, and the patient's mustache.

The drape was removed. The surgical field was cleaned. Dexamethasone-neomycin-polymyxin-b ointment was placed over the incisions. Atropine was placed in the left eye along with dexamethasone-neomycin-polymyxin-b ophthalmic ointment and a sterile eye pad and shield were placed. The patient was extubated. The patient tolerated the procedure well without any complications.

49.4.1 Surgical Exploration and Repair: Pearls

- Complicated stellate corneal wounds may require extensive suturing and re-suturing.
- In complex wounds with significant uveal prolapse, placing some sutures (that may ultimately be removed) to re-approximate the lacerated tissue can help decrease uveal prolapse and ease the process of repair.
- Utilization of an adjustable suture technique can greatly facilitate the efficiency and efficacy of wound closure in long and complicated corneal wounds. The sutures are left in an adjustable state until most or all of the sutures are placed.

Then the tension is adjusted on all of the sutures and only permanently tied when they are all at the appropriate tension.

- The surgeon should consider intraoperative repair of any additional traumatic injuries, and additional consulting services may be necessary to perform such repairs.

49.5 Post-operative Course

The patient completed a 48 hour course of intravenous antibiotics. On post-operative day one he still had light perception vision with no view to the posterior pole. The corneal wounds were intact and the bandage contact lens was in place (Fig. 49.4). B-scan ultrasound revealed poorly organized intraocular contents.

Follow up seven days later with the trauma service and the retina service showed continued light perception vision and continued pain. There was no view posteriorly, but B-scan ultrasound revealed a total funnel retinal detachment with some retinal incarceration in the scleral wounds (Fig. 49.5). The patient was

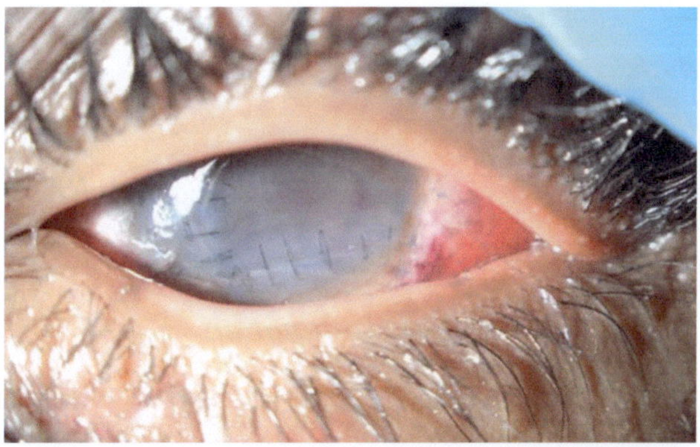

Fig. 49.4 External photograph of the left eye taken at post-operative week 1 after globe repair showing at least 16 of the 28 10-0 nylon corneal sutures with a hazy, edematous cornea and a poor view of the anterior chamber

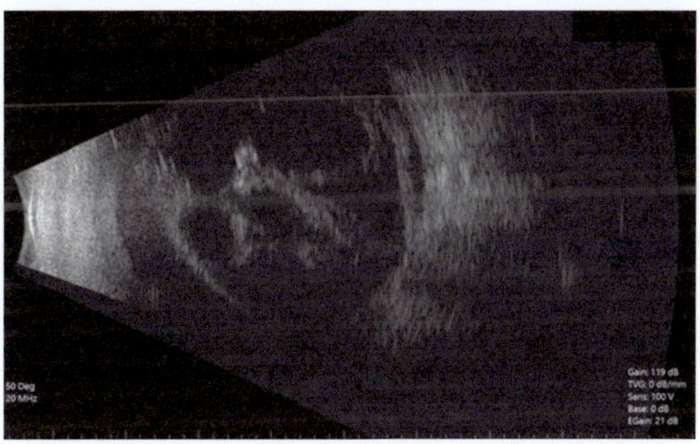

Fig. 49.5 B-scan ultrasound of the left globe at post-operative week 1 showing intact globe but total funnel retinal detachment

counseled on poor visual and functional outcomes associated with the total retinal detachment, however, he was offered surgical repair with vitrectomy, retinectomy, and temporary keratoprosthesis as an opportunity for potential preservation or improvement of his light perception vision. The patient was not interested in further surgeries and continued to have significant pain in this eye. He later opted for enucleation.

The patient did not subsequently follow up at our institution, but arranged for follow up near his home in a different state, where he ultimately underwent enucleation.

49.6 Final Trauma Evaluation

49.6.1 Final Visual Acuity

OD: 20/30+2
OS: Light Perception

49.6.2 Pupils

OD: Reactive
OS: No view to pupil, afferent pupillary defect by reverse

49.6.3 Slit Lamp Examination

	OD	OS
Lids and lashes	Healing lower eyelid laceration	Normal
Sclera and conjunctiva	Normal	Mild conjunctival injection, subconjunctival hemorrhage
Cornea	Normal	Bandage contact lens in good position, 28 corneal sutures over complex corneal laceration
Anterior chamber	Normal	No clear view, hemorrhage and uveal tissue posterior to cornea, poor view
Iris	Normal	Inferior 1/2 to 2/3 of iris missing, though some superior iris still present, poor view
Lens	Normal	Not seen
Vitreous	Normal	No view

49.6.4 *Dilated Examination*

Macula/Nerve OD: Normal
Periphery OD: Normal
Macula/Nerve: OS: No view
Periphery OS: No view

49.7 Review and Lessons Learned

In cases of suspected open globe injury where adequate pre-operative examination is impaired due to patient intoxication, young age, or intractable emotional distress, it may be prudent to defer examination until the globe can be examined under general anesthesia. While this limits the surgeon's ability to perfectly predict which special instruments or suture material may be necessary ahead of time, it prevents placing undue stress on the patient, which can lead to exacerbation of the ocular trauma (e.g. further extrusion of intraocular contents due to patient straining or squeezing the eye shut). Collateral methods of ocular examination, such as CT imaging (which should be ordered for all patients), should be used as another source of pre-operative information gathering.

Additional trauma, such as our patient's full-thickness lip laceration, may necessitate close collaboration with additional specialties for combined repair. While this may not be possible at all institutions, one important consideration is ensuring timely repair of the globe despite the schedules of other consultants. While it may be preferable to have the patient undergo combined surgery at one time, it is always appropriate to consider multiple staged repairs in the operating room in order to ensure timely closure of the eye. Delay in open globe repair increases the risk of endophthalmitis by up to 400% and should be avoided if at all possible [1].

In cases where lacerations cross the limbus, and especially in cases such as ours with complex corneal lacerations, it is important to first re-approximate the limbus [2]. Stellate wounds can be very challenging to repair as discussed in earlier cases. Early sutures can be used to re-approximate the lacerated tissue and prevent uveal prolapse. One should then first work to re-approximate the limbus and all of the apices of stellate corneal wounds. Apices of corneal lacerations are often the site of wound leaks and therefore need to be carefully positioned. Multiple techniques have been described to suture the complex stellate wound apices, such as butterfly sutures, star-shaped sutures, and purse string sutures. Ultimately, the choice depends on surgeon preference.

Many open globes require multiple surgeries and procedures in order to provide the patient the best chance for post-operative visual recovery. Retinal detachment (RD) in the setting of open globe injury can be addressed by vitreoretinal surgeons and should be offered to patients, as failure to correct the RD may result in progressive loss of vision, chronic low grade inflammation, and ultimately phthisis bulbi. Our patient's B-scan revealed a total funnel retinal detachment with retinal incarceration. Our patient was offered repair by a retina surgeon, although the poor prognosis was discussed at length with the patient. Ultimately, our patient refused further surgical procedures for retinal repair and requested evisceration or enucleation of his painful eye.

While it is natural for the ophthalmologist to desire an outcome resulting in a formed globe and retained vision, it is important to understand that the patient's desired outcome may be different based on their personal goals. Enucleation or evisceration of the injured eye is sometimes preferable to patients even with some low level of vision. The risks and benefits of enucleation versus retention of the eye should be discussed with patients, and the goals of patients should be thoroughly explored. In our case, the patient maintained light perception vision and an intact globe but ultimately opted for secondary enucleation. This decision was likely driven by multiple factors, including pre- and post-operative pain, low vision with poor prognosis for significant improvement, hesitation to undergo further surgery, perceived physical disfigurement, and psychological trauma. All options should be discussed with the patient.

49.8 Key Learning Points

- Intraoperative examination under anesthesia may be required prior to repair of an open globe when the initial pre-operative clinical exam is severely limited.
- It is important to extensively counsel and support patients both pre- and post-operatively after eye trauma. All options should be discussed with the patient including enucleation in the setting of poor prognosis and persistent pain.

References

1. Ahmed Y, Schimel AM, Pathengay A, et al. Endophthalmitis following open-globe injuries. Eye (Lond). 2012;26(2):212–7.
2. Sullivan P. The open globe: Surgical techniques for the closure of ocular wounds. London: Eyelearning Ltd; 2013.

Chapter 50
Case 45: Endophthalmitis After Open Globe Injury Repair

Katherine E. Talcott, Yewlin E. Chee, Roberto Pineda, and John B. Miller

50.1 History of Present Illness

A 45-year-old previously healthy man presented after being hit in the right eye with a rock.

- The patient was hammering at work when he was struck in the right eye with a rock.
- He noticed immediate decrease in vision, tearing, and pain.
- The patient presented immediately to the Massachusetts Eye and Ear.

K. E. Talcott, M.D. (✉)
Vitreoretinal Surgery, Wills Eye Hospital, Philadelphia, PA, USA

Y. E. Chee, M.D.
Vitreoretinal Surgery, Department of Ophthalmology, University of Washington, Seattle, WA, USA

R. Pineda, M.D.
Cornea and Refractive Surgery, Department of Ophthalmology, Harvard Medical School, Massachusetts Eye and Ear, Boston, MA, USA

J. B. Miller, M.D.
Vitreoretinal Surgery, Department of Ophthalmology, Harvard Medical School, Massachusetts Eye and Ear, Boston, MA, USA

S. Grob, C. Kloek (eds.), *Management of Open Globe Injuries*,
https://doi.org/10.1007/978-3-319-72410-2_50

50.2 Initial Trauma Evaluation

50.2.1 Visual Acuity (Without Correction)

OD: Count fingers at 1 foot
OS: 20/20

50.2.2 Pupils

OD: Peaked nasally, no afferent pupillary defect
OS: Round

50.2.3 External Examination

Normal. No lacerations or other trauma noted.

50.2.4 Slit Lamp Examination

	OD	OS
Lids and lashes	Normal	Normal
Sclera and conjunctiva	Injection without obvious extension of laceration onto sclera	Normal
Cornea	Large (7 mm), curvilinear corneal laceration extending to nasal limbus and with significant uveal prolapse	Normal
Anterior chamber	Vitreous and uvea to wound	Normal
Iris	Peaked nasally	Normal
Lens	Limited view	Normal
Vitreous	Vitreous to wound, limited view	Normal

50.2.5 Dilated Examination

Macula/Nerve OD: No view
Periphery OD: No view
Macula/Nerve: OS: Normal
Periphery OS: Normal

50.2.6 Radiographic Imaging

Computed tomography (CT) of the orbits showed an irregular globe contour of the right eye. There were no intraocular foreign bodies or fractures.

50.3 Surgeon's Initial Assessment and Pre-operative Plan

The patient presented soon after injury with a large Zone I open globe injury of the right eye with significant uveal and vitreous prolapse.

Large open globe lacerations are at increased risk of endophthalmitis and should be repaired promptly. To decrease the risk of endophthalmitis in open globe patients at Massachusetts Eye and Ear (MEE), we take them to the operating room for surgical repair as soon as possible after anesthesia clearance and operating room availability. We have support to repair these patients within 24 hours from the time of the injury, even if this means operating overnight. We also start intravenous antibiotics (typically vancomycin and ceftazidime) as soon as their open globe injury is diagnosed, whether the patient is at MEE or being transferred from a different facility. It is important to check with anesthesia or post-operative nursing care team about continuing intravenous antibiotics according to schedule. There is risk for missed or delayed antibiotic doses given multiple phases of care. At MEE, we have instituted an antibiotic checklist to be completed by the nursing staff and reviewed by the surgeon to ensure that all doses have been given.

Repairing open globe injuries promptly, especially extensive corneal ones, often facilitates closure. Even within hours of the injury, the cornea becomes edematous and uveal tissue sticky. This can make it harder to visualize intraocular tissues in the operating room, reposit the uveal tissue and achieve good closure of the wounds. Edematous corneal wounds may be Seidel negative at the time of repair but can leak with resolution of the edema. Care should also be taken in the operating room not to incorporate uvea or vitreous. We start by using a blade to carefully de-epithelialize prolapsed tissue and perform Weck-cel vitrectomy as necessary. Nylon sutures can be placed to first approximate the wound before using a cyclodialysis spatula and filtered air or balanced salt solution to reposit the uvea. There is often iridodialysis present so care should be taken to avoid additional iris trauma while using the cyclodialysis spatula. If this is unsuccessful, ophthalmic viscosurgical devices can be used to push back iris and longer suture passes can be used.

In this case, we expedited the patient and were able to get him to the operating room within 7 hours of his injury. Despite this timely intervention, we counseled the patient that he was still at high risk for infection or intraocular damage given his large injury and contact with organic material.

50.4 Surgical Exploration and Repair: Operative Note

The risks, benefits, and alternatives were discussed with the patient pre-operatively, and consent was obtained for open globe exploration and repair of the right eye. The patient was brought to the operating room where the anesthesia team induced general anesthesia. A careful timeout was observed, and the correct patient and the right eye were identified.

The right eye was prepped and draped in the usual sterile ophthalmic fashion, using a Jaffe lid speculum to provide adequate exposure. On inspection of the globe, it was noted that there was a full-thickness corneal laceration with significant uveal and vitreous prolapse. The prolapsed iris was gently irrigated with balanced salt solution and de-epithelialized with a crescent blade. A paracentesis was made with a supersharp blade at 8 o'clock and balanced salt solution was injected into the anterior chamber. Multiple 10-0 nylon sutures were placed in an interrupted fashion to close the corneal wound with care taken not to incorporate the uvea. Significant vitreous was encountered and careful Wekcel vitrectomy was performed to prevent vitreous incarceration into the wounds. The anterior chamber was again reformed with balanced salt solution through the paracentesis. The paracentesis wound was hydrated and found to be water tight. Fluoroscein was used to check the corneal laceration site and it was found to be Seidel negative at this time. Calipers were used to measure the laceration, which was found to be 7 mm in length. A subconjunctival injection of cefazolin and dexamethasone was placed.

50.4.1 Surgical Exploration and Repair: Pearls

- Eyes with large corneal lacerations are at increased risk of endophthalmitis. It is important to promptly start systemic antibiotics and surgically repair the wound.
- Removal of vitreous prolapse from the corneal laceration or rupture site is important to relieve vitreous traction. This can be done with a gentle Weck-cel vitrectomy. Care should also be taken to reposit the uvea without incorporation into the wound.

50.5 Post-operative Course

The patient was admitted to MEE to complete a 48 hour course of intravenous antibiotics. On post-operative day (POD) 1, he had count fingers vision, significant pain, and an intraocular pressure of 52 mmHg. There was fibrin in the anterior chamber and although the view of the lens was hazy, there was no obvious lens violation seen. He was given oral acetazolamide and intraocular pressure (IOP) lowering drops hourly. He was discharged on POD 2 with improved pain and IOP 29 mmHg. He returned POD 3 for an IOP check on maximum medical therapy. While his vision was stable, he reported increased pain. His IOP was elevated to

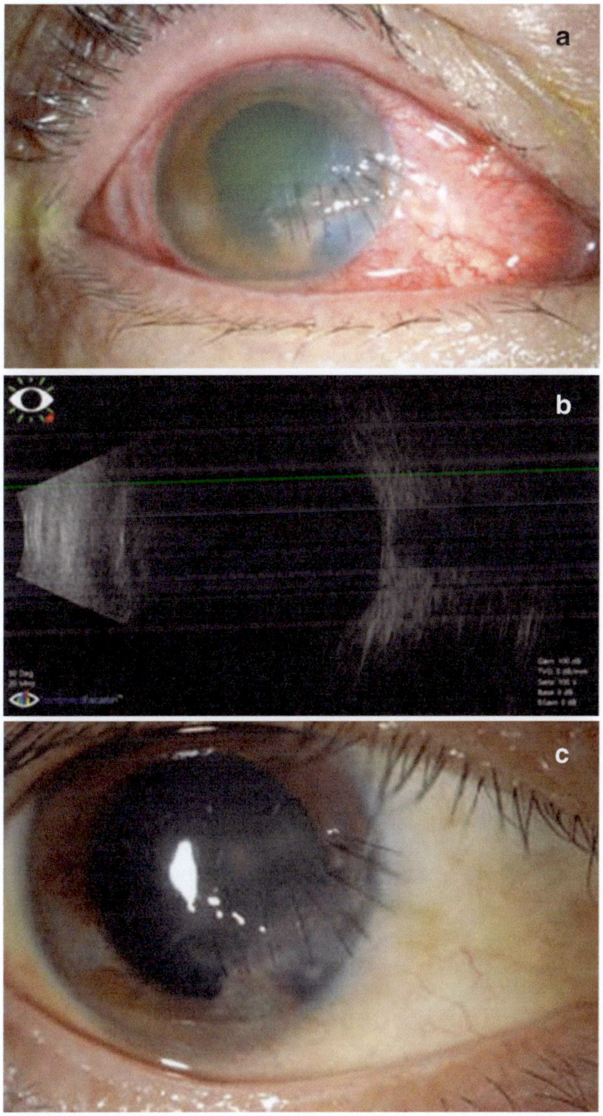

Fig. 50.1 (**a**) Slit lamp photograph showing sutured corneal laceration on POD 3 with conjunctival injection, fibrin, small hypopyon and iridodialysis. (**b**) Ultrasound with moderate vitreous debris on POD 3. (**c**) Slit lamp photograph at post-operative month 2 showing resolved inflammation

40 mmHg and his exam was notable for a new 0.2 mm hypopyon. An ultrasound showed annular-shaped membranes with debris (Fig. 50.1a, b). The Retina Service was consulted given concern for endophthalmitis and the patient underwent an anterior chamber tap and intravitreal injection of vancomycin and ceftazidime. He was started on a course of oral moxifloxacin. His cultures did not grow any organisms. Over the next month, he was carefully monitored by the Retina and Trauma Services. His inflammation subsided and vision improved to 20/50+1. He was weaned off intraocular pressure-lowering medications.

Approximately 2 months after the injury, the patient's corneal sutures were carefully removed over two sessions (Fig. 50.1c). One deep limbal suture was

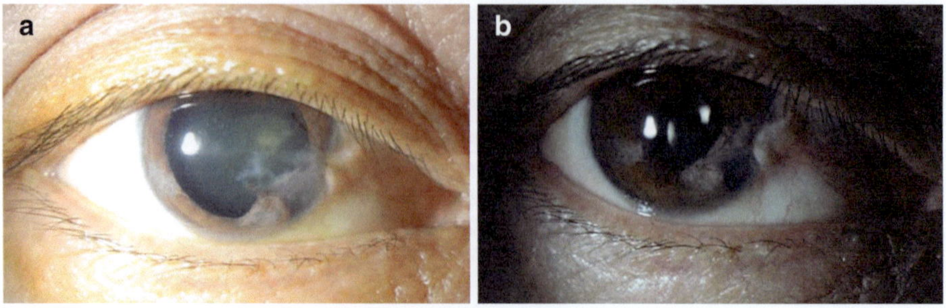

Fig. 50.2 (**a**) Slit lamp photograph of the right eye at post-operative month 6 showing progressive traumatic cataract and residual scar and iridodialysis. (**b**) Slit lamp photograph of the right eye at post-operative month 12 after cataract extraction and pupilloplasty

unable to be safely removed. His exam was still notable for significant nasal iridodialysis as well as an early traumatic cataract. His vision improved to 20/50 pinhole 20/30–2, but he reported distorted vision and significant photophobia. He was referred to the Contact Lens Service. They evaluated the patient with a gas permeable lens to help correct astigmatism as well as a tinted soft contact lens to help with glare and photophobia. The gas permeable lens did not significantly improve his visual acuity. He was bothered by loss of peripheral vision with the tinted soft contact lens and elected against it.

Six months after the injury, the patient was noted to have worsening vision with a visual acuity of 20/50. On exam, his traumatic cataract including a posterior subcapsular cataract had progressed (Fig. 50.2a). He was referred to the Cornea Service given his multiple anterior segment abnormalities. He underwent a successful cataract extraction with synechiolysis, pupilloplasty and posterior chamber intraocular lens implantation. At 1 year after his injury, his vision was 20/20 with refraction (Fig. 50.2b).

50.6 Final Trauma Evaluation

50.6.1 Final Visual Acuity

OD: 20/20
OS: 20/20

50.6.2 Pupils

OD: More round, transillumination defect nasally with slight irregularity nasally
OS: Normal

50.6.3 Slit Lamp Examination

	OD	OS
Lids and lashes	Normal	Normal
Sclera and conjunctiva	Normal	Normal
Cornea	Corneal scar inferonasally with deep corneal suture	Normal
Anterior chamber	Normal	Normal
Iris	Transillumination defect nasally	Normal
Lens	Posterior chamber intraocular lens	Normal
Vitreous	Mild debris	Normal

50.6.4 Dilated Examination

Macula/Nerve OD: Normal, C/D 0.3
Periphery OD: Normal
Macula/Nerve: OS: Normal, C/D 0.3
Periphery OS: Normal

50.7 Review and Lessons Learned

It is important to always have a high suspicion for infection in open globe patients and to take measures to minimize risk. Endophthalmitis can be a devastating complication of open globe injury, occurring in up to 12% of cases [1]. Most cases occur several days after injury and can progress rapidly, even when treatment is given promptly. Visual prognosis can be poor. The most common organisms in posttraumatic endophthalmitis including coagulase-negative Staphylococci, Streptococci and Bacillus species, which can have a fulminant course [2, 3]. Preventative measures should be taken to decrease the risk of endophthalmitis. At our institution, a standardized protocol is followed in all open globe injuries. This includes institution of prophylactic intravenous antibiotics (typically vancomycin and ceftazidime) on first suspicion of open globe injury and continuation for 48 hours while admitted. Additionally, surgical repair is performed as soon as possible and certainly within 24 hours of the injury if the patient is stable. Patients are then maintained on topical antibiotic drops (fluoroquinolone) for 7 days or until the corneal epithelial defect is healed. Intravitreal antibiotics are sometimes given in high-risk populations. A retrospective review of our open globe cases over 7 years was associated with a low rate of endophthalmitis of 0.9%. Risk factors for endophthalmitis included intraocular foreign body and primary intraocular lens placement [4].

Additionally, it is important to have a high suspicion for endophthalmitis in open globe patients and to treat aggressively once diagnosed. Our patient had risk factors for endophthalmitis, namely a large laceration from a dirty object. His elevated intraocular pressure after surgery was likely an early sign of infection and the decision was made to carefully follow the patient even after discharge from the hospital. After diagnosis of endophthalmitis in the presence of a hypopyon, the patient was promptly treated with intravitreal antibiotics and had a good visual outcome. In ocular trauma, it is important to have good relationships with other ophthalmic subspecialties and to have a low threshold to request their consultation. Finally, counseling the patient is important. We always counsel pre-operative trauma patients about the risk of infection. This conversation continues post-operatively, especially if there are unexpected findings or complications. It is important to communicate findings, concerns and why it is important that they adhere to the treatment plan. In our case, the patient returned nearly daily to our institution over the first 2 weeks for management of his trauma and endophthalmitis, but was fortunate to have an excellent visual outcome despite his complicated course.

50.8 Key Learning Points

- Open globe injury patients are at high risk for endophthalmitis. A standardized protocol involving systemic antibiotics and prompt surgical repair should be adhered to in order to minimize its risk.
- Even after uncomplicated surgical repair of open globe injuries, suspicion should always be high for infection and endophthalmitis. These patients should be promptly referred to retinal specialists comfortable treating endophthalmitis with intravitreal antibiotics and consideration of further surgery as needed.

References

1. Zhang Y, Zhang MN, Jiang CH, Yao Y, Zhang Z. Endophthalmitis following open globe injury. Br J Ophthalmol. 2010;94:111–4.
2. Cebulla CM, Flynn HW. Endophthalmitis after open globe injuries. Am J Ophthalmol. 2009;147:567–8.
3. Essex RW, Yi Q, Charles PGP, Allen PJ. Post-traumatic endophthalmitis. Ophthalmology. 2004;111:2015–22.
4. Andreoli CM, Andreoli MT, Kloek CE, Ahuero AE, Vavvas D, Durand ML. Low rate of endophthalmitis in a large series of open globe injuries. Am J Ophthalmol. 2009;147:601–8.

Chapter 51
Case 46: Wound Leak After Open Globe Repair Requiring Corneal Glue and Re-suturing

Natalie Wolkow, Katherine E. Talcott, and Seanna Grob

51.1 History of Present Illness

A 28-year-old healthy male electrician presents with an open globe injury of the left eye 21 hours after the time of injury.

- The patient had been hammering a piece of metal the previous night, was not wearing eye protection, and felt something fly into his left eye.
- He was evaluated at an outside hospital and was found to have a full-thickness corneal laceration and an intraocular foreign body. He was then referred to Mass Eye and Ear for further management.

51.2 Initial Trauma Evaluation

51.2.1 Visual Acuity (Without Correction)

OD: 20/20
OS: 20/70 pinhole 20/30−2

N. Wolkow, M.D., Ph.D. (✉) • S. Grob, M.D., M.A.S.
Department of Ophthalmology, Harvard Medical School, Massachusetts Eye and Ear, Boston, MA, USA
e-mail: natalie_wolkow@meei.harvard.edu

K. E. Talcott, M.D.
Vitreoretinal Surgery, Wills Eye Hospital, Philadelphia, PA, USA

S. Grob, C. Kloek (eds.), *Management of Open Globe Injuries*,
https://doi.org/10.1007/978-3-319-72410-2_51

51.2.2 Pupils

OD: Round, no afferent pupillary defect
OS: Round, no afferent pupillary defect

51.2.3 Intraocular Pressure with Tono-Pen

OD: 16
OS: Deferred

51.2.4 External Examination

Normal. No signs of external trauma.

51.2.5 Slit Lamp Examination

	OD	OS
Lids and lashes	Normal	Normal
Sclera and conjunctiva	Normal	2+ diffuse injection
Cornea	Normal	Vertical 1.5 mm laceration inferiorly at 6 o'clock with iris strands coming to wound
Anterior chamber	Normal	Very shallow, metallic foreign body present between cornea and iris
Iris	Normal	Inferior transillumination defect with iris strands extending to the wound, foreign body at the transillumination defect
Lens	Normal	Normal (undilated—due to foreign body sitting on the iris)
Vitreous	Normal	Normal (undilated)

51.2.6 Dilated Examination

Macula/Nerve OD: Normal, sharp nerve
Periphery OD: Normal
Macula/Nerve: OS: Undilated due to foreign body on the iris, limited view
Periphery OS: Undilated due to foreign body on the iris

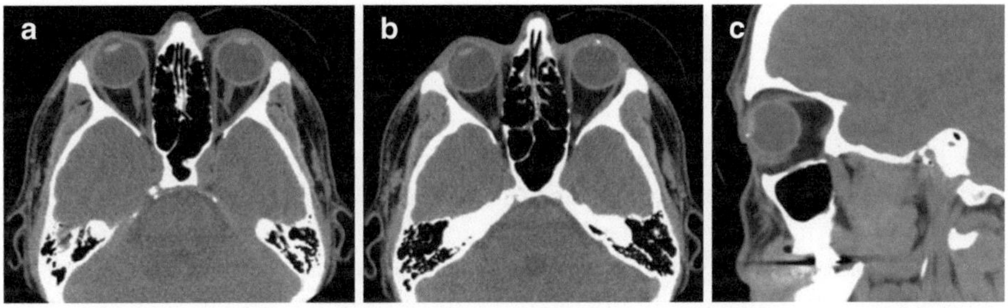

Fig. 51.1 Non-contrast CT scan of the orbits, demonstrating a shallow left anterior chamber as well as an inferior metallic foreign body in the anterior chamber. (**a**) Axial view demonstrating the shallow left anterior chamber. (**b**) Axial view demonstrating the metallic foreign body. (**c**) Sagittal view demonstrating the metallic foreign body in the anterior chamber

51.2.7 Radiographic Imaging

Computed tomography (CT) of the orbits showed a flat left anterior chamber with a 2-mm hyperdense focus, likely metallic foreign body, in the inferior left cornea and anterior chamber. No posterior foreign bodies were noted (Fig. 51.1a–c).

51.2.8 Surgeon's Initial Assessment and Pre-operative Plan

The patient presented 21 hours after the time of injury, but this is still within the recommended 24 hour window for open globe injury repair. The wound should therefore be repaired expediently. As discussed previously, it is often helpful to evaluate a corneal laceration as close as possible to the time of the injury, since corneal edema usually progresses with time. For surgeons who are new to corneal laceration repair, it may be useful to draw a diagram of the corneal laceration in order to plan the location of suture placement prior to taking the patient to the operating room. Not only is this useful for intraoperative planning, but is also helpful if there is a delay in getting the patient to the operating room, as significant corneal edema may sometimes obscure the exact location and extent of the laceration.

There are very few times when dilation is not recommended prior to open globe repair, and this case is a good example. When there is a foreign body in the anterior chamber that could potentially migrate posteriorly, the pupil should not be dilated until the foreign body has been removed. This is usually more of a concern with small foreign bodies that are no longer within the cornea and are sitting free on the iris or in the anterior chamber, rather than larger, embedded, foreign bodies. If the foreign body penetrates the iris, the decision to dilate depends on the specific case, but often it is still permissible to dilate to evaluate for posterior pathology.

Removal of the foreign body can be approached several ways. If the foreign body is still within the cornea, one can make a paracentesis and use microsurgical technology (MST) forceps to grasp the foreign body and push it up through the corneal wound. If the foreign body is free in the anterior chamber, MST forceps may be used through a paracentesis to grasp the foreign body and pull it out through the paracentesis. The wound may need to be enlarged depending on the size of the foreign body. An ophthalmic viscosurgical device (OVD) can be used to maintain anterior chamber depth and also to sequester the foreign body away from the pupillary border, so that it does not fall posteriorly. Cohesive OVDs, such as Healon 5 or Provisc, are easier to remove from the anterior chamber (compared to dispersive OVDs) once the foreign body has been retrieved.

51.3 Surgical Exploration and Repair: Operative Note

Informed consent was obtained prior to the procedure. The patient was then taken to the operating room and general anesthesia was induced. The eye was prepped and draped in the usual sterile manner for ophthalmic surgery. Jaffe lid specula were placed. The metal foreign body was removed from the wound using MST curved forceps and sent for pathology. The eye was dilated with phenylephrine-tropicamide. A paracentesis port was made with a supersharp blade at 4 o'clock. Balanced saline solution was injected to inflate the anterior chamber and two 10-0 nylon sutures were used to close the wound that measured approximately 3 mm and was located around 6 o'clock in the inferior peripheral cornea. The area where the iris transillumination defect had been seen pre-operatively was inspected more closely; a Kuglin hook was used to lift the iris to inspect the lens; a focal lens opacity without disruption of the anterior capsule was noted in the area. The paracentesis was hydrated. It was noted that the wound had a slow leak due to a small wound gape from the foreign body entry site. The decision was made to place a bandage contact lens (Kontour, base curve 8.9, diameter 16). The anterior chamber remained stable and maintained pressure with the contact lens in position. A subconjunctival injection of antibiotic and steroid were administered. The speculum was removed and the eye was cleaned. Antibiotic drops were instilled. The eye was then patched and a Fox shield was placed. The patient tolerated the procedure well without any complications.

51.3.1 Surgical Exploration and Repair: Pearls

- If pre-operative iris transillumination defects are noted, the lens capsule may be violated and should be carefully inspected intraoperatively to ensure that there are no lenticular foreign bodies or injuries.

- To minimize corneal wound leaks, every effort should be made to ensure that corneal sutures are at 80–95% depth and long enough to produce sufficient tension on the wound. Shallow, short sutures lead to wound gape and wound leak.
- If there is a brisk wound leak intraoperatively, it is best to try to place new sutures to address the leak. If there is a slow leak, then there are several options to consider. First, however, it is important to determine where the leak is emanating from. Slow leaks from suture tracks often will resolve on their own, and do not require intervention beyond a bandage contact lens. If there is a slow leak from the main wound, a bandage contact lens may be placed at the conclusion of the case, and may be sufficient in many situations. In cases where there is slightly higher concern about wound stability and healing, corneal glue may be applied to seal the leak, with a bandage contact lens placed over it. Sutures may also be replaced for slow leaks, but repeated suture passes can macerate the corneal tissue making it even more difficult to close and more prone to wound leak. When closing a wound where there was a corneal foreign body, sutures may need to be placed tighter than usual to close a gaping wound and prevent wound leak. Tighter than typical sutures are especially important when significant corneal edema is noted intraoperatively because as the edema improves post-operatively, sutures loosen.

51.4 Post-operative Course

On post-operative day 1 the patient's vision was count fingers in the left eye. The bandage contact lens was still in place, but the anterior chamber was extremely shallow with peripheral irido-corneal touch, suggesting a wound leak. The decision was made to place corneal glue in the procedure room.

51.4.1 Post-operative Day 1 Procedure Note

The risks and benefits of applying corneal glue and reforming the anterior chamber were discussed and informed consent was obtained. The patient was taken to the minor procedure room, where topical anesthesia was applied. The eye was prepped in the sterile ophthalmic fashion with betadine drops and gatifloxacin and the bandage contact lens was removed. A 1020 drape was used to make a round disc using a 3-mm derm punch. A drop of polysporin ointment was placed on the tip of the wooden end of a Q-tip, and then the round punched-out disc was placed on top of the ointment. A drop of corneal glue was then placed on top of the disc. The wound was dried with a Wek-cel and the disc with the glue was applied to the wound with the glue facing the wound and the plastic disc on the outside surface.

The glue was allowed to dry for 3 min and then a Wek-cel was used to dry the wound. It was noted that there was a residual small superior leak on the wound and another disc was prepared and applied. After this the wound was noted to be dry. The anterior chamber was reformed with balanced salt solution and appeared to be holding its form. A bandage contact lens was reapplied to cover the rough surface of the glue, and a drop of gatifloxacin was placed. The patient was re-examined after an hour at the slit lamp to ensure that the anterior chamber remained formed prior to discharge home.

51.5 Post-operative Course

In addition to the standard post-operative drops of prednisolone, atropine and gatifloxacin, the patient was also started on timolol drops twice daily in the surgical eye to decrease aqueous production and therefore slow the wound leak in order to help wound healing. On post-operative week 1, the anterior chamber was still formed and the glue and bandage lens were in place and his vision was improving. He complained of minor discomfort and photophobia.

On post-operative week 2, the glue no longer appeared adherent under the bandage contact lens despite a formed anterior chamber. The bandage contact lens and loose glue were removed. The two corneal sutures were still intact, but the wound was Seidel positive. Glue was re-applied in the procedure room and a bandage contact lens was placed again.

In subsequent post-operative weeks, his vision continued to improve steadily, the anterior chamber remained well-formed and the glue and contact lens remained in place. He did continue to note constant discomfort and photophobia in the surgical eye. He remained on gatifloxacin, timolol, and prednisolone.

On post-operative week 8 the visual acuity in the left eye was 20/20−2 without correction. The corneal glue had loosened again by this time and was easily removed. After the corneal glue was removed, the two corneal sutures were visible and were found to be very loose, and therefore were removed. After the corneal sutures were removed, the wound was observed to be briskly Seidel positive. The epithelium around the corneal laceration was noted to be very irregular and it was difficult to determine the exact location of the laceration and leakage site.

51.6 Surgeon's Assessment and Pre-operative Plan

The possible reasons for this otherwise healthy patient's inadequate wound healing were discussed. In patients who have a persistently leaking wound, despite tight corneal sutures or corneal glue, formation of a fistula should be considered. Corneal wound fistulas may form when there is either ingrowth of surface epithelium onto the wound edges, or when there is necrosis and inflammation of the wound edges, preventing normal wound healing [1]. Fistulas are more common in patients with delayed presentation after injury, as the increased time prior to repair allows the epithelium to grow over the wound surface and wound edges [1]. Alternatively a poorly sutured wound that is persistently leaking may give epithelium the opportunity to establish along the wound edges and form a fistula. Although frequently one thinks of epithelial downgrowth or ingrowth as a devastating situation where there is elevated intraocular pressure and visible tissue growth onto the corneal endothelium and the iris, epithelial downgrowth may also occur to a lesser degree, presenting mainly as the inability of a wound to close [1]. In situations of poor wound closure due to epithelial downgrowth, the epithelium must be excised prior to repeat wound closure. Some advocate wound scraping, others elliptical excision of wound edges with primary wound closure, while others recommend trephination of the wound with patch graft [1]. Wounds may also leak if they presented with delay and there was edema at the wound edges, which subsequently deturgesced [2]. They may also leak in delayed open globe injuries if the wound edges are infected [2]. And finally, wounds leak more frequently when they are stellate or complex [2].

Several options were discussed with the patient, including a third attempt at corneal gluing, a return to the operating room for wound exploration and re-suturing, or return to the operating room with excision of the leaking wound edges by trephination and then suturing of a patch graft. Given that the wound did not heal after primary suturing and two attempts with corneal glue, it did not seem likely that it would heal with a third attempt as there was likely a fistulous tract. Moreover, the patient preferred to return to the operating room for re-suturing. A new bandage contact lens was placed and the patient was scheduled for surgical repair the following day.

A surgical plan was formulated. The irregular surface epithelium would first be debrided with a flat blade, such as a #57 Beaver blade or a flat blade, to clearly visualize the corneal laceration. The edges of the corneal laceration would be scraped to freshen the wound edges and remove any potential epithelial ingrowth, in order to create healthy edges that would promote healing. Tight corneal sutures would be placed to re-approximate the wound edges. Should the wound appear to be not amenable to scraping and primary closure, trephination and corneal patch graft would be considered.

51.7 Second Surgical Repair: Operative Note

In the pre-operative area, the patient was identified and the left eye was marked. The bandage contact lens was removed and the eye was examined with a slit lamp. The wound edges were gaping and the wound was leaking. The patient was brought into the operating room where a time out was performed. General anesthesia was induced. The patient was prepped and draped in the standard sterile ophthalmic fashion. Jaffe lid specula were used to distract the eyelids without putting pressure on the globe. Under the operating microscope the eye was examined, and a small vertical wound with slightly gaping edges, overlying loose epithelium and mild neovascularization was seen inferiorly near the 6 o'clock limbus. A temporal paracentesis was made with a 15° super sharp blade. Next, the super sharp blade was used to gently debride the corneal wound edges in order to freshen the surface and to remove any potential epithelial ingrowth that may have been preventing wound healing. The superficial loose epithelium that was surrounding the wound was gently removed with a Beaver blade. The anterior chamber was then filled with filtered air. Three 10-0 nylon sutures were used to tightly suture the wound and approximate the wound edges. The air in the anterior chamber was replaced with BSS. The wound was tested with fluorescein and found to be Seidel negative. The paracentesis wound was also closed with a 10-0 nylon suture. An injection of subconjunctival cefazolin-dexamethasone was administered. A 16 mm Kontour bandage contact lens was then placed, given the epithelial defect and the prior history of wound leak. The eyelid specula were removed. Atropine and tobramycin 0.3%/dexamethasone 0.1% drops were administered and the eye was patched. The patient tolerated the procedure well without complications.

51.7.1 Surgical Repair: Pearls

- In delayed corneal lacerations or wounds with persistent leaks, corneal epithelium may grow onto the wound edges, preventing normal wound healing. It is helpful to debride the abnormal corneal epithelium from the corneal surface and the wound edges. This allows better visualization of the corneal laceration, so the sutures can be placed appropriately and also helps prevent and/or eliminate epithelial ingrowth.
- Corneal lacerations from foreign bodies can be prone to wound leak, in part because the foreign bodies may cause local tissue necrosis. Slight scraping of the wound edges, and placement of tighter corneal sutures can help appose the wound edges and prevent wound leaks.

51.8 Post-operative Course

On post-operative day 1 after resuturing the corneal laceration, the patient's visual acuity was 20/400, pinhole 20/80, and intraocular pressure was 26 mmHg. The inferior corneal wound had three tightly placed sutures. The vision was affected by corneal edema and astigmatism from the sutures.

On post-operative week 1, his acuity was 20/200, pinhole to 20/25−1. The bandage contact lens was removed and the wound was Seidel negative. The patient was much more comfortable and was followed closely over the following weeks (Fig. 51.2).

At post-operative week 8, two sutures were removed from the main wound, followed by the final corneal suture at post-operative week 10. The wound was found to be Seidel negative after the final suture removal and visual acuity was 20/25+3, pinhole 20/15−1. Over the subsequent 9 months his vision remained excellent without the need for corrective glasses or a contact lens (Fig. 51.3). There were no signs of epithelial downgrowth on follow-up examination and his eye remained comfortable.

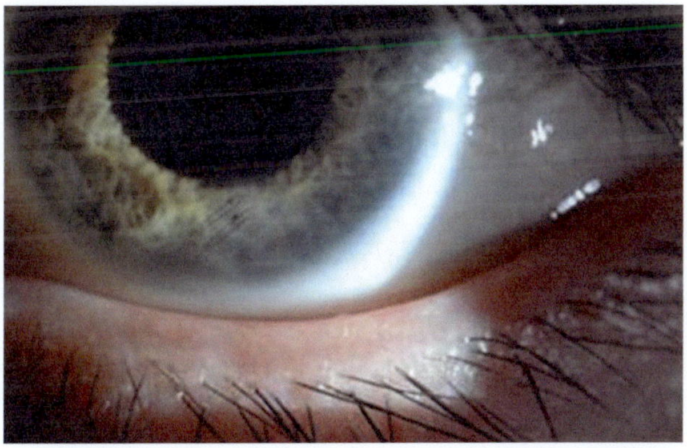

Fig. 51.2 Slit lamp photograph of the left eye 4 weeks after the second surgical repair, demonstrating three evenly spaced corneal sutures of adequate depth. Mild corneal stromal scarring noted

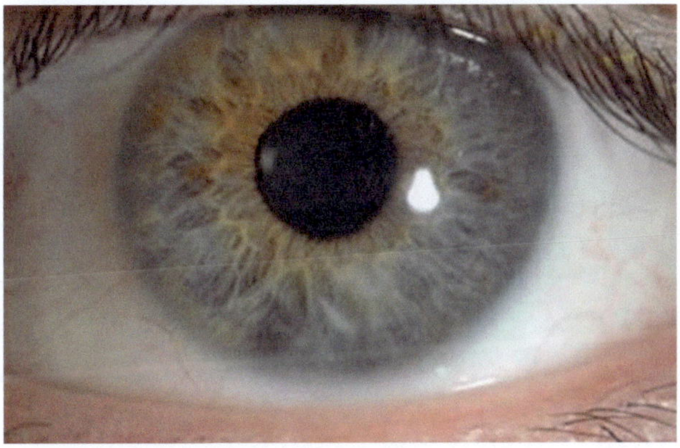

Fig. 51.3 Slit lamp photograph of the left eye taken 5 months after the second surgical repair, demonstrating a well-healed cornea with minimal residual corneal scarring

51.9 Final Trauma Evaluation

51.9.1 Final Visual Acuity sc

OD: 20/15
OS: 20/15−2

51.9.2 Pupils

OD: Round, no afferent pupillary defect
OS: Round, no afferent pupillary defect

51.9.3 Slit Lamp Examination

	OD	OS
Lids and lashes	Normal	Normal
Sclera and conjunctiva	Normal	Normal
Cornea	Normal	Stromal scar inferiorly from 5 to 6 o'clock with overlying epithelium well healed. Seidel negative.
Anterior chamber	Normal	Deep and quiet
Iris	Normal	Transillumination defect at 6 o'clock
Lens	Normal	Normal
Vitreous	Normal	Normal

51.9.4 Dilated Examination

Macula/Nerve OD: Normal
Periphery OD: Normal
Macula/Nerve: OS: Normal
Periphery OS: Normal

51.10 Review and Lessons Learned

Wound leaks are unfortunately not an uncommon complication after open globe injury repairs. Given the complex nature of open globe injuries, the variable presentation time to medical care, wounds repaired after open globe injury are naturally more prone to such complications than those after standard planned ocular surgeries. A recent large review of 267 open globe injuries from 2009 to 2011 at the Royal Victoria Eye and Ear Hospital found that wound leak after open globe repair occurred in 16.4% of cases [2]. Risks for developing post-surgical wound leak included the presence of concomitant microbial keratitis, delay in open globe presentation and stellate wound shape [2]. Of those wounds that leaked, 59% were treated successfully with conservative therapy, including bandage contact lenses, aqueous suppressants or corneal glue [2]. Forty-one percent of wound leak cases (18 patients total) required return to the operating room for re-suturing [2]. Of those that returned to the operating room eight patients (18%), like the patient illustrated in the current chapter, had failed prior conservative measures [2].

As illustrated in prior cases in this text, corneal lacerations from foreign bodies may cause round corneal defects or gaping wounds that may be difficult to close or may be prone to leaks. Foreign bodies may also contribute to local tissue necrosis at wound edges, making wound healing more difficult, or may cause infection leading to wound leak. Placing tight corneal sutures can help to appose the wound edges and prevent post-operative leaks, as can gently scraping necrotic tissue from the wound edges prior to suturing. In situations where tight sutures are placed, it is important to inform the patient that he or she will have blurry vision from the sutures. We have found that after corneal sutures are removed, much of the corneal astigmatism relaxes, and the visual outcome may be quite good, as in this case with 20/15 vision.

At the end of wound closure, it is best to ensure that corneal wounds are not leaking. If a wound is Seidel positive, additional sutures may need to be placed in the area of leakage, or shallow and/or loose sutures may need to be replaced. Sometimes very slow leaks may be addressed with a bandage contact lens, but there is a risk of the anterior chamber becoming shallow post-operatively if the wound leak persists, or the leak becoming more brisk as corneal edema resolves and the sutures loosen. In situations of a slow wound leak, the patient may be placed on an aqueous suppressant, such as timolol, to slow the rate of flow through the wound, allowing for wound healing. The use of aqueous suppressants is based mostly on theoretical considerations and clinical anecdotes, and large studies of their use in wound leaks have not been performed.

Corneal glue is relatively easy to apply in a clinic setting, and is quite effective at immediately sealing a corneal wound, as seen in our case; however, glue is not ideal and is best avoided if possible. Corneal glue produces an irregular surface, which then is uncomfortable for the patient and requires the use of a bandage contact lens. Patients may have significant discomfort and photophobia with the glue in position. It can also lead to more scarring than would be seen with sutures only. Additionally, although corneal glue may patch or cover a leak on the surface, the underlying tissue still needs to be well enough apposed and healthy to heal under the glue. If the wound underneath is not well approximated, the wound may still leak after the glue is removed, as illustrated in our case. If a wound continues to leak, even after repeat gluing, it may be best to try another approach, such as re-suturing, as we did in this case.

In delayed presentation open globes, open globe with uveal extrusion, or open globes with persistent wound leaks, one needs to remember the epithelium and its ability to quickly grow over surfaces and edges and potential to prevent normal wound healing. Normal corneal epithelium grows quickly and can often fill epithelial defects within 24 hours [3], thus especially in injuries that are close to 24 hours from presentation, epithelium may be present on the wound surface and edges and may prevent normal suturing and wound apposition. In primary repairs, it may be beneficial to gently debride the epithelial surface and the wound edges with a Beaver blade. Abnormal epithelium can obscure the view of the exact configuration of the laceration. By removing the abnormal epithelium the structure of the wound becomes more apparent, allowing for correct placement of corneal sutures. In our case, the corneal epithelium was irregular after the corneal glue was removed, and scraping off the abnormal corneal epithelium prior to re-suturing helped to define the laceration. Lightly scraping the edges of the corneal wound may also eliminate epithelial ingrowth that could be preventing wound healing [3].

In delayed wound presentation, where there is also uveal extrusion, epithelium may also grow over and coat the uvea [3]. Thus, if uveal tissue is to be reposited, it is important to also remove epithelial overgrowth meticulously from the uveal tissue prior to repositing it into the eye, or even to consider excision of the tissue [3]. Some advocate scraping the epithelium off the uveal tissue, while others recommend application of absolute ethanol, although ethanol is toxic to the anterior chamber if any is inadvertently introduced [3]. Despite careful removal of epithelial tissue from the corneal surface, wound edges and extruding uvea, in traumatic cases epithelium may still be introduced in to the anterior chamber with devastating consequences of epithelial downgrowth [3].

Epithelial downgrowth is classically thought of as a post-surgical condition where epithelium grows through the wound and into the anterior chamber, coating surfaces such as the endothelium, iris and angle structures, and resulting in glaucoma, ocular pain and decreased vision [4]. Epithelial downgrowth is typically described as forming sheets, epithelial pearls or epithelial cysts [4], and often its presence may be confirmed with application of argon laser to the iris, where the epithelial tissue will whiten [4]. Epithelial downgrowth, however, may often present insidiously, and may have minimal symptoms. It may be present on wound edges in histologic samples, creating a fistula, without producing clinically visible growth on the endothelium, and without growing on the iris, with a negative argon laser test [1, 4].

Suspicion for epithelial downgrowth in post-traumatic cases should always be quite high, as after cataract surgery, ocular trauma is the situation in which epithelial downgrowth is most commonly found [4–6]. In a 50-year retrospective review of 207 cases of epithelial downgrowth at the Wilmer Ophthalmological Institute, 48 cases occurred after trauma [5]. Similarly, in a 30-year retrospective review of cases of epithelial downgrowth at the Massachusetts Eye and Ear Infirmary, 18 of 124 cases of epithelial downgrowth were post-traumatic [6]. In the post-traumatic cases, histologic examination revealed a fistulous tract in 50% [6].

Symptoms and signs in patients presenting with epithelial downgrowth were variable, and included glaucoma, fistula, Seidel positivity, retro-corneal membrane, pain, vision loss, photophobia, iris cyst, hypotony, leukoma, corneal ulcer, band keratopathy, distorted pupil, red eye, tearing, foreign body sensation, and even no symptoms [5, 6]. In the Mass Eye and Ear series, 20% of patients presented with Seidel positivity, while in the Wilmer series, 16% of patients presented with a fistula [5, 6]. Only 17% of patients presented with glaucoma in the Wilmer series and 41% in the Mass Eye and Ear series [5, 6].

Interestingly, in the Wilmer series, epithelial downgrowth was not suspected clinically in a large proportion of patients (up to 50% of patients seen from 1990 to 1994) prior to histologic diagnosis [5]. This highlights the difficulty in diagnosis of epithelial downgrowth, the insidious nature of the signs and symptoms, and the need to maintain high suspicion of it in post-traumatic cases with poor wound healing or other unusual post-operative symptoms.

51.11 Key Learning Points

- Post-operative wound leak is more common in delayed-presentation open globes, open globe injuries with stellate wounds, and injuries with microbial keratitis.
- Delayed presentation corneal lacerations with significant corneal edema or corneal lacerations with persistent wound leaks, may benefit from debridement of the superficial corneal epithelium and wound edges to help define the corneal laceration and remove any epithelial ingrowth or necrotic unhealthy tissue.
- Tight corneal sutures may be helpful in gaping corneal lacerations, especially in situations where a corneal foreign body was involved. Sutures may loosen over time as corneal edema subsides, leading to a wound leak.
- A corneal wound with a slow leak may be covered with a bandage contact lens, but a corneal wound with a brisk leak is unlikely to resolve with a contact lens alone. If there is a brisk leak, it is best to evaluate the location of the leak and determine if additional sutures or replacement of sutures is necessary. Corneal glue is an option, but is best avoided if possible.
- If a wound continues to leak, especially after repeated corneal gluing or repeated suturing, formation of a fistulous tract should be suspected, and it is best to try a different approach.
- Trauma is the second most common cause of epithelial downgrowth, and there should be a high level of suspicion for it in cases where there is poor wound healing, or unexpected symptoms or findings.
- If significant epithelial downgrowth is suspected, confirmation may be attempted with argon laser to the iris.
- Scraping of the corneal surface and wound edges may be sufficient in mild cases of epithelial downgrowth, but in some cases elliptical excision of wound edges or trephination of the wound with a patch graft may be needed.

References

1. Soong HK, Meyer RF, Wolter JR. Fistula excision and peripheral grafts in the treatment of persistent limbal wound leaks. Ophthalmology. 1988;95(1):31–6.
2. Kong GY, Henderson RH, Sandhu SS, Essex RW, Allen PJ, Campbell WG. Wound-related complications and clinical outcomes following open globe injury repair. Clin Exp Ophthalmol. 2015;43(6):508–13.
3. Orlin SE, Farber MG, Brucker AJ, Frayer WC. The unexpected guest: problem of iris reposition. Surv Ophthalmol. 1990;35(1):59–66.
4. Chen SH, Pineda R 2nd. Epithelial and fibrous downgrowth: mechanisms of disease. Ophthalmol Clin North Am. 2002;15(1):41–8. Review
5. Küchle M, Green WR. Epithelial ingrowth: a study of 207 histopathologically proven cases. Ger J Ophthalmol. 1996;5(4):211–23.
6. Weiner MJ, Trentacoste J, Pon DM, Albert DM. Epithelial downgrowth: a 30-year clinicopathologic review. Br J Ophthalmol. 1989;73(1):6–11.

Chapter 52
Case 47: Zone I/II Open Globe Repair with Post-Operative Elevated Intraocular Pressure

Jonathan C. Chou, Veena Rao, and Seanna Grob

52.1 History of Present Illness

A 58-year-old man with history of hypertension and hyperlipidemia presents with concern for open globe of the left eye.

- While pulling up a screw that was malpositioned with a screwdriver in the same hand, his hand slipped and the handle of the screwdriver hit his left eye.
- He noticed a sudden decrease in vision and was taken to the nearest emergency department for evaluation.
- He was evaluated at an outside hospital where a computed tomography (CT) scan was concerning for a left open globe with posterior displacement of the lens. He was sent to Mass Eye and Ear for further management.

52.2 Initial Trauma Evaluation

52.2.1 Visual Acuity (Without Correction)

OD: 20/20
OS: Light perception

Electronic Supplementary Material The online version of this chapter (https://doi.org/10.1007/978-3-319-72410-2_52) contains supplementary material, which is available to authorized users.

J. C. Chou, M.D. (✉) • V. Rao, M.D. • S. Grob, M.D., M.A.S.
Department of Ophthalmology, Harvard Medical School, Massachusetts Eye and Ear, Boston, MA, USA

S. Grob, C. Kloek (eds.), *Management of Open Globe Injuries*,
https://doi.org/10.1007/978-3-319-72410-2_52

52.2.2 Intraocular Pressure (mmHg)

OD: 15
OS: Deferred

52.2.3 Pupils

OD: Reactive
OS: Irregular, no afferent pupillary defect by reverse

52.2.4 External Examination

No evidence of facial lacerations or other trauma.

52.2.5 Slit Lamp Examination

	OD	OS
Lids and lashes	Normal	Mild edema
Sclera and conjunctiva	Normal	Diffuse injection
Cornea	Normal	Full-thickness curvilinear rupture from 5 to 8 o'clock following the limbus with significant iris prolapse
Anterior chamber	Normal	Shallow with hyphema
Iris	Normal	Temporal iris avulsed and prolapsed through the rupture site inferonasally
Lens	Normal	Posterolaterally displaced
Vitreous	Normal	Noted anteriorly

52.2.6 Dilated Examination

Macula/Nerve OD: Normal
Periphery OD: Normal
Macula/Nerve: OS: No view
Periphery OS: No view

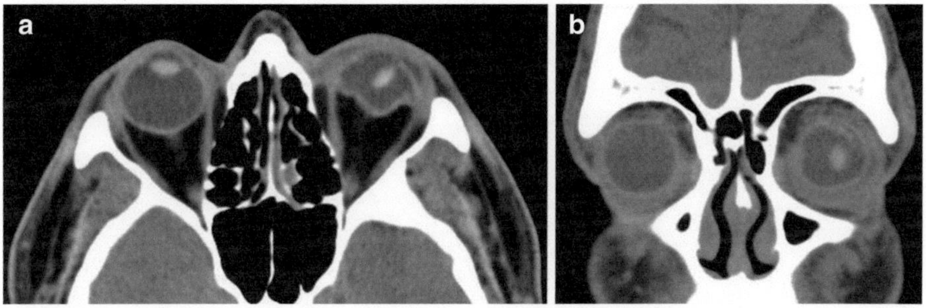

Fig. 52.1 Non-contrast CT scan of the orbits (**a**) Axial CT image demonstrating the significant irregularity of the globe contour on the left with a displaced intraocular lens. (**b**) Coronal CT image showing irregularity to the scleral contour nasally and a displaced lens

52.2.7 Radiographic Imaging

CT of the orbits showed ruptured left globe with postero-lateral displacement of lens. There was no evidence of an intraocular foreign body. No fractures were noted (Fig. 52.1a, b).

52.3 Surgeon's Initial Assessment and Pre-Operative Plan

The patient had a Zone I/II open globe injury of the left eye with associated lens dislocation.

Surgical plan was to repair the ruptured globe primarily and then address the dislocated lens at a later date after a post-operative ultrasound, which would give us more information about the status of the lens and the retina. Please refer to earlier chapters for details regarding pre-operative considerations in Zone I and/or II injuries. Specifically for this globe, since the rupture site followed the limbus, our plan was to place radial nylon sutures to re-approximate the limbus.

52.4 Surgical Exploration and Repair: Operative Note

In the pre-operative area, the patient was identified and the left eye was marked. He was brought into the operating room where a time out per standard protocol was performed. General anesthesia was induced. The left eye was then prepped and draped as per standard ophthalmic fashion, taking care to be very gentle as there was extruded uveal tissue that was touching the eyelid margin. Jaffe lid specula were inserted for better visualization. The eye was inspected under the surgical microscope. A shelved full-thickness rupture was seen curving along the limbus from 5 to 9

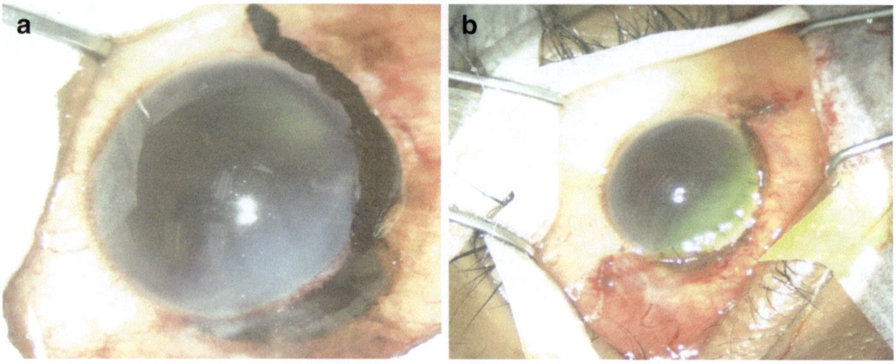

Fig. 52.2 (**a**) Pre-operative photo showing significant iris avulsion inferiorly; (**b**) Post-operative photo after iris repositioning and corneal limbal wound closure

o'clock. There appeared to be iris avulsion from 2:30 to 9:00, but the view into the anterior chamber was hazy due to hemorrhage. A long segment of iris was extruding though the corneal laceration at 6 o'clock (Fig. 52.2a). Areas of hemorrhage were noted in the anterior chamber, which obscured the view of the lens.

An iris spatula was used to gently reposit the iris into the anterior chamber. Westcott scissors were used to initiate a peritomy at 11 o'clock and to bluntly dissect the conjunctiva and Tenon's from the underlying sclera toward the direction of the limbal wound. The other side of the peritomy was initiated at approximately 4 o'clock and blunt dissection was continued to expose the scleral rupture further. Next, the limbal wound was closed with eight 10-0 nylon interrupted sutures directed radial to the limbus, using an iris spatula with each pass to prevent uveal incarceration in the wound. The wound was tested with fluorescein and was found to be Seidel negative. The globe was further explored and no additional rupture sites were found. 8-0 Vicryl sutures were then used to close the conjunctival peritomy (Fig. 52.2b). A subconjunctival injection of cefazolin and dexamethasone was then administered. The lid specula were removed under visualization. The patient tolerated the procedure well, without complication.

52.4.1 Surgical Exploration and Repair: Pearls

- For ruptures that follow the curvature of the limbus, radial sutures can be placed to re-approximate the limbus.
- Minimize intraocular tissue loss, repositing uveal tissue when possible and only excising tissue that is necrotic, infected, or not viable tissue.

52.4.2 Surgical Video

Please see Video 52.1

52.5 Post-Operative Course

The patient was admitted to complete the 48 hour course of intravenous antibiotics. On post-operative day one, visual acuity was hand motion and intraocular pressure (IOP) was 24 mmHg in the left eye. The wound was well-approximated and Seidel negative. There was a layered hyphema and loss of iris tissue noted temporally (Fig. 52.3a). A B-scan ultrasound showed posterior displacement of the lens (Fig. 52.3b). He was started on routine post-operative drops including moxifloxacin, 1% prednisolone and atropine. Subsequently, the patient underwent a pars plana vitrectomy and lensectomy 2 weeks after open globe repair (Fig. 52.4). Intraoperatively, the retina was found to be completely attached and the free-floating lens fragments were removed.

His IOP was 14 mmHg the following day. At his 1 week post-operative visit, his IOP had increased to 31 mmHg and he was started on dorzolamide hydrochloride—timolol maleate (2%/0.5%) twice a day and a prednisolone taper

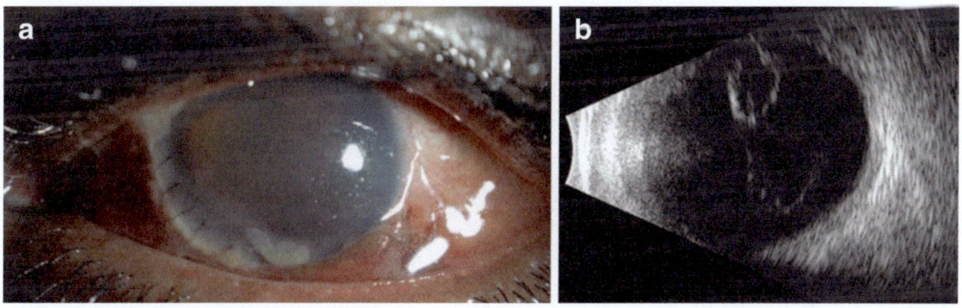

Fig. 52.3 (**a**) Slit lamp photograph of the left eye at post-operative day 1. Radial nylon sutures are seen inferonasally, with a layering hyphema and loss of iris tissue temporally; (**b**) B-scan ultrasound showing lens dislocation posteriorly into the vitreous

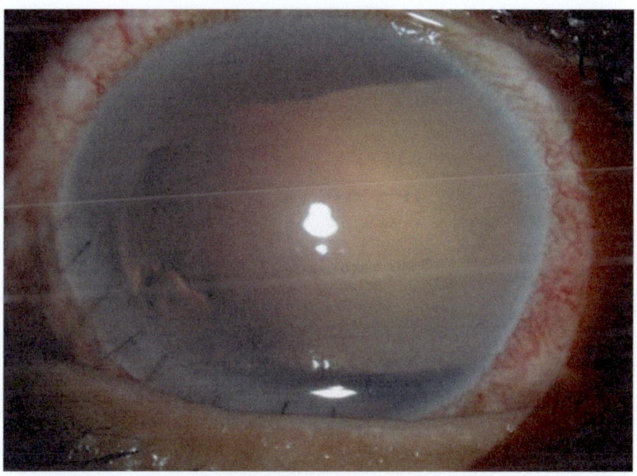

Fig. 52.4 Slit lamp photograph of the left eye after pars plana vitrectomy and lensectomy. The eye is now aphakic with notable loss of iris tissue temporally

was initiated. Two weeks later his pressure was 36 mmHg with good compliance. Gonioscopy revealed diffuse anterior synechiae nasally and inferiorly with no angle structures identified in these quadrants as well as angle recession superiorly and temporally in the left eye. He was evaluated by a glaucoma specialist and brimonidine tartrate 0.2% three times a day and latanoprost 0.005% at night were added. His IOP improved to the mid-teens after 1 week. Dilated funduscopic exam showed normal optic nerves and the retinal nerve fiber layer optical coherence tomography (OCT) was within normal limits. Initial visual field testing using a + 15.00 D lens for aphakic correction showed possible superior and inferior nasal depressions (Fig. 52.5a–c). After corneal suture removal, the patient was fitted for an aphakic

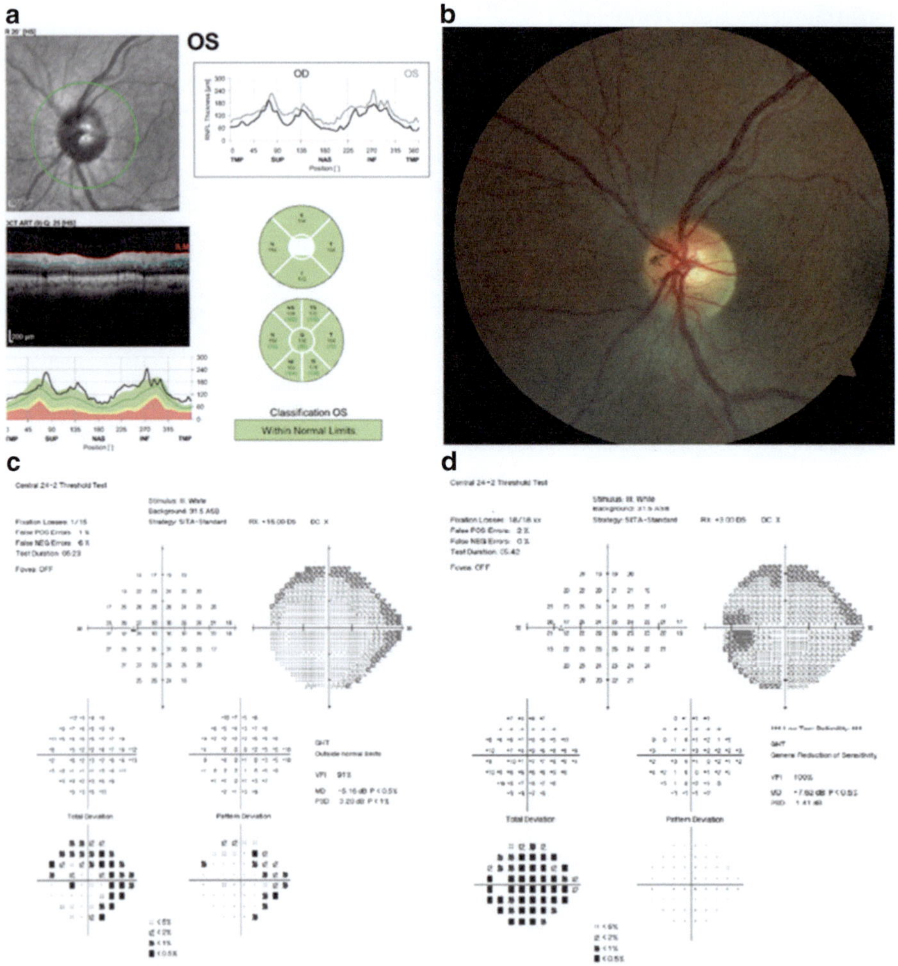

Fig. 52.5 (**a**) Optic nerve OCT of the left eye showing healthy nerve fiber layer. (**b**) Disc photo of the left eye showing a pink and healthy nerve with a cup to disc ratio of 0.3; (**c**) 24-2 Humphrey Visual Field performed with a + 15.0 lens showing possible superonasal and inferonasal depression of the left eye 1 month after open globe repair; (**d**) Repeat 24-2 Humphrey Visual Field performed 6 months later, after contact lens fitting, showing normal pattern standard deviation without gross defect

contact lens and vision improved to 20/60-2. Follow up visual fields showed no evidence of visual field defects (Fig. 52.5d).

52.6 Final Trauma Evaluation

52.6.1 Final Visual Acuity

OD: 20/20-
OS: 20/60-2 (best corrected with contact lens)

52.6.2 Intraocular Pressure (mmHg)

OD: 15
OS: 17

52.6.3 Pupils

OD: Normal
OS: Loss of iris tissue temporally, no afferent pupillary defect

52.6.4 Slit Lamp Examination

	OD	OS
Lids and lashes	Normal	Normal
Sclera and conjunctiva	Normal	Trace injection inferiorly
Cornea	Normal	Mild corneal haze inferonasally, mild pannus inferonasally, trace epithelial edema inferiorly
Anterior chamber	Normal	Rare mixed pigment/old cell, deep
Iris	Normal	Iridodialysis with loss of iris tissue temporally (Fig. 52.6)
Lens	Normal	Aphakia
Vitreous	Normal	Normal

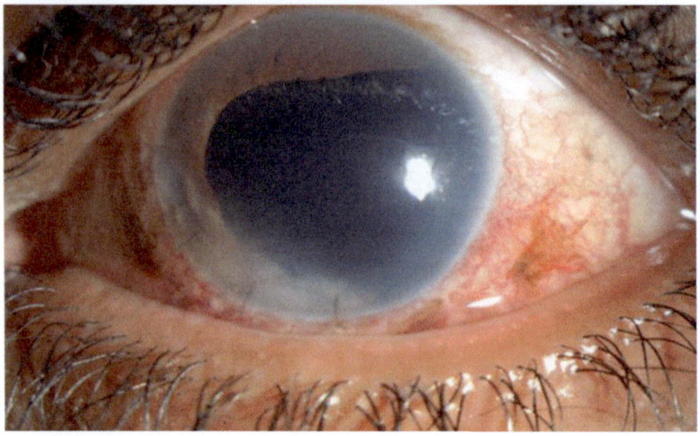

Fig. 52.6 Final slit lamp photograph of the left eye showing three remaining radial nylon sutures with mild corneal scarring inferonasally and an otherwise clear cornea with loss of iris tissue temporally and aphakia

52.6.5 Dilated Examination

Macula/Nerve OD: Normal
Periphery OD: Normal
Macula/Nerve: OS: Rim intact, cup to disc ratio 0.3, trace epiretinal membrane
Periphery OS: Attached retina, condensed vitreous inferiorly

52.7 Review and Lessons Learned

Patients with ruptured globe injuries are at risk of post-operative IOP elevation due to multiple possible mechanisms, several of which are illustrated here. In one case-control study, 17% of patients developed an IOP $\geq$ 22 mmHg after an open globe injury with an average maximum IOP of 33.4 mmHg at a median follow-up of 21 days. Risk factors found were age, hyphema, lens injury and Zone II injury [1]. The United States Eye Injury Registry indicates an overall 2.67% risk of developing glaucoma following trauma; glaucoma risk was correlated with age, poor visual acuity at presentation, lens involvement, and inflammation [2]. IOP elevation can present early in the post-operative course or even years later, requiring long-term monitoring. An initial low or normal IOP is not reassurance that the IOP will not elevate later in the post-operative course.

Let us review factors that may have played a role in this case. First, at the time of surgery, the patient was treated with subconjunctival and topical steroids, placing him at risk for steroid-induced glaucoma. Steroid-related IOP elevation is thought to be related to decreased trabecular meshwork outflow; some studies show degradation of the extracellular matrix causing accumulation of mucopolysaccharides in the trabecular meshwork [3]. Second, his significant iris trauma led to scarring of the angle with development of peripheral anterior synechiae, which can increase resistance to aqueous outflow. Third, this patient showed signs of angle recession, which is common after trauma and can lead to glaucoma months or years after the initial trauma. Glaucoma related to angle recession tends to develop either in the first year or greater than 10 years after injury [4]. The proposed mechanism is that damage to the iris and ciliary body leads to fibrosis and scarring of the trabecular meshwork and/or Schlemm's canal. A hyaline membrane has also been reported to grow over the trabecular meshwork, which can also cause decreased aqueous outflow [5]. Also notable in this case is the presence of lens dislocation and lens fragments that were removed during pars plana vitrectomy; it is possible for lens particles to disrupt the trabecular meshwork and increase IOP. Although not present in this case, it is important to assess for any evidence of pupillary block which might cause IOP elevation.

Treatment of the elevated intraocular pressure depends on the underlying mechanism(s) and, for the most part, is managed similarly to non-traumatic glaucomas. In our case, the topical steroid was tapered and the patient was started on topical IOP-lowering medications. In the acute phase of trauma, the clinician should be cautious when using prostaglandin analogues as they tend to be pro-inflammatory. Cholinergic agonists (e.g. pilocarpine) should be avoided in cases of angle recession and may incite inflammation. Goniosynechialysis can be considered in cases where there is extensive peripheral anterior synechiae and iridotomy and/or lens removal can be useful in cases involving pupillary block. If the IOP continues to be elevated despite conservative treatment with medications, glaucoma filtration surgeries may need to be considered.

In traumatic lens dislocation cases with associated globe rupture, it is important to address the open globe first. This helps minimize tissue loss and possible extrusion from intraocular surgery. Allowing the corneal and scleral tissue to heal can be helpful prior to additional secondary surgeries. In cases where a dislocated lens cannot be safely retrieved via an anterior approach, a pars plana technique is required (see earlier cases for further discussion). It is important to counsel all patients with ruptured globe trauma that they will require careful, often life-long, monitoring of their intraocular pressure.

52.8 Key Learning Points

- Elevated intraocular pressure can occur after ruptured globe and has multiple mechanisms (e.g. angle recession, steroid-induced, peripheral anterior synechiae).
- It is important that patients are counselled regarding the importance of long-term follow up (at least on a yearly basis) after post-operative recovery, especially if they have risk factors for glaucoma after the trauma.

References

1. Turalba AV, Shah AS, Andreoli MT, Andreoli CM, Rhee DJ. Predictors and outcomes of ocular hypertension after open-globe injury. J Glaucoma. 2014;23(1):5–10.
2. Girkin CA, McGwin G Jr, Long C, Morris R, Kuhn F. Glaucoma after ocular contusion: a cohort study of the United States Eye Injury Registry. J Glaucoma. 2005;14(6):470–3.
3. Kersey JP, Broadway DC. Corticosteroid-induced glaucoma: a review of the literature. Eye (Lond). 2006;20(4):407–16.
4. Blanton FM. Anterior chamber angle recession and secondary glaucoma. A study of the aftereffects of traumatic hyphemas. Arch Ophthalmol. 1964;72:39–43.
5. Jensen OA. Contusive angle recession. A histopathological study of a Danish material. Acta Ophthalmol. 1968;46(6):1207–12.

Chapter 53
Case 48: Zone I/II/III Open Globe and Eyelid Lacerations from a Box Cutter with Post-Operative Wound Dehiscence

Seanna Grob and Alice C. Lorch

53.1 History of Present Illness

A 43-year-old man with history of substance abuse presents with concern for open globe of the left eye.

- The patient reports he was attacked by a known assailant who first hit him in the head and then cut his left eye and face with a box cutter. The patient denied any other trauma or loss of consciousness.
- He was seen at an outside hospital and computed tomography (CT) imaging was consistent with an open globe injury so he was transferred to Massachusetts Eye and Ear (MEE).
- He reports decreased vision and only being able to discern light from dark in the left eye.

53.2 Initial Trauma Evaluation

53.2.1 Visual Acuity (Without Correction)

OD: 20/40
OS: Light perception

S. Grob, M.D., M.A.S. (✉) • A. C. Lorch, M.D., M.P.H.
Department of Ophthalmology, Harvard Medical School, Massachusetts Eye and Ear, Boston, MA, USA

S. Grob, C. Kloek (eds.), *Management of Open Globe Injuries*,
https://doi.org/10.1007/978-3-319-72410-2_53

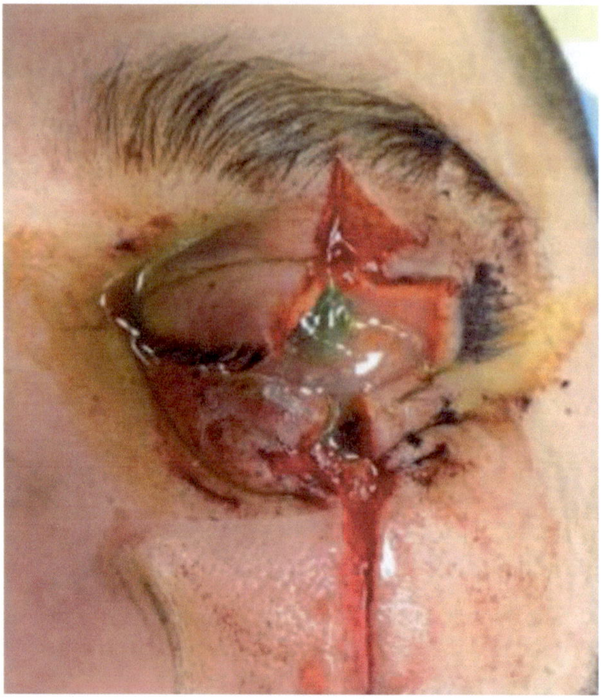

Fig. 53.1 A clinical image of the left eye on presentation showing the vertical laceration from the box cutter through the upper and lower eyelids

53.2.2 Pupils

OD: Round, no afferent pupillary defect
OS: Irregular, no afferent pupillary defect by reverse

53.2.3 External Examination

Vertical facial laceration extending from the brow through the left upper eyelid, left lower eyelid, and face to the lateral commissure of the mouth (Fig. 53.1).

53.2.4 Slit Lamp Examination

	OD	OS
Lids and lashes	Normal	Upper and lower eyelid marginal lacerations
Sclera and conjunctiva	Normal	Subconjunctival hemorrhage, with temporal vertical corneal-scleral laceration
Cornea	Normal	Temporal vertical corneal laceration extending from superior to inferior limbus with uveal and vitreous prolapse

	OD	OS
Anterior chamber	Normal	Flat, with iridocorneal touch
Iris	Normal	Iridocorneal touch, otherwise intact
Lens	Normal	No view
Vitreous	Normal	No view

53.2.5 Dilated Examination

Macula/Nerve OD: Normal
Periphery OD: Normal
Macula/Nerve: OS: No view
Periphery OS: No view

53.2.6 Radiographic Imaging

CT of the orbits showed a ruptured globe of the left eye (Fig. 53.2), without evidence of an intraocular foreign body. There was a small left inferior orbital rim chip fracture and associated soft tissue laceration with facial swelling. No intracranial injury was identified.

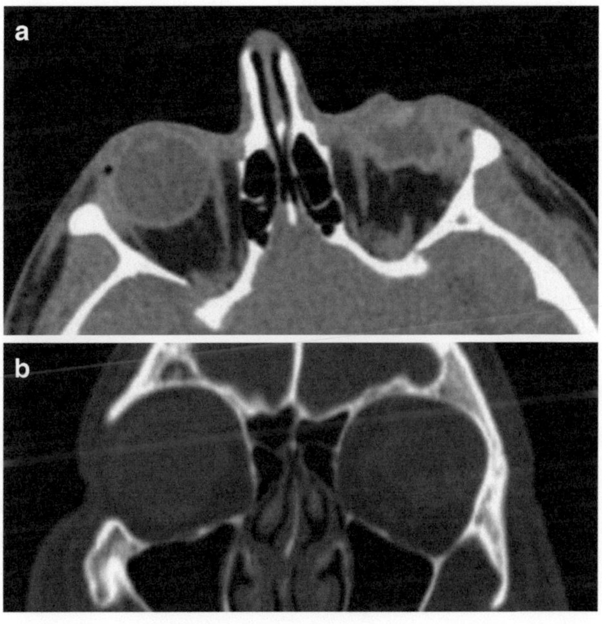

Fig. 53.2 Axial (**a**) and coronal (**b**) CT images showing a normal globe on the right and a markedly deformed globe on the left

53.3 Surgeon's Initial Assessment and Pre-Operative Plan

The patient had a Zone I/II/III open globe injury of the left eye and a large vertical facial laceration caused by a box cutter requiring surgical repair.

This case illustrates three important areas of discussion beyond the standard repair of a Zone I/II/III laceration (see earlier cases in this book for examples). These are: the management of concomitant periocular lacerations, pain control in a patient with substance abuse, and post-operative wound dehiscence.

Open globes with concomitant facial lacerations require special attention. Lid lacerations should be examined thoroughly, but with care not to put any pressure on the eye. Lids should be everted and fornices evaluated if the mechanism of laceration was dirty—an example might be a car accident in which gravel presents on the lids. All foreign bodies should be removed. The type of laceration should then be identified; specifically, it should be noted whether or not the margin is involved. Lacerations near the medial canthus should prompt a low threshold for probing and irrigation to ensure that the lacrimal apparatus is not involved. At MEE, we involve the oculoplastics service for closure of complex lacerations, but this option is not available in many other medical facilities. We always plan to close the open globe wound before the facial lacerations, prioritizing protection of the globe from any external pressure.

The Zone I/II/III laceration pre-operative plan would not differ from standard (see earlier cases in this book for examples) despite the extensive periocular lacerations.

For straightforward globe injuries, patients generally receive post-operative narcotics for pain control for 2 days while they remain inpatient, with the goal to wean them off of narcotics to acetaminophen as soon as possible. A few require prescriptions for pain control on discharge and are generally given prescriptions for 3–5 days. In the absence of complications like high intraocular pressure that cause significant pain, most patients should be fairly comfortable using acetaminophen alone after open globe repair. Patients that request narcotic prescriptions for longer than a few days, in the absence of any significant signs of pain, are asked to see their primary care physician. This patient had a history of substance abuse, most recently using heroine and suboxone by his report. Given this, we anticipated a higher requirement for pain medications. At MEE, we consult our pain management service for guidance, but this service is not available at all medical facilities.

53.4 Surgical Exploration and Repair: Operative Note

Informed consent was obtained and the operative eye was verified and marked. The uninjured right eye was taped and shielded for protection. The left eye was then prepped and draped in the usual sterile ophthalmic fashion. Since the left upper eyelid was completely transected, the usual Jaffe lid speculum was not able to be used for retraction of the upper eyelid. In this case, two 4-0 silk sutures were used to retract the two sections of the upper eyelid. A Jaffe lid speculum was inserted into the lower eyelid. A 360° peritomy was initiated nasally away from the laceration and then extended circumferentially. Gentle dissection was continued into the superotemporal and inferotemporal quadrants with blunt Westcott scissors. A linear laceration extending from approximately the 2:00 o'clock position near the limbus extending vertically down through the cornea, continuing inferiorly through the sclera up to the insertion of the inferior rectus muscle was noted. The laceration measured 13-mm and extended 6.5-mm inferior to the limbus. The inferior rectus muscle was hooked with a Gass muscle hook and was isolated using a 2-0 silk suture. The limbus was then approximated with a 9-0 nylon suture both at 2 o'clock and 4:30 o'clock. The corneal wound was then closed using 10-0 nylon and the scleral wound was closed using 8-0 nylon. An iris spatula was used throughout the closure of the laceration to ensure complete repositioning of uveal tissue inside the eye without causing any entrapment within the sutures or wound. Then multiple corneal sutures were replaced to ensure a relatively uniform corneal contour and then the suture knots were rotated so the knot would be buried and located away from the visual axis. The wound was then checked for leaks with fluorescein strips and was found to be watertight. The silk suture was removed from the inferior rectus. The peritomy was closed using an 8-0 Vicryl suture on a spatulated needed. An episcleral bite was taken nasally and superiorly to prevent draping of the conjunctiva over the cornea. A subconjunctival injection of cefazolin and dexamethasone was given inferonasally away from the laceration. The lid margin traction sutures were removed. Atropine drops and neomycin and polymyxin B sulfates and dexamethasone ophthalmic ointment were instilled in the eye. The drape was removed and the left facial laceration area was prepped and drapped in the usual sterile manner.

The left upper and lower eyelid margins were re-approximated in a similar fashion. A vertical mattress 6-0 silk suture was passed to re-align the eyelid margin, specifically the gray line and the tarsus. Multiple interrupted partial thickness Vicryl sutures were used to re-approximate the tarsus. An additional vertical mattress silk suture was placed at the lid margin to re-align the eyelashes. The margin sutures were tied resulting in good eversion at the margin and the tails were left long. Silk interrupted sutures were used to re-align the skin of the eyelid laceration and the tails of the margin sutures were incorporated into these knots to keep them directed away from the cornea. Deep 5-0 Vicryl sutures were used to close the facial laceration extending from the eyelids followed by 5-0 Prolene interrupted sutures to close the skin.

53.4.1 Surgical Exploration and Repair: Pearls

- In cases with eyelid lacerations that prevent the use of a Jaffe lid speculum, 4-0 silk sutures can be placed through the lid margin and can be affixed using steri-strips or mosquito locking forceps.

- Careful examination of the eyelids in the operating room is key as patients are often too uncomfortable pre-operatively to allow for adequate evaluation. Look carefully at the medial eyelid and consider probing of the canaliculi to rule out canalicular trauma that could potentially hide in edematous eyelids. Intraoperatively, you can take time to remove small shards of glass or gravel or other small foreign bodies. If the wound is dirty, thorough irrigation with sterile saline solution is recommended prior to closure.

53.5 Post-Operative Course

The patient was admitted to MEE to complete a 48 hour course of intravenous antibiotics. On post-operative day one he still had light perception vision, with no view to the posterior pole. A B-scan ultrasound showed shallow uveal effusions with an attached retina on the left.

He then followed up 5 days after repair with a retina specialist and visual acuity was 20/800 pinhole 20/200 and there was still minimal view posteriorly. The options were discussed with the patient who agreed to proceed with a pars plana vitrectomy, lensectomy, and endolaser.

This took place 23 days later. Intraoperatively, the patient was found to have multiple retinal folds, but no clear retinal breaks. Endolaser was applied to the inferior retina to an inferior retinal fold associated with a vitreoretinal stalk. (See earlier cases for further discussion of vitreoretinal surgery after open globe repair.)

The patient was followed closely by the retina and trauma service over the following weeks. Six weeks after his injury, the corneal sutures were removed in the trauma clinic, per standard practice and the wound appeared well healed. On follow up, the temporal cornea was noted to be very thin, so an aphakic contact lens evaluation was deferred, so as to minimize manipulation of the cornea by the patient at that time. The patient followed up 2 weeks later with intermittent pain and floaters in the left eye and was found to have a dehisced corneal wound with an iris plug that had epithelialized and was seidel negative. The patient was consented for immediate surgical repair of his dehisced corneal wound.

53.6 Second Surgical Repair: Operative Note

A paracentesis was made at 1 o'clock directed temporally towards the corneal wound. A cyclodialysis spatula was inserted through the paracentesis and was used to release the iris tissue from the corneal wound. A Beaver blade was then used to scrape the epithelial cells adjacent to the wound edge and along the edges of the laceration to remove any possible epithelial ingrowth that would prevent would healing. The laceration was then closed with 10-0 nylon sutures using an iris spatula to keep the iris out of the wound until the wound was well-approximated and water tight.

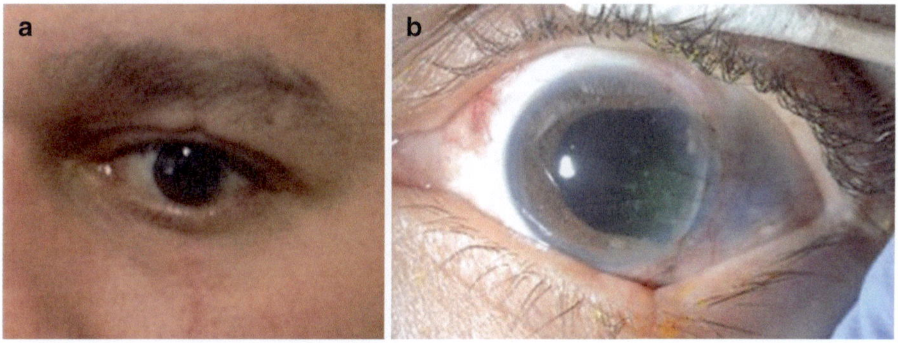

Fig. 53.3 (**a**) External photograph showing a well healed vertical scar (**b**). Anterior segment slit lamp photograph showing three remaining radial nylon sutures temporally and one limbal suture superotemporally, with loss of temporal iris tissue

53.6.1 Second Surgical Repair: Pearls

- In wounds that have either dehisced, or continue to leak, we have found it helpful to return to the operating room and scrape the adjacent epithelium and the wound edges gently, as well as any exposed iris tissue, to remove any epithelial ingrowth that might be preventing wound healing or cause formation of intraocular epithelial membranes. The wound is then re-approximated with 10-0 nylon sutures.

Due to the wound dehiscing, we planned to leave the corneal sutures in position for an extended period of time and to remove them in a staged fashion. After 4 months, we started to remove the corneal sutures and they were removed over two visits with a gap of 2 months in between due to issues with patient follow up (Fig. 53.3).

53.7 Final Trauma Evaluation

53.7.1 Final Visual Acuity

OD: 20/15
OS: 20/30-2 with +12.00 D lens

53.7.2 Pupils

OD: Round, no afferent pupillary defect by reverse
OS: Irregular, with loss of iris tissue temporally, no afferent pupillary defect by reverse

53.7.3 Slit Lamp Examination

	OD	OS
Lids and lashes	Normal	Upper and lower eyelid scars from laceration (Fig. 53.3a)
Sclera and conjunctiva	Normal	White and quiet
Cornea	Normal	Temporal vertical corneal scarring (Fig. 53.3b)
Anterior chamber	Normal	Formed, quiet
Iris	Normal	Loss of iris tissue temporally from 1–5 o'clock
Lens	Normal	Aphakic
Vitreous	Normal	Status post pars plana vitrectomy

53.7.4 Dilated Examination

Macula/Nerve OD: Normal
Periphery OD: Normal (Fig. 53.4a)
Macula/Nerve: OS: Normal
Periphery OS: Trace old vitreous hemorrhage inferiorly, retina attached, inferior laser and inferior retinal folds nearly resolved, no posterior vitreoretinopathy (Fig. 53.4b)

53.8 Review and Lessons Learned

In cases that present with periocular trauma, it is important to address the open globe first. Facial lacerations and fracture repair should be postponed if at all possible. Manipulation of the periocular tissues can lead to expulsion of intraocular contents if the eye has not been closed. It is important for the ophthalmologist to stress this point directly to any primary trauma, emergency department, or surgery team as other specialists are not as aware of the consequences of pressure on an open globe.

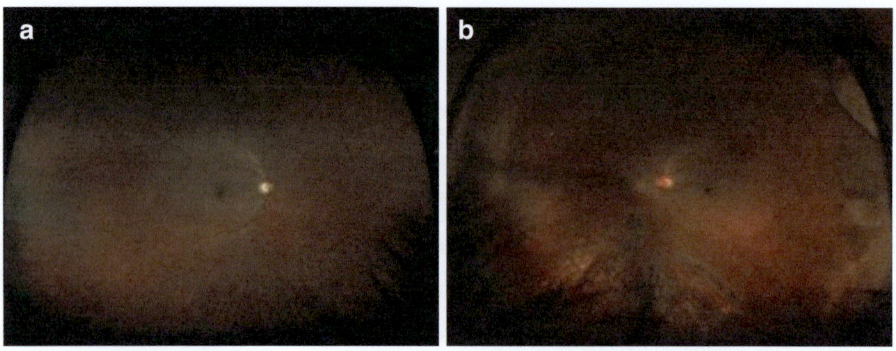

Fig. 53.4 Fundus photos of the (**a**) Right normal eye and (**b**) Left eye with inferior laser scars, but otherwise attached retina

Jaffe lid speculums are the specula of choice in open globe surgery since they place minimal pressure on the globe. However, if these cannot be placed appropriately due to eyelid or periocular lacerations, then a silk suture can be used through the eyelid margin or pieces of the lid margin and retracted back with a mosquito forcep, hemostat, or steri-strips.

Cornea sutures are usually removed at 6 weeks to avoid corneal scarring. However, with limbus to limbus lacerations, complex stellate corneal wounds, or delayed presentation corneal lacerations, one should consider staged removal. These wounds are prone to leak and may require more time to heal in order to avoid wound dehiscence [1]. We often remove alternating (every other) suture at 6 weeks for these patients, and then proceed slowly at subsequent appointments. One should take into account also the location of the limbus to limbus laceration- the temporal position of this laceration may have caused more traction and led to dehiscence. Patient manipulation of the eye and rubbing can often cause dehiscence as well and so patients should be counseled about this, and encouraged to wear an eye shield at all times while sutures are in place, particularly while sleeping. We have found also that if an open globe patient requires a second surgery, like retina surgery, it is often helpful to push out the suture removal longer than the 6-week period or only remove a portion of the sutures at this visit and then have the patient return in 2–3 weeks for additional suture removal. Sutures can be removed over several visits if needed.

If a patient has a wound dehiscence, it is important to carefully coach them through the follow up care and repair. After the repair of the dehisced corneal wound, we recommend leaving the sutures in much longer the second time around and taking the sutures out in a staged fashion. These patients can often still do very well. Even with the prolonged course, this patient went from only light perception vision on presentation to 20/30 with correction.

53.9 Key Learning Points

- In cases that present with periocular trauma, it is important to address the open globe first.
- If you cannot use Jaffe speculums for intraoperative eyelid retraction due to eyelid lacerations, you can use a silk suture through the eyelid margin and then retract the lids.
- Remove sutures slowly on long or irregular wounds. If a wound does dehisce, consider leaving the sutures in place for at least a couple of months and then remove them in a staged fashion.

Reference

1. Kong GYX, Henderson RH, Sandhu SS, et al. Wound-related complications and clinical outcomes following open globe injury repair. Clin Exp Ophthalmol. 2015;43(6):508–13.

Chapter 54
Case 49: Corneal Ulcer Associated with Sutures After Zone I/II Open Globe Injury

Liza M. Cohen and Katherine E. Talcott

54.1 History of Present Illness

An 80-year-old man with history of hypertension and hyperlipidemia presented with concern for open globe of the left eye.

- The patient reported he was trying to repair a chair when a metal clip attached to a coiled spring flew off the chair and hit him in the left eye.
- He presented to an outside hospital where computed tomography (CT) imaging was consistent with an open globe injury. He was given a tetanus booster, intravenous vancomycin, and intravenous cefepime and was transferred to the Massachusetts Eye & Ear for further management.
- He reported decreased vision in the left eye and was only able to see shadows. He was also experiencing throbbing pain in the left eye.

54.2 Initial Trauma Evaluation

54.2.1 Visual Acuity (Without Correction)

OD: 20/30-1
OS: Hand motion

L. M. Cohen, M.D. (✉)
Department of Ophthalmology, Harvard Medical School, Massachusetts Eye and Ear, Boston, MA, USA
e-mail: liza_cohen@meei.harvard.edu

K. E. Talcott, M.D.
Vitreoretinal Surgery, Wills Eye Hospital, Philadelphia, PA, USA

S. Grob, C. Kloek (eds.), *Management of Open Globe Injuries*,
https://doi.org/10.1007/978-3-319-72410-2_54

54.2.2 Pupils

OD: Round and reactive
OS: No view, no relative afferent pupillary defect by reverse

54.2.3 Slit Lamp Examination

	OD	OS
Lids and lashes	Normal	Normal
Sclera and conjunctiva	Normal	Minimal extension of superior corneal laceration onto conjunctival surface at 11 o'clock, 5 mm extension of inferotemporal corneal laceration into the sclera at 5 o'clock, subconjunctival hemorrhage inferotemporally
Cornea	Normal	Full-thickness shelved curvilinear corneal laceration from 11 o'clock peripherally extending inferiorly and bifurcating into two lacerations (one extending toward 7 o'clock and the other extending toward 5 o'clock passing through the limbus), Descemet membrane folds
Anterior chamber	Normal	Shallow with blood clots and fibrin inferonasally and inferotemporally
Iris	Normal	Incarcerated in corneal wound, transillumination defects superonasally and temporally
Lens	2+ Nuclear sclerosis	Hydropic, subluxed superotemporally and tilted on axis, loss of zonules temporally
Vitreous	Normal	No view

54.2.4 Dilated Examination

Macula/Nerve OD: Normal
Periphery OD: Normal
Macula/Nerve OS: No view
Periphery OS: No view

54.2.5 Radiographic Imaging

CT of the orbits demonstrated a ruptured globe of the left eye with a shallow anterior chamber and dislocated lens, without evidence of an intraocular foreign body. No intracranial injury was identified.

54.3 Surgeon's Initial Assessment and Pre-Operative Plan

This patient had a Zone I/I open globe injury of the left eye caused by a metal chair clip requiring surgical repair.

This case illustrates two important areas of discussion beyond the standard repair of a Zone I/II laceration: the management of complex stellate corneal lacerations and suture abscesses/corneal infections after open globe repair.

As with any standard corneal laceration, prior to closure, the laceration should be explored to determine if there is scleral involvement as well, and any prolapsed intraocular contents should be appropriately managed. Repair should begin at the limbus and proceed with the placement of 10-0 nylon sutures in an interrupted fashion, as this provides the most uniform approximation of corneal tissue, allowing for faster healing and removal of sutures separately. Sutures should be trimmed close to the knot and buried to prevent exposure.

As discussed in earlier chapters, stellate lacerations in particular present a challenge to the surgeon, as these wounds are often difficult to close due to the need to approximate many pieces of tissue. Tissue apposition of stellate lacerations can be suboptimal, especially at the apices where there can be malposition of wound edges and/or leakage from the wound. After re-approximating the apex, it can be helpful to place sutures beginning peripherally and proceeding centrally, directing them toward the apex in order to push corneal tissue into the apex and prevent tissue gap. This helps reduce tension at the stellate component and the risk of leaking. Additionally, special suture techniques including buried purse-string sutures and crossing sutures, as well as cyanoacrylate adhesive or patch grafts, are sometimes used to repair these wounds, with the goal of creating a watertight closure [1]. A "star-shaped suture" technique has also been described, in which the first needle pass occurs inside one of the wound lips in a clockwise direction with subsequent sutures proceeding with the adjacent wound limb in a counter-clockwise direction, while the suture passes are in a clockwise direction [2]. This continuous suture technique may provide a more even distribution of tension with tractional forces directed toward the center of the wound [2]. However, disadvantages of this technique are increased manipulation of fragile tissue, the inability to remove sutures in a step-wise fashion, and the potential for more severe infection if one part of the suture develops an abscess. Regardless of the technique utilized, the repair of stellate corneal lacerations requires close attention to approximating the wound edges, particularly at the apices.

54.4 Surgical Exploration and Repair: Operative Note

Informed consent was obtained and the operative eye was verified and marked. The uninjured right eye was taped and shielded for protection. The left eye was then prepped and draped in the usual sterile ophthalmic fashion.

On examination under the microscope, the patient was found to have a full-thickness corneal laceration, extending from the superior limbus around 12 o'clock inferiorly and then bifurcating into two lacerations; one extending toward 7 o'clock but not crossing the limbus and the other extending toward 5 o'clock passing the limbus and extending into the sclera. A significant amount of vitreous was found to be prolapsed from the corneal laceration. A gentle Weck-Cel vitrectomy was performed to clear the vitreous from the wound. A peritomy was initiated to explore the extent of the superior laceration, which did not extend beyond the limbus. Then, a second peritomy was initiated to explore the extent of the inferior laceration. The patient was found to have a full-thickness scleral laceration that extended 4 mm past the limbus. The limbus was re-approximated with a 9-0 nylon suture at approximately 5 o'clock, taking care not to incarcerate uvea. The corneal laceration was repaired with multiple 10-0 nylon sutures. A paracentesis was made at 2 o'clock and balanced salt solution was injected to re-inflate the globe. The inferior lacerations were re-approximated with slightly more vertically placed sutures (starting peripherally and proceeding centrally) in order to carefully re-approximate the apices of the stellate corneal laceration to prevent wound leak in this area. The full-thickness scleral laceration inferiorly was repaired with 8-0 nylon sutures. The whole length of the laceration was approximately 17 mm, with approximately 12 mm on the cornea and 5 mm on the sclera. Attention was then turned to re-examine the lens that appeared to be displaced anteriorly into the anterior chamber, and lens violation was suspected; however, given the poor view and concern for a displaced dense lens, a lensectomy was not performed. Fluorescein was applied and the wounds were found to be Seidel negative with provocation. The conjunctiva was then closed with interrupted 8-0 Vicryl (polyglactin) sutures. A subconjunctival steroid and antibiotic injection was performed nasally away from the laceration. The patient tolerated the procedure well, without any complications.

54.4.1 Surgical Exploration and Repair: Pearls

- Careful exploration prior to the repair of corneal lacerations is important in order to determine the full extent of injuries and evaluate whether there are concomitant limbal and/or scleral lacerations present.
- Careful attention to the forces in a complex stellate wound is necessary to achieve optimal closure. Initiating corneal closure peripherally to work toward the apex or re-orienting suture placement to combat slippage can be helpful.
- Consider the use of special suture techniques, such as buried purse-string sutures, crossing sutures, and star-shaped sutures, to repair complex stellate corneal lacerations. If there is loss of tissue or difficulty maintaining wound closure, cyanoacrylate adhesive and patch grafts can be used as well.

54.5 Post-Operative Course

The patient was admitted to complete a 48 hour course of intravenous antibiotics. On post-operative day one he still had hand motion vision with no view to the posterior pole (Fig. 54.1a). Gentle B-scan ultrasound was performed which showed a dislocated lens, posterior capsule violation, and small choroidal detachment. He was started on gatifloxacin, prednisolone, atropine, and timolol drops. On post-operative day five he underwent pars plana vitrectomy and lensectomy. He continued to follow with the retina service and recovered well from surgery, although his vision remained hand motion.

Approximately 1 month later (5.5 weeks after his open globe repair), he was seen by the trauma service. He reported pain, a "pulling" sensation in the middle of the left eye, and decreased vision for 2 weeks, although he did not seek urgent evaluation until his scheduled appointment. He had been off all antibiotic and steroid drops for 1 week. His vision was still hand motion and he was noted to have a corneal ulcer around two loose sutures just superior to the connected apices of the stellate wound (Fig. 54.1b). The ulcer was cultured, and he was started on fortified

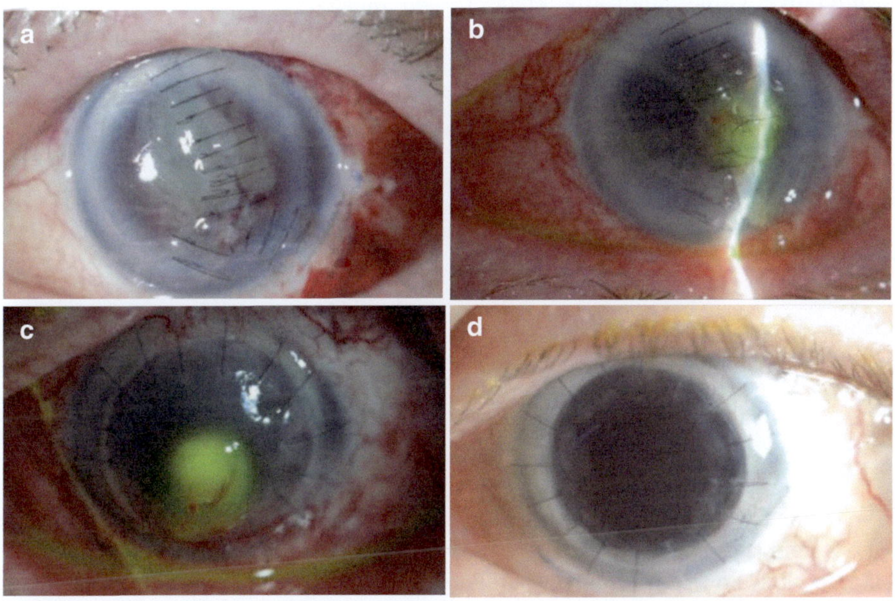

Fig. 54.1 Slit lamp photographs of the left eye. (**a**) Post-operative day 1: Corneal sutures of complex stellate wound intact. (**b**) Post-operative week 5.5: Development of a central corneal ulcer at the apex of the wound around two loose sutures. (**c**) Post-operative month 14: Corneal ulcer that formed in the penetrating keratoplasty graft. (**d**) Post-operative month 24: Clear corneal graft 3 months status-post repeat penetrating keratoplasty

vancomycin and tobramycin drops every 1 hour. Two days later, the loose sutures were removed and the wound was found to be Seidel positive. The wound leak was slow, however, so in conjunction with the cornea service, the decision was made to observe. Two additional days later, the infiltrate was improving but the wound remained Seidel positive, so it was glued. Antibiotics were tapered. Cultures grew rare staphylococcus aureus sensitive to levofloxacin; therefore, once the epithelial defect had healed, he was transitioned to moxifloxacin drops, which were eventually tapered.

Although the infection resolved, he developed kissing choroidals, requiring choroidal drainage, and then developed a total retinal detachment, requiring placement of a scleral buckle, pars plana vitrectomy, choroidal drainage, retinectomy, and silicone oil placement. Four months following his initial open globe repair, he began to undergo gradual corneal suture removal. A large central corneal scar formed, requiring penetrating keratoplasty, and at the same time he underwent placement of a scleral-fixated intraocular lens. Subsequently, he developed a corneal ulcer in the graft (Fig. 54.1c) leading to formation of another scar and underwent repeat penetrating keratoplasty. Three months status-post repeat penetrating keratoplasty (2 years following open globe repair), the corneal graft was clear (Fig. 54.1d). He then developed a tractional macula-off retinal detachment and proliferative vitreoretinopathy grade C and underwent pars plana vitrectomy, membrane peel, retinectomy, endolaser, and C3F8 placement. On most recent follow-up, the retina remains attached.

54.6 Final Trauma Evaluation

54.6.1 Final Visual Acuity

OD: 20/20-2
OS: Count fingers at face

54.6.2 Pupils

OD: Round and reactive
OS: No view, no relative afferent pupillary defect by reverse

54.6.3 Slit Lamp Examination

	OD	OS
Lids and lashes	Normal	Mild left upper eyelid ptosis
Sclera and conjunctiva	Normal	Trace injection, haptic seen under conjunctiva inferonasally and superonasally with 10-0 nylon sutures
Cornea	Normal	Penetrating keratoplasty graft intact, no infiltrate, all 16 sutures intact and buried
Anterior chamber	Normal	Deep and formed
Iris	Normal	Scarred and dilated, peripheral anterior synechiae
Lens	2+ Nuclear sclerosis	Scleral-fixated intraocular lens well-centered
Vitreous	Normal	Status-post pars plana vitrectomy, clear

54.6.4 Dilated Examination

Macula/Nerve OD: Normal
Periphery OD: Normal
Macula/Nerve: OS: Laser scars in inferotemporal macula, attached, nerve normal
Periphery OS: Laser scars inferotemporally around retinectomies/membranes, laser scars 360°, attached

54.7 Review and Lessons Learned

This patient's post-operative course was complicated by the development of a suture-related corneal ulcer 5.5 weeks after open globe repair. Suture-related infections typically present as suture abscesses around a loose suture. If left untreated, these can progress to become a larger corneal ulcer, which can have vision-threatening complications such as endophthalmitis or perforation of the cornea. It is therefore important to prevent infections from occurring and know how to manage them when they do occur.

Patients at risk for developing suture-related infections should be identified as early as pre-operatively, and care should be taken to attempt to mitigate the risk of infection. Stellate-shaped wounds are associated with post-operative wound leak and the development of microbial keratitis [3].

Suture-related infections can occur at any time post-operatively. Those occurring within the first 3–6 months are typically caused by suture loosening with increased exposure and subsequent mucus accumulation, whereas those that occur more than 12 months post-operatively are typically due to biodegradation of suture material [4]. Loose sutures can result from uneven suture tension at the time of surgery, [4] which is why it is important to take great care in repairing corneal lacerations, especially those that are complex. Sutures can loosen as a result of eye rubbing, and patients should be counseled to avoid rubbing their eyes and wear an eye shield at all times while sutures remain in place, especially while sleeping. Patients with loose sutures may present with symptoms of foreign-body sensation or mechanical discomfort [4]. If a loose or broken suture is discovered, it should be removed immediately to prevent accumulation of mucus and development of an infection. A short course of treatment with a topical broad-spectrum antibiotic should be initiated to guard against the possibility of introducing bacteria into the cornea at the time of suture removal [5]. Likewise, if a suture abscess is present, the offending suture should be removed and treatment with topical broad-spectrum antibiotics should be initiated, perhaps for a longer course of treatment with more frequent monitoring to ensure resolution of the infection [6]. In the case of development of a serious corneal ulcer, at Massachusetts Eye & Ear we routinely obtain cultures and start fortified vancomycin and tobramycin drops every hour. Patients should have frequent visits until the infection completely resolves. Tissue adhesives may play a role in sealing infected perforations, such as in the case of this patient, and it is important to remove any mucus prior to applying the adhesive [1].

Having a plan in place for suture removal can also help prevent the development of suture-related infections. If corneal lacerations are uncomplicated and the post-operative course uneventful, the first sutures are typically removed at 6 weeks post-operatively in adults to prevent scarring and the development of loose or broken sutures with associated complications [1]. In cases of large or complex stellate wounds, sutures may be removed in a stepwise manner to prevent wound dehiscence. At Massachusetts Eye & Ear, we often remove alternating sutures at 6 weeks post-operatively and then proceed with further suture removal at subsequent visits as determined by the wound length and healing. For this patient, the development of infection occurred prior to six-weeks post-operatively and was likely due to uneven wound tension caused by a difficult-to-close complex stellate wound.

54.8 Key Learning Points

- The repair of complex stellate corneal lacerations requires a pre-operative plan. Closure can typically be achieved by careful individual suture placement. However, techniques such as the use of buried purse-string sutures, crossing sutures, or star-shaped sutures, as well as cyanoacrylate adhesive or patch grafts, can also be used to repair complex wounds.

- Patients with complex corneal lacerations should be followed closely and monitored for evidence of loose sutures and suture abscesses. If either of these occurs, remove the offending suture immediately.
- If there is an infection, it is important to treat aggressively with broad-spectrum antibiotic drops. Consider obtaining cultures and the use of fortified antibiotics in cases of corneal ulcers. Always check the integrity of the wound, and if there is a leak, consider the use of cyanoacrylate adhesive to seal the leak. Continue to follow the patient closely and taper antibiotics accordingly until the infection completely resolves.
- Suture-related infections due to loose sutures may be prevented by appropriately counseling patients to avoid eye rubbing and wear a shield, as well as having a plan to remove sutures once the wound has healed.

References

1. Lin DT, Webster RG, Abbott RL. Repair of corneal lacerations and perforations. Int Ophthalmol Clin. 1988;28(1):69–75.
2. Akkin C, Kayikcioglu O, Erakgun T. A novel suture technique in stellate corneal lacerations. Ophthalmic Surg Lasers. 2001;32(5):436–7.
3. Kong GY, Henderson RH, Sandhu SS, et al. Wound-related complications and clinical outcomes following open globe injury repair. Clin Exp Ophthalmol. 2015;43(6):508–13.
4. Acheson JF, Lyons CJ. Ocular morbidity due to monofilament nylon corneal sutures. Eye. 1991;5:106–12.
5. Heaven CJ, Davison CRN, Cockcroft PM. Bacterial contamination of nylon corneal sutures. Eye. 1995;9:116–8.
6. Leahey AB, Avery RL, Gottsch JD, Mallette RA, Stark WJ. Suture abscesses after penetrating keratoplasty. Cornea. 1993;12(6):489–92.

Chapter 55
Case 50: Sympathetic Ophthalmia After Open Globe Repair

Cindy Ung, Katherine E. Talcott, Shizuo Mukai, and Lucia Sobrin

55.1 Case Presentation

A 53 year-old man with no prior ocular history presents with a ruptured open globe injury of the left eye.

- The patient reports he was working on an antique car door when a spring-loaded piece hit him in the left eye.
- He reports decreased vision in the left eye.

55.2 Initial Trauma Evaluation

55.2.1 Visual Acuity (Without Correction)

OD: 20/20
OS: Light perception

55.2.2 Pupils

OD: Round and reactive
OS: +Afferent pupillary defect

C. Ung, M.D. (✉) • S. Mukai, M.D. • L. Sobrin, M.D., M.P.H.
Department of Ophthalmology, Harvard Medical School, Massachusetts Eye and Ear, Boston, MA, USA
e-mail: cindy_ung@meei.harvard.edu

K. E. Talcott, M.D.
Vitreoretinal Surgery, Wills Eye Hospital, Philadelphia, PA, USA

S. Grob, C. Kloek (eds.), *Management of Open Globe Injuries*,
https://doi.org/10.1007/978-3-319-72410-2_55

55.2.3 External Examination

Minor abrasions and well apposed 0.5 cm laceration above left eyebrow and lateral to left canthus.

55.2.4 Slit Lamp Examination

	OD	OS
Lids and lashes	Normal	Normal
Sclera and conjunctiva	Normal	Bullous subconjunctival hemorrhage for 360° with temporal conjunctival laceration
Cornea	Normal	Central abrasion with scattered Descemet's folds
Anterior chamber	Normal	5 mm layered hyphema
Iris	Normal	No view
Lens	Normal	No view
Vitreous	Normal	No view

55.2.5 Dilated Examination

Macula/Nerve OD: Normal
Periphery OD: Normal
Macula/Nerve: OS: No view
Periphery OS: No view

55.2.6 Radiographic Imaging

Computed tomography of the orbits showed deformity of the left globe (Fig. 55.1).

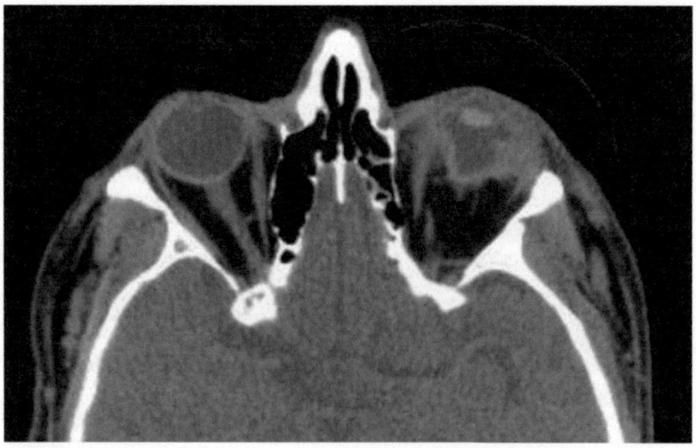

Fig. 55.1 Axial orbital computed tomography scan taken on presentation demonstrates a markedly irregular left globe

55.3 Surgical Exploration and Repair

The patient underwent primary repair of this open globe injury. Intraoperatively, the patient was found to have a Zone III open globe injury with a full-thickness scleral rupture that spanned from the insertion of the superior rectus to the insertion of the lateral rectus, approximately 20 mm in length. Uvea and vitreous were found to protrude through the scleral rupture laterally. He underwent repair of the scleral rupture, which involved disinsertion and re-attachment of the superior rectus muscle of the left eye. The scleral rupture was reapproximated with 8-0 nylon sutures in interrupted fashion with care taken not to incorporate the uvea.

55.4 Post-operative Course

On the first day after surgery, the patient was light perception in the left eye. The patient followed up with a retina specialist 1 week after open globe repair. B-scan ultrasonography revealed vitreous hemorrhage, hemorrhagic choroidals and concern for retinal detachment. He underwent a pars plana vitrectomy (PPV) a week later where intra-operative examination revealed extensive retinal incarceration into the wound and a retinal detachment with a giant retinal tear in the superotemporal and superior periphery extending four clock hours. A 360° relaxing retinectomy, lensectomy, silicone oil tamponade and scleral buckling were performed.

Two months after his PPV, his best corrected visual acuity in the left eye improved to 20/80. At this time, he underwent silicone oil removal and secondary implantation of an anterior chamber intraocular lens. He developed diffuse hemorrhage on the anterior surface of his anterior chamber intraocular lens (ACIOL) over the following month, which reduced his visual acuity to hand motion (Fig. 55.2).

Two months following his second PPV, the patient returned with decreased vision and metamorphopsia in his right eye.

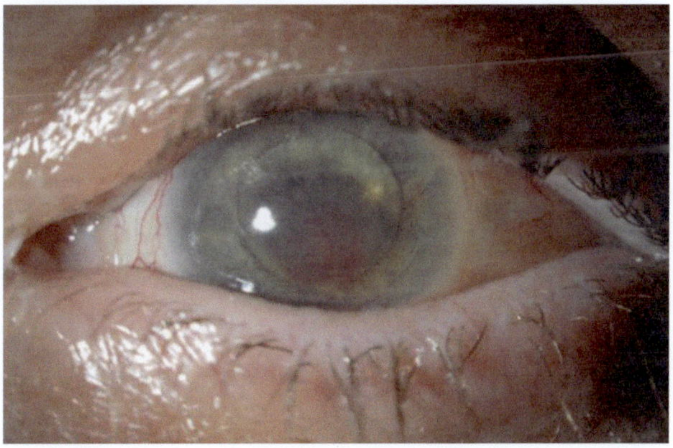

Fig. 55.2 (**a**) External photograph of the left eye revealing corneal edema, ACIOL with diffuse fibrin and heme overlying lens, and a surgical pupil

55.5 Follow Up Evaluation

55.5.1 *Visual Acuity*

OD: 20/400
OS: Light perception

55.5.2 *Pupils*

OD: Round and reactive
OS: +Afferent pupillary defect

55.5.3 *IOP*

OD: 27
OS: 8

55.5.4 *Slit Lamp Examination*

	OD	OS
Lids and lashes	Normal	Normal
Sclera and conjunctiva	Normal	Normal
Cornea	Keratic precipitates inferiorly	1+ Descemet's folds
Anterior chamber	2+ cell	1+ pigmented cell and flare, heme on anterior surface of ACIOL
Iris	Normal	Normal
Lens	Normal	ACIOL with diffuse red blood cells and membrane on anterior surface
Vitreous	1–2+ cell	No view

55.5.5 *Dilated Examination*

Macula/Nerve OD: Mild edema
Periphery OD: Serous retinal detachment, Dalen-Fuchs nodules throughout (Fig. 55.3a)
Macula/Nerve: OS: No view
Periphery OS: No view

55.5.6 Further Studies

Fluorescein angiography (FA) demonstrated multiple pinpoint areas of hyperfluorescence and pooling of the dye in the area of serous retinal detachments (Fig. 55.3b). Optical coherence tomography (OCT) showed serous retinal detachments in the posterior pole (Fig. 55.3c). B-scan ultrasonography revealed thickening of the choroid bilaterally (Fig. 55.4).

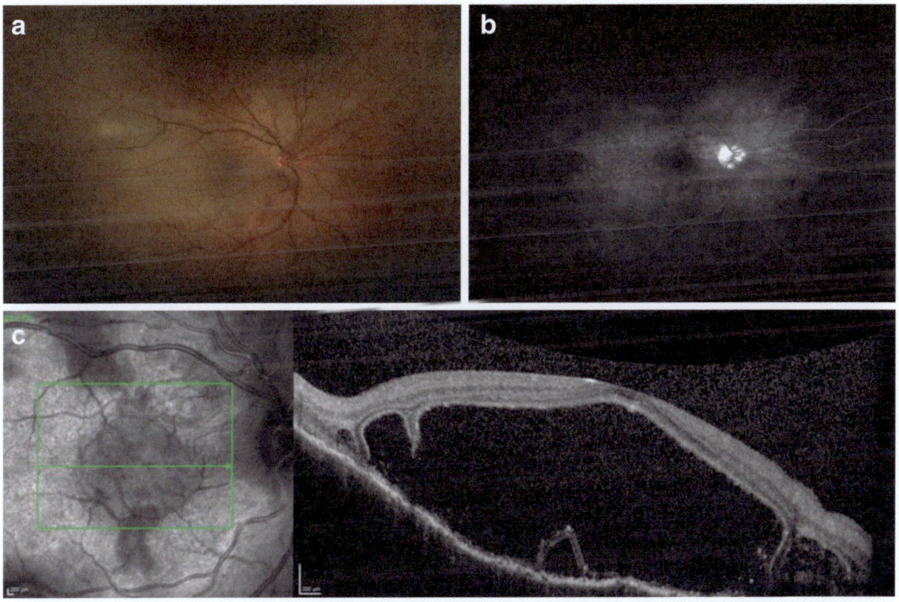

Fig. 55.3 (**a**) Optos photograph of the right eye shows mild vitritis, multiple foci of serous retinal detachments, and Dalen-Fuchs nodules throughout. (**b**) Fluorescein angiogram of the right eye in the late phase reveals pooling of fluid pockets in the posterior pole. (**c**) OCT of the right eye reveals a large pocket of subretinal fluid

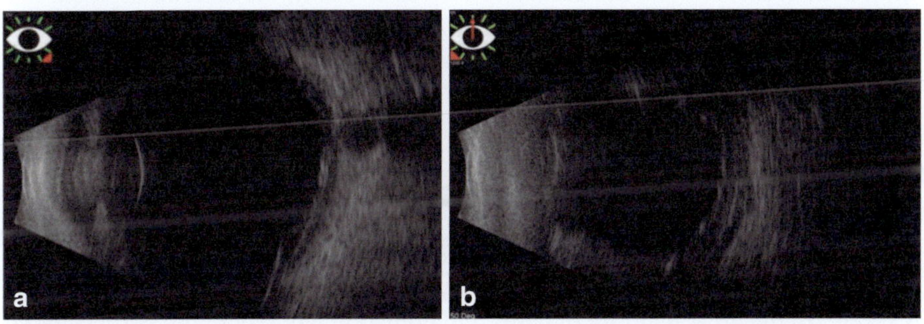

Fig. 55.4 (**a**) B-scan ultrasonography of the right eye revealing thickened choroid. (**b**) B-scan ultrasonography of the left eye showed thickened choroid

55.6 Clinical Course

Serologic work up was ordered with negative results. These included rapid plasma reagent, fluorescent treponemal antibody absorption test, angiotensin-converting enzyme, lysozyme, QuantiFERON TB. Given the panuveitis, subretinal fluid, and multiple leakage points on angiography in the setting of recent ocular trauma and surgery, the patient was diagnosed with sympathetic ophthalmia.

The patient was treated with three doses of intravenous methylprednisolone daily and then started on prednisone 80 mg daily and mycophenolate 1 g twice a day. The inflammation in the patient's right eye improved, and his best-corrected visual acuity returned to 20/20 in the right eye. The patient remained stable without evidence of ocular inflammation. No systemic features developed.

55.7 Review and Lessons Learned

Sympathetic ophthalmia (SO), a diffuse bilateral granulomatous panuveitis, is a serious potential complication after either eye surgery or penetrating or perforating eye injury. The eye with a history of injury or surgery is referred to as the "inciting" eye, whereas the contralateral eye is said to be "sympathizing". The time from surgery or trauma to onset of SO varies from days to decades, with 80% of the cases occurring within 3 months, and 90% within 1 year [1, 2].

Although the pathogenesis of SO is not completely understood, it is believed to be a cell-mediated autoimmune response to a retinal, retinal pigment epithelial or choroidal antigen [3]. A wound with uveal prolapse may permit sequestered ocular antigens to sensitize the host and abrogate tolerance to these antigens, resulting in intraocular inflammation. Repeated ocular surgery, particularly vitreoretinal surgery, is recognized as a likely risk factor for SO. Incidence following non-surgical penetrating wounds is 0.19%, after intraocular surgeries is 0.007% and after pars plana vitrectomy is 0.001% [3–5].

The diagnosis of sympathetic ophthalmia is based on the patient's history and clinical examination. The inflammatory response seen in the anterior segment is a granulomatous anterior uveitis with mutton-fat keratic precipitates. In the posterior segment, SO can manifest itself in the form of moderate to severe vitritis, inflammation of the ciliary body, chorioretinal spots known as Dalen-Fuchs nodules, and optic nerve edema. Serous retinal detachment and macular edema may also be present.

Systemic corticosteroids are the cornerstone of therapy and are recommended on a daily basis, beginning with high dose oral steroids with dosages ranging from 0.5 to 2 mg/kg/day or a combination of topical and oral steroids (50–75 mg/day) [6]. Intravenous pulse steroid therapy (1.0 g/day × 3 days) can be initiated if the disease is severe. In the great majority of cases, inflammation will recur with corticosteroid tapering, and therapy with steroid-sparing immunosuppressive therapy will be necessary.

Our patient had a ruptured open globe with uveal prolapse and repeat vitreoretinal surgery, all contributing to the increased risk for sympathetic ophthalmia. He was initially treated with intravenous methylprednisolone for 3 days and started on prednisone and mycophenolate. His visual acuity returned to 20/20 in the right eye. Prompt evaluation and management with systemic immunosuppressive agents help to control the disease and retain good visual acuity.

Sympathetic ophthalmia, though rare, is a potentially blinding condition and warrants prompt treatment to maintain a favorable visual outcome. It is appropriate to counsel patients with open globe injuries about the risks of sympathetic ophthalmia.

55.8 Key Learning Points

- Sympathetic ophthalmia following uveal trauma is a rare but potentially blinding condition.
- Thorough examination of anterior and posterior segment of the normal eye in cases of ocular trauma and at follow-up appointments should be conducted.
- Prompt evaluation and management with systemic immunosuppressive agents may control the disease and help maintain a favorable visual outcome.
- It is important to counsel trauma patients about the risk of sympathetic ophthalmia and encourage them to seek immediate evaluation with visual changes in either eye.

References

1. Zaharia MA, Lamarche J, Laurin M. Sympathetic uveitis 66 years after injury. Can J Ophthalmol. 1984;19:240–3.
2. Lubin JR, Albert DM, Weinstein M. Sixty-five years of sympathetic ophthalmia. A clinicopathologic review of 105 cases (1913–1978). Ophthalmology. 1980;87:109–21.
3. Marak GE Jr. Recent advances in sympathetic ophthalmia. Surv Ophthalmol. 1979;24:141–56.
4. Kilmartin DJ, Dick AD, Forrester JV. Sympathetic ophthalmia risk following vitrectomy: should we counsel patients? Br J Ophthalmol. 2000;84:448–9.
5. Makley TA Jr, Azar A. Sympathetic ophthalmia. A long-term follow-up. Arch Ophthalmol. 1978;96:257–62.
6. Chang GC, Young LH. Sympathetic ophthalmia. Semin Ophthalmol. 2011;26:316–20.

Index

S. Grob, C. Kloek (eds.), *Management of Open Globe Injuries*,
https://doi.org/10.1007/978-3-319-72410-2

MIX
Papier aus verantwortungsvollen Quellen
Paper from responsible sources
FSC® C105338

If you have any concerns about our products,
you can contact us on
ProductSafety@springernature.com

In case Publisher is established outside the EU,
the EU authorized representative is:
Springer Nature Customer Service Center GmbH
Europaplatz 3, 69115 Heidelberg, Germany

Printed by Libri Plureos GmbH
in Hamburg, Germany